FOUNDATIONS OF
ADULT
NURSING

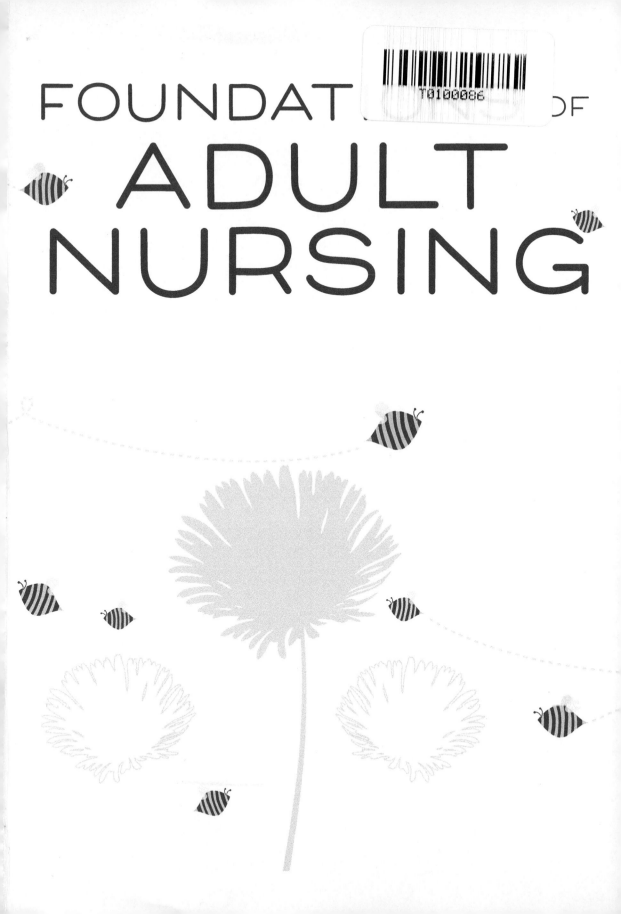

FOUNDATIONS OF ADULT NURSING

EDITED BY

Dianne Burns

3RD EDITION

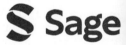

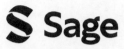

1 Oliver's Yard
55 City Road
London EC1Y 1SP

2455 Teller Road
Thousand Oaks, California 91320

Unit No 323-333, Third Floor, F-Block
International Trade Tower Nehru Place
New Delhi – 110 019

8 Marina View Suite 43-053
Asia Square Tower 1
Singapore 018960

Editor: Martha Cunneen
Editorial Assistant: Sahar Jamfar
Production Editor: Gourav Kumar
Copyeditor: Clare Weaver
Proofreader: Derek Markham
Indexer: KnowledgeWorks Global Ltd
Marketing Manager: Ruslana Khatagova
Cover Design: Sheila Tong
Typeset by KnowledgeWorks Global Ltd
Printed and bound by CPI Group (UK) Ltd,
Croydon, CR0 4YY

Library of Congress Control Number: 2023935661

British Library Cataloguing in Publication data

A catalogue record for this book is available from the British Library

ISBN 978-1-5297-7598-3
ISBN 978-1-5297-7597-6 (pbk)

At Sage we take sustainability seriously. Most of our products are printed in the UK using responsibly sourced papers and boards. When we print overseas, we ensure sustainable papers are used as measured by the Paper Chain Project grading system. We undertake an annual audit to monitor our sustainability.

This book is dedicated to Dorothy Needham (1930–2023) whose love, guidance and determined spirit will be remembered forever.

Contents

About the Editor and Contributors

Editor

Dianne Burns, BSc (Hons) Nurse Practitioner, MSc (Clinical Leadership), PGCert T&L, RGN, RNT, SFHEA (Senior Fellow Higher Education Academy), is a Senior Lecturer in Adult Nursing at the University of Manchester. She is the Programme Director of the PG Cert in Medical and Health Education, and Academic Lead for LEAP (Leadership in Education and Awards Programme) and Staff Development Programmes within the Faculty of Biology, Medicine, and Health. She also leads the postgraduate Leadership in Professional Practice module within the Division of Nursing, Midwifery and Social Work. A Registered General Nurse since 1984, Dianne worked in a variety of acute clinical settings (Acute Medical/Surgical, Orthopaedics, Accident and Emergency) before moving into community nursing to work as a practice nurse then Nurse Practitioner/Nursing Team Co-Ordinator within a large semi-rural GP (General Practitioner) practice. Each of these roles provide a perfect opportunity for her to draw upon her enthusiasm and passion for engaging with students, colleagues, and healthcare practitioners to enhance teaching and learning within the university and the wider community.

Contributors

Greg Bleakley, BSc (Hons), PG Cert (Critical Care), DProf, DipN, RN, RNT, AFHEA, has worked in critical care and as a Specialist Nurse (Organ Donation) for a decade. His research interests include critical illness management, organ donation and transplantation, critical care, and end of life care.

Sarah Booth, RN BSc (Hons), Community Health (with District Nursing Qualification), PGCE, PG Cert in Business and Executive Coaching (Distinction), has always been passionate to support learners in practice. She has worked for 30 years in the NHS, both as a District Nurse and Practice Education Facilitator. More recently, she worked as Preceptorship Lead at Stockport NHS Foundation Trust.

Jane Brooks, RN, PhD is a senior lecturer at the University of Manchester. She is a historian of nursing and author of many articles and books in the discipline. She is currently Editor in Chief for *Nursing History Review,* the peer-reviewed academic journal of the American Association for the History of Nursing.

Christine Brown Wilson, PhD RN a Professor of Nursing (Education) at Queen's University Belfast. She leads the Education and Practice Research Theme for the School of Nursing and Midwifery and is a Principal Fellow of Advance HE. Christine has an international profile in ageing and dementia research.

Claire Burns, MSc, BSc (Hons), SFHEA, PGCE, RN, is a lecturer at the University of Manchester.

Janice Christie, PhD, MA, PgDip, PgCert, BSc, RN, RSCPHN, is a senior lecturer at the University of Manchester.

Mark Cole, BA (Hons), MSc, PhD, RNT, RGN, RMN, is a Senior Lecturer in Adult Nursing at the University of Manchester.

Dawn Dowding, PhD, RN, FAAN is Professor in Clinical Decision Making at the University of Manchester, is Co-Chair of the Royal College of Nursing eHealth Forum and lead for digital health and social care research for the Division of Nursing, Midwifery and Social Work.

Morgan Evans, graduated from the University of Cambridge in medicine and is currently working as a junior doctor in Jersey.

Sam Freeman, PhD, RN, MSc, BSc (Hons), PGCE, SFHEA is a senior lecturer in adult nursing and the Director of Education in the Division of Nursing, Midwifery and Social Work at the University of Manchester.

Brendan Garry, MSc, BSc, PgDip, PgCert, RN, DN, QN, RNT, MAcadMEd, SFHEA is a lecturer in nursing at the University of Manchester

Laura Green, BSc (Hons), MSc, PhD, RGN, SFHEA, PgCert is a lecturer in Adult Nursing at the University of Manchester. She is Programme Director for the Bachelor of Nursing and Master of Nursing and writes a regular column for the *International Journal of Palliative Nursing.*

Trudy Hadcroft, MSc, BSc (Hons), NMP, DPSN, RGN is a Clinical Nurse Specialist in Pain management at Bolton Hospital NHS Foundation Trust. Trudy has worked in pain management for twelve years and prior to this worked for many years in Critical Care.

Karen Heggs, MA, PGCert, PGDip, FHEA, BSc (Hons), RN, RSCPHN (HV) is Director of Nursing and Midwifery in the School of Health and Society, at the University of Salford. She has had an extensive and varied clinical and academic career over the last 25 years, working across a range of specialisms including Specialist Palliative Care, Emergency Nursing and Health Visiting.

Heather Iles-Smith, MSc, PhD, RGN, was Head of Nursing Research and Innovation at Leeds Teaching Hospitals Trust (LTHT) and Honorary Clinical Associate Professor, Faculty of Health, University of Leeds. She is currently a Clinical Academic holding a Joint Chair of Nursing with the Northern Care Alliance (NCA) NHS Group and the School of Health and Society, University of Salford.

Karen Iley, BSc (Hons), MSc, RN, RNT, is a Lecturer in Adult Nursing at the University of Manchester.

Caroline Jagger, BSc (Hons), MSc, Dip HE, RN, NMP, qualified as a nurse in 2001 and works as a Clinical Nurse Specialist at Manchester University NHS Foundation Trust.

Elizabeth Lee-Woolf, BSc, MSc (BOE), DipN, RN, RM, RNT, was, until retirement, a Lecturer at the University of Manchester. Her experience in nursing education spans the last 30 years and she has been involved in the development and delivery of several curricula, with particular emphasis on the biosciences applied to nursing and the development of e-learning strategies.

Judith Ormrod, BEd, BSc, MA, MSc, PhD, RGN, has spent most of her clinical nursing experience working as a staff nurse and senior ward sister in intensive care units and acute admission wards in central London Hospitals.

Janet Roberts, MSc, BSc (Hons), DPSN, NMP, RGN is the Lead Pain Nurse Specialist at Bolton Hospital NHS Foundation Trust. Janet has been a qualified nurse since 1987 and has specialised in pain management for over twenty years.

Jean Rogers, BSc (Hons), MSc, CertEd (FE (Further Education)), RGN, is an associate lecturer at the Open University. Jean has been a qualified nurse for over 35 years and has worked in various clinical and educational areas before embarking on her current role.

Gillian Singleton, MRes, BSc (Hons), PGCE, RM, is a Lecturer in Midwifery at the University of Manchester.

Emma Stanmore, BNurs (Hons), MRes, PhD, DN, RN, is a Reader and Lead for the Healthy Ageing Research Group in the Division of Nursing, Midwifery and Social Work at the University of Manchester. She has taken several ageing and technology research projects from concept through to implementation such as gamified telerehabilitation and an NHS approved digital falls prevention platform.

Colin Steen, MSc, PGCE, RN, FHEA, is a Lecturer in the Division of Nursing, Midwifery and Social Work at the University of Manchester.

Joanne Timpson, BA(Hons) Nurs Ed, MSc Nursing, Nurse Tutor, Dip, Oncology, Cert Counselling, is a Senior Lecturer and Directorate Lead for Adult Nursing within the Division of Nursing, Midwifery and Social Work at the University of Manchester.

Ann Wakefield, MSc, PhD, Cert Ed, RGN, RMN, RCNT, RNT, Dip Nursing Part A (London), PFHEA, is a Professor of Nursing Education at the University of Manchester.

Acknowledgements

We are particularly grateful to all the practitioners, educators, students, and others we have met over the years who have helped and guided us in our own nursing and teaching practice. We would like to thank families, friends, and colleagues for their support.

On behalf of the authors, SAGE would like to thank all the academics who provided original material for the previous edition or reviewed the content of the book, helping to shape and influence it for the better:

Lesley Andrews
Darren Brand
Beryl Cooledge
Kevin Crimmons
Helen Davidson
Yvonne Dexter
Julie Fletcher
Catherine Hill
Angela Hudson
Jan Hunter
Julia Jones
Mhairi Kidd
Erin King
Scott Macpherson
Carole McGlone
Susan Ramsdale
Georgia Taylor
Suzan Thompson

Publisher's Acknowledgements

On behalf of the Editor and the Contributors, the publisher would like to extend their thanks to all third parties who granted us permission to reproduce the following material:

Figure 6.3 Hierarchies of evidence, adapted from Porzsolt, F., Ohletz, A., Thim, A., Gardner, D., Ruatti, H., Meier, H., Schlotz-Gorton, N. & Schrott, L. (2003) 'Evidence-based decision making – the six step approach,' *BMJ Evidence-Based Medicine*, 8(6): 165–6. © 2001–2017, The Board of Regents of the University of Wisconsin System.

Table 6.8 Examples of database information related to nursing and healthcare, reproduced with permission from Wakefield, A. (2014) 'Searching and critiquing the research literature,' *Nursing Standard*, 28(39): 49.

Figure 7.1 A hypothetico-deductive approach to clinical decision making, Tanner, C., Padrick, K., Westfall, U. and Putzier, D. (1987) 'Diagnostic reasoning: strategies for nurses and nursing students', *Nursing Research*, 36: 358–63. Wolters Kluwer.

Figure 7.2 From novice to expert, 1982 Benner, P. (1982) 'From novice to expert', *American Journal of Nursing*, 82: 402–7. Wolters Kluwer.

Figure 7.4 Carper's interconnected 'patterns of knowing,' Carper (1978) 'Fundamental patterns of knowing in nursing', *Advanced Nursing Science*, 1(1): 1113–23. Wolters Kluwer.

Figure 7.6 Schematic representation of the Situated Clinical Decision-Making Framework, Gillespie, M., and Paterson, B.L. (2009) 'Helping novice nurses make effective clinical decisions: the situated clinical decision-making framework', *Nursing Education Perspectives*, May/June, 9(3): 165–70. Wolters Kluwer.

Figure 8.4 Grol's (1997) 5-stage implementation process, Grol, R. (1997), Beliefs and evidence in changing clinical practice, *BMJ*, 315: 418–25.

Figure 8.5 Illustrative tools and methods in improvement, Batalden, P.B. and Davidoff, F. (2007) 'What is "quality improvement" and how can it transform healthcare?', *Quality and Safety in Healthcare*, 16: 2–3. BMJ Publishing Group Ltd and the Health Foundation.

Table 8.2 Stakeholder engagement approaches, reproduced with permission of stakeholder-map.com.

Figure 8.8 Plan, Do, Study, Act Cycle, Langley, G.L., Nolan, K.M., Nolan, T.W., Norman, C.L. and Provost, L.P. (2009) *The Improvement Guide: A Practical Approach to Enhancing Organizational Performance*, 2nd edition. San Francisco, CA: Jossey-Bass.

Figure 9.2 Valuing older workers (RCN, 2012) 'Valuing older workers', Royal College of Nursing: London.

Figure 11.2 The overlap between long-term conditions and mental health problems, Naylor, C., Parsonage, M., McDaid, D., Knapp, M., Fossey, M. and Galea, A. (2012) *Longterm Conditions and Mental Health: The Cost of Co-morbidities*. London: The King's Fund.

Figure 11.3 The NHS and Social Care Long Term Conditions Model (2007) Department of Health: London. © Crown copyright.

Figure 11.5 The House of Care Model, Coulter, A., Roberts, S. and Dixson, A. (2013) Delivering Better Services for People With Long-Term Conditions: Building the House of Care. London: The King's Fund.

Figure 11.7 Continuum strategies to support self-management, de Longh, A., Fagan, P., Fenner, J. and Kidd, L. (2015) A practical guide to self-management support. Available from: www.health.org.uk/publication/practical-guide-self-management-support.   London: The Health Foundation.

Table 12.4 NEWS score and Table 12.5 Outline clinical response to NEWS triggers, Royal College of Physicians, 2012.

Figure 16.1 The Eatwell Guide, Public Health England in association with the Welsh government, Food Standards Scotland, and the Food Standards Agency in Northern Ireland.

Figure 16.2 Influences on health, Dahlgren, G. and Whitehead, M. (1991) *Policies and Strategies to Promote Social Equity in Health*. Stockholm: Institute for Future Studies. World Health Organization: Denmark.

Figure 16.3 Herd immunity, National Institute of Allergy, and Infectious Diseases.

Introduction

This book aims to provide a concise, easy-to-read introductory text for those individuals who are undertaking their studies focusing on *adult nursing at undergraduate level* (i.e., students on the Nursing and Midwifery Council [NMC] approved undergraduate programmes) leading to Registered Nurse status. However, we recognise that it will be of interest to learners undertaking *nursing associate* programmes and *nursing apprenticeships* along with those from other fields of nursing. Practice supervisors, assessors, mentors, coaches, and those involved in supporting such learners (e.g., lecturers, nurse teachers and academic assessors) will also find the book and accompanying resources useful.

As a core text for 'beginners,' the book is written in an easy-to-access, user-friendly style and examines in detail the essential knowledge and skills needed to provide therapeutic care to adults with a range of health needs. Taking a broad rather than a deep approach, we will be encouraging you as the reader to explore the core principles and key aspects of an adult nurse's role, reflecting upon current nursing theory and the factors that underpin high-quality, evidence-based care delivery in practice. By incorporating a variety of activities and case scenarios we intend to bring to life many of the contemporary issues faced by adult nurses today. By also guiding you to other resources as appropriate, our primary aim is to assist you in the development of an understanding of the importance of *person-centered care* using an *evidence-based approach* to inform adult nursing. In doing so, we hope not only that this will help you demonstrate your knowledge in written assignments and examinations, but also more importantly that you will use your knowledge and understanding of each of these fundamental aspects to underpin the care you provide for all those in your care.

The *Modernising Nursing Careers Framework* (Department of Health, Social Services and Public Safety or DHSSPS, 2006) identifies the changing context for healthcare and a need for the current nursing workforce to reflect those changes and become more adaptable. This approach will be illustrated throughout this book in terms of its relevance to current UK healthcare provision and policy, namely regarding:

- An expanding older population;
- The increasing incidence of long-term conditions;
- The growing impact of preventable conditions due to lifestyle choices (i.e., smoking, obesity, alcohol intake, etc.);
- The need for nurses to demonstrate skills in caring for people in a variety of settings.

The content of the book is underpinned throughout by the Nursing and Midwifery Council's *Future Nurse: Standards of Proficiency for Registered Nurses* (NMC, 2018a), which clearly defines what nursing students must achieve before entering the professional register (and what regis-tered nurses must continue to meet throughout their professional career), and *The Code* (NMC, 2018b), which presents the professional standards that nurses and midwives must uphold in order to be registered to practice in the UK. It will also reflect current UK policy, since contem-porary adult nursing is delivered to a diverse client group in a variety of settings.

Focusing primarily on the top morbidity and mortality indicators across the UK (i.e., circula-tory disease, cardiovascular disease, respiratory disease, diabetes, cancer, infectious disease, and dementia), it includes specific content to support the development of knowledge and skills related to the EU Directive 2005/36EC (European Commission, 2011) which demands that adult nurses gain exposure to the following:

- General and specialist medicine;
- General and specialist surgery;
- Childcare and paediatrics;
- Maternity care;
- Mental health and psychiatry;
- Care of the older person;
- Home nursing (community nursing).

The book is composed of two parts.

Part 1: Theory and Context in Relation to Adult Nursing

Made up of Chapters 1–10, this part of the book introduces the overarching theoretical and contemporary practice issues faced by adult nurses today.

Chapter 1: Essentials of nursing: values, knowledge, skills, and practice

This chapter introduces you to the key principles, core values, and legal and professional issues that inform contemporary nursing practice, recognising the importance of self-awareness and professional regulation in developing your own practice. The significance of core values is explored (i.e., empathy, compassion, dignity, respect, cultural competence and communication) to help you develop an appreciation of how such values must underpin your nursing practice. We also briefly introduce the importance of evidence-based care and nursing research.

Chapter 2: Nursing therapeutics

In this chapter we encourage you to consider appropriate philosophies, models, and frameworks for the delivery of safe and competent care. We identify the factors that contribute to the devel-opment of therapeutic partnerships, exploring the concept of safe and effective person-centred care. The overall focus of the chapter is on challenging routine and tradition in nursing practice and the importance of effective communication, which assists in the development of a therapeutic relationship with individuals and their families, including those who are vulnerable and therefore most at risk.

Chapter 3: Fundamental aspects of adult nursing

This chapter introduces you to the application of systematic approaches to nursing care, the nature of nursing interventions and the mechanisms by which interventions can be selected and evaluated. Focusing on the activities of daily living (Roper et al., 2000), we explore ways in which nurses can undertake a holistic nursing assessment, considering requirements for making reasonable adjustments and identifying some of the clinical nursing skills needed to be able to provide high-quality nursing care. In doing so, we also consider the key concepts of *'confidentiality,' 'informed consent,' 'mental capacity'* and *'infection control.'*

Chapter 4: Interprofessional and Multidisciplinary Team Working

This chapter explores how multi-agency working has the potential to positively impact on health, highlighting the importance of accurate record keeping, effective communication, accountability, and delegation. You will begin to understand the significance and the benefits of teamwork in the provision of effective healthcare. We also identify useful strategies for overcoming common barriers to interprofessional and multidisciplinary working in practice settings.

Chapter 5: Digital literacy

This chapter considers the role of digital technologies in healthcare, and how their implementation and use can support professional nursing practice. It discusses the factors you need to be aware of when using digital technology and the skills you need to practice as a nurse in a digitally enabled healthcare environment.

Chapter 6: Medicines management

This chapter provides an overview of the nurses' responsibilities related to the safe administration of medications, considering the key components of the medicines management process. Understanding the key principles in this chapter will help you to become a safe, conscientious, and ethical nurse.

Chapter 7: Evidence-based practice and the importance of research

This chapter aims to nurture your ability to critically appraise evidence to help you to make informed decisions about the care you administer. It begins by exploring the origins of evidence-based practice and examines why evidence-based medicine (EBM) and research are important in today's healthcare systems. It goes on to examine how you can implement evidence-based principles into your own clinical practice, by supporting the development of critical appraisal skills, and outlining strategies that can also be employed to encourage others to use evidence as part of their everyday work.

Chapter 8: Clinical decision making

This chapter considers the nature of judgement and decision making in professional nursing practice. It explores concepts such as uncertainty in healthcare practice and provides an overview of different theories related to judgement and decision making in healthcare contexts. The chapter will give you understanding and insight into how you use knowledge (information) to inform the judgements and decisions you take in clinical practice. It will also help you to appraise and critically evaluate your judgment and decision-making skills, as well as how to ensure individuals and their families are also involved in decisions about their care.

Chapter 9: Leadership and management

This chapter reviews current leadership approaches within contemporary healthcare settings and encourages you to reflect upon the importance of leadership and management skills, recognising potential areas for personal improvement to enhance your own leadership skills. It also seeks to explain the difference between 'risk aversion' and 'risk management' and explores effective strategies for risk assessment and management to provide a safe and healthy environment for service-users and staff.

Chapter 10: Developing practice and managing change

In this chapter we appraise the concept of quality, focusing on quality assurance frameworks and methods of monitoring and improving the quality of care and service provision. We outline current legal, ethical, and professional drivers for change/service improvement and critically discuss the role of a change agent(s) in developing and leading teams to effective change. We also discuss barriers to service improvement implementation, appraising effective strategies for change management and sustaining service improvements.

Part 2: Caring for Adults in a Variety of Settings

This section of the book highlights specific areas of care that are commonly encountered within adult nursing practice.

Chapter 11: Supporting and promoting health

This chapter introduces you to the principles and practice of epidemiology, public health, health promotion/health education and preventative healthcare, thereby enabling you to gain a basic understanding of how demographic health information and epidemiological data inform national and global priorities for health and health promotion/public health initiatives. Here, we explore the role of the adult nurse in contemporary public health practice, the interrelationship of the health of the public, the social determinants influencing health, and the tools and structures that underpin the assessment of health and healthcare needs. We look at the impact of 'risky behaviours' (i.e. unhealthy eating, physical inactivity, alcohol and substance misuse, and sexual health), focusing on national health promotion initiatives and services to provide a clear overview of both the government agenda and legislative practice. We also consider the range of opportunities available to promote health within any contemporary healthcare setting, emphasising the requirements of adult nurses to be able to recognise and respond appropriately to the various health needs of individuals, for example: babies, children and young people (CYP); pregnant and postnatal women; people living with mental health problems; people living with disabilities; older people; and those with long-term problems such as cognitive impairment.

Chapter 12: Specialist care of the older person: a person-centred, biographical approach

This chapter considers the knowledge, skills and attitudes required by nurses for the optimum care of the older person, and explores how we might promote individualised, person-centered care in our everyday practice. You will develop an understanding of the principles of health promotion, quality of life, dignity in care, independence, empowerment, and choice in relation to older people. We explore the needs of older people and their carers in a variety of care settings, considering the nature of care that older people may require. A key focus of the chapter is promoting an understanding of the principles of anti-discriminatory practice with reference to age and considering how this is applied in practice with an emphasis on the 'frail' older person. We look at the challenges faced by those living with dementia with reference to physical activity and fall prevention.

Chapter 13: Caring for adults with long-term conditions

This chapter examines the bio-psychosocial impact of living with and caring for individuals experiencing long-term ill health, exploring ways in which you can work effectively to support individuals and their families/carers by promoting self-care and empowerment within a variety of settings. It identifies the common problems encountered by individuals living with a long-term condition and the relevant government policies that aim to support self-management, personalised care planning, and partnership working with individuals, families, and carers. It seeks to help you to develop a greater understanding of how the concepts of *empowerment, shared decision making,* and *concordance* can be used to inform the adult nurse's role.

Chapter 14: Caring for the acutely ill adult

This chapter considers the impact of acute illness on normal daily functioning and explores the principles of working towards recovery from acute illness, utilising contemporary medical and surgical approaches with a particular focus on acute assessment. Highlighting the significance of risk assessment, prioritising care and the prevention of deterioration, the importance of the application of critical thinking, evaluation, and timely communication to provide safe, knowledgeable, and competent person-centred care competently is explored.

Chapter 15: Caring for the critically ill adult

This chapter focuses on the comprehensive assessment of a critically ill adult who requires specialist care within a critical care environment. We provide an outline of the nurse's role in recognising and responding to critically ill adults using appropriate evidence-based strategies and an ABCDE approach (Resuscitation Council UK, 2021). We also explore some of the legal and ethical issues relating to the individual in critical care settings, including consent, confidentiality, best interest principles, after-care rehabilitation, and organ donation.

Chapter 16: Palliative care

This chapter provides an overview of some of the contemporary challenges in palliative care, outlining the role of the nurse and offering an overview of approaches to care to assist the development of therapeutic relationships required in order to profoundly enhance nursing practice.

Chapter 17: Managing the transition to registered nursing practice

This closing chapter explores the challenge of managing role transition to help you to prepare for the start of a professional registered nursing career. We consider how best to approach your final practice learning experience, describe the process of application for employment and explain how best to promote yourself to prospective employers. We also explain how preceptorship can support you in your transition from student nurse to registrant, outline the process of revalidation and consider the role of a registered nurse when responding to a major incident.

References

Department of Health, Social Services and Public Safety (2006) *Modernising Nursing Careers: Setting the Direction*. Belfast: DHSSPS.

European Commission (2011) *European Union Directive 2005/36/EC* (consolidated version). Available at: https://eur-lex.europa.eu/legal-content/EN/TXT/?uri=celex%3A32005L0036 (last accessed 29th March 2023).

Nursing and Midwifery Council (2018a) *Future Nurse: Standards of Proficiency for Registered Nurses*. London: NMC.

Nursing and Midwifery Council (2018b) *The Code: Professional Standards of Practice and Behaviour for Nurses and Midwives*. London: NMC.

Resuscitation Council UK (2021) *Resuscitation Guidelines*. Available at: www.resus.org.uk/library/2021-resuscitation-guidelines (last accessed 29th March 2023).

Roper, N., Logan, W.W., and Tierney, A.J. (2000) The Roper–Logan–Tierney Model of Nursing: Based on Activities of Living. London: Churchill-Livingstone.

NMC Proficiencies Map for Registered Nurses

Platform 1: Being an accountable professional Registered nurses act in the best interests of people, putting them first and providing nursing care that is person-centred, safe, and compassionate. They act professionally at all times and use their knowledge and experience to make evidence-based decisions about care. They communicate effectively, are role models for others and are accountable for their actions. Registered nurses continually reflect on their practice and keep abreast of new and emerging developments in nursing, health, and care. The outcomes set out below reflect the proficiencies for accountable professional practice that must be applied across the standards of proficiency for registered nurses, as described in platforms 2-7, in all care settings and areas of practice. At the point of registration, the registered nurse will be able to:

NMC Proficiencies for Registered Nurses	Main Chapter/s (But also referred to in other chapters as appropriate)
1.1 Understand and act in accordance with The Code: Professional standards of practice and behaviour for nurses and midwives and fulfil all registration requirements	Chapters 1 & 11-16
1.2 Understand and apply relevant legal, regulatory and governance requirements, policies, and ethical frameworks to all areas of practice, differentiating where appropriate between the devolved legislatures of the United Kingdom	Chapters 1 & 11-16
1.3 Understand and apply the principles of courage, transparency, and the duty of candour, recognising and reporting any situations, behaviours or errors that could result in poor care outcomes	Chapters 1 & 9
1.4 Demonstrate an understanding of and the ability to challenge discriminatory behaviour	Chapter 1
1.5 Understand the demands of professional practice and demonstrate how to recognise signs of vulnerability in themselves or their colleagues and the action required to minimise risks to health	Chapters 1, 2 & 9
1.6 Understand and maintain the level of health, fitness and wellbeing required to meet people's needs for mental and physical care	Chapters 1 & 17
1.7 Demonstrate an understanding of research methods, ethics, and governance in order to critically analyse, safely use, share, and apply research findings to promote and inform best nursing practice	Chapters 7 & 8
1.8 Demonstrate the knowledge, skills, and ability to think critically when applying evidence and drawing on experience to make evidence-informed decisions in all situations	Chapters 7 & 11-16

1.9 Understand the need to base all decisions regarding care and interventions on people's needs and preferences, recognising and addressing any personal and external factors that may unduly influence decisions	All Chapters
1.10 Demonstrate resilience and emotional intelligence and be capable of explaining the rationale that influences judgements and decisions in routine, complex and challenging situations	Chapters 1, 7 & 9
1.11 Communicate effectively using a range of skills and strategies with colleagues and people at all stages of life and with a range of mental, physical, cognitive, and behavioural health challenges	Chapters 3, 5 & 11-16
1.12 Demonstrate the skills and abilities required to support people at all stages of life who are emotionally or physically vulnerable	Chapters 2 & 11-16
1.13 Demonstrate the skills and abilities required to develop, manage, and maintain appropriate relationships with people, their families, carers, and colleagues	All Chapters
1.14 Provide and promote non-discriminatory, person-centred, and sensitive care at all times, reflecting on people's values and beliefs, diverse backgrounds, cultural characteristics, language requirements, needs and preferences, taking account of any need for adjustments	Chapters 3 & 11-16
1.15 Demonstrate the numeracy, literacy, digital and technological skills required to meet the needs of people in their care to ensure safe and effective nursing practice	Chapters 3, 5, 6 & 11-16
1.16 Demonstrate the ability to keep complete, clear, accurate and timely records	Chapters 4 & 11-16
1.17 Take responsibility for continuous self-reflection, seeking and responding to support and feedback to develop their professional knowledge and skills	Chapters 1 & 17
1.18 Demonstrate the knowledge and confidence to contribute effectively and proactively in an interdisciplinary team	Chapters 4, 9 & 11-16
1.19 Act as an ambassador, upholding the reputation of the profession and promoting public confidence in nursing, health, and care services	Chapters 1 & 17
1.20 Safely demonstrate evidence-based practice in all skills and procedures stated in Annexes A and B	Chapters 2, 3, 6 and 11-16
Platform 2: Promoting health and preventing ill health Registered nurses play a key role in improving and maintaining the mental, physical, and behavioural health and wellbeing of people, families, communities, and populations. They support and enable people at all stages of life and in all care settings to make informed choices about how to manage health challenges in order to maximise their quality of life and improve health outcomes. They are actively involved in the prevention of and protection against disease and ill health and engage in public health, community development and global health agendas and in the reduction of health inequalities. The proficiencies identified below will equip the newly registered nurse with the underpinning knowledge and skills required for their role in health promotion and protection and prevention of ill health. At the point of registration, the registered nurse will be able to:	
2.1 Understand and apply the aims and principles of health promotion, protection and improvement and the prevention of ill health when engaging with people	Chapter 11
2.2 Demonstrate knowledge of epidemiology, demography, genomics and the wider determinants of health, illness and wellbeing and apply this to an understanding of global patterns of health and wellbeing outcomes	Chapter 11

2.3 Understand the factors that may lead to inequalities in health outcomes	Chapter 11
2.4 Identify and use all appropriate opportunities, making reasonable adjustments when required, to discuss the impact of smoking, substance and alcohol use, sexual behaviours, diet and exercise on mental, physical, and behavioural health and wellbeing, in the context of people's individual circumstances	Chapter 11
2.5 Promote and improve mental, physical, behavioural, and other health-related outcomes by understanding and explaining the principles, practice and evidence base for health screening programmes	Chapter 11
2.6 Understand the importance of early years and childhood experiences and the possible impact on life choices, mental, physical, and behavioural health, and wellbeing	Chapter 11
2.7 Understand and explain the contribution of social influences, health literacy, individual circumstances, behaviours, and lifestyle choices to mental, physical, and behavioural health outcomes	Chapter 11
2.8 Explain and demonstrate the use of up-to-date approaches to behaviour change to enable people to use their strengths and expertise and make informed choices when managing their own health and making lifestyle adjustments	Chapters 11 & 13
2.9 Use appropriate communication skills and strength-based approaches to support and enable people to make informed choices about their care to manage health challenges in order to have satisfying and fulfilling lives within the limitations caused by reduced capability, ill health, and disability	Chapters 2 & 11-16
2.10 Provide information in accessible ways to help people understand and make decisions about their health, life choices, illness, and care	Chapters 2 & 11-16
2.11 Promote health and prevent ill health by understanding and explaining to people the principles of pathogenesis, immunology and the evidence base for immunisation, vaccination, and herd immunity	Chapter 11
2.12 Protect health through understanding and applying the principles of infection prevention and control, including communicable disease surveillance and antimicrobial stewardship and resistance	Chapter 3
Platform 3: Assessing needs and planning care Registered nurses prioritise the needs of people when assessing and reviewing their mental, physical, cognitive, behavioural, social, and spiritual needs. They use information obtained during assessments to identify the priorities and requirements for person-centred and evidence-based nursing interventions and support. They work in partnership with people to develop person-centred care plans that take into account their circumstances, characteristics, and preferences. The proficiencies identified below will equip the newly registered nurse with the underpinning knowledge and skills required for their role in assessing and initiating person-centred plans of care. At the point of registration, the registered nurse will be able to:	
3.1 Demonstrate and apply knowledge of human development from conception to death when undertaking full and accurate person-centred nursing assessments and developing appropriate care plans	Chapters 3 & 11-16
3.2 Demonstrate and apply knowledge of body systems and homeostasis, human anatomy and physiology, biology, genomics, pharmacology, social and behavioural sciences when undertaking full and accurate person-centred nursing assessments and developing appropriate care plans	Chapters 3 & 11-16

3.3 Demonstrate and apply knowledge of all commonly encountered mental, physical, behavioural, and cognitive health conditions, medication usage and treatments when undertaking full and accurate assessments of nursing care needs and when developing, prioritising, and reviewing person-centred care plans	Chapters 3, 6 & 11–16
3.4 Understand and apply a person-centred approach to nursing care, demonstrating shared assessment, planning, decision making and goal setting when working with people, their families, communities, and populations of all ages	Chapters 2, 3 & 11–16
3.5 Demonstrate the ability to accurately process all information gathered during the assessment process to identify needs for individualised nursing care and develop person-centred evidence-based plans for nursing interventions with agreed goals	Chapters 3 & 11–16
3.6 Effectively assess a person's capacity to make decisions about their own care and to give or withhold consent	Chapters 3 & 11–16
3.7 Understand and apply the principles and processes for making reasonable adjustments and best interest decisions where people do not have capacity	Chapters 3 & 11–16
3.8 Recognise and assess people at risk of harm and the situations that may put them at risk, ensuring prompt action is taken to safeguard those who are vulnerable	Chapters 3, 9 & 11–16
3.9 Undertake routine investigations, interpreting and sharing findings as appropriate	Chapters 3 & 11–16
3.10 Interpret results from routine investigations, taking prompt action when required by implementing appropriate interventions, requesting additional investigations, or escalating to others	Chapters 3 &11–16
3.11 Demonstrate an understanding of co-morbidities and the demands of meeting people's complex nursing and social care needs when prioritising care plans	Chapters 3 & 11–16
3.12 Identify and assess the needs of people and families for care at the end of life, including requirements for palliative care and decision making related to their treatment and care preferences	Chapter 16
3.13 Demonstrate the ability to work in partnership with people, families, and carers to continuously monitor, evaluate and reassess the effectiveness of all agreed nursing care plans and care, sharing decision making and readjusting agreed goals, documenting progress and decisions made	Chapters 3 & 11–16
3.14 Demonstrate knowledge of when and how to refer people safely to other professionals or services for clinical intervention or support	Chapters 4, 9 & 11–16
Platform 4: Providing and evaluating care Registered nurses take the lead in providing evidence-based, compassionate, and safe nursing interventions. They ensure that care they provide, and delegate is person-centred and of a consistently high standard. They support people of all ages in a range of care settings. They work in partnership with people, families, and carers to evaluate whether care is effective, and the goals of care have been met in line with their wishes, preferences, and desired outcomes. The proficiencies identified below will equip the newly registered nurse with the underpinning knowledge and skills required for their role in providing and evaluating person-centred care. At the point of registration, the registered nurse will be able to:	

4.1 Demonstrate and apply an understanding of what is important to people and how to use this knowledge to ensure their needs for safety, dignity, privacy, comfort, and sleep can be met, acting as a role model for others in providing evidence-based person-centred care	Chapters 2, 3 & 10-16
4.2 Work in partnership with people to encourage shared decision making, in order to support individuals, their families and carers to manage their own care when appropriate	Chapters 2, 3, 4, 6, 7 & 11-16
4.3 Demonstrate the knowledge, communication and relationship management skills required to provide people, families and carers with accurate information that meets their needs before, during and after a range of interventions	Chapters 2, 3 & 11-16
4.4 Demonstrate the knowledge and skills required to support people with commonly encountered mental health, behavioural, cognitive, and learning challenges, and act as role model for others in providing high-quality nursing interventions to meet people's needs	Chapters 3, 9 & 11-16
4.5 Demonstrate the knowledge and skills required to support people with commonly encountered physical health conditions, their medication usage and treatments and act as role model for others in providing high-quality nursing interventions when meeting people's needs	Chapter 3, 6 & 11-16
4.6 Demonstrate the knowledge, skills, and ability to act as a role model for others in providing evidence-based nursing care to meet people's needs related to nutrition, hydration, and elimination	Chapters 3 & 11-16
4.7 Demonstrate the knowledge, skills, and ability to act as a role model for others in providing evidence-based, person-centred nursing care to meet people's needs related to mobility, hygiene, oral care, wound care, and skin integrity	Chapters 3 & 11-16
4.8 Demonstrate the knowledge and skills required to identify and initiate appropriate interventions to support people with commonly encountered symptoms including anxiety, confusion, discomfort, and pain	Chapters 3 & 11-16
4.9 Demonstrate the knowledge and skills required to prioritise what is important to people and their families when providing evidence-based person-centred nursing care at end of life including the care of people who are dying, families, the deceased and bereaved	Chapter 16
4.10 Demonstrate the knowledge and ability to respond proactively and promptly to signs of deterioration or distress in mental, physical, cognitive, and behavioural health and use this knowledge to make sound clinical decisions	Chapters 7 & 11-16
4.11 Demonstrate the ability to manage commonly encountered devices and confidently carry out related nursing procedures to meet people's needs for evidence-based, person-centred care	Chapters 3 & 11-16
4.12 Demonstrate the knowledge, skills, and confidence to provide first-aid procedures and basic life support	Chapters 14 & 17
4.13 Understand the principles of safe and effective administration and optimisation of medicines in accordance with local and national policies and demonstrate proficiency and accuracy when calculating dosages of prescribed medicines	Chapter 6

4.14 Demonstrate knowledge of pharmacology and the ability to recognise the effects of medicines, allergies, drug sensitivities, side effects, contraindications, incompatibilities, adverse reactions, prescribing errors, and the impact of polypharmacy and over the counter medication usage	Chapter 6
4.15 Demonstrate knowledge of how prescriptions can be generated, the role of generic, unlicensed, and off label prescribing and an understanding of the potential risks associated with these approaches to prescribing	Chapter 6
4.16 Apply knowledge of pharmacology to the care of people, demonstrating the ability to progress to a prescribing qualification following registration	Chapter 6
4.17 Demonstrate the ability to coordinate and undertake the processes and procedures involved in routine planning and management of safe discharge home or transfer of people between care settings	Chapters 12-16
Platform 5: Leading and managing nursing care and working in teams Registered nurses provide leadership by acting as a role model for best practice in the delivery of nursing care. They are responsible for managing nursing care and are accountable for the appropriate delegation and supervision of care provided by others in the team including lay carers. They play an active and equal role in the interdisciplinary team, collaborating and communicating effectively with a range of colleagues. The proficiencies identified below will equip the newly registered nurse with the underpinning knowledge and skills required for their role in leading and managing nursing care and working effectively as part of an interdisciplinary team. At the point of registration, the registered nurse will be able to:	
5.1 Understand the principles of effective leadership, management, group and organisational dynamics and culture and apply these to team working and decision making.	Chapters 9 & 10
5.2 Understand and apply the principles of human factors, environmental factors and strength-based approaches when working in teams.	Chapters 4, 9 & 10
5.3 Understand the principles and application of processes for performance management and how these apply to the nursing team.	Chapters 9 & 10
5.4 Demonstrate an understanding of the roles, responsibilities, and scope of practice of all members of the nursing and interdisciplinary team and how to make best use of the contributions of others involved in providing care.	Chapters 4, 9 & 10
5.5 Safely and effectively lead and manage the nursing care of a group of people demonstrating appropriate prioritisation, delegation, and assignment of care responsibilities to others involved in providing care.	Chapter 9
5.6 Exhibit leadership potential by demonstrating an ability to guide, support and motivate individuals and interact confidently with other members of the care team.	Chapter 9
5.7 Demonstrate the ability to monitor and evaluate the quality of care delivered by others in the team and lay carers.	Chapters 9 & 10
5.8 Support and supervise students in the delivery of nursing care, promoting reflection, and providing constructive feedback and evaluating and documenting their performance.	Chapter 9
5.9 Demonstrate the ability to challenge and provide constructive feedback about care delivered by others in the team and support them to identify and agree individual learning needs.	Chapter 9
5.10 Contribute to supervision and team reflection activities to promote improvements in practice and services.	Chapters 9 & 10

5.11 Effectively and responsibly use a range of digital technologies to access, input, share and apply information and data within teams and between agencies.	Chapters 4, 5, 9, 10 & 11-16
5.12 Understand the mechanisms that can be used to influence organisational change and public policy, demonstrating the development of political awareness and skills.	Chapter 9
Platform 6: Improving safety and quality of care Registered nurses make a key contribution to the continuous monitoring and quality improvement of care and treatment in order to enhance health outcomes and people's experience of nursing and related care. They assess risks to safety or experience and take appropriate action to manage those, putting the best interests, needs and preferences of people first. The proficiencies identified below will equip the newly registered nurse with the underpinning knowledge and skills required for their role in contributing to risk monitoring and quality of care improvement agendas. At the point of registration, the registered nurse will be able to:	
6.1 Understand and apply the principles of health and safety legislation and regulations and maintain safe work and care environments.	Chapters 3, 9 & 11-16
6.2 Understand the relationship between safe staffing levels, appropriate skills mix, safety, and quality of care, recognising risks to public protection and quality of care, escalating concerns appropriately.	Chapters 9 & 10
6.3 Comply with local and national frameworks, legislation, and regulations for assessing, managing, and reporting risks, ensuring the appropriate action is taken.	Chapters 6, 9 & 11-16
6.4 Demonstrate an understanding of the principles of improvement methodologies, participate in all stages of audit activity and identify appropriate quality improvement strategies.	Chapter 10
6.5 Demonstrate the ability to accurately undertake risk assessments in a range of care settings using a range of contemporary assessment and improvement tools.	Chapters 3, 9 & 11-16
6.6 Identify the need to make improvements and proactively respond to potential hazards that may affect the safety of people.	Chapters 9, 10 & 11-16
6.7 Understand how the quality and effectiveness of nursing care can be evaluated in practice and demonstrate how to use service delivery evaluation and audit findings to bring about continuous improvement.	Chapter 10
6.8 Demonstrate an understanding of how to identify, report and critically reflect on near misses, critical incidents, major incidents, and serious adverse events in order to learn from them and influence their future practice.	Chapters 5, 9 & 10
6.9 Work with people, their families, carers, and colleagues, to develop effective improvement strategies for quality and safety, sharing feedback and learning from positive outcomes and experiences, mistakes and adverse outcomes and experiences.	Chapters 4 & 10
6.10 Apply an understanding of the differences between risk aversion and risk management and how to avoid compromising quality of care and health outcomes.	Chapter 9
6.11 Acknowledge the need to accept and manage uncertainty and demonstrate an understanding of strategies that develop resilience in self and others.	Chapters 1, 7 & 17
6.12 Understand the role of registered nurses and other health and care professionals at different levels of experience and seniority when managing and prioritising actions and care in the event of a major incident.	Chapter 17

Platform 7: Coordinating care

Registered nurses play a leadership role in coordinating and managing the complex nursing and integrated care needs of people at any stage of their lives, across a range of organisations and settings. They contribute to processes of organisational change through an awareness of local and national policies. The proficiencies identified below will equip the newly registered nurse with the underpinning knowledge and skills required for their role in coordinating and leading and managing the complex needs of people across organisations and settings. At the point of registration, the registered nurse will be able to:

7.1 Understand and apply the principles of partnership, collaboration, and interagency working across all relevant sectors	Chapters 4 & 11-16
7.2 Understand health legislation and current health and social care policies, and the mechanisms involved in influencing policy development and change, differentiating where appropriate between the devolved legislatures of the United Kingdom	Chapters 1 & 10
7.3 Understand the principles of health economics and their relevance to resource allocation in health and social care organisations and other agencies	Chapter 10
7.4 Identify the implications of current health policy and future policy changes for nursing and other professions and understand the impact of policy changes on the delivery and coordination of care	Chapters 9, 10 & 11-16
7.5 Understand and recognise the need to respond to the challenges of providing safe, effective, and person-centred nursing care for people who have co-morbidities and complex care needs	Chapters 11-16
7.6 Demonstrate an understanding of the complexities of providing mental, cognitive, behavioural, and physical care services across a wide range of integrated care settings	Chapters 11-16
7.7 Understand how to monitor and evaluate the quality of people's experience of complex care	Chapters 9, 10 & 15
7.8 Understand the principles and processes involved in supporting people and families with a range of care needs to maintain optimal independence and avoid unnecessary interventions and disruptions to their lives	Chapters 3 & 11-16
7.9 Facilitate equitable access to healthcare for people who are vulnerable or have a disability and demonstrate the ability to advocate on their behalf when required and make necessary reasonable adjustments to the assessment, planning and delivery of their care	Chapters 3 & 11-16
7.10 Understand the principles and processes involved in planning and facilitating the safe discharge and transition of people between caseloads, settings, and services	Chapters 3 & 11-16
7.11 Demonstrate the ability to identify and manage risks and take proactive measures to improve the quality of care and services when needed	Chapters 2, 10 & 11-16
7.12 Demonstrate an understanding of the processes involved in developing a basic business case for additional care funding, by applying knowledge of finance, resources, and safe staffing levels	Chapter 10

7.13 Demonstrate an understanding of the importance of exercising political awareness throughout their career, to maximise the influence and effect of registered nursing on quality of care, patient safety, and cost effectiveness	Chapter 10

Annexe A: Communication and relationship management skills

The communication and relationship management skills that a newly registered nurse must be able to demonstrate in order to meet the proficiency outcomes outlined previously are set out in this annexe. Effective communication is central to the provision of safe and compassionate person-centred care. Registered nurses in all fields of nursing practice must be able to demonstrate the ability to communicate and manage relationships with people of all ages with a range of mental, physical, cognitive, and behavioural health challenges. This is because a diverse range of communication and relationship management skills is required to ensure that individuals, their families, and carers are actively involved in and understand care decisions. These skills are vital when making accurate, culturally aware assessments of care needs and ensuring that the needs, priorities, expertise, and preferences of people are always valued and taken into account. Where people have special communication needs or a disability, it is essential that reasonable adjustments are made in order to communicate, provide, and share information in a manner that promotes optimum understanding and engagement and facilitates equal access to high-quality care. The communication and relationship management skills within this annexe are set out in four sections. For the reasons above, these requirements are relevant to all fields of nursing practice and apply to all care settings. It is expected that these skills would be assessed in a student's chosen field of practice. Those skills outlined in Annexe A, Section 3: Evidence-based, best practice communication skills and approaches for providing therapeutic interventions also apply to all registered nurses, but the level of expertise and knowledge required will vary depending on the chosen field of practice.

Registered nurses must be able to demonstrate these skills to an appropriate level for their intended field(s) of practice. At the point of registration, the registered nurse will be able to safely demonstrate the following skills:

1 Underpinning communication skills for assessing, planning, providing and managing best practice, evidence-based nursing care

1.1 Actively listen, recognise and respond to verbal and non-verbal cues	Chapter 3
1.2 Use prompts and positive verbal and non-verbal reinforcement	Chapter 3
1.3 Use appropriate non-verbal communication including touch, eye contact and personal space	Chapter 3
1.4 Make appropriate use of open and closed questioning.	Chapter 3
1.5 Use caring conversation techniques.	Chapter 3
1.6 Check understanding and use clarification techniques.	Chapter 3
1.7 Be aware of own unconscious bias in communication encounters.	Chapter 3
1.8 Write accurate, clear, legible records and documentation.	Chapter 4
1.9 Confidently and clearly share and present verbal and written reports with individuals and groups.	Chapter 4
1.10 Analyse and clearly record and share digital information and data.	Chapter 4
1.11 Provide clear verbal, digital or written information and instructions when delegating or handing over responsibility for care.	Chapters 4, 9 & 14
1.12 Recognise the need for and facilitate access to translator services and material.	Chapters 2 & 3

2 Evidence-based, best practice approaches to communication for supporting people of all ages, their families, and carers in preventing ill health and in managing their care	
2.1 Share information and check understanding about the causes and implications and treatment of a range of common health conditions including anxiety, depression, memory loss, diabetes, dementia, respiratory disease, cardiac disease, neurological disease, cancer, skin problems, immune deficiencies, psychosis, stroke, and arthritis.	Chapters 11–16
2.2 Use clear language and appropriate written materials, making reasonable adjustments where appropriate in order to optimise people's understanding of what has caused their health condition and the implications of their care and treatment.	Chapters 2 & 11–16
2.3 Recognise and accommodate sensory impairments during all communications.	Chapters 2, 3 & 11–16
2.4 Support and manage the use of personal communication aids.	Chapters 2 & 11–16
2.5 Identify the need for and manage a range of alternative communication techniques.	Chapters 2 & 11–16
2.6 Use repetition and positive reinforcement strategies.	Chapters 3 & 11–16
2.7 Assess motivation and capacity for behaviour change and clearly explain cause and effect relationships related to common health risk behaviours including smoking, obesity, sexual practice, alcohol, and substance use.	Chapter 11
2.8 Provide information and explanation to people, families and carers and respond to questions about their treatment and care and possible ways of preventing ill health to enhance understanding.	Chapters 11–16
2.9 Engage in difficult conversations, including breaking bad news and support people who are feeling emotionally or physically vulnerable or in distress, conveying compassion and sensitivity.	Chapters 2 & 11–16
3 Evidence-based, best practice communication skills and approaches for providing therapeutic interventions	
3.1 Motivational interview techniques.	Chapter 3
3.2 Solution focused therapies.	Chapter 3
3.3 Reminiscence therapies.	Chapter 3
3.4 Talking therapies.	Chapter 3
3.5 De-escalation strategies and techniques.	Chapters 2 & 3
3.6 Cognitive behavioural therapy techniques.	Chapter 3
3.7 Play therapy.	Chapters 3 & 11
3.8 Distraction and diversion strategies	Chapters 3 & 14
3.9 Positive behaviour support approaches	Chapter 11
4 Evidence-based, best practice communication skills and approaches for working with people in professional teams	
4.1 Demonstrate effective supervision, teaching and performance appraisal through the use of:	
4.1.1 clear instructions and explanations when supervising, teaching, or appraising others	Chapters 9, 10 & 17

4.1.2 clear instructions and check understanding when delegating care responsibilities to others	Chapter 9
4.1.3 unambiguous, constructive feedback about strengths and weaknesses and potential for improvement	Chapters 9, 10 & 17
4.1.4 encouragement to colleagues that helps them to reflect on their practice	Chapters 9, 10 & 17
4.1.5 unambiguous records of performance	Chapters 9 & 10
4.2 Demonstrate effective person and team management through the use of:	
4.2.1 strengths-based approaches to developing teams and managing change	Chapter 10
4.2.2 active listening when dealing with team members' concerns and anxieties	Chapters 9 & 10
4.2.3 a calm presence when dealing with conflict	Chapter 9
4.2.4 appropriate and effective confrontation strategies	Chapter 9
4.2.5 de-escalation strategies and techniques when dealing with conflict	Chapter 9
4.2.6 effective coordination and navigation skills through:	Chapter 9
4.2.6.1 appropriate negotiation strategies	Chapter 9
4.2.6.3 appropriate approaches to advocacy	Chapters 9 & 11-16

Annexe B: Nursing procedures

The nursing procedures that a newly registered nurse must be able to demonstrate in order to meet the proficiency outcomes, outlined previously above are set out in this annexe. The registered nurse must be able to undertake these procedures effectively in order to provide, compassionate, evidence-based person-centred nursing care. A holistic approach to the care of people is essential and all nursing procedures should be carried out in a way which reflects cultural awareness and ensures that the needs, priorities, expertise, and preferences of people are always valued and taken into account. Registered nurses in all fields of practice must demonstrate the ability to provide nursing intervention and support for people of all ages who require nursing procedures during the processes of assessment, diagnosis, care, and treatment for mental, physical, cognitive, and behavioural health challenges. Where people are disabled or have specific cognitive needs it is essential that reasonable adjustments are made to ensure that all procedures are undertaken safely. The nursing procedures within this annexe are set out in two sections. These requirements are relevant to all fields of nursing practice although it is recognised that different care settings may require different approaches to the provision of care. It is expected that these procedures would be assessed in a student's chosen field of practice where practicable.

Those procedures outlined in Annexe B, Part I: Procedures for assessing needs for person-centred care, sections 1 and 2 also apply to all registered nurses, but the level of expertise and knowledge required will vary depending on the chosen field(s) of practice. Registered nurses must therefore be able to demonstrate the ability to undertake these procedures at an appropriate level for their intended field(s) of practice.

At the point of registration, the registered nurse will be able to safely demonstrate the following procedures:

Part I: Procedures for assessing people's needs for person-centred care	
1 Use evidence-based, best practice approaches to take a history, observe, recognise and accurately assess people of all ages	Chapter 3
1.1 Mental health and wellbeing status	Chapter 3

1.1.1 signs of mental and emotional distress or vulnerability	Chapter 3
1.1.2 cognitive health status and wellbeing	Chapter 3
1.1.3 signs of cognitive distress and impairment	Chapter 3
1.1.4 behavioural distress-based needs	Chapter 3
1.1.5 signs of mental and emotional distress including agitation, aggression, and challenging behaviour	Chapter 3
1.2 Physical health and wellbeing	Chapters 3 & 11–16
1.2.1 symptoms and signs of physical ill health	Chapters 3 & 11–16
1.2.2 symptoms and signs of physical distress	Chapters 3 & 11–16
1.2.3 symptoms and signs of deterioration and sepsis	Chapters 14 & 15
2 Use evidence-based, best practice approaches to undertake the following procedures	
2.1 Take, record and interpret vital signs manually and via technological devices	Chapters 3 & 11–16
2.2 Undertake venepuncture and cannulation and blood sampling, interpreting normal and common abnormal blood profiles and venous blood gases	Chapters 3, 14 & 15
2.3 Set up and manage routine electrocardiogram (ECG) investigations and interpret normal and commonly encountered abnormal traces	Chapters 14–15
2.4 Manage and monitor blood component transfusions	Chapters 14–15
2.5 Manage and interpret cardiac monitors, infusion pumps, blood glucose monitors and other monitoring devices	Chapters 3 & 14–16
2.6 Accurately measure weight and height, calculate body mass index, and recognise healthy ranges and clinically significant low/high readings	Chapter 3
2.7 Undertake a whole-body systems assessment including respiratory, circulatory, neurological, musculoskeletal, cardiovascular, and skin status	Chapter 3
2.8 Undertake chest auscultation and interpret findings	Chapter 3
2.9 Collect and observe sputum, urine, stool, and vomit specimens, undertaking routine analysis and interpreting findings	Chapter 3
2.10 Measure and interpret blood glucose levels	Chapter 3
2.11 Recognise and respond to signs of all forms of abuse	Chapters 3 & 11–16
2.12 Undertake, respond to, and interpret neurological observations and assessments	Chapter 3
2.13 Identify and respond to signs of deterioration and sepsis	Chapters 14–15
2.14 Administer basic mental health first aid	Chapter 11
2.15 Administer basic physical first aid	Chapters 14 & 17
2.16 Recognise and manage seizures	Chapter 17
3 Use evidence-based, best practice approaches for meeting needs for care and support with rest, sleep, comfort, and the maintenance of dignity, accurately assessing the person's capacity for independence and self-care and initiating appropriate interventions	
3.1 Observe and assess comfort and pain levels and rest and sleep patterns	Chapters 3 & 11–16

3.2 Use appropriate bed-making techniques including those required for people who are unconscious or who have limited mobility	Chapter 3
3.3 Use appropriate positioning and pressure relieving techniques	Chapters 3 & 11–16
3.4 Take appropriate action to ensure privacy and dignity at all times	Chapters 3 & 11–16
3.5 Take appropriate action to reduce or minimise pain or discomfort	Chapters 3 & 11–16
3.6 Take appropriate action to reduce fatigue, minimise insomnia and support improved rest and sleep hygiene	Chapters 3 & 11–16
4 Use evidence-based, best practice approaches for meeting the needs for care and support with hygiene and the maintenance of skin integrity, accurately assessing the person's capacity for independence and self-care and initiating appropriate interventions	
4.1 Observe, assess, and optimise skin and hygiene status and determine the need for support and intervention	Chapter 3
4.2 Use contemporary approaches to the assessment of skin integrity and use appropriate products to prevent or manage skin breakdown	Chapter 3
4.3 Assess need for and provide appropriate assistance with washing, bathing, shaving, and dressing	Chapter 3
4.4 Identify and manage skin irritations and rashes	Chapter 3
4.5 Assess need for and provide appropriate oral, dental, eye and nail care and decide when an onward referral is needed	Chapter 3
4.6 Use aseptic techniques when undertaking wound care including dressings, pressure bandaging, suture removal and vacuum closures	Chapter 3
4.7 Use aseptic techniques when managing wound and drainage processes	Chapter 3
4.8 Assess, respond, and effectively manage pyrexia and hypothermia	Chapters 3 & 11–16
5 Use evidence-based, best practice approaches for meeting needs for care and support with nutrition and hydration, accurately assessing the person's capacity for independence and self-care and initiating appropriate interventions	
5.1 Observe, assess, and optimise nutrition and hydration status and determine the need for intervention and support	Chapters 3 & 11–16
5.2 Use contemporary nutritional assessment tools	Chapters 3 & 11–16
5.3 Assist with feeding and drinking and use appropriate feeding and drinking aids	Chapters 3 & 12–16
5.4 Record fluid intake and output and identify, respond to, and manage dehydration or fluid retention	Chapters 3 & 12–16
5.5 Identify, respond to, and manage nausea and vomiting	Chapters 3 & 12–16
5.6 Insert, manage and remove oral/nasal/gastric tubes	Chapters 3 & 12–16
5.7 Manage artificial nutrition and hydration using oral, enteral, and parenteral routes	Chapters 14 & 15
5.8 Manage the administration of IV fluids	Chapters 14 & 15
5.9 Manage fluid and nutritional infusion pumps and devices	Chapters 14 & 15
6 Use evidence-based, best practice approaches for meeting needs for care and support with bladder and bowel health, accurately assessing the person's capacity for independence and self-care and initiating appropriate interventions	

6.1 Observe and assess level of urinary and bowel continence to determine the need for support and intervention assisting with toileting, maintaining dignity and privacy, and managing the use of appropriate aids	Chapter 3
6.2 Select and use appropriate continence products; insert, manage, and remove catheters for all genders; and assist with self-catheterisation when required	Chapters 3 & 12-16
6.3 Manage bladder drainage	Chapters 12-16
6.4 Assess elimination patterns to identify and respond to constipation, diarrhoea, and urinary and faecal retention	Chapter 3
6.5 Administer enemas and suppositories and undertake rectal examination and manual evacuation when appropriate	Chapters 3 & 12-16
6.6 Undertake stoma care identifying and using appropriate products and approaches	Chapter 3
7 Use evidence-based, best practice approaches for meeting needs for care and support with mobility and safety, accurately assessing the person's capacity for independence and self-care and initiating appropriate interventions	
7.1 Observe and use evidence-based risk assessment tools to determine need for support and intervention to optimise mobility and safety, and to identify and manage risk of falls using best practice risk assessment approaches	Chapters 3 & 12-16
7.2 Use a range of contemporary moving and handling techniques and mobility aids	Chapters 3 & 12-16
7.3 Use appropriate moving and handling equipment to support people with impaired mobility	Chapters 3 & 12-16
7.4 Use appropriate safety techniques and devices	Chapters 3 & 11-16
8 Use evidence-based, best practice approaches for meeting needs for respiratory care and support, accurately assessing the person's capacity for independence and self-care and initiating appropriate interventions	
8.1 Observe and assess the need for intervention and respond to restlessness, agitation and breathlessness using appropriate interventions	Chapters 3 & 12-16
8.2 Manage the administration of oxygen using a range of routes and best practice approaches	Chapters 13, 14 & 15
8.3 Take and interpret peak flow and oximetry measurements	Chapter 3
8.4 Use appropriate nasal and oral suctioning techniques	Chapters 3 & 14-15
8.5 Manage inhalation, humidifier, and nebuliser devices	Chapter 3
8.6 Manage airway and respiratory processes and equipment	Chapters 14-15
9 Use evidence-based, best practice approaches for meeting needs for care and support with the prevention and management of infection, accurately assessing the person's capacity for independence and self-care and initiating appropriate interventions	
9.1 Observe, assess, and respond rapidly to potential infection risks using best practice guidelines	Chapter 3
9.2 Use standard precautions protocols	Chapter 3
9.3 Use effective aseptic, non-touch techniques	Chapter 3
9.4 Use appropriate personal protection equipment	Chapter 3

9.5 Implement isolation procedures	Chapter 3
9.6 Use evidence-based hand hygiene techniques	Chapter 3
9.7 Safely decontaminate equipment and environment	Chapter 3
9.8 Safely use and dispose of waste, laundry, and sharps	Chapter 3
9.9 Safely assess and manage invasive medical devices and lines	Chapters 3, 14 & 15
10 Use evidence-based, best practice approaches for meeting needs for care and support at the end of life, accurately assessing the person's capacity for independence and self-care and initiating appropriate interventions	
10.1 Observe and assess the need for intervention for people, families, and carers, identify, assess, and respond appropriately to uncontrolled symptoms and signs of distress including pain, nausea, thirst, constipation, restlessness, agitation, anxiety, and depression	Chapters 12-16
10.2 Manage and monitor effectiveness of symptom relief medication, infusion pumps and other devices	Chapters 12-16
10.3 Assess and review preferences and care priorities of the dying person and their family and carers	Chapter 16
10.4 Understand and apply organ and tissue donation protocols, advanced planning decisions, living wills and health and lasting powers of attorney for health	Chapters 15 & 16
10.5 Understand and apply DNACPR (do not attempt cardiopulmonary resuscitation) decisions and verification of expected death	Chapters 15 & 16
10.6 Provide care for the deceased person and the bereaved respecting cultural requirements and protocols	Chapter 16
11 Procedural competencies required for best practice, evidence-based medicines administration and optimisation	
11.1 Carry out initial and continued assessments of people receiving care and their ability to self-administer their own medications	Chapter 6
11.2 Recognise the various procedural routes under which medicines can be prescribed, supplied, dispensed, and administered; and the laws, policies, regulations, and guidance that underpin them	Chapter 6
11.3 Use the principles of safe remote prescribing and directions to administer medicines	Chapter 6
11.4 Undertake accurate drug calculations for a range of medications	Chapter 6
11.5 Undertake accurate checks, including transcription and titration, of any direction to supply or administer a medicinal product	Chapter 6
11.6 Exercise professional accountability in ensuring the safe administration of medicines to those receiving care	Chapter 6
11.7 Administer injections using intramuscular, subcutaneous, intradermal, and intravenous routes and manage injection equipment	Chapter 6
11.8 Administer medications using a range of routes	Chapter 6
11.9 Administer and monitor medications using vascular access devices and enteral equipment	Chapter 6
11.10 Recognise and respond to adverse or abnormal reactions to medications	Chapter 6
11.11 Undertake safe storage, transportation, and disposal of medicinal products	Chapter 6

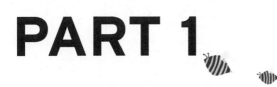

PART 1

THEORY AND CONTEXT IN RELATION TO ADULT NURSING

1

ESSENTIALS OF NURSING: VALUES, KNOWLEDGE, SKILLS, AND PRACTICE

Joanne Timpson, Jane Brooks, Elizabeth Lee-Woolf, and Dianne Burns

Chapter objectives

- Outline the landmarks of nursing history and highlight how these have influenced nursing practice across the UK;
- Explain how legal and ethical principles provide a core framework for professional practise;
- Define the core values that underpin nursing and recognise their application to practise;
- Understand the principles of *The Code* (Nursing and Midwifery Council or NMC, 2018a) by which we practise and how these define our fitness to practise;
- Highlight the challenges to modern nursing and relate these to our professional values regarding cultural competence, emotional intelligence, and professional resilience.

Nursing is a unique privilege born of presence and predicated on the partnerships we construct to meet the needs of the people we care for. As you begin your studies in nursing, we hope that you will be as curious as you are enthusiastic for your chosen profession and trust that you are prepared for the exciting challenge ahead. Our aim is to engage you with our own passion for nursing and to instill an ethos of nursing as a privilege. Together, we will review key landmarks in nursing history, debate the core facets of nursing knowledge and values, and explore how these will underpin your practice in a way that we hope will excite your professional imagination, intelligence, and intent.

Related Nursing and Midwifery Council (NMC) proficiencies for Registered Nurses

The overarching NMC requirement is that all nurses act in the best interests of people, putting them first and providing nursing care that is person-centred, safe, and compassionate. Both students and registered nurses should always act professionally, applying their knowledge and experience to make evidence-based decisions about care. Nurses communicate effectively, are role models for others and are accountable for their actions. Registered nurses continually reflect on their practice and keep abreast of new and emerging developments in nursing, health, and social care (NMC, 2018b). When unsure, nurses stop and thoughtfully revisit their preparedness and competency to act (Seedhouse and Peutherer, 2020). This is an essential professional attribute and one that requires self-awareness, moral judgement, and confidence. Never be afraid to question planned interventions if you feel they are outside of *The Code* (NMC, 2018a) or at variance with the current evidence base. It is your duty to challenge yourself when you are unsure of yourself or others.

TO ACHIEVE ENTRY TO THE NMC REGISTER YOU MUST BE ABLE TO

- Understand and act in accordance with *The Code: Professional Standards of Practice and Behaviour for Nurses and Midwives* and fulfil all registration requirements (NMC, 2018a);
- Act as an ambassador, upholding the reputation of your profession and promoting public confidence in nursing, health, and care services;
- Understand and apply relevant legal, regulatory and governance requirements, policies, and ethical frameworks to all areas of practice, differentiating where appropriate between the devolved legislatures of the United Kingdom;
- Demonstrate professional resilience and emotional intelligence and be capable of explaining the rationale that influences your judgements and decisions in routine, complex and challenging situations;
- Understand and maintain the level of health, fitness and wellbeing required to meet people's needs for mental and physical care;
- Understand the demands of professional practise and demonstrate how to recognise signs of vulnerability in yourself or your colleagues and the action required to minimise risks to health;
- Understand and apply the principles of courage, transparency, and the duty of candour, recognising and reporting any situations, behaviours or errors that could result in poor care outcomes;

- Demonstrate an understanding of and the ability to challenge discriminatory behaviour;
- Take responsibility for continuous self-reflection, seeking and responding to support and feedback to develop your professional knowledge and skills.

(Adapted from NMC, 2018b)

To understand the role of the contemporary adult nurse in the UK, it is important to know a little of nursing's history and to recognise key landmarks over the last 150 years that signal the development towards the professional nursing practice we have today. However, it is not our intention to provide a detailed history of nursing here and you are advised to explore 'Further Reading' at the end of this chapter, which illustrates in more detail the historical threads that bring us to this point.

Although caring, and the role of carer, has existed throughout history, nursing in its modern sense is a recent concept. It is recognised that the words 'nurse' and 'nursing' are derived from the Old French *nourice* and the Late Latin *nutrire*, meaning to nourish and care (*Oxford English Dictionary*, 2014), but their use in today's sense has occurred only from the seventeenth century onwards. It is often suggested that nursing can be traced back through history to its earliest times. If you accept that this reflects the act of caring, then this is undoubtedly true. The themes that run through the earliest annals of history involve those who provided succour (i.e., assistance and support in times of hardship or distress) for families, communities or for those injured in battle, for example. What is perhaps more important here for modern notions of nursing are those involved with what Reverby (1987), O'Brien D'Antonio (1993) and Mann Wall (1998) have called 'professed-nursing', namely the care of sick strangers This distinction is crucial because, if we understand modern professional nursing as caring for those who are not friends or family, this means that it is a very different undertaking from caring for those who are. Nevertheless, often the carers who nursed 'sick strangers' were influenced by religious values and altruism, believing that it would be wrong to gain monetarily from their work. There was, however, a more insidious ideology at work: once a lady worked for money, she was no longer considered a lady. To cite historian Hawkins, '*they forfeited their respectability*' (Hawkins, 2010: 29). Given that nursing reformers in the nineteenth century wished to increase the number of educated middle-class women in the occupation this was clearly a problem. Hence, the vocation or calling to nurse has been the province of those who had a desire to care with little thought of reward or, more pertinently, were felt not to want such financial reward because they were respectable. Either way, whilst philanthropy may indeed be admirable, such notions influenced the status of the nurse and some might argue, limited the evolution of nursing as a highly skilled profession (Helmstadter, 1993, 1996).

Throughout the eighteenth century we can see the appearance of what might be termed the 'modern hospital' in Britain. This was also the Age of Enlightenment – a movement made up of intellectuals who wished to see development in many areas of life through reasoned argument and science rather than adhering to traditions without thought. This influence can be seen in the funding of modern 'voluntary hospitals' by wealthy benefactors such as Thomas Guy who funded

Guy's Hospital in London (1719), followed by the Edinburgh Royal Infirmary (founded in 1729), St Bartholomew's Hospital (opened in 1730, funded by public subscription), the Middlesex Hospital (opened in 1745, funded by public subscription) and the Manchester Royal Infirmary (in 1752). These hospitals had a charitable remit to provide treatment for the poor which was recognised by an Act of Parliament in 1836. However, they needed to provide care only for the 'deserving poor,' and all voluntary hospitals tended to focus on acute illnesses that could be treated and would therefore provide excellent advertisements for potential future benefactors. This system excluded the chronically sick, the elderly and infirm, the mentally ill and those with learning disabilities. The last two types of people were cared for in separate 'asylums for the insane' whereas the elderly and chronically sick were cared for in Poor Law Hospitals. The Poor Law Hospitals were described as 'murderous pesthouses' into which 'the dense mass of living creatures were crammed' (cited in White, 1978: 18).

- How do people today consider the work carried out by nurses in intensive care units in acute hospitals?
- How do people view the nursing of older people with dementia?
- What sort of facilities do we offer to each of these groups of people?
- The thing about history is that there are often reasons in our past that go some way to explaining the ways in which services develop over time.
- Are you able to identify any links with history for the care of older people that exist today?

Modern nursing has its roots in the nineteenth century (please note, we do not wish to ignore the notion that there were significant examples of nursing-type activities in earlier times, but it would be difficult to present their importance here without sounding superficial). As the Industrial Revolution changed the face of our national landscape the need to care for and manage the sick faced equal challenges. The choices surrounding who did what were primarily influenced by industry and the developing urban communities employed therein, but also by gender role. As a result, those individuals who nursed tended to be women. Living conditions were often crowded, unsanitary and polluted. Disease flourished and work-based accidents were common.

Some Early Nursing Pioneers in Britain

Florence Nightingale was born in 1820 to a wealthy family. She was encouraged and taught to think and question in a way that was unusual for a girl of those times. Her parents did not approve of her wish to nurse, which they deemed unconventional. However, in 1851 she travelled to Kaiserswerth for three months to learn to be a nurse and two years later Nightingale became superintendent of a hospital for gentlewomen in Harley Street. The outbreak of the Crimean War, and the plight of wounded soldiers in terrible conditions, saw her initiate a campaign to take a team of nurses to military hospitals in Turkey where, despite relentless opposition, she improved the care and conditions for those in her care. Even before her return to Britain in 1856 the Nightingale Fund – which the grateful public of Britain had established in her name following her work in the Crimea – had accrued significant monies. Although initially not enthused by the project, in 1860 the Nightingale Training School for nurses at St Thomas's Hospital in London was established in her name (Baly, 1997; Bostridge, 2008). The purpose of the school was to train nurses who would then establish similar schools based on her principles. By 1867 probationer nurses were able to pay to attend and this facilitated a two-tier system of nurses where, by the turn of the twentieth century, only those who had paid for their training would be offered a post as Sister.

Mary Seacole was another Crimean pioneer (Alexander and Dewjee, 1984; Griffon, 1998). Born in Jamaica in 1805 (her father was a Scot and her mother Jamaican), Seacole was well travelled and had gained perspectives on medicines and care wherever she went. Like Florence Nightingale, in 1854 Seacole asked the British government to send her to the Crimea to assist in the army hospital. In her autobiography, Seacole recalled being turned down. However, she did then fund her own travel to the Crimea, where she cared for soldiers. On returning to the UK her health was poor and she had little money and no family to support her. She achieved a great deal but died in 1881 and thus did not live to see the achievement of nurse registration.

Ethel Gordon Manson (who later became known as Mrs Bedford Fenwick) was passionate about the improvements to nursing and nurse training. She trained as a nurse at the Nottingham Children's Hospital and then at Manchester's Royal Infirmary between 1878 and 1879. She became the matron of St Bartholomew's Hospital in London at the age of only 24 years. In 1888 she married Dr Bedford Fenwick, retired from nursing, and devoted her life to national and international nursing matters. As the founder of the Royal British Nurses' Association (1887) and the International Council of Nurses (1899), and editor of the first professional nursing journal *The Nursing Record/The British Journal of Nursing*, from 1893 to 1946, she staunchly advocated that nursing should be regulated and every nurse should be registered. She is considered to have contributed to phenomenal achievements in the development of nursing (Griffon, 1995). She died on 13 March 1947.

Activity 1.1

Find out more about the pioneers of nursing practice and identify their contribution to the development of nursing and nurse education.

You can start by accessing the UK Association for the History of Nursing at http://ukahn.org/wp/

We should not deny the fact that, while nursing was struggling for recognition, this aspect also reflects an earlier period in medicine where doctors had little recognisably organised training as such. The Medical Act of 1858 responded to a need for the public to be able to determine whether a doctor was qualified to practise and resulted in the inauguration of the General Medical Council. This professional body was (and remains to this day) charged with registering practitioners and ensuring that the public have access to that information (although this is now governed under the Medical Act of 1983). Following on from this, many recognised the logic for nurses to be registered in a similar fashion. The debate and will for this became more organised, especially after the beginning of nursing training in 1860.

By 1880 the Hospitals' Association (HA) agreed that some form of nurse registration was a necessity and therefore voluntary registration was introduced. Ethel Bedford Fenwick (a member of the Matrons' Committee) passionately believed in professionalism and that nurses should be registered in a similar fashion to doctors. She set up the British Nurses' Association, which provided an alternative voluntary register that noted completion of a programme of study, but also more importantly aligned itself with a remit to protect the public.

The First World War provided the pivotal impetus for registration. Many women had answered a call to go and nurse which had, incidentally, raised the profile of nursing with the public. Women's role in society was changing and their contribution to working life while soldiers were away generally noted and applauded. Meanwhile, the College of Nursing was founded in 1916 (later to become the Royal College of Nursing). This organisation led and supported initiatives to further develop and raise the profile of nursing and the need for a nursing register. In 1919 one MP (Major Barnet) was persuaded to propose a Private Members' Bill which resulted in the Nurse Registration Act. This called upon the General Nursing Council to maintain and monitor a nursing register, as well as provide central guidance to inform nurse training programmes. It was replaced by the United Kingdom Central Council in 1983 and subsequently by the Nursing and Midwifery Council in 2002. All had similar duties in their role to maintain the register, provide educational guidance and ensure protection of the public. In the same year nursing became a registrable profession, women over the age of 30 were given the right to vote. However, this would have excluded many nurses. It would not be until 1928 that women had the same rights of franchise as men.

The NHS was created in 1948, which again reflected the changes that war had brought to society. However, and despite the work of many groups, nurse education and the role of the nurse were slow to evolve. Graduate education for nurses was embryonic although several university medical schools began offering some form of nurse education at degree level. The University of Edinburgh offered the first degree in nursing in 1960 (Brooks, 2011) and the University of Manchester's Bachelor of Nursing degree soon followed (Hallett, 2005). It was at the University of Manchester that the first Professor of Nursing was appointed – Jean Kennedy McFarlane, later to become Baroness McFarlane of Llandaff. Other 'experimental' courses were tried throughout the 1960s and 1970s, with some at degree and some at diploma level.

The Birth of Modern Nursing

Several reports during the twentieth century culminated in the Briggs Committee's remit to consider various concerns surrounding the methods, content and quality of nurse education and its interface with the NHS. Margaret Scott Wright was an influential member of this committee and the report that followed in 1972 recommended a step change resulting in a move away from training towards professional education and the development of research into all aspects of education and nursing practice. After much wrangling the Nurses, Midwives and Health Visitors Act (passed in 1979) saw the beginnings of a modern-day nursing education.

Project 2000 was introduced in 1988 and diploma education for nurses was piloted in several schools prior to it being rolled out across the UK. Student nurses now had student status and were no longer employees of the hospital in which the School of Nursing was based. This created some challenges for nursing practice, but these were not insurmountable and many nurses at all levels engaged with this innovative approach to education with enthusiasm. Between 1990 and 2010 diploma and degree courses in nursing ran side by side, but in 2010 legislation was enacted to ensure that every nurse in England would be educated to degree level, reflecting previous changes already effected in Scotland, Northern Ireland, and Wales, for both nursing and other allied health professions such as physiotherapy, radiography, and occupational therapy.

Twentieth-Century Pioneers in Nursing

Lisbeth Hockey was born Lisbeth Hochsinger on 17 October 1918 in Graz, Steiermark, Austria. In 1936, at the age of 18, she commenced her medical studies at the Karl-Franzens University of Graz. However, following the Nazi occupation of Austria in 1938 she left for England (Brooks, 2011). Hockey was not able to recommence her medical studies in England for three reasons: she was a woman (and few British women went to university at that time); she did not speak English; and she had no money. British friends recommended nursing as an alternative and so Hockey began her training at the London Hospital in Whitechapel in 1939 (Mason, 2005: 2-5). Her importance to the nursing profession came from her natural desire to ask questions. However, during her training this was to cause her problems with those in authority:

> *What intrigued me or alarmed me was the number of pressure sores and bed sores of course in those days. But what interested me more, was why some patients did not get bed sores ... And I went to the sister one day and said, 'please explain to me why some patients have got bed sores and others didn't' seeing as I was interested in the ones that did not, and she said, 'it's not your place to ask questions, go back and do your work.'* (Hockey, 2001)

She was not put off, and after qualifying as a nurse she trained as both a district nurse and then a health visitor before becoming a tutor at the Royal College of Nursing. In 1971, Hockey became the Director of the first Nursing Research Unit at the University of Edinburgh (Weir, 2004). She was awarded her PhD on 3 December 1979 and on 4 December the same year was invested Order of the British Empire in recognition of her contribution to nursing research (Mason, 2005: 2). She died on 15 June 2004.

Baroness Jean McFarlane of Llandaff (Jean Kennedy McFarlane) was born on 1 April 1926. The youngest child of a large family, she did well at school and went to study sciences at London University. However, her voluntary work with people experiencing difficult life situations led her to undertake a nursing course at Manchester Royal Infirmary, and then later she qualified as both a midwife and health visitor. Her career in nursing saw her lead a project, sponsored by the then Department of Health and Social Security and the RCN (Royal College of Nursing), to research nursing care in depth and provide evidence for quality care. McFarlane's role was to summarise the project and produce a literature review on '*The proper study of the nurse*' (McFarlane, 1970). She returned to Manchester in the early 1970s to work with the Department of Community Medicine, her vision being that nurses' education should be of graduate standing and prepare them to work equally in a hospital or a community setting. This resulted in the development of a bachelor's degree in nursing with additional health visiting and district nursing qualifications. Her work was renowned on both the national and the international stage. McFarlane was awarded a chair in nursing at Manchester in 1974 – the first in England – and her subsequent work for the Royal Commission on the NHS led to her parliamentary seat in the House of Lords and further influence on several select committees. Although Baroness McFarlane died in 2012, her influence on people and undergraduate nurse education continues to evolve and respond to the dynamic world of healthcare provision.

Margaret Scott Wright (a contemporary of both Jean McFarlane and Lisbeth Hockey) enjoyed significant nursing and nurse management roles at St George's and the Middlesex Hospitals in London before embarking on a challenging career as a nursing researcher in both Edinburgh and several Canadian universities (Brooks, 2011). Her clinical work spanned a period of immense development of the nursing role in care, the advance of technology in diagnostics and treatment, and a stronger dialogue between medical practitioners and nurses, which would evolve into clinical specialist nursing opportunities. Scott Wright was passionate about the development of nursing research because she believed it would enhance the quality-of-care provision by adding academic rigour to the clinical nurse's expertise. She was also one of the first UK nurses to study for a Doctor of Philosophy (1961) and in 1971 was awarded the first chair of nursing studies in Europe while at Edinburgh University. Her desire to see nursing research as a central theme in nurse education was helped by her role in the influential Briggs Committee which reported to government in 1972 and strongly supported the development of nursing research units across the UK. Her career finally took her to Canada where she continued to have international influence on the development of nursing research.

So, What Can We Learn From Our Nursing History?

We can learn that nursing has, at its roots, nurture, caring, comfort, and compassion, ministered by those committed to humanitarian values and often enduring significant hardship in the process. Several conflicts have given rise to ground-breaking innovations and discoveries in medical technology and treatment (as necessity has driven invention), and the evolution of nursing has taken place alongside these. As a result, advances in nursing practice, and more recently nursing research, have often followed the development of medical practice. One thing that we can be sure of is that as a nursing student you will study, learn, practise and develop your knowledge and skills in the light of new discoveries and treatments. Indeed, nursing in the future will surely be different from what it is today. However, in this regard we must advise caution: we must be careful not to live in our history because this can distract us from the importance of our present and the potential for nursing's future. A healthy interest in events that have shaped the profession will often provide the impetus and courage to ensure that our nursing practice continues to evolve and can meet the needs of service users in a dynamic world.

- Are you able to identify your reasons for becoming a nurse?
- What is it that you wish to achieve?
- What skills and attributes do you feel you can offer the profession?

Keep a note of your answers to these questions because we shall revisit this topic later in the chapter.

Where Are We Now?

Today, those aspiring to be professional nurses can access the benefits of established educational programmes which are both validated and monitored by a professional body, the Nursing and Midwifery Council (NMC), and the Higher Education Institutions (HEI) in which they take place. As new registrants launch their careers, learning continues. Nurses grow in knowledge and skill while experience, reflective practice, and professional discussion facilitate the delivery of effective, compassionate care to those who need it and for colleagues alike. Strategies such as *Modernising Nursing Careers* (Department of Health, Social Services and Public Safety or DHSSPS, 2006) and *Preceptorship Frameworks* (NHS Wales, 2014; NHS Education for Scotland, 2021; NHS England 2022; Northern Ireland Practice and Education Council for Nursing and Midwifery, 2022) support this development.

The role of the nurse has extended, and nurses are now significant partners with other health professionals and service users in care provision. Increasingly, specialist nurses are the leaders of care and take on additional responsibilities in areas such as prescribing, implementing complex care interventions, performing minor surgery and other invasive treatments. It is clear that nursing as a profession is facing an unprecedented rate of change. This is partly in response to the changing face of healthcare itself as we move towards a more community-based focus of care. However, it is also because of improvements in treatments and emergent technologies. We face targets and the competitive aspects of a free-market economy, which has been introduced to the NHS where it is almost impossible to put a price on the time you spend with a frightened person waiting for uncertain news in the Accident & Emergency department for example. We continue to face increased scrutiny from our service users and those who provide carer support. Increased media coverage has led to an atmosphere of alarm, ambiguity, and a perception of neglect, especially in the context of ongoing chronic disease and end of life care. This lack of compassion and kindness was highlighted in its starkest form in various reports and enquiries (Parliamentary and Health

Service Ombudsman, 2011; Department of Health, 2012a; Francis, 2013), provoking a necessary period of professional introspection, an avowed reclaiming of core values and the emergence of the seven principles of the NHS Constitution (NHS England, 2015), which will be explored and discussed in more detail later in the chapter.

It is our hope that as a registered nurse you will develop the knowledge, skills, and confidence to enable you to provide high-quality, evidence-based nursing in a variety of settings. Furthermore, we hope that you will always be sensitive to the needs of those in your care, their families and/or carers, and to your multidisciplinary colleagues with whom you work and communicate in the provision of holistic care.

The parameters for your programme of study are laid down by the NMC in *Future Nurse: Standards of Proficiency for Registered Nurses* (NMC, 2018b). These standards provide a framework to which your university or higher educational institution (HEI) will add the appropriate knowledge and experience that will help you meet these essential requirements. During your studies you will undoubtedly learn about nursing theory and practice, anatomy and physiology in health and illness, psychology and communication, sociology, pharmacology, microbiology, health promotion and education, law, and ethics. When applied to nursing these topics will form the building blocks that will then inform your practice. As you move through several learning experiences you will begin to appreciate the diverse nature of adult nursing and the various specialist roles of those who work within it. There may well be some aspects that you will find more difficult to learn than others and some areas where you will feel more at home. The point here is that you will be exposed to an essential variety of care settings that will facilitate your development and help you make decisions about where you will want to focus your own practice when registered.

Your experience will also be influenced by both local and national developments in policy and practice; for example, National Service Frameworks, Clinical Guidelines or Plans for Care and/or Care Pathways (which will be referred to regularly throughout the chapters that follow).

Then, wherever you undertake your learning it will reflect the fact that contemporary adult nursing takes place in various settings where care is often delivered to a diverse client group. This might seem a tall order if you are new to a nursing programme, but you will bring knowledge and experience with you as you start a course of study, and gradually you will be encouraged and guided to build and extend that knowledge and understanding over the three years of your programme and beyond, thereby embarking on a lifelong learning journey.

This is where a professional portfolio or profile and your skills of reflective practice will prove invaluable. Completing a programme of study in a practice discipline such as nursing is akin to learning to climb a mountain. There are strict protocols and procedures to assimilate and follow. When you first set off the terrain is unfamiliar and you will find yourself concentrating on your feet so that you do not fall over. Sometimes you will get out of breath if you try to climb too quickly or if you are trying to keep up with colleagues. At some point you will stop to catch your breath, turn around and admire the view, just in time to realise how far you have come. This then gives you the confidence to look up and out rather than down as the terrain has become more familiar. You will build sufficient stamina to keep going and navigate each new challenge. Occasionally, you will have to walk round or even down to be able to carry on climbing and that is fine because that is the safest route, for you and those in your care.

Professional practise can, on occasion, feel very uncertain. We traverse unfamiliar territory every day. Successful safe and self-aware practice is as reliant upon the interpretation and enactment of protocols and procedures as it is personal judgement, self-awareness, resilience, resourcefulness, and courage. All are necessary attributes. Your professional portfolio or profile is a comprehensive record of your professional achievements and developing reflective skills. It is a requirement of registration with the Nursing and Midwifery Council that every nurse can demonstrate that they have met the requirements for practice and continuing professional development (NMC, 2018c). Keeping a professional portfolio will help you adopt a 'lifelong learning' approach to both your professional and your personal development in addition to supporting the revalidation process.

Within any portfolio it is important to provide evidence of that development. This evidence will help you demonstrate to others that you have achieved the required learning outcomes in practice. During your studies you will acquire both study and practice skills to prepare you for your role as a qualified nurse. These skills will include those that are necessary to become a reflective practitioner, i.e., a professional individual who challenges practice in a constructive and helpful way.

Hence your portfolio is a record of your development as a nurse throughout every aspect of your course. It is a means of demonstrating your ongoing achievement and recording your development throughout your course and beyond. It is also a tool to help you develop the skills of critical awareness, reflective practice, rational decision making and clinical judgement. In summary, your portfolio is your showcase. It gives value to both the practical and the academic work you have completed.

Reflection is a process by which you can think about and achieve better knowledge and understanding of your practice, learning from your own experiences to improve the care you provide to those who need it. Reflecting on our experiences and interactions with others enables us, as caring professionals, to establish what we have learnt and the influence we may have had on others. The key message about reflection here is that it is purposeful and has meaning when it is undertaken and, just as with nursing practice, is constantly evolving. Reflection is often also referred to as "reflexivity, acting as an internal monitor or check for an individual's ever-changing self" (Todd, 2002: 62). As individuals we learn and evolve through education and a range of professional, personal, and third-party experiences; this then influences our behaviours and actions. Reflexivity is an integral part of developing as an effective nurse and is crucial whether we are caring for a dying person, someone who is suffering from an acute illness or a person who needs additional support to manage a chronic condition.

Schön (1983) suggests that there are two types of reflective practice: reflection in action (in the moment) and reflection on action (looking back on the moment), and purports that experienced nurses can reflect while in action and if necessary, change and adapt, whereas the novice reflects retrospectively. However, it is likely that these actions occur simultaneously, partly due to the evolution of nurse education and development since the 1980s. Most healthcare professionals are introduced to the concept of reflection and are encouraged throughout their course and professional life to apply reflexivity to their practice. Reflection is an active, purposeful act intended to make us challenge the world around us. It is a lifelong process of learning about ourselves and how things that happen to us can be thought about, deliberated, and acted on. This does not have to be a significant life-changing episode that you may have witnessed when providing care (e.g., communicating a terminal diagnosis); it may be something that has made you stop and consider the impact this has had on you.

There are many different models of reflection that can be used depending on your individual learning style and personal preference. One such example is the Gibbs reflective cycle (Gibbs, 1988) illustrated in Figure 1.1 which describes reflection as a process with distinct steps, i.e., as a description of what happened and the feelings evoked, followed by your evaluation and analysis of the situation, concluding with a review of the situation, including consideration of what you might do differently and the provision of an action plan based on your learning and aspirations for your future practice.

By documenting in your professional portfolio the things you have learned, the challenges you have faced (both the good and bad experiences encountered) and the wide range of people you have met in possibly heart-breaking circumstances, you will not only make a record of your professional journey and provide evidence of your achievements, but also build your reflexive aptitude and a capacity for self-awareness which should help you engage more effectively in order to improve people's healthcare outcomes. The important thing is that you can learn from your experiences and apply what you have learnt to your future practice. By using reflective practice and your portfolio in this way you should be able to trace the development of your knowledge base and skills for practice, your clinical judgement and decision making, and your leadership and management approaches as you prepare to nurse adults irrespective of their age, health status, culture, or disability. The ability to reflect upon practice in this way is something that we will revisit in subsequent chapters.

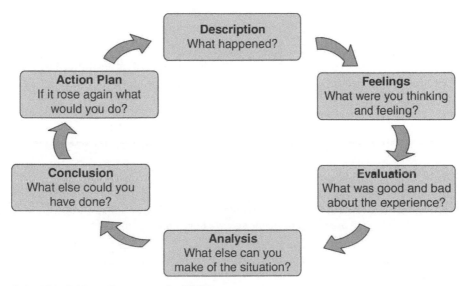

Figure 1.1   The Gibbs reflective cycle (1988)

'Profession,' 'Professional' and 'Professionalism'

Throughout this chapter we use the words 'profession' and 'professional' quite liberally. However, it is important to understand the difference between the two.

- What does being professional mean to you?
- Can you describe what professionalism means?

Entering or belonging to a profession means that you have undertaken a specific area of study (at degree level), and the way in which you carry out your work is governed by a set of codes and standards that is regulated by legislation (law). As a professional, you have a certain level of autonomy, and you are both responsible and accountable for all your actions. Belonging to a profession affords a status; being professional describes how you conduct yourself in that status. 'Professionalism' describes a set of values and behaviours that influence not just what you do but also how and when you do it. Professionalism is also framed in terms of awareness, attitudes and behaviours and relates to having sufficient professional judgement to identify the attitude and type of behaviour that are appropriate in any given situation. This is a distinction that may sometimes be missed. In all the caring professions, professionalism includes the ability to demonstrate the following values:

- Integrity;
- Honesty;
- Transparency;
- A sense of duty;
- Decency.

These are the values that will dictate how you should behave as a professional and therefore will have a direct impact on care provision. Indeed, being an accountable professional is the first platform of the NMC (2018b) proficiencies.

Activity 1.2

1   Go to the Nursing and Midwifery Council website and access the '*Enabling professionalism in nursing and midwifery practice*' document at: www.nmc.org.uk/globalassets/sitedocuments/ other-publications/enabling-professionalism.pdf
    Write down the key elements that are thought to be important and keep these handy. You will need to compare these later.
2   Now access the Professional Standards Authority website and review the following blog: www. professionalstandards.org.uk/news-and-blog/blog/detail/blog/2022/07/14/what-is-fitness-to-practise

Identify the key concepts that are related to 'Fitness to Practise' and make a list of issues that 'Fitness to Practise' committees are likely to be concerned about.

Why do you think 'Fitness to Practise' panel hearings are important?

3 Now look at the *'Professionalism in Healthcare Professionals'* report (HCPC, 2011) available at: www.hcpc-uk.org/globalassets/resources/reports/professionalism-in-healthcare-professionals.pdf

In the previous *'Professionalism in Healthcare Professionals'* report you may have noticed a trend in cases linked to a broad range of behaviours which were distinct from technical capability and termed 'professionalism' and the report provides an excellent summary of what professionalism entails. It also puts this in the context of healthcare in terms of relevant examples.

The key findings were that:

1 The concept of what professionalism is remains common regardless of the professional group, status, or training route;
2 Regulations are basic guidance and signposting on what is appropriate and what is unacceptable behaviour (acting as a baseline for behaviour rather than a specification) (HCPC, 2011).

An appropriate set of moral values and personal qualities must be the foundation to which we would add specialist knowledge and clinical skills. The above report supports the view that it is both possible and desirable to *'be* professional' before acquiring the necessary knowledge and skills to become a registered professional. This is particularly crucial in the context of healthcare students who, unlike many other undergraduate students, must be professional from day one because they must interact with individuals receiving care, their families and qualified healthcare professionals while working within a variety of health and social care learning environments. Professionalism is the consequence of qualities that an individual brings to the profession – indeed many of those questioned in the study felt that this was an essential part of themselves. Yet how does this manifest itself?

Consider the examples in the following activity.

The way in which we present ourselves is significant because it is the first impression people will get. What does it say about you if:

- You regularly turn up on time for lectures or shifts?
- You respond to a text on your mobile device during your first meeting with your practice assessor or supervisor?
- You often appear dishevelled and unkempt?
- You turn up to pre-arranged meetings with your supervisor or assessor having undertaken some preparation beforehand?
- You are sometimes rude or brusque?
- You listen carefully and act upon feedback?

How might an individual receiving care interpret each of the above behaviours in terms of the standard of care they think they will receive?

Obviously, there will always be the odd occasion when we are running late and even with the best of intentions our plans can sometimes go wrong. However, turning up on time to meetings, lectures or shifts in practice is one way of demonstrating our ongoing commitment – to those we care for, colleagues, and other professionals. Similarly, being rude to or about our colleagues gives an extremely poor impression to those we care for and their families, not only of ourselves as individuals but of the whole team providing care. Faulkner (1998) argues that those who find it difficult to communicate effectively with each other are less likely to be effective when interacting with people and their families. This is also demonstrated by HCPC UK (2011) who found that individuals who are professional have an innate sense of decency towards others and suggest that they are polite, courteous, non-condescending, and act honestly and with integrity.

How Do Legal and Ethical Principles Underpin Our Professional Practice?

The law may be broadly defined as:

> *The system of rules which a particular country or community recognises as regulating the actions of its members and which it may enforce by the imposition of penalties.* (Oxford Reference, 2023)

This is clearly reflected in *The Code* (NMC, 2018a: 18) where it states that, as a nurse:

- *You should uphold the reputation of your profession at all times;*
- *You should display a personal commitment to the standards of practice and behaviour set out in The Code;*
- *You should be a model of integrity and leadership for others to aspire to.*

This should lead to trust and confidence in the profession from those receiving care, other healthcare professionals and the public.

As our professional roles develop alongside innovations in healthcare knowledge and practice, associated technologies and increasing public demand, Wheeler (2012: 3) reminds us that 'moral values guide our thinking and behaviour and impact on our ethical decision making in relation to caring'. Therefore, as a student of nursing you are a developing professional and it is essential that you understand *The Code* (NMC, 2018a) to which you aspire and how this relates to all aspects of your everyday life and work.

Activity 1.3

Access and read the latest copy of the NMC **Code**, available at www.nmc.org.uk/standards/code

- What do you consider to be the aims of *The Code*?
- Which elements do you consider to be the most important and why?

The Code (NMC, 2018a) is designed to ensure that your practice is safe and that you do not leave your actions open to challenge. However, you are also expected to explore topics such as moral values, ethical theories, attitude development, accountability, confidentiality, integrity, and trust, to mention but a few. Each of these will underpin the relationships you form with individuals receiving care and their families, colleagues, the profession, and society in general. Developing your knowledge base to include these aspects will help you increase your appreciation of how legal requirements affect your work and be alert to situations where you should gain further advice and support.

If an understanding of the law helps us to have better understanding of what is legally right and wrong within the parameters of our nursing practice, then an appreciation of ethical principles helps us determine, through a process of structured reasoning, the morally 'good' course of action from the 'bad.' In both cases the perception of what is right and what is good will be influenced by your personal beliefs and values. For example, in a previous activity when asked to reflect on why you want to become a nurse, you may have considered that your desire is driven by your own moral compass, including your personal beliefs and values. Is this related to a belief in the centrality of integrity, compassion, and a willingness to be kind and caring, and a wish to empathise with those in need? However, what happens if your impulse is not based on a willingness to care? What if you are not empathic or non-judgemental?

It is important for nurses to be open-minded and able to care equally for all individuals, irrespective of their illness, age, sexuality, race, or religion. As an adult nurse you will be required to adhere to the ethical principles enshrined within *The Code* (NMC, 2018a), including the intention to do good, the insight to do no harm, the capacity to ensure justice, and the competence to promote dignity by respecting autonomy and affording participation and choice (Beauchamp and Childress, 2013). This is a complex and complicated process that relies on commitment and conviction and will require discipline and an enduring capacity to explore your own impulses. You will need to foster an ability to justify and articulate your choices in terms of both your actions and your omissions. You will often be called on to balance your private understandings against public expectations and professional requirements, and to promote the best interests of individuals, society, and the profession. You will need to accept shared professional parameters and role model professional values. You will also need to understand and be able to articulate your obligations to clients and colleagues alike.

It is vital to your own development – and more specifically to those in receipt of your care – that you are sure of the moral basis of your impetus to nurse. You may remember the answers you gave to the previous activity above. However, we would invite you to expand on these here and reflect upon the following questions:

- What informs your impulse to care?
- Why have you deliberately opted to work with individuals experiencing illness?
- How would you define nursing?
- What makes a '*good*' nurse and what kind of nurse do you want to be?
- As a conduit through which caring is facilitated, what skills do you possess/would you like to foster to best enact your nursing role?
- How might these skills be best secured and articulated?
- How can you give yourself the best chance of success?
- What are your goals?
- What are your sources of motivation and inspiration?

When reflecting upon how you might define nursing you may wish to consider three definitions of nursing that have evolved over the last 150 years:

> *Nature alone cures … and what nursing has to do … is to put the patient in the best condition for nature to act upon him.* (Nightingale, 1859)

> *The unique function of the nurse is to assist the individual – sick or well – in the performance of those activities contributing to health or its recovery (or to peaceful death) that he would perform unaided if he had the necessary strength, will or knowledge. And to do this in such a way as help him gain independence as rapidly as possible.* (Henderson, 1960)

> *Nursing is the use of clinical judgement in the provision of care to enable people to improve, maintain, or recover health, to cope with health problems and to achieve the best possible quality of life – whatever their disease or disability until death.* (RCN, 2014)

As a registered nurse you will inevitably face a range of ethical dilemmas during your studies and indeed throughout your professional life. As the conduit of care, your moral compass will dictate your actions and inform your choices. People deserve to always be nursed by someone who is careful, compassionate, and considerate. This calls for purposeful moral engagement combined with emotional intelligence based on a deliberate intention to place them at the centre of all your care, a personal philosophy of nursing as privilege and the facilitation of candour in terms of truthfulness and transparency. We work in partnership with those we care for, fostering a deliberate shared-care ethos whereby we recognise the autonomy and inner resources of those we nurse (Price, 2019).

The concept of moral engagement arises from social cognitive theory (Bandura, 1986; 1991) and requires you to stand firm in your moral behaviour, despite the possibility of peer or social pressure to act differently. This takes moral courage. Bandura suggests that a sure way to demonstrate this concept is through empathy. This means that you must accept responsibility for your behaviours and demonstrate a humane concern for others at all times. This ability to self-govern our behaviours ensures that we can consider best practice and best interest for those in our care.

In April 2015, the Criminal Justice and Courts Act (www.legislation.gov.uk/ukpga/2015/2/contents/enacted) made it an offence for 'an individual who has the care of another individual by virtue of being a care worker to ill-treat or willfully to neglect that individual'. It relates to the conduct of the individual and applies to healthcare workers (such as nurses, doctors, dentists etc) and exposes what that person did, or did not do, for the individual cared for rather than specifically any harm caused. Offences under this and associated legislation extend to all individuals irrespective of mental capacity or age. Griffith (2015) reports that neglect is said to occur where a healthcare worker does not do what is expected of them in relation to care provision, and can include omission of medication, incorrect recording of care or failing to assist a person in difficulty. Nurses must be honest and truthful at all times and meet the standards of law and the NMC by understanding the need to follow good practice. Nurses must be able to justify the reasons for their actions and duty of care, and all verbal engagement and records must reflect their precise involvement in any care provision.

Emotional intelligence (EI) is defined by Goleman (2005) as the ability to perceive and regulate your own emotions and those of others in a way that positively influences communication, motivation, and teamwork. Snowden et al. (2015) comment that, although elements of EI may be trait based, it can also be learned. The concept has gained popularity in a nursing context and appears to have links with quality-of-care provision, supports reflective practice and thus facilitates an increase in nurse resilience. Fernandez et al. (2012) explored the notion that higher levels of EI might link to increased performance and, although there are limited available studies as to whether EI can influence academic intelligence, Codier and Odell (2014) found a positive correlation between academic performance and EI in Year 1 student nurses. According to Goleman (2005), there are five integrated EI domains: self-awareness, self-regulation, motivation, empathy, and social skills. An interesting longitudinal study from Snowden et al. (2015) found that previous caring experiences did not mean that EI was heightened but rather that over time specific strategies to support the development of EI were helpful. Most recently, Carragher and Gormley (2016) have explored the link between EI and leadership, demonstrating the importance of this quality to the promotion of effective and supportive leadership. We will be revisiting the importance of EI again in subsequent chapters.

Resilience is defined as an ability to adapt to, or recover from, change or challenging situations (McAllister and McKinnon, 2009) and where you learn new skills to address similar situations in the future. It originates from Latin, *to rebound*. Nurses meet both joy and grief in their everyday work and must be able to respond to and support those we care for in joy and adversity. In addition, they must manage the demands of professionals working alongside the current constraints on the care provision workforce and regulatory changes. These challenges are complex, and Hart et al. (2014) link the lack of resilience to increased stress, dissonance, and the likelihood that healthcare workers will leave their profession for work of lesser emotional and ethical challenge. This requires nurse educators to be proactive in the facilitation of your learning and to include resilience as part of your professional and personal development. You may ask why this is important but, as Stephens (2013) suggests, you will inevitably meet new situations that challenge your existing views and beliefs, such that you must review the basis of your existing knowledge and be prepared to explore further. You will learn these skills, not just from a theoretical perspective but also during your practice learning together with clinical colleagues and via your reflections. Thomas and Revell (2016) suggest that this aspect of development will not just benefit you in the longer term but will help to create an environment in which your wish to learn will flourish.

The 10 Commitments of Nursing

We have established that caring and compassion have been fundamental aspects of a nurse's role since nursing's inception, and that good moral values and personal qualities are central to who a person is and will directly impact on their behaviour towards others. You will note that the title of this chapter begins with values and is followed by knowledge and skills, which, in their entirety, underpin nursing practice and give rise to the best possible healthcare outcomes. Without the appropriate set of values and personal qualities, there is no foundation on which to add the building blocks of clinical skills, education, professional standards, codes, and ethics.

In 2012, and in recognition of the importance of these values, the Chief Nursing Officer of England and the Director of Nursing at the Department of Health launched a strategy (DH, 2012b) based on six core values (the 6Cs), which were adopted to determine effective care. This followed similar standards previously outlined in Northern Ireland (DHSSPS, 2006; 2008). These include moral values, professionalism and aspects of dedication that are used to define the basis of decent quality nursing care.

The key elements identified within this framework are outlined below (Figure 1.2):

- *Care*: the care we deliver helps the individual and improves the health of the whole community. Caring defines us in our work. The people receiving care expect it to be right for them consistently throughout every stage of their life.
- *Compassion*: this is how care is given through relationships based on respect.
- *Communication*: this is central to successful caring relationships and effective teamwork. All successful interactions between individuals are based on effective communication, which comes in many formats and encompasses multiple means, such as non-verbal, verbal and written.
- *Courage*: this relates to us as nurses having the courage to do the right thing for the people we care for, to speak up when we have concerns, and to have the personal strength and vision to embrace new ways of working.
- *Commitment*: commitment to individuals and populations is the cornerstone of what we do, and we need to build on this to improve the care and experience of those we care for.

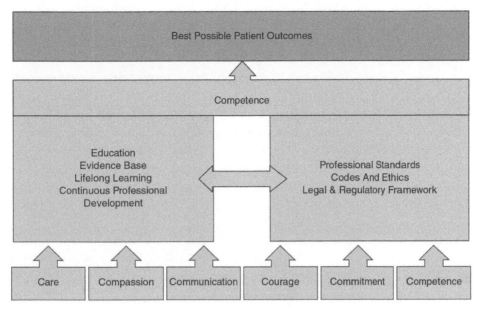

Figure 1.2   The 6Cs: the foundations of professional nursing practice

- *Competence*: all those in caring roles must have the ability to understand an individual's health and social needs and have the clinical expertise and technical knowledge to deliver effective care and treatments based on research and evidence.
- *Candour*: In 2015, 'candour' was an additional C added by the NMC and relates to 'a professional responsibility to be honest [with individuals] when things go wrong'.

In 2016, Cummings, in her role as CNO for England, played a key role in the publication of *Leading Change, Adding Value* (NHS England, 2016), which enhanced her concept of the 6Cs and introduced the 10 commitments as described here:

1   We will promote a culture where improving the population's health is a core component of the practice of all nursing, midwifery, and care staff (health improvement);
2   We will increase the visibility of nursing and midwifery leadership and input in prevention;
3   We will work with individuals, families, and communities to equip them to make informed choices and manage their own health;
4   We will be centered on individuals experiencing high value care;
5   We will work in partnership with individuals, their families, carers, and others important to them;
6   We will actively respond to what matters most to our staff and colleagues;
7   We will lead and drive research to evidence the impact of what we do;
8   We will champion the use of technology and informatics to improve practice, address unwarranted variations and enhance outcomes;

9   We will have the right education, training, and development to enhance our skills, knowledge and understanding;

10 We will have the right staff in the right places and at the right time.

As you may realise, the core values and 10 commitments, as outlined here, are not new. They are based on the key fundamental principles of what have always been considered vital to the role of nurse. Florence Nightingale, for example, always tried to strive for accessibility and simplicity of expression and to stress the importance of enacting core values. However, there is now a need to be more specific and explicit in terms of what these are and how they underpin practice.

The 7Cs and 10 commitments highlighted above resonate with the values needed to support the development of a therapeutic relationship. You will notice that all the elements enshrined in both are framed within *The Code* (NMC, 2018a), and all are used by nurses in tandem to help them refine their appreciation of the complexity that is nursing.

Remember, nothing you will ever do as a nurse should be considered basic. Nursing is a complex and purposeful endeavour that relies on you as the conduit of care to meet the needs of people in your care. Everything you do as a nurse relies on a myriad of technical and interpersonal skills, which are themselves underpinned by multiple intelligences, including intellectual, moral, social, and aesthetic ways of knowing and seeing the world.

Upholding the Professional Reputation of Nursing

Thus far we have outlined the fundamental values and principles of nursing practise. However, let us now stop and think about contemporary nursing practise.

- What is the image of nursing today?
- How is the nursing profession perceived by those in need of care, carers and/or members of the public?

Activity 1.4

Follow the link as detailed below which will take you to the personal account of Christina Patterson, a well-known and respected journalist: www.bbc.co.uk/programmes/b010mrzt (this highlights a programme recorded for BBC Radio 4 (2011), entitled *'Care to be a nurse*?', in which she describes her experiences while undergoing six operations for breast cancer over a period of eight years at different hospitals).

While listening consider the following questions and make a note of your answers:

- What were the key issues here?
- Why do you think this happened?
- How did Christina feel?
- How does this account make **you** feel?
- As a nurse involved in Christina's care what would you have done differently?
- Were there any barriers – and if so – how might you have overcome them?
- What were the key positive nursing actions important to her?

The Code (NMC, 2018a) requires us to 'be open and honest, act with integrity and uphold the reputation' of our profession, and therefore it would be disingenuous if we did not acknowledge the gravity and extent of the challenges to the nursing profession's reputation in previous years. Although it is important to recognise that in some areas there are excellent standards of nursing care, we must acknowledge the evidence that demonstrates that in other areas the current opinion of the nursing profession is low. At this point we should look at events that have brought into question the professional reputation of nurses over the last few years. We need to try to work out why and how these events have been allowed to happen and then create a strategy of both reform and support to ensure that they will not do so again. One of the key aspects that Christina focuses on is a lack of care, compassion, and basic human kindness. Crucially, before Christina went into hospital for the first time, she was not worried about her care since she did not think she would have to. Yet she experienced poor care consistently throughout her healthcare journey. Why was this? Where was the effective communication, care and compassion for her situation, the competence and commitment to provide the best evidence-based care and the courage to ensure that the nurses who worked with her understood her personal journey through ill health? As her case clearly demonstrates, somewhere along the way the nurses involved in the delivery of her care seemed to have lost sight of the art of nursing. This example indicates that vulnerability and personal status constitute universal features of illness experience.

Hallett (2012) considers a range of potential factors that may have contributed to Christina's poor experience, including:

- The changing emphasis towards more technical skills and knowledge;
- The shift in roles between what doctors used to have sole responsibility for and the extended role of the nurse;
- The professionalisation of the nursing role;
- The delegation of fundamental (sometimes refered to as basic) care provision to healthcare assistants;
- Bureaucracy and box ticking given priority over compassion;
- The wider social, economic, and political factors.

Christina's account also adds to revelations from the Care Quality Commission's (CQC's) inspection of over 150 hospitals and care homes (CQC, 2013), the events at Winterbourne View Hospital (DH, 2012a), the Princess of Wales and Neath Port Talbot hospitals (Andrews and Butler, 2014) and the publication of the Francis Reports (Francis, 2013) highlighting the abuse and suffering of many individuals at the Mid Staffordshire Foundation NHS Trust.

Activity 1.5

Access and read the following documents:

1   The Francis Report. You can find this information on the Executive Summary and recommendations at: www.midstaffs publicinquiry.com/report:
2   Care Quality Commission (CQC), Nursing and Midwifery Council (NMC) and NHS Wales responses to the Francis Report. You can find this information at the following websites:

- www.cqc.org.uk/content/care-quality-commission-response-francis-report
- www.cqc.org.uk/content/cqc-highlights-changes-following-francis-report
- www.nmc-uk.org/About-us/Our-response-to-the-Francis-Inquiry-Report

Make a list of all factors identified in each report.

The original report into events at Mid Staffs (Francis, 2013) noted that *'It was striking how many accounts related to basic nursing care as opposed to clinical errors leading to injury or death'*. Jane Cummings (Chief Nursing Officer for England) noted that *'such poor care is a betrayal of all that we stand for'* (DH, 2012b: 7). Francis (2013) went on to highlight 290 recommendations for stakeholders to consider across a wide and enduring spectrum of concern including the neglect, negligence, and abuse of individuals, along with a wide range of associated factors including organisational structures, staff shortages, management policies, bonus payments for managers and the imposition of targets devoid of any research evidence base. Nor did the CQC emerge from the Francis Report unscathed because it was clear that their criteria for inspection were not sufficiently robust. A response issued by the CQC (2013) acknowledged these shortcomings, highlighting a schedule of changes including the appointment of an Inspector of Hospitals, a more searching assessment process in profiling institutions and an expert base for their inspection teams. They also reaffirmed their remit to monitor the quality of healthcare environments for the people who matter most – service users.

Although most nurses would find these behaviours and actions to be as abhorrent as they are incomprehensible, you will by now have recognised that nurses have a personal duty of care that includes obligations and promises to adhere to the standards as espoused within *The Code* (NMC, 2018a). This means that we are personally and collectively responsible and accountable for the decisions we make and the actions we take, regardless of the pressures or environment within which we are working. This therefore calls upon us to display courage and commitment, acting as advocates for those we care for to ensure that we always act in their 'best interest.'

The Challenges to Contemporary Practice

At the outset of this chapter, we outlined the challenges faced by nurses, whether they be some of the very personal aspects of the work, the issues of gender, the fight for recognition as a profession, the emotional labour involved or the hardships of nursing during wartime. Some of these challenges remain ever present whereas others will change and evolve. Many of these are covered in more depth in later chapters but this chapter highlights some of the key issues facing nurses today. The most significant challenge is that of public perception, namely the image of nursing and the prevailing culture of care within our profession.

Advances in technology and the changing emphasis in recent years on nurses becoming more technically specialised (Hallett, 2012; Law and Aranda, 2010), inequalities, inadequate working conditions and chronic excessive work pressures (The Kings Fund, 2020) have all been blamed for the loss of care and compassion. However, we should consider whether these two must be mutually exclusive. We would be failing ourselves and our profession if we did not maintain our competence and continue to develop as techniques and technology improve. Hallett (2007) suggests that core values are constant whereas technology is a tool to be wielded in the services of health.

When people require any kind of medical intervention, it is the level of empathic and compassionate care they receive that makes the difference between a good and an unpleasant experience: it is effective communication (especially listening carefully), kindness, caring and empathy and not the technical intervention that really make the difference. It is also clear that such values, qualities, and behaviours are crucial to good nursing. In one study, Smith (2012) found that 44 different words or phrases were used by those receiving care to describe 'ideal' and 'real' nurses. Interestingly, only six of these related to functional attributes such as efficient, observant, and capable of doing their job. The caring and emotional aspects of nursing were clearly seen as distinct but complementary to and, more importantly, underpinning the functional aspects of everything we do as nurses. Kindness, helpfulness, and patience were the attributes most frequently used. Talking, listening, and showing interest and sympathy also featured heavily as aspects of the ideal nurse. It is clear how these attributes align closely with *The Code* (NMC, 2018a), 7Cs and 10 commitments (DH, 2012b; GMC/NMC, 2015; NHS England, 2016), but all of this is best expressed by one individual who concluded:

> A nurse has to be aware of the patient's (sic) condition and how to tackle it. She has to have a nursing manner which requires a lot of patience and forethought and to try and relieve pain and suffering not by medical means but by compassion. (Smith, 2012: 27)

Furthermore, with easier access to the internet, the public are much better informed and have access to a huge amount of information and related data about their health. They will often have high expectations in terms of openness and transparency, and the right to be included and informed. As a result, as nurses we must work hard to keep our own knowledge up to date and ensure that our practice is firmly based on sound evidence. We must also demonstrate care and compassion not only in how we treat individuals and their families, but also in respecting their right to be involved in all the decisions affecting them. Respect, privacy, and dignity should feature strongly in every aspect of our care delivery. We must ensure that we listen to their concerns, needs, and wants, acting as their advocates when required. This requires commitment to ensure that we are continually updating our knowledge and that we maintain our competency. It also requires effective communication to ensure that we listen to concerns and answer questions, making sure that we explain ourselves clearly and that we have been understood (a topic that will be focused on in more detail in subsequent chapters).

Fitness to Practise

Part of the NMC's role as a professional regulator is to maintain the professional register and ensure that the public are protected from poor practice. The NMC takes these aspects of their work most seriously to maintain the reputation of the profession and promote public confidence that nurses on the register meet the necessary standards of a competent practitioner and pose no risk. There are procedures in place to guide employers, colleagues and the public who wish to raise concerns about any nurse's fitness to practise and the NMC investigates these concerns thoroughly, to promote learning and prevent issues from arising again.

So, what does the term 'fitness to practise' mean? The current NMC guidance (NMC, 2022) states that a nurse or nursing associate who is fit to practise is someone who makes sure that 'their skills, knowledge, education, or behaviour do not fall below the standards needed to deliver safe, effective, and kind care' as set out in *The Code* (NMC, 2018a). In practical terms this means that, as a nurse, you maintain appropriate standards of proficiency, ensure that you are of good health and good character, and that you adhere to the principles of good practice that are set out in the various standards, guidance, and advice.

The notion of being suitably prepared by your educational programme to undertake the nurse registrant's role, and that you should have valid and current registration with the regulatory body, is quite straightforward. Demonstrating that you are of good health and good character is intricately linked to the ways in which you work and live and ensuring that these are aligned to *The Code* (NMC, 2018a).

Activity 1.6

Follow the links on the NMC website (www.nmc.org.uk/) and read the current version of *The Code* and the information related to fitness to practise and good health and good character.

Make note of any questions that occur to you as you read this and consider where or to whom you might go for help in answering your questions.

Some of your questions may well be 'How do I prepare for this responsibility?' or 'What happens if something occurs that means I question my own fitness to practise?'

It is important that we explore this concept of 'fitness to practise' with you and what it means to be of good health and good character. You will soon appreciate that during your programme of study you will normally be well prepared to face the challenges of professional life and demonstrate the knowledge, skills, behaviours and standards of care that the public would expect from nurses.

During your programme of study there will be information and opportunities for discussion which will enable you to develop a better understanding of these concepts and recognise the implications for those who fail to study appropriately and/or fail to abide by *The Code* (NMC, 2018a) to which you aspire. Although you are not expected to enter your pre-registration education with all the required professional attributes, it is important to ensure that you are made aware of these concepts, that you understand them, and that you grow in competence and confidence regarding these skills alongside other areas of your development.

We will start with the concept of good health. You may wonder why demonstrating good health is an essential component of a nurse's fitness to practise. If we can demonstrate that we lead a healthy lifestyle, then the benefits of this are that we may be better able to guide those in our care. However, there will be occasions for all of us where we become temporarily incapacitated such that we are unable to work or study. In these circumstances our professional behaviour is to follow the relevant sickness and absence policies. There may be some conditions that challenge our ability to undertake our role safely and competently. At these times it is vital that we seek appropriate support in a timely way to make certain that we have the right help and that we do not endanger our colleagues or those in our care. Often it is not the event or incidence of ill health that becomes an issue but rather what we have done about it. Have we been honest with ourselves and others? Have we sought appropriate professional support and guidance?

The NMC (2018b: 8) proficiencies state that nurses

"…must understand the professional responsibility to adopt a healthy lifestyle to maintain the level of personal fitness and wellbeing required to meet people's needs for mental and physical care".

How does this proficiency relate to the situations highlighted above?

How are we to interpret this competency in relation to going to work even though we are not well enough; a nurse living with diabetes not taking regular breaks for food or medication; another who feels that they never have a hangover so they can drink heavily before going on duty? All these actions demonstrate a lack of insight into our health, wellbeing, and professional obligations. Health issues can catch us all out.

- Should a nurse smoke or be over or underweight?
- Should nurses always role model healthy behaviour?
- Are nurses policing or promoting health?

You may recall from engaging in some of the previous activities that there are four principal areas from which an individual's fitness to practise can be called into question. These are criminal behaviour, dishonesty, unprofessional behaviour and ill health (Ellis et al., 2011). Here you will see that honesty and integrity figure highly in the professional equation, i.e., our ability to know right from wrong and thus act appropriately.

In considering these four areas again it may be that some activities feel easier to identify than others: for example, harm to another person; stealing; misuse of or dealing in illegal substances; fraudulent activity; and the abuse of vulnerable people. These are unacceptable behaviours and ones that do not adhere to *The Code* (NMC, 2018a). However, by reading this chapter you should also be aware that other unprofessional behaviours (e.g., ongoing poor time management, rudeness to others, breach of confidentiality, examination cheating or plagiarism, and bullying) are equally relevant.

Activity 1.7

Visit the NMC website (www.nmc.org.uk/concerns-nurses-midwives/hearings/) and access the recent case hearings presented to the NMC Fitness to Practise Committee. Identify one that relates to out-of-work activities compromising their professionalism:

- How do you feel about these circumstances?
- Which circumstances were work related and which occurred in their own personal time?

What is particularly significant here is the notion that what happens in your personal life is just as important as events in your professional, registrant and/or student life.

Whether you are a student or a registrant, sit back for a minute and think about the things you do in terms of email correspondence, being out with friends or engaging in online social media:

- How do you speak to people?
- Does this vary depending on who it is?
- Do you use a form of shorthand in text or on social media?
- Is this appropriate?
- Does it matter?

These are the sorts of questions you must be able to answer. You can discuss this with fellow colleagues, teachers, or line managers. As students we can seek advice and feedback from teachers, supervisors, and assessors to support our professional development and, since 2004, students have been asked to affirm that they are of good health and good character in line with the NMC Quality Assurance (QA) Framework requirements for pre-registration courses (NMC, 2016: 2018c).

As registrants we also affirm our good health and character each year when our registration is renewed, and it is clearly stated in *The Code* (NMC, 2018a) that we have a duty to inform both our employer and the NMC of any concerns we have about our ability to practice safely or any involvement with the police as soon as possible after a concern has been highlighted. Do remember that any caution or conviction recorded by the police remains on your personal record for life and is viewed by employers through the Disclosure and Barring Service.

Further information about this service can be accessed at the following website: www.gov.uk/government/organisations/disclosure-and-barring-service

What are the processes for investigating 'fitness to practise' in your school of nursing and how are these issues addressed in your programme of study?

Now visit www.nmc.org.uk/concerns-nurses-midwives/hearings and compare your university process with that of the NMC when investigating allegations of professional misconduct.

- What differences have you highlighted?
- Does your university process mirror that of the NMC?

Most students and registrants do not have their fitness to practise challenged in such a way that requires investigation and sanction. David and Bray (2009) acknowledge that the percentage of students investigated via these procedures is thought to be low. The reason for this is that, although each university is charged with having a 'fitness to practise' procedure for students, there is no central collation of the number of students investigated or the outcomes of such investigations. However, from half a million registered nurses and midwives less than 1% of registrants had concerns raised against them (NMC, 2018).

David and Lee-Woolf (2010) also point out that student nurses are still learning and therefore the seriousness of any given situation may vary dependent on the stage reached in the programme of study. However, it is necessary that you are aware of the potential pitfalls that can sometimes catch you unaware and you must not close your eyes to the subject. You should be careful to be self-aware and not self-righteous in respect of this concept, ensuring that by safe practice and reflective development you are able to recognise any problems or challenges to your practice and act appropriately. Similarly, as a registrant, although there is an expectation that you will adhere to *The Code* (NMC, 2018a), there is also an acknowledgement of varying degrees of experience that may impact on any allegation that questions your fitness to practise as a nurse.

Both student and registrant processes that examine fitness to practise have several sanctions that can be applied to any given situation. These can range from there being no case to answer, through varying levels of supervision or suspension, to a student's place on their course being withdrawn or a registrant removed from the register permanently. Whatever the outcome in relation to the sanctions applied, there must be robust evidence in support of any allegations made and the probability of the event reoccurring must be balanced against the sanction chosen.

In most cases – as either student or registrant – there will be evidence of mitigation to be considered alongside an allegation. It is important to realise that such mitigation can never condone an unprofessional action, but it may be used to determine the outcome and level of sanction imposed.

Activity 1.8

Let us now revisit the '*Enabling Professionalism*' document we reviewed in Activity 1.2 earlier in the chapter   (www.nmc.org.uk/globalassets/sitedocuments/other-publications/enabling-professionalism. pdf) and re-consider the questions below:

Are you ready to be a professional?
What does be 'professional' mean to you?
How will you ensure that you model professional behavior from the onset of your studies and beyond?

The Importance of Evidence-based Practice

We have acknowledged growing public awareness and the perennial challenge that nurses should be able to justify their actions. *The Code* (NMC, 2018a) also tells us to ensure that our nursing practice should be based on the best available evidence. Therefore, as adult nurses we must learn how to find this evidence and ascertain whether it is good.

Good, evidence-based, person-centred care is vital to modern healthcare and will underpin the expertise and sensitivity of care strategies, thus demonstrating the quality-of-care provision (Emanuel et al., 2011). Evidence-based practice is an essential component in defining the efficacy of our nursing practice, though it is worthwhile realising that we will not find a research base for every aspect of care. However, the increasing breadth of knowledge and technology available to inform our decisions adds weight to the explanations of why we do what we do. Our knowledge base for nursing is influenced by knowledge from other disciplines such as the physical and social sciences, law, and ethics. We must be able to work with these different elements and apply them to all the clinical situations we encounter.

The capacity to know what is the right thing to do in any nursing situation relies on our ability to explore the relevant and current knowledge in a certain area, to understand what that is trying to tell us, and for us to utilise our research appreciation skills to distil whether or not this knowledge can be applied to a particular situation. Although this is a tall order, we as professional nurses are committed to lifelong learning that will facilitate our clinical development over our working lives.

Therefore, during your programme of study or as a registrant you will be expected to learn and develop the skills of research appraisal (see Chapter 7). These will enable you to reflect critically on research worthiness and not only to understand the implications of research for nursing care but also to play your part in ensuring that appropriate research-based care strategies are implemented in practice.

Developing Your Nursing Skills

We all enter nursing with diverse levels of life experience and emotional maturity, and these can differ widely regardless of age. The concept of emotional intelligence is often associated with experiential learning and learning from the lessons of life, and this will evolve as we are exposed to more such experiences and gain experience in the nursing context (Bulmer Smith et al., 2009).

- Are you ready to practise nursing?
- Are you fit to practise?

Pause for a moment and reflect on whether these questions are asking the same thing.

- How would you answer these questions if asked?

Chapter Summary

Throughout this chapter we have introduced you to the complexity of the nursing role and hopefully posed challenging questions that will help you to scrutinise and interpret your impulse to nurse and aspirations for your future nursing practise. We have drawn your attention to the evolution of nursing by highlighting noteworthy events and people who have helped to shape the profession we have today. In so doing, we have asked you to reflect upon your motivation to nurse and your own philosophy on caring, and to that end we have explored some of the legal, moral, and ethical issues that can challenge our fitness to practise. We have also discussed some of the challenges faced by nurses today and the tension that exists between the technical expertise of caring and its softer, yet vital skill counterpart – compassion.

As you begin your journey in the nursing profession, we trust that this chapter has helped you to share our passion for nursing and has stimulated your interest to read and explore the concepts and issues highlighted in subsequent chapters of this book.

Further Reading

Craig, J.V. and Dowding, D. (2019) *Evidence-Based Practice in Nursing*, 4th edn. London: Elsevier.

Goleman, D. (1995) *Emotional Intelligence*. New York: Bantam.

Griffith, R. and Dowie, I. (2019) *Dimond's Legal Aspects of Nursing, A Definitive Guide to Law for Nurses*, 8th edn. London: Pearson

Hallett, C. (2014) *Veiled Warriors: Allied Nurses of the First World War*. Oxford: Oxford University Press.

Rafferty, A.M., Philipou, J., Fitzpatrick J.M. and Ball, J. (2015) *'Culture of Care' Barometer*. National Nursing Research Unit, London, Kings College.

Timmins, F. and Duffy, A. (2011) *Writing Your Nursing Portfolio: A Step-by-Step Guide*. Maidenhead: Open University Press.

References

Alexander, Z. and Dewjee, A. (1984) *The Wonderful Adventures of Mary Seacole in Many Lands*. Bristol: Falling Wall Press.

Andrews, A. and Butler, M. (2014) *Trusted to Care. An Independent Review of the Princess of Wales Hospital and Neath Port Talbot Hospital at Abertawe Bro Morgannwg University Health Boards (Executive Summary)*. Available at: www.gov.wales/sites/default/files/publications/2019-04/trusted-to-care.pdf (last accessed 3 March 2023).

Baly, M. (1997) *Florence Nightingale and the Nursing Legacy*. London: Whurr.

Bandura, A. (1986) *Social Foundations of Thought and Action: A Social Cognitive Theory*. Englewood Cliffs, NJ: Prentice Hall.

Bandura, A. (1991) 'Social cognitive theory of self-regulation', *Organizational Behavior and Human Decision Processes*, 50: 248–87. http://dx.doi.org/10.1016/0749-5978 (91)90022-LBBC

Radio 4 (2011) *Four Thought Series 2: Christina Patterson: Care To Be a Nurse?* Available at: www.bbc.co.uk/programmes/b010mrzt (last accessed 3 March 2023).

Beauchamp, T. and Childress, J. (2013) *Principles of Biomedical Ethics*, 6th edn. Oxford: Oxford University Press.

Bostridge, M. (2008) *Florence Nightingale: The Woman and Her Legend*. London: Penguin.

Brooks, J. (2011) 'The first undergraduate nursing students: A quantitative historical study of the Edinburgh degrees, 1960–1985', *Nurse Education Today*, 31(6): 633–7.

Brooks, J. (2020) 'My questionable status as a friendly enemy alien: British responses to Jewish refugee nurses 1933 to 1948', *Nursing History Review*, 29: 202–22.

Bulmer Smith, K., Profetto-McGrath, J., and Cummings, G.G. (2009) 'Emotional intelligence and nursing: an integrative literature review', *International Journal of Nursing Studies*, 46: 1624–36.

Care Quality Commission (2013) *Care Quality Commission Response to Francis Report*. Available at: www.cqc.org.uk/content/care-quality-commission-response-francis-report (last accessed 3 March 2023).

Carragher, J. and Gormley, K. (2016) 'Leadership and emotional intelligence in nursing and midwifery education and practice: a discussion paper', *Journal of Advanced Nursing*, 73(1): 85–96.

Codier, E. and Odell, E. (2014) 'Measured emotional intelligence ability and grade point average in nursing students', *Nurse Education Today*, 34(4): 608–12.

David, T.J. and Bray, S.A. (2009) 'Healthcare student fitness to practise cases: reason for referral and outcomes', *Education Law Journal*, 196–203.

David, T.J. and Lee-Woolf, E. (2010) 'Fitness to practise for student nurses: principles, standards and procedures', *Nursing Times*, 106 (39): 23–6.

Department of Health (2012a) *Transforming Care: A National Response to Winterbourne Hospital*. London: HMSO. Available at: https://assets.publishing.service.gov.uk/government/uploads/system/uploads/attachment_data/file/213215/final-report.pdf (last accessed 3 March 2023).

Department of Health (2012b) *Compassion in Practice: Nursing, Midwifery and Care Staff: Our Vision and Strategy*. London: HMSO.

Department of Health, Social Services and Public Safety (2006) *Modernising Nursing Careers: Setting the Direction*. Belfast: DHSSPS.

Department of Health, Social Services and Public Safety (2008) *Improving the Patient and Client Experience*. Belfast: DHSSPS.

Ellis, J., Lee-Woolf, E. and David, T. (2011) 'Supporting nursing students during fitness to practise hearings', *Nursing Standard*, 25(32): 38–43.

Emanuel, V., Day, K. and Diegnan, L. (2011) 'Developing evidence-based practice amongst students', *Nursing Times*, 107(49/50): 21–3.

Faulkner, A. (1998) 'The ABC of palliative care: communication with patients, families and other professionals', *British Medical Journal*, 316(7125): 130–2.

Fernandez, R., Salamonson, Y. and Griffiths, R. (2012) 'Emotional intelligence as a predictor of academic performance in first year accelerated graduate entry nursing students', *Journal of Clinical Nursing*, 21: 3485–92.

Francis, R. (2013) *The Mid Staffordshire NHS Foundation Trust Public Enquiry*. Available at: https://assets.publishing.service.gov.uk/government/uploads/system/uploads/attachment_data/file/279124/0947.pdf (last accessed 3 March 2023).

Gibbs, G. (1988) *Learning by Doing, A Guide to Teaching and Learning Methods*. Oxford: Further Education Unit, Oxford Brookes University.

GMC/NMC (2015) *Openness and Honesty When Things Go Wrong: The Professional Duty of Candour*. London: GMC/NMC.

Goleman, D. (1995) *Emotional Intelligence. Why it can matter more than IQ:* New York: Bantam Dell.

Griffith, R. (2015) 'Patient protection: ill-treatment and willful neglect', *British Journal of Nursing*, 12 June 24(11). Available at: www.magonlinelibrary.com/doi/abs/10.12968/bjon.2015.24.11.600 (last accessed 3 March 2023).

Griffon, D.P. (1995) '"Crowning the edifice": Ethel Fenwick and state registration', *Nursing History Review*, 3: 201–12.

Griffon, D.P. (1998) '"A somewhat duskier skin": Mary Seacole in the Crimea', *Nursing History Review*, 6: 115–27.

Hallett, C.E. (2005) 'The "Manchester scheme": a study of the Diploma in Community Nursing, the first pre-registration nursing programme in a British university,' *Nursing Inquiry*, 12(4): 287–94.

Hallett, C.E. (2007) 'Editorial: a "gallop" through history: nursing in social context', *Journal of Clinical Nursing*, 16(3): 429–30.

Hallett, C.E. (2012) *Nursing: the lost art?* Conference paper presented at the International History of Nursing Conference, Kolding, Denmark, 11 August.

Hart, P.L., Brebban, J.D. and Chesney, M. (2014) 'Resilience in nursing: an Integrative review', *Journal of Nursing Management*, 22(6): 720–34.

Hawkins, S. (2010) *Nursing and Women's Labour in the Nineteenth Century*. London: Routledge.

Health and Care Professions Council UK (2011) *Research Report: Professionalism in Healthcare Professionals*. London: HCPC. Available at: www.nmc.org.uk/globalassets/sitedocuments/other-publications/enabling-professionalism.pdf (last accessed 3 March 2023).

Helmstadter, C. (1993) 'Old nurses and new: nursing in the London teaching hospitals before and after the mid-nineteenth century reforms', *Nursing History Review*, 1: 43–70.

Helmstadter, C. (1996) 'Nurse recruitment and retention in the 19th century London teaching hospitals', *International History of Nursing Journal*, 2(1): 58–69.

Henderson, V. (1960) *Basic Principles of Nursing Care*. London: International Council of Nurses.

Hockey, L. (2001) *Oral history interview by Jane Brooks in Edinburgh on 8 August 2001*. UK Centre for the History of Nursing and Midwifery, School of Nursing, Midwifery and Social Work, University of Manchester.

Law, K. and Aranda, K. (2010) 'The shifting foundations of nursing', *Nurse Education Today*, 30: 544–7.

Mann Wall, B. (1998) 'Called to a mission of charity: the sisters of St Joseph in the Civil War'. *Nursing History Review*, 6: 85–113.

Mason, K. (2005) *Dr Lisbeth Hockey, 1918–2004: Biography*. Available at: www.yumpu.com/en/document/view/40373697/lisbeth-hockey-full-biography-school-of-nursing-midwifery-and-. (last accessed 3 March 2023).

McAllister, M. and McKinnon, J. (2009) 'The importance of teaching and learning resilience in the health disciplines: a critical review of the literature', *Nurse Education Today*, 29(4): 371–9. http://dx.doi.org/10.1016/j.nedt.2008.10.011

McFarlane, J.J. (1970) *The Proper Study of the Nurse*. London: Royal College of Nursing.

NHS Education for Scotland (2021) *Preceptorship*. Available at: www.nes.scot.nhs.uk/our-work/preceptorship/ (last accessed 3 March 2023).

NHS Employers (2014) *Simplified Knowledge and Skills Framework (KSF)*. Available at: www.nhsemployers.org/system/files/2021-07/The-NHS-Knowledge-and-Skills-Framework.pdf (last accessed 3 March 2023).

NHS England (2015) *The NHS Constitution*. London: DH.

NHS England (2016) *Leading Change: Adding Value*. Available at: www.england.nhs.uk/wp-content/uploads/2016/05/nursing-framework.pdf (last accessed 7 March 2023).

NHS England (2022) *National Preceptorship Framework for Nursing*. Available at: www.england.nhs.uk/publication/national-preceptorship-framework-for-nursing/ (last accessed 3 March 2023).

NHS Wales (2014) *Preceptorship for Newly Registered Nurses and Midwives Policy*. Available at: https://cavuhb.nhs.wales/files/policies-procedures-and-guidelines/corporate-policy/p-q-corporate-policy/11-4-preceptorship-policy-and-ehia-pdf/ (last accessed 3 March 2023).

Nightingale, F. (1859) *Notes on Nursing: What It Is and What It Is Not*. London: Harrison.

Northern Ireland Practice and Education Council for Nursing and Midwifery (2022) *Preceptorship Framework*. Available at: https://nipec.hscni.net/wpfd_file/preceptorship-framework-final-31-8-22-df/ (last accessed 3 March 2023).

Nursing and Midwifery Council (2016) *Health and Character Guidance for AEIs*. Available at: www.nmc.org.uk/education/what-we-expect-of-educational-institutions/good-health-and-good-character-for-aeis (last accessed 3 March 2023).

Nursing and Midwifery Council (2018a) *The Code: Professional Standards of Practice and Behaviour for Nurses and Midwives*. Available at: www.nmc.org.uk/globalassets/sitedocuments/nmc-publications/nmc-code.pdf (last accessed 27 March 2023).

Nursing and Midwifery Council (2018b) *Future Nurse: Standards of Proficiency for Registered Nurses*. London: NMC.

Nursing and Midwifery Council (2018c) *Quality Assurance Framework*. Available at: www.nmc.org.uk/globalassets/sitedocuments/edandqa/pre-2018-nmc-quality-assurance-framework.pdf (last accessed 7 March 2023).

Nursing and Midwifery Council (2022) *An Introduction to Fitness to Practise*. Available at: www. kingsfund.org.uk/publications/courage-compassion-supporting-nurses-midwives (last accessed 3 March 2023).

O'Brien D'Antonio, P. (1993) 'The legacy of domesticity: nursing in early nineteenth-century America', *Nursing History Review*, 1: 229–46.

Oxford English Dictionary (2014) Available at: http://dictionary.reference.com/browse/nurse (last accessed 3 March 2023).

Oxford Reference (2023) Available at: subject/law#:~:text=Law%20is%20the%20study%20of,the%20 actions%20of%20its%20members l (Last accessed 7 March 2023).

Parliamentary and Health Service Ombudsman (2011) *Care and compassion? Report of the Health Service Ombudsman on ten investigations into NHS care of older people*. Available at: https://assets.publishing. service.gov.uk/government/uploads/system/uploads/attachment_ data/file/247493/0778.pdf (last accessed 3 March 2023).

Price, B. (2019) *Delivering Person-Centred Care in Nursing*. London: Macmillan.

Reverby, S. (1987) *Ordered to Care: The Dilemma of America Nursing*. New York: Cambridge University Press.

Royal College of Nursing (2014) *Defining Nursing*. London: RCN.

Schön, D. (1983) *The Reflective Practitioner: How Professionals Think in Action*. London: Temple Smith.

Seedhouse, D. and Peutherere, V. (2020) *Using Personal Judgement in Nursing and Healthcare*. London: Sage.

Smith, P. (2012) *The Emotional Labour of Nursing Revisited*, 2nd edn. Basingstoke: Palgrave Macmillan.

Snowden, A., Stenhouse, R., Young, J., Carver, H., Carver, F. and Brown, N. (2015) 'The relationship between emotional intelligence, previous caring experience and mindfulness in student nurses and midwives: a cross sectional analysis', *Nurse Education Today*, 35(1): 152–8. Available at: www.sciencedirect.com/science/article/pii/S0260691714003025 (last accessed 3 March 2023).

Stephens, T. (2013) 'Nursing student resilience: a concept clarification,' *Nursing Forum*, 48(2): 125–33.

The Kings Fund (2020) *The Courage of Compassion: supporting nurses and midwives to deliver high-quality care*. Available at: www.kingsfund.org.uk/publications/courage-compassion-supporting-nurses-midwives (last accessed 3 March 2023).

Thomas, L.J. and Revell, S.H. (2016) 'Resilience in nursing students: an integrative review', *Nurse Education Today*, 36: 457–62.

Todd, G. (2002) 'The role of the internal supervisor in developing therapeutic nursing'. In: D. Freshwater (ed.), *Therapeutic Nursing*. London: Sage, pp. 58–82.

Weir, R.I. (2004) *Educating Nurses in Scotland: A History of Innovation and Change, 1950–2000*. Penzance: The Hypatia Trust.

Wheeler, H. (2012) *Law, Ethics and Professional Issues for Nursing: A Reflective and Portfolio Building-Approach*. London: Routledge.

White, R. (1978) *Social Change and the Nursing Profession: A Study of the Poor Law Nursing Service, 1848–1948*. London: Henry Klimpton.

2

NURSING THERAPEUTICS

Dianne Burns, Caroline Jagger, and Heather Iles-Smith

Chapter objectives

- Explain underpinning theories used to define a therapeutic approach in nursing;
- Identify key communication skills that assist in the development of a therapeutic relationship with adults and their families;
- Discuss the importance of person-centred care and how this can be achieved in practice;
- Assist you to recognise your duty of care and any actions that you may need to take in relation to the safeguarding of vulnerable adults.

The term 'nursing therapeutics' encompasses the therapeutic relationship that exists between a nurse, an individual in their care and the key elements that influence that relationship. Influencing factors include the notion of person-centred care and the use of systematic approaches in planning, implementing, and evaluating nursing care provision. The application of effective interpersonal skills and an ability to critically reflect upon the care we have provided, along with consideration of the underpinning professional values and the legal and ethical frameworks outlined in Chapter 1, are of the utmost importance.

Nursing therapeutics is not a new concept. It has been an integral part of nursing throughout history, although it has not always been well defined, or its importance clearly articulated in the nursing literature.

Throughout this chapter the concept of a therapeutic relationship will be explored in more depth. The overarching aim of this chapter is to define what we deem to be a therapeutic relationship, to identify the components of such a relationship, and to explore how this can be developed further using frameworks and reflection. Examples from practice will be used to highlight how a therapeutic relationship is established and maintained in practice.

Related Nursing and Midwifery Council (NMC) Proficiencies for Registered Nurses

The overarching requirement of the NMC is that all registered nurses must act in the best interests of those in their care, putting them first and providing nursing care that is person-centred, safe, and compassionate. They must communicate effectively, act as role models for others and be accountable for their actions. Registered nurses must prioritise the needs of people when assessing and reviewing their mental, physical, cognitive, behavioural, social, and spiritual needs (NMC, 2018a).

■■■■■■■■ TO ACHIEVE ENTRY TO THE NMC REGISTER
YOU MUST BE ABLE TO ■■■■■■■■

- Communicate effectively using a range of skills and strategies with colleagues and people at all stages of life, and with a range of mental, physical, cognitive, and behavioural health challenges;
- Understand the need to base all decisions regarding care and interventions on individual needs and preferences, recognising and addressing any personal and external factors that may unduly influence your decisions;
- Always provide and promote non-discriminatory, person-centred, and sensitive care, reflecting on individual values and beliefs, diverse backgrounds, cultural characteristics, language requirements, needs and preferences, taking account of any need for adjustments;
- Demonstrate and apply an understanding of what is important to people and how to use this knowledge to ensure that their needs for safety, dignity, privacy, comfort, and sleep can be met, acting as a role model for others in providing evidence-based person-centred care.

(Adapted from NMC, 2018a)

Therapeutic Relationships

A therapeutic relationship in nursing involves working in partnership with individuals to help speed up the recovery process and enhance their care experience (Peplau, 1991). However, due to the complexity of disease processes and the human body's resourcefulness, it is important to acknowledge that people may recover in spite of, rather than because of, what nurses do. Nevertheless, the therapeutic relationship enables us to maximise the likelihood that an individual will recover because we have helped them in some way.

There is no single definition of a therapeutic relationship. Likewise, there is no single means of defining the role of a nurse, other than a fundamental wish to make a positive difference to the life of a person receiving care. However, there are numerous models detailing the key elements of a therapeutic relationship.

Therapeutic Relationship Models

Watson (1979) suggested that the therapeutic relationship is seen as a two-way reciprocal relationship. Considering the mind, body and soul to be interlinked, she describes ten factors that could provide a framework for nursing care: formation of an altruistic system of values; instillation of faith–hope; cultivation of sensitivity to self and others; development of a help–trust relationship; acceptance of positive and negative feelings; use of the scientific problem-solving method for decision making; promotion of interpersonal teaching–learning; provision for a supportive, protective and/or corrective mental, physical, sociocultural and spiritual environment; assistance with the gratification of human needs; and the allowance of existential-phenomenological forces.

Benner (1984) explained that the nurse should view people receiving care with an unconditional positive regard, also known as 'mutuality'.

Peplau (1987) identified three essential attitudes of the therapeutic relationship: genuineness, respect, and empathy.

Muetzel's (1988) model of activities and factors in the therapeutic relationship includes intimacy, reciprocity, and a partnership between the person receiving care and the nurse. Intimacy includes 'spirit' closeness, vulnerability, and atmosphere, such as security and freedom, with dynamics such as control, contact and communication.

Rogers (1996) suggested five client-related outcomes of nursing presence: achievement of client goals; satisfaction with nursing care; comfort; growth; and enhancing care. These all encompass what is viewed as the therapeutic relationship.

Sundeen et al. (1998) suggested that therapeutic nursing involves four key stages:

1 A *pre-interaction* stage requires planning and includes a review such as an individual's medical notes, past medical history, and social circumstances;
2 An *orientation* stage describes the first meeting with the person receiving care laying down the foundation of the relationship where effective communication is imperative. A 'contract' is developed (either formal or informal)
3 A *maintenance* phase where both the nurse and person receiving care are progressing towards the agreed goal, each of which involves effective communication and leads to 'feelings' being exchanged;
4 A *termination* phase which leads to the ending of the relationship.

A therapeutic relationship is two-way, with both the individual receiving care and the care giver positively benefiting from the experience (McKlindon and Barnsteiner, 1999). This falls within the notion of *emphasize* which is defined as a positive act being returned via another positive deed between two individuals. Sociological studies have shown that such positive or 'kind' endeavours lead individuals to behave in a more friendly and cooperative way (Ernst and Gächter, 2000). A nurse's acts of kindness can give rise to feelings of wellbeing for both the person receiving care and the nurse, which are likely to help build trust and aid the development of a positive therapeutic relationship. Muetzel (1988) developed a theory of partnership, intimacy and reciprocity that enveloped three circles with the recipient of care at the centre (Figure 2.1).

Intimacy includes spirit closeness, vulnerability, and atmosphere, such as security and freedom, encompassing dynamics such as control, contract, and communication. Although Muetzel's theory may seem dated, it is still reflected in government policies today. Putting people at the heart of care is considered a fundamental principle aimed at ensuring that people and their families are involved in the decision-making aspects of care provision.

The therapeutic relationship is concerned with both the science and the art of nursing and how we transfer our knowledge and skills into meaningful exchanges with individuals and their important others. The science of nursing is conceptualised by a scientific understanding of the human body (including normality and symptoms) and knowledge of the latest medications, treatments, and evidence-based care. Conversely, the art of nursing includes the practitioner's elevated levels of emotional intelligence, expert interpersonal and communication skills, and values-based care, which encompass notions of compassion, empathy, trust, dignity, and respect. The ability to engage in judiciously intimate interactions is a key part of the therapeutic relationship (Williams, 2001). Nursing is dependent on a thorough understanding of its science and a mastery of its art. Factors such as experience and learning will influence the ease

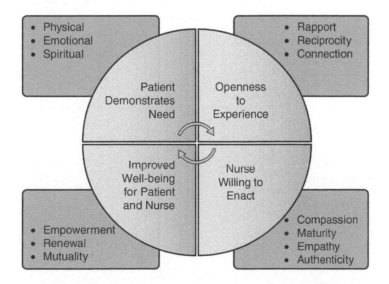

Figure 2.1   Presence model: implications for practice. (*Source:* Boeck, 2014)

with which you are able to build effective therapeutic relationships Yet compassion, empathy, emotional intelligence, and excellent communication skills are at times far more important than experience. Adult nursing requires commitment, intellectual intelligence, emotional intelligence, and the inherent capacity to care.

Moral Dimensions of Nursing Care

By previously focusing on nursing history and the development of professional nursing in Chapter 1 you will have already explored the societal expectation that all nurses will possess characteristics associated with strong moral virtues or values – sometimes being referred to by the public as 'angels'. The expectation to do good, to be compassionate at all times, express empathy, and sympathy, and treat people with dignity and respect – these qualities are a fundamental requirement of the adult nursing role. They lie at the heart of delivering good nursing care and are the foundation of a therapeutic relationship (Von Dietze and Orb, 2000).

Compassion is a complex concept and is often discussed alongside associated notions such as empathy, sympathy, respect, and dignity (Dewar et al., 2011). In fact, it is often difficult to separate these concepts because they are all interconnected, resulting in ill-defined definitions of compassion. However, Schantz (2007) believes that compassion goes further than pure sympathy and pity and involves actions to relieve distress. Other authors suggest that compassion is a basic human-to-human understanding, and a need to receive and give comfort and alleviate someone's suffering, distress, or pain (Straughair, 2012). A great deal of emphasis has been placed on the integral part compassion plays in the delivery of good nursing care and effective therapeutic relationships by both government and professional bodies. The NHS Constitution (DH, 2021), Northern Ireland's Strategy for Nursing and Midwifery (Department of Health, Social Services and Public Safety or DHSSPS, 2010), the Scottish Government's Strategy (Scottish Government, 2017) and NHS Wales (2016) all outline pledges that people can expect to be treated with compassion, humanity, and kindness by-healthcare professionals. Likewise, compassion is a consistent thread throughout the Nursing and Midwifery Council's *Code* (2018b) and *Proficiencies* (2018a).

Empathy, often described as the ability to walk in another's shoes, has also been widely accepted as an essential part of effective nursing care and is at the heart of the therapeutic relationship. It is an essential attribute – not only to understand a person's emotional state but also to have the ability to remain professional. Empathy is different from sympathy because sympathy is more emotionally charged (Peplau, 1987). According to Kunyk and Olson (2001), there are five conceptualisations of empathy:

1   A human trait;
2   A professional state;
3   A communication process;
4   A caring relationship;
5   A special relationship.

That is not to say that, when a person receives sad news, you should remain stoic and motion-less, but as a nurse you will still need to be able to function and support their emotional needs, having an ability to put their needs above your own. Presence can also be linked with empathy because it entails sensitivity along with other traits such as holism, intimacy, vulnerability, and the ability to adapt to unique circumstances. Finfgeld-Connett (2006) suggests that there are six features of presence:

1 Uniqueness;
2 Connecting with another individual's experience;
3 Sensing;
4 Going beyond the science;
5 Knowing;
6 Being with the individual.

Fredriksson (1999) argues that the value of presence lies in a nurse's ability to create a space where a person can be in deep contact with their suffering, thereby allowing them to share with a caring individual and assisting them in finding their own way forward. The act of being pre-sent allows that individual to perceive a meaningful exchange. Boeck (2014) clearly illustrates the meaning and value of 'presence' in contemporary nursing practice (Figure 2.1).

The importance of reflective practice and emotional intelligence (EI) has already been established (see Chapter 1). The use of reflection enables a therapeutic relationship to be developed and sustained through the assessment of our behaviours and our impact on care provision. Goleman (1995) suggests that it is vital to recognise that personal qualities such as self-awareness, self-confidence, self-control, self-knowledge, personal reflection, resil-ience, and determination are the foundation of how we behave.

Activity 2.1

- Access the following YouTube clip where emotional intelligence is explained further: www.youtube.com/watch?v=-Gpn_06NT9w What personal qualities do you have that you would associate with emotional intelligence?
- How might you use these positively to develop therapeutic relationships with those in your care?

A nurse's work is clearly set within a rollercoaster of human emotions whether these be fear, pain, sadness, and despair, or, at the other end of the spectrum, joy, relief, and hope. It is under-standable that people want empathic and emotionally competent nurses, but it is equally clear that these aspects are often lacking, along with effective communication skills (Williams and Stickley, 2010).

A defining quality in being able to establish a therapeutic relationship is the ability to recognise what others are feeling. Although this in part is being able to empathise, we must first recognise that there are some concerns or problems. As described below, in terms of communication, more than 90% of messages are transmitted non-verbally and as a result we must use our emotional intelligence to identify those feelings.

Activity 2.1 might have prompted you to include some of the following:

- Sensitivity;
- Awareness;
- Perceptive;
- Thoughtful;
- Anticipatory;
- Intuitive;
- In tune;
- Insightful.

It is often through the application of these attributes and skills that we can identify the significant issues faced by those receiving care. By having a sensitive awareness and/or intuition, or by simply 'being interested,' we can often notice something wrong. Our own life experience of the same or similar situations enhances our ability to do this. However, previous experience in a similar situation that we have observed, reflected upon, and learnt from also provides us with increasing perceptiveness or anticipation of what may occur. By listening carefully to what is being said, the tone or verbal expression that is used – and more importantly what is *not* said (along with facial expressions and body language) – can reveal more information to us.

The Importance of Effective Communication

It is widely accepted that words form only a small percentage of our communication (Hargie et al., 2004). Over 90% of communication is via non-verbal messages transmitted through our body language, tone, and facial communication.

Reflecting on the role that we ourselves play in our interactions is integral to understanding how effective we are as practitioners at communicating with others. Awareness of our own values and beliefs and how these influence our behaviours can also lead to us being more attentive to another person's needs and help us to develop productive therapeutic relationships (we will revisit this concept again later in the chapter). To make our interactions with others meaningful we must consider what we wish to achieve. For example, if we intend to advise how to take a medication, this is likely to be achieved by using a more formal, verbal interaction with written information supplied to aid *concordance*. How we transmit meaningful information in a way that others can process and understand is crucial to prevent misunderstanding, misinterpretation, and confusion. This is dependent on our ability to combine non-verbal and the most

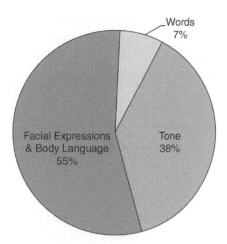

Figure 2.2 It is not just what you say, it is very much how you say it

appropriate verbal communication using jargon-free language coupled with active listening, questioning, clarification and summarising the conversation to ensure that we have been understood (Figure 2.2).

Active listening is defined by Mobley (2005) as the primary way of conveying empathy because it demonstrates that we are giving a person our full attention. According to Webb (2011), active listening is important for several reasons. When people are worried, they will often experience difficulties in communicating their ideas or problems clearly. It can help people who are in a stressful situation to get their ideas across so that their problems can be resolved more easily. Active listening has as much to do with body language as it is to do with verbal skills, and such skills are particularly useful when people are angry or highly emotional. The skills of active listening include the following:

- Attending and acknowledging, e.g., providing verbal or non-verbal awareness of the other person;
- Restating and paraphrasing, e.g., responding to the person using their basic verbal message;
- Reflecting, e.g., feelings, experiences or content that has been heard or perceived through cues;
- Summarising, e.g., bringing together feelings and experiences to provide a focus;
- Checking perceptions, e.g., if your perceptions and interpretations are accurate;
- Being quiet, e.g., giving the other person time to think as well as to talk.

Hilda

Hilda, an elderly person being cared for in hospital, is tearful and upset. You think this could be due to an imminent major surgical procedure. How would you respond to this situation?

Freshwater (2004: 93) asserts that 'One sigh may be communicating a lifetime of emotions'. Having picked up that something is wrong, we then must engage. It is the emotionally intelligent practitioner who hears the sigh, makes eye contact, communicates understanding and demonstrates human care. This basic human contact – achieved through engaging with the eyes together with a knowing look or a smile – could in that moment have the most profound and healing effect (Freshwater and Stickley, 2004).

As an emotionally intelligent nurse in this situation, you would speak to Hilda and try to elicit the reason for distress. You might consider that there could be another reason behind this (other than the obvious one) and would then actively explore the possibility. One way of earning Hilda's trust and respect would be by demonstrating genuine interest and care or as Rogers (1961) describes 'being present'. Active listening requires a nurse to listen very carefully to what is being said so they can understand the position from another person's point of view. Egan (2019) argues that it also requires an ability to convey to the person that they understand what has been said, not by repeating their words but by *being present* – psychologically, socially, and emotionally.

Hilda is far more likely to open up to you if she thinks that you will actively listen. By taking the time and care to find out more you might learn, for example, that Hilda had lost a precious wedding ring and that her husband of more than 40 years had died only 3 months previously. You would therefore have a deeper understanding that the emotions expressed by Hilda were manifested in raw grief. As an emotionally intelligent nurse you would use the whole spectrum of communication and interpersonal skills to allow Hilda to talk about and express her feelings and emotions, taking into account that fear of impending surgery might be a factor but that this has been compounded by the loss of her husband and now, further compounded, by not having the comfort of her wedding ring and all that it represented. Demonstrating this understanding could have a profound impact – even if the ring could not be found.

Verbal Communication

Communicating effectively enables a nurse to establish whether a person has understood what their care involves. This is clearly illustrated in the scenario below.

Harsha and Peter

Harsha (a district nurse) is undertaking one of her weekly visits to Peter whose HbA1c (glycated haemoglobin) blood glucose readings have been consistently higher than normal despite being prescribed medication to control diabetes. Harsha suspects that this might be because Peter has stopped taking prescribed medication regularly.

To understand if Peter takes the prescribed medication appropriately, further information is required. In nursing there are different purposes for our questioning and so we must use a series of open, closed, or probing questions. If we consider whether Peter is taking medication as prescribed, we may use closed questions such as 'Have you taken your diabetes medication today?' This is factual and can be used in an emergency or to give structure to a conversation. However, leading questions are unhelpful because they may prompt and influence an answer. This in turn may skew the information given when Peter is replying to the question. Open questions, on the other hand, are a way to allow Peter to give additional information. For example, asking what time of day prescribed medication is taken allows for further discussion. A probing question would allow time and help Harsha develop a deeper understanding of Peter's perceptions. Therefore , questioning in the right format is crucial to communicating successfully with those in our care.

Questioning styles and active listening

The types of questions Harsha may use when interacting with Peter about medication may include closed or open questions such as the following:

> Closed question: 'Do you understand how to take your medication?' (Peter's response would be 'yes' or 'no.')
> Open question: 'What do you understand about taking your medication?'
> Searching question: 'How are you feeling today?'

Paralanguage is concerned with the way something is said such as the pitch and tone, and the softness or loudness of words, all of which can support or contraindicate what is being said (Thompson, 2011). Therefore, it is important to consider not only what you are going to say but how you are going to say it. Of equal importance is the environment in which the communication takes place. The need to consider the scene for an interaction also plays a part in successful communication. In a study undertaken by Swayden et al. (2012), participants perceived that a physician spent more time with them when they sat down next to the bedside than when they stood up, demonstrating how the perception of time can be affected and lead to an increased satisfaction with the information received.

Non-verbal communication is concerned with anything that is communicated without the use of verbal language, such as the way we nod appropriately. Argyle (1988) suggests that non-verbal communication is up to five times more effective than verbal communication. During any interaction it is crucial that we consider how we are positioned in relation to a person. Egan (2019) advocates using the acronym SOLER:

> S = sit squarely in relation to the person
> O= in an open position
> L = lean slightly towards the person (at approximately 45°)
> E = maintain eye contact
> R = remain relaxed.

Applying the SOLER framework during a clinical interview when breaking unwelcome news, or during any other communicative contact with individuals and/or relatives, will help set the scene and put them at ease. If managed well it can also help us transmit empathy and compassion to those with whom we are interacting.

Can you think of a conversation you have had with someone who has not given you their full attention or was there a contrast between what they are saying and what they are doing?

- How did it make you feel?

Consider dealing with a person who feels that they have not been listened to:

- How could you make this different?
- How could the environment, your body language, vocabulary, pitch, and tone, as well as the content of your conversation, affect the outcome of the situation?
- What could you do to show that you are attentive to their needs?
- How could you frame the interaction so that it helps to build a positive mutual relationship?

It may be that the inferences made through inflections in the voice or body language, or the lack of eye contact were main elements leading to dissatisfaction. Professional communication is a skill that can be enhanced by being aware of your own interactions. It differs from social communication because it is purposeful, ethical and has boundaries. Effective communication is a vital component in any workplace and professional role. Moreover, in nursing, excellent communication and advanced interpersonal skills are crucial for successful interactions with other people: they are the bedrock for formulating and maintaining therapeutic relationships. However, unfortunately, 16.8% of all written hospital complaints arise from communication difficulties (NHS Digital, 2022) and therefore the use of communication as an effective tool should never be underestimated. Recognising and actively listening to other people can be beneficial. By making every interaction with people count, one small act of kindness or just being 'present' in the moment can make all the difference.

However, it is important to recognise that there are many potential barriers to effective communication. These include the following:

- Use of jargon, slang terms or abbreviations;
- Foreign languages, dialect, or difficulties with speech;
- Sensory deprivation (i.e., blindness, deafness, or difficulty hearing);
- Cultural differences;
- Emotional difficulties, anxiety, or distress;
- Environmental issues (i.e., poor lighting, noisy environments, or physical barriers).

Anxiety and Hospital Admission

Admission to hospital is a major event in many peoples' lives and can cause varying levels of anxiety because of fear of the unknown, fear arising from adverse media reports of poor hospital care and a perception that hospitals may be dangerous places.

Anxiety is a multisystem response to a perceived threat or danger. It reflects a combination of biochemical changes in the body, an individual's personal history and memory, and the social situation. An anxious person may present with an increased heart and respiratory rate and feelings of nausea. They can appear to be aggressive or demanding and require a lot of attention. Elevated levels of nervousness and apprehension may also hinder the ability to understand or follow simple instructions.

All health professionals should be able to identify those individuals who are at risk of anxiety or depression and respond appropriately with effective and supportive care. For example, in adult nursing there is a professional responsibility to ensure that people are adequately prepared for surgery both physically and psychologically.

What would you do to ensure that you could communicate effectively in the following scenarios?

- Asefa, a 26-year-old refugee who does not speak English;
- Alice, a 40-year-old who is partially sighted and deaf;
- Bobby, a young person living with a learning disability;
- Victor, an 85-year-old living with dementia.

All of these individuals could face huge challenges because their situation or conditions can affect their ability to understand or use language to communicate effectively. In all circumstances it would be important to consider their own preferred communication methods and cultural background, dealing with each issue sensitively. Speaking clearly using short sentences – not giving too much information or asking too many questions – using simple vocabulary and avoiding jargon will help in most situations.

Ensuring that they have access to necessary aids and equipment (e.g., glasses or hearing aids) is also crucial. It might be necessary to request interpreter services or use other visual, auditory, and tactile or signing methods to help them make effective use of alternative means of communication appropriate to their needs. Bobby, for example, may require information about available treatments in accessible formats, such as pictures, symbols or short videos.

Making reasonable adjustments to services requires the possession of knowledge of the health vulnerabilities that are specific to individuals, coupled with an assessment of their communication abilities, views and preferences (Doukas et al., 2017). Public Health England (2018) suggest the adoption of the following reasonable adjustments where applicable:

- *Use of health passports*: These documents contain an outline of the individual's health and illness history, health problems and treatments which should help you to provide the right care and treatment;
- *Allowing extra time*: Find a quiet environment to hold uninterrupted conversations. Talk to the individual receiving care rather than the supporting carer or professional if possible. Ensure that communication is effective by speaking slowly and clearly, using simple language, photographs, symbols, or other accessible communication aids as needed and stopping to check understanding at regular points;

• *Informed decision making*: Ensure that the 5 key principles of the Mental Capacity Act legislation (gov.uk/ukpga/2005/9/contents) are followed at all times.

Activity 2.2

Find out more about how you might effectively communicate with vulnerable people by accessing the following websites:

1   Alzheimer's Society: www.alzheimers.org.uk/about-dementia/symptoms-and-diagnosis/symptoms/how-to-communicate-dementia
2   MENCAP: www.mencap.org.uk/learning-disability-explained/communicating-people-learning-disability
3   Royal National Insitute for the Blind-Communicating with someone with a sensory loss: www.rnib.org.uk/sites/default/files/AOHL%20Toolkit%20%28English%29.pdf

---

The Importance of Cultural Competence in Nursing

Cultural competence can be defined as having the attitude, knowledge, and skills necessary for providing quality care to diverse populations: ensuring that everyone's needs are addressed, irrespective of their ethnicity or cultural background (Seeleman et al., 2009). The term 'cultural competence' is often used to describe an ability to consider how social and cultural factors influence individual attitudes towards health and healthcare (Black and Purnell, 2002). At an interpersonal level, this includes having an ability to bridge cultural differences in order to build an effective therapeutic relationship. The key features of cultural competence are:

• A diverse workforce that reflects the population;
• Healthcare facilities that are convenient for the community;
• Language assistance available for people with limited English proficiency;
• Ongoing staff training regarding the delivery of culturally and linguistically appropriate services;
• Exploring and respecting an individual's beliefs, values, preferences, and their understanding of the meaning of illness;
• Building rapport and trust;
• Finding common ground;
• Being aware of own biases/assumptions;
• Being knowledgeable about other cultures;
• Being aware of disparities and discrimination affecting minority groups;
• Using an interpreter when needed.

Saha et al. (2008)

The essence of cultural competence lies in a nurse's ability to consider a person's individual needs. Whilst cultural context and effective communication are relevant to the provision of care, cultural competence has the capacity to enhance person-centeredness and improve care quality for all, not just those from a different ethnic, racial, or cultural background to our own.

Think carefully about how you might demonstrate cultural competence in your daily nursing practice:
- What will this involve?
- How does this influence the outcome of the care that you deliver?

First, you will need the ability to learn about yourself (i.e., be self-reflective), a skill that is linked to emotional intelligence (Goleman, 1995).

Cultural awareness is defined as having the ability to acknowledge one's own culture, but also to recognise the potential for prejudice, bias, and stereotyping. To recognise and reflect upon how our own culturally specific beliefs, customs and values influence not only our practice but also the behaviours of those we care for is crucial. Having the capacity to alter our behaviour in response to this deeper understanding is defined as cultural sensitivity. Matteliano and Street (2012) describe this as learning about unfamiliar cultures and then adapting the way we deliver care to account for these differences. This involves:

- Building trust and conveying unconditional positive regard by never making assumptions about cultural practices or beliefs and showing respect for a person's support group (e.g., their family, friends, religious leaders);
- Asking questions about cultural practices in a professional and thoughtful manner if necessary;
- Addressing any communication or language barriers (e.g., using interpreter services if appropriate).

Activity 2.3

Find out more about how to enhance your own cultural competence by accessing guidance material at the following website:

- Gov UK: Cultural Competence Guidance: www.gov.uk/guidance/culture-spirituality-and-religion

Unconscious and Conscious Bias

Unconscious bias can happen when we make decisions or assumptions based on our own background, values, beliefs, and experiences without realising it. There is evidence to suggest that healthcare professionals unfortunately exhibit the same levels of unconscious bias as the general population, and that such bias is likely to influence diagnosis, decisions about treatment and levels of care in some circumstances (Fitzgerald and Hurst, 2017). *Conscious* bias or *explicit* bias refers to the attitudes and beliefs that we have about individuals or groups at a conscious level. Stockwell (1972) concluded that people who behave in a certain manner (e.g., grumbling, complaining or otherwise demanding attention) could at times be considered difficult or unpopular (conscious bias). Certainly, there will be times when some individuals project challenging behaviour due to many complex reasons. It could be that they are in pain, anxious or distressed; they may be incapacitated or feel that they have a lack of control due to their illness. Nevertheless, it is the nurse's role to reflect on their own behaviours and find a way to develop a therapeutic relationship and remain professional. Look at the following case scenarios. As you read them, make a mental note of any feelings, thoughts, and views that you are experiencing.

Alice

76-year-old Alice is admitted on to a busy medical unit for routine investigations. Several days after admission Alice becomes more demanding and especially during handover, repeatedly summons help for various things, e.g., requesting fresh water, asking for replacement pillows, and requesting help from someone to straighten the bed sheets as they are uncomfortable and are not 'sitting right' on the bed.

Andre

Andre, a 42-year-old, is admitted to a surgical ward directly from the theatre. Information given at handover is that Andre has suffered several deep lacerations from a knife injury. The allocated nurse has taken baseline observations and has completed a nursing assessment. Andre has many wounds to his abdomen and when checking the wound dressings, the nurse asks Andre how the injuries were sustained. Andre describes a confrontation with another person resulting in numerous lacerations and stab wounds. It later transpires that Andre had been attacked by another relative for allegedly sexually assaulting a younger family member.

Lou

Lou is admitted to a busy surgical unit post-surgery to recover from injuries sustained after an attempted suicide. Lou has previously undergone gender re-assignment surgery and is very withdrawn and unhappy having been subjected to persistent verbal and physical abuse. On admission Lou is very reluctant to speak other than to confirm the essential information, and when providing any information speaks very quietly.

- How were your feelings, thoughts and views provoked by each of the scenarios above?
- How would you manage each situation?
- What are the challenges you would face?
- How would you develop a therapeutic relationship with individuals who exhibit challenging behaviour or are unpopular? For example, would you be able to ensure your body language remained unchanged?
- How could the culture on the ward influence the reactions of members of staff to each of these individuals?
- How might these affect each person's recovery?
- How would you ensure that you are non-judgemental and engage with each of the individuals here to ensure that they each receive the best care?

Rogers' (1961) core condition of unconditional positive regard is simply having an attitude that enables us to be non-judgemental and always to act without bias or prejudice. In this way, the emotionally intelligent practitioner will not see or pre-judge any of these individuals. Indeed, the NMC (2018b) makes it clear that all nurses must practice in a holistic, non-judgemental, caring, and sensitive manner that avoids assumptions, supports social inclusion, recognises and respects individual choice, and acknowledges diversity. Where necessary you must provide the highest standard of practice and person-centred care possible at all times; in addition, you must put aside your own personal and cultural preferences when considering the needs of those in your care.

Certainly, there are many aspects of care to consider in each of the above scenarios, not just physical but also emotional and ongoing mental health. For example, some lesbian, gay, bisexual, transgender, queer or questioning, intersex, asexual, +PLUS people (LGBTQIA+) feel discriminated against by healthcare staff with around one in seven people avoiding getting help for conditions due to fear of discrimination (Bachmann and Gooch, 2018). It is essential that nurses are aware of their own implicit biases and prejudices because this can affect the way people are perceived and can impact on interaction between certain groups of individuals (Fitzgerald and Hurst, 2017). Indeed, current legislation (The Equality Act 2010 – see www.legislation.gov.uk/ukpga/2010/15/contents) means that it is against the law to discriminate against a person on the grounds of age, disability, gender reassignment, race, religion or belief, sex, sexual orientation, and pregnancy or maternity. The Royal College of Nursing (2016, 2020) has produced useful guidance in relation to the care of LGBTQIA+ individuals, aiming to ensure that as nurses we can challenge stigma and address unlawful discrimination in healthcare.

The Use of Therapeutic Touch

Consideration should be given to the use of therapeutic touch as a means of non-verbal communication. There are formal ways of using touch (e.g., massage) but the act of laying hands on a person (e.g., hand holding) can also have a positive effect; it is a means of communication at a basic human level. As children, we are often nurtured and given lots of hugs by our parents and families. As adults there are fewer opportunities to continue with this, with the loss of partners and grown-up children. The appropriate use of touch can cut through culture, race, and nationalities, and help us to connect with people. It can be considered a visible sign of caring (Busch et al., 2012), although as healthcare professionals it is important to remain cognisant of cultural differences, certain settings, and particular circumstances where touch is not appropriate (Davidhizar and Giger, 1997). Muliira and Muliira (2013) propose the use of an acronym 'TOUCH' which should be considered before using a therapeutic touch:

- **T:** Talk to people, identify preferences, and comfort levels before touch.
- **O:** Observe a person's verbal and non-verbal cues to guide their preference, such as avoiding eye contact.
- **U:** Understand and show understanding when touch is rejected.
- **C:** Care provider's touch as an intervention is more likely to be acceptable if considered to be the same gender as the receiver.
- **H:** Handedness (e.g., touch with the right hand is preferred by some following a Muslim faith, as some believe the left hand is unclean).

Although Clark and Clark (1984) argue that empirical support for the use of therapeutic touch is weak, some studies have shown that individuals have benefited from the use of touch. These benefits can show a reduction in anxiety, a decrease in perceived pain, and a reduction in heart rate and blood pressure (Tabatabaee et al., 2016; Maksum et al., 2019; Alp et al., 2021).

Person-centred Care

In recent years there has been a shift from the doctrine of a *patient* being at the mercy of healthcare professionals to one where the *person* is at the centre of all decisions. Person-centred care (PCC) is considered the bedrock of good care and the opposite of disease or task-based care, something that has been extensively implemented throughout nursing and medical history. PCC plays a key role in developing and maintaining a therapeutic relationship because it enables both the person and nurse to establish trust and understanding. Although there are numerous definitions of PCC and differing terminologies for similar outcomes-based care, Rogers (1961) was one of the first to develop a form of PCC known as 'client-centred therapy'. This is not a technique, but an approach based on a small set of core conditions that are required to facilitate therapeutic relationships, requiring high-level skills of emotion, intellect, attitude, and behaviour, which encapsulate the concept of emotional intelligence discussed earlier. These conditions are:

- Empathy;
- Unconditional positive regard;
- Congruence.

Unconditional positive regard is having an attitude that enables us to be non-judgemental and to act without bias or prejudice. Congruence relates to sincerity, genuineness and 'being present' in the relationship because you genuinely care. It is the difference between caring *for* a person and caring *about* a person. Corbin (2008) describes this as putting caring into practice through behaviours that address the specific needs of individuals by getting 'in touch' with the person to discover and understand those needs.

The overarching goal of PCC is to include individuals in the assessment and planning of their care to meet their agreed physical and psychological needs, ensuring that they feel valued, listened to, and included. This method elicits trust between the nurse and individual and empowers someone to make decisions about their own care and future health requirements, thereby fostering a productive therapeutic relationship. During PCC, the locus of control or power between nurse or healthcare professional and individual is likely to be equally distributed (Parley, 2001). Conversely, 'disease-' or 'task-based' care involves a nurse delivering care according to someone's disease or symptoms. In such cases, assumptions about a person's requirements can often be made by those delivering care. Task-based care was constructed around Parsons' (1951) 'sick role', which theorised that a person was dependent on a nurse, doctor or carer who was the most knowledgeable participant in the relationship. The power of the relationship was firmly within the remit of the healthcare professional and people were often discouraged from asking about or questioning the care delivered by nurses or doctors. Historically, task or disease-based nursing care was often delivered according to a nurse's schedule, focused on their need to 'get the job done' by the end of their shift rather than based on the needs of an individual person. This kind of care often involves the allocation of basic nursing care tasks as separate duties, with nursing staff focusing on a task or several tasks during their shift (e.g., observations, toileting, changing dressings, escorting a person to theatre). Unfortunately, there are still elements of task-based nursing care visible in modern-day nursing, particularly where time pressures are prevalent.

In general, PCC is the care model of choice in mainstream nursing, with its advantages leading to effective relationships between those individuals receiving care and healthcare professionals.

Activity 2.4

Access and read the following publications:

1   Wong, E., Mavondo, F. and Fisher, J. (2020) 'Patient feedback to improve quality of patient-centred care in public hospitals: a systematic review of the evidence', *BMC Health Services Research* 20. doi:10.1186/s12913-020-05383-3.
2   National Voices (2017) *Person-centred care in 2017*. Evidence from service users. Available at: www.nationalvoices.org.uk/publications/our-publications/person-centred-care-2017

What could you do to ensure that all individuals feel included in their care?

Safeguarding Vulnerable Adults

It is the duty of every qualified nurse to promote safety and to recognise and assess people at risk of harm and situations that may put them at risk, ensuring that prompt action is taken to safeguard those who are vulnerable (NMC, 2018a, 2018b). An adult's capacity for self-care will be affected by their own personal circumstances such as physical ability, learning disability, mental health, illness, and frailty, as well as factors within the local environment, personal strengths, and social contacts and support (DH, 2011). Harm or abuse may be physical, sexual, psychological, discriminatory, financial, or neglectful in nature (DH, 2011). Nurses are in a key position to identify possible safeguarding concerns; for example, when a vulnerable adult is admitted to hospital with unexplained injuries, or when a community nurse makes a home visit and suspects abuse within the family unit. In both cases local protocols and procedures will provide guidance on what action to take. Whatever the response, it is likely to involve a range of professionals and agencies. Local authorities hold statutory responsibility for the safeguarding of adults, but equally all staff working within health and social care settings have a duty of care to ensure the safety and wellbeing of those in their care. That duty is outlined by key principles outlined in The Care Act 2014 (see www.legislation.gov.uk/ukpga/2014/23/contents):

1   *Empowerment*: people being supported and encouraged to make their own decisions and informed consent;
2   *Protection*: ensuring support and representation for those in greatest need;
3   *Prevention*: taking action before harm occurs;
4   *Proportionality*: ensuring that any response is the least intrusive and is appropriate to the risk presented;
5   *Partnership*: working in partnership with other services and communities to prevent, detect and report neglect and abuse;
6   *Accountability*: accountability and transparency in safeguarding practice.

(Social Care Institute for Excellence, 2017)

As a registered nurse, you will need to ensure that you are familiar with procedures for safeguarding vulnerable adults in your area and know who to contact to express any concerns you might have. If you suspect the abuse of an adult, you should report your concerns to a more experienced colleague, who can refer the matter to the named nurse for safeguarding adults, who in turn can make a referral to social services. You must record your concerns – exactly what you observed and heard from whom and when. You should also record why this is of concern and what you did about your concerns. Excellent communication and record keeping are crucial. The Mental Capacity Act 2005 (see www.legislation.gov.uk/ukpga/2005/9/contents) provides a framework to empower and protect adults who may lack the capacity to make decisions for themselves. This might be because of an illness such as dementia, a brain injury, a learning disability, or mental health problems. The Act aims to provide a balance between an individual's right to make their own decisions and their right to protection from harm if they lack such capacity. Accordingly, every adult must be assumed to have capacity unless proved otherwise – you cannot assume someone lacks capacity based on a diagnosis. If an adult in hospital needs continuous supervision and lacks the capacity to consent to treatment or care arrangements, extra safeguards may be needed such as Liberty Protection Safeguards (LPS) (which form part of the Mental Capacity Act) to be able to restrict or restrain individuals if it is deemed to be in their own best interests.

Activity 2.5

Find out more about safeguarding and Liberty Protection Safeguards (LPS) at the Social Care Institute for Excellence website: https://www.scie.org.uk/safeguarding

---

Emotional resilience

Compassionate care is central to nursing practice. As an adult nurse you will no doubt be faced with many challenging situations in the future, which you will need to reflect upon and then consider how these experiences might influence or change your future practice. As healthcare professionals we learn to put the needs of others before our own. Nurses will often spend their working day exposed to the emotional strain of dealing with people who are sick or dying, and those who have extreme physical and/or emotional needs. However, with an ever-increasing workload and an unprecedented demand for resources, nurses can often feel 'stressed' and begin to suffer from physical and mental fatigue. One American physician (Remen, 2006: 52) suggests that

> "the expectation that we can be immersed in suffering and loss daily and not be touched by it is as unrealistic as expecting to be able to walk through water without getting wet".

This emotional strain, coupled with other stress factors inherent in the healthcare work environment, results in healthcare professionals being especially vulnerable to stress and burnout; this is more likely to occur when a nurse struggles with their work–life balance, job uncertainty, a lack of control in the workplace and feeling undervalued (Garrosa et al., 2011).

Activity 2.6

Access the following webpages and articles and then write down your answers to the questions that follow:

- www.psychologytoday.com/us/basics/compassion-fatigue
- Cavanagh, N., Cockett, G., Heinrich, C., Doig, L., Fiest, K., Guichon, J.R., Page, S., Mitchell, I. and Doig, C.J. (2020) 'Compassion fatigue in healthcare providers: a systematic review and meta-analysis', *Nurs Ethics*. May; 27(3): 639–65. doi: 10.1177/0969733019889400. Epub 2019 Dec 12. PMID: 31829113.
- How might we recognise compassion fatigue in ourselves and/or our colleagues?
- What are the contributory factors?

Now access and look at the following website materials before considering what you can do to reduce the risks: www.edumed.org/resources/compassion-fatigue-online-guide/. It is important to develop some strategies to cope with such stressors. Maksum et al. (2004) found that both short- and long-term coping strategies, such as taking part in self-care activities (e.g., going to the gym, walking, and having a sense of humour and a positive mental attitude) were useful. Longer-term strategies included having an awareness of the various triggers and developing coping strategies, e.g., having both professional and personal supportive relationships.

Access the NMC (2018a) *Future Nurse: Standards of Proficiency for Registered Nurses* document, identifying all the clinical competencies required of registered nurses.

Focusing particularly on effective communication skills, what do you need to do to ensure that you can develop your skills to meet the required competencies outlined?

Chapter Summary

Contemporary nursing practise demands an ability to build therapeutic relationships with all those in our care. The development of an effective therapeutic relationship, and the ability to demonstrate empathy, compassion and caring, foster reciprocity and uphold the professional values of nursing are what remain central to the delivery of good nursing care. To do this well you will need to be able to communicate effectively, putting those in your care at the heart of your decision-making processes; listening to their views and involving them in decisions about their care as long as they are willing and able to do so. In addition, the use of empathy and compassion are vital elements of nursing therapeutics that should be realised and put into practice by all nurses.

Further Reading

Arnold, E. and Underman-Boggs, K. (2011) *Interpersonal Relationships: Professional Communication Skills for Nursing*, 6th edn. St Louis, MO: Elsevier Saunders.

Egan, G. (2017) *The Skilled Helper. A Client Centred Approach*, 2nd edn. Belmont, CA: Brooks Cole Cengage Learning.

Freshwater, D. (2002) *Therapeutic Nursing: Improving Patient Care through Self Awareness and Reflection.* London: Sage.

Skills for Health, Health Education England, and Skills for Care (2015) *Dementia Core Skills Education and Training Framework.* (Updated 2018) Available at: www.skillsforhealth.org.uk/info-hub/dementia-2015-updated-2018/

Skills for Care (2022) *Learning Disability.* Available at: www.skillsforcare.org.uk/Developing-your-workforce/Care-topics/Learning-disability/Learning-disability.aspx

Skills for Health, Health Education England, and Skills for Care (2016) *Mental Health Core Skills Education and Training Framework.* Available at: www.skillsforhealth.org.uk/info-hub/mental-health-2016/

References

Alp, F.Y. and Yucel, S.C. (2021) 'The effect of therapeutic touch on the comfort and anxiety of nursing home residents', *Journal of Religion and Health*, 60, 2037–50. doi:10.1007/s10943-020-01025-4

Argyle, M. (1988) *Bodily Communication*, 2nd edn. London: Methuen.

Bachmann, C.L. and Gooch, B. (2018) *LGBT in Britain Health Report.* Stonewall/You Gov. Available at: www.stonewall.org.uk/system/files/lgbt_in_britain_health.pdf. (last accessed 19 August 2022).

Benner, P. (1984) *From Novice to Expert: Excellence and Power in Clinical Nursing Practice.* Menlo Park, CA: Addison Wesley.

Black, J.D. and Purnell, L.D. (2002) 'Cultural competence for the physical therapy professional', *Journal of Physical Therapy Education*, 16: 3–10.

Boeck, P.R. (2014) 'Presence: a concept analysis', *SAGE Open*, 4. doi:10.1177/2158244014527990. Available at: https://journals.sagepub.com/doi/10.1177/2158244014527990. (last accessed 22 August 2022).

Busch, M., Visser, A., Eybrechts, M., Komen, R., Oen, I., Olff, M., Dokter, J. and Boxma, H. (2012) 'The implementation and evaluation of therapeutic touch in burn patients: an instructive experience of conducting a scientific study within a non-academic nursing setting', *Patient Education and Counselling*, 89: 439–46.

Clark, P.E. and Clark, M.J. (1984) 'Therapeutic touch: is there a scientific basis for the practice?', *Nursing Research*, 33(1): 37–41.

Corbin, J. (2008) 'Guest editorial: is caring a lost art in nursing?', *International Journal of Nursing Studies*, 45: 163–5.

Davidhizar, R. and Giger, J.N. (1997) 'When touch is not the best approach', *Journal of Clinical Nursing*, 6: 203–6.

Department of Health (2011) *Safeguarding Adults: The Role of Health Service Practitioners*. London: DH. Available at: www.gov.uk/government/publications/safeguarding-adults-the-role-of-health-services. (last accessed 23 August 2022).

Department of Health and Social Care (2021) *The NHS Constitution,* London: DH. Available at: https://www.gov.uk/government/publications/the-nhs-constitution-for-england/the-nhs-constitution-for-england (last accessed 19th June 2023).

Department of Health, Social Services and Public Safety (2010) *A Partnership for Care, Northern Ireland Strategy for Nursing and Midwifery 2010–2015*. Belfast: DHSSPS.

Dewar, B., Pullin, S. and Tocheris, R. (2011) 'Valuing compassion through definition and measurement', *Nursing Management*, 17(9): 32–7.

Doukas, T., Fergusson, A., Fullerton, M. and Grace, J. (2017) *Supporting People with Profound and Multiple Learning Disabilities. Core and Essential Service Standards* (1st edn). PMLD Link. Available at: www.pmldlink.org.uk/wp-content/uploads/2017/11/Standards-PMLD-h-web.pdf. (last accessed 19 August 2022).

Egan, G. (2019) *The Skilled Helper. A Client Centred Approach*, 2nd edn. Belmont, CA: Brooks Cole Cengage Learning.

Ernst, F. and Gächter, S. (2000) 'Fairness and retaliation: the economics of reciprocity', *Journal of Economic Perspectives*, 14(3): 159–81.

Finfgeld-Connett, D. (2006) 'Meat-synthesis of presence in nursing', *Journal of Advanced Nursing*, 55(6): 708–14.

Fitzgerald, C. and Hurst, S. (2017) 'Implicit bias in healthcare professionals: a systematic review', *BMC Medical Ethics*, 18: 19.

Fredriksson, L. (1999) 'Modes of relating in a caring conversation: a research synthesis on presence, touch and listening', *Journal of Advanced Nursing*, 30(5): 1167–76.

Freshwater, D. and Stickley, T. (2004) 'The heart of the art: emotional intelligence in nurse education', *Nursing Enquiry*, 11(2): 91–8.

Garrosa, E., Moreno-Jimenez, B., Rodriguez-Munoz, A. and Rodriguez-Carvajal, R. (2011) 'Role stress and personal resources in nursing: a cross-sectional study of burnout and engagement', *International Journal of Nursing Studies*, 48(4): 479–89.

Goleman, D. (1995) *Emotional Intelligence*. New York: Bantam.

Hargie, O., Dickson, D. and Tourish, D. (2004) *Communication Skills for Effective Management*. Basingstoke: Palgrave.

Kunyk, D. and Olson, J.K. (2001) 'Clarification of conceptualizations of empathy', *Journal of Advanced Nursing*, 35(3): 317–25.

Maksum, Sujianto, U. and Johan, A. (2019) 'Effects of therapeutic touch to reduce anxiety as a complementary therapy: a systematic review', in *Selection and Peer-review under the responsibility of the ICHT Conference Committee*, KnE Life Sciences: 162–175. DOI 10.18502/kls.v4i13.5237

Matteliano, M.A. and Street, D. (2012) 'Nurse practitioners' contributions to cultural competence in primary care settings', *Journal of the American Academy of Nurse Practice*, 24(7): 425–35.

McKlindon, D. and Barnsteiner, J.H. (1999) 'Therapeutic relationship', *American Journal of Maternal and Child Health Nursing*, 5: 237–43.

Mobley, J. (2005) *An Integrated Existential Approach to Counseling Theory and Practice*. Lewiston, NY: Edwin Mellon.

Muetzel, P.A. (1988) 'Therapeutic nursing'. In A. Pearson (ed.), *Primary Nursing: Nursing in the Burford and Oxford Nursing Development Units*. Beckenham: Croom Helm, pp. 89–116.

Muliira, J. and Muliira, R. (2013) 'Teaching culturally appropriate therapeutic touch to nursing students in the sultanate of Oman: reflections on observations and experiences with Muslim patients', *Holistic Nursing Practice*, 27(1): 45–8.

NHS Digital (2022) *Data on Written Complaints in the NHS 2021-22* Quarter 3 and 4. Available at: https://digital.nhs.uk/data-and-information/publications/statistical/data-on-written-complaints-in-the-nhs/2021-22-quarter-3-and-quarter-4. (last accessed 19 August 2022).

NHS Wales (2016) *The Core Principles of NHS Wales*. Available at: www.wales.nhs.uk/nhswalesaboutus/ thecoreprinciplesofnhswales. (last accessed 13 September 2022).

Nursing and Midwifery Council (2018a) *Future Nurse: Standards of Proficiency for Registered Nurses*. London: NMC.

Nursing and Midwifery Council (2018b) *The Code: Professional Practice and Behaviour: Standards of Nurses and Midwives*. London: NMC.

Parley, F. (2001) 'Person-centred outcomes: are outcomes improved where a person-centred care model is used?', *Journal of Intellectual Disabilities*, 5(4): 299–308.

Parsons, T. (1951) *The Social System*. London: Routledge & Kegan Paul.

Peplau, H.E. (1987) 'Interpersonal constructs for nursing practice', *Nurse Education Today*, 7: 201–8.

Peplau, H.E. (1991) *Interpersonal Relations in Nursing*. New York: Springer. (Original work published 1952).

Public Health England (2018) *Learning Disabilities: Applying All Our Health*. Available at: www.gov. uk/government/publications/learning-disability-applying-all-our-health/learning-disabilities-applying-all-our-health#core-principles-for-health-professionals. (last accessed 19 August 2022).

Remen, R.N. (2006) *Kitchen Table Wisdom: Stories that Heal*, 10th anniversary edn. London: Penguin.

Rogers, C. (1961) *On Becoming a Person: A Therapist's View of Psychotherapy*. Wiltshire: Redwood Books.

Rogers, S. (1996) 'Facilitative affiliation: nurse–client interactions that enhance healing', *Issues in Mental Health Nursing*, 17(3): 171–84.

Royal College of Nursing (2016) *Caring for Lesbian, Gay, Bisexual or Trans Clients or Patients: Guide for nurses and health care support workers on next of kin issues*, London: RCN (Royal College of Nursing). Available at www.rcn.org.uk/library/subject-guides/lgbtq-health. (last accessed 22 August 2022).

Royal College of Nursing (2020) *Fair Care for Trans and Non-binary People: An RCN guide for nursing and health care professionals*, 3rd edn. London: RCN. Available at: www.rcn.org.uk/library/ subject-guides/lgbtq-health. (last accessed 22 August 2022).

Saha, S., Beach, M.C. and Cooper, L.A. (2008) 'Patient centeredness, cultural competence and healthcare quality', *Journal of Natural Medicine Association*, 100(11): 1275–85.

Schantz, M. (2007) 'Compassion: a concepts analysis', *Nursing Forum*, 42: 48–55.

Scottish Government, The (2017) *The Healthcare Quality Strategy for NHS Scotland*. Edinburgh: The Scottish Government. Available at: www.gov.scot/binaries/content/documents/govscot/publications/strategy-plan/2017/07/nursing-2030-vision-9781788511001/documents/00522376-pdf/00522376-pdf/govscot%3Adocument/00522376.pdf (last accessed 18 August 2022).

Social Care Institute for Excellence (2017) *Safeguarding Adults*. Available at: www.scie.org.uk/safeguarding/adults/introduction/highlights#principles (last accessed 13 August 2022).

Stockwell, F. (1972) *The Unpopular Patient. The Study of Nursing Care Project Reports*. London: Royal College of Nursing.

Straughair, C. (2012) 'Exploring compassion: implications for contemporary nursing, Part 2', *British Journal of Nursing*, 21(4): 239–44.

Sundeen, S.J., Stuart, G.W., Rankin, E.A.D. and Cohen, S.A. (1998) *Nurse–Client Interaction: Implementing the Nursing Process*, 6th edn. St Louis, MO: Mosby.

Swayden, K., Anderson, K., Connelly, L., Moran, J., McMahon, J. and Arnold, P. (2012) 'Effect of sitting versus standing on perception of provider time at bedside: a pilot study', *Patient Education and Counselling*, 86(2): 166–71.

Tabatabaee, A., Tafreshi, M., Rassouli, M., Aledavood, S., Alavimajd, H., and Farahmand, A. (2016) 'Effect of therapeutic touch on pain related parameters in patients with cancer: a randomized clinical trial', *Materia Socio Medica* Jun; 28(3): 220–3. doi: 10.5455/msm.2016.28.220-223. Epub 2016 Jun 1. PMID: 27482166; PMCID: PMC4949034.

Thompson, N. (2011) *Effective Communication: A Guide for People Professions*, 2nd edn. Basingstoke: Palgrave Macmillan.

Von Dietze, E. and Orb, A. (2000) 'Compassionate care: a moral dimension of nursing', *Nursing Inquiry*, 7(3): 166–74.

Watson, J. (1979) *Nursing: The Philosophy and Science of Caring*. Boulder, CO: University of Colorado Press.

Webb, L. (2011) *Nursing: Communication Skills in Practice*. Oxford: Oxford University Press.

Williams, A. (2001) 'A literature review on the concept of intimacy in nursing', *Journal of Advanced Nursing*, 33(5): 660–7.

Williams, J. and Stickley, T. (2010) 'Empathy and nurse education', *Nurse Education Today*, 30: 752–5.

3

FUNDAMENTAL ASPECTS OF ADULT NURSING

Dianne Burns and Mark Cole

— Chapter objectives —

- Explain the concepts of informed consent, mental capacity and confidentiality;
- Describe how systematic approaches can be used to assess a person's capacity for independence and self-care;
- Identify appropriate evidence-based assessment tools to determine the need for support and intervention to optimise mobility and safety;
- Make relevant links to core nursing skills;
- Outline the basic principles of infection control and wound care practices.

The previous chapter highlighted the importance of a nurse's ability to develop and build a therapeutic relationship with individuals and their families. It also identified some of the key skills needed by nurses to communicate effectively with people to identify their wishes and needs when planning care. Here we will begin to explore ways in which nurses can undertake a holistic nursing assessment, identifying more of the core nursing skills needed to be able to provide high-quality nursing care. It is important to point out here that we are not intending to provide specific instruction on how to carry out various clinical skills since there are plenty of other excellent resources that can help you with this aspect of your development. Instead, our intention is to utilise a series of activities and case scenarios to help you to consider some of the fundamental aspects of adult nursing practice. The chapter will also help to set the scene for Part 2 of this book, which will examine specific aspects of nursing and care provision commonly encountered when caring for adults and their families.

Related Nursing and Midwifery Council (NMC) Proficiencies for Registered Nurses

The overarching NMC requirement is that registered nurses must use information obtained during assessments to identify the priorities and requirements for person-centred and evidence-based nursing interventions and support. They must work in partnership with people to develop person-centred care plans that consider their circumstances, characteristics, and preferences (NMC, 2018a).

TO ACHIEVE ENTRY TO THE NMC REGISTER
YOU MUST BE ABLE TO

- Understand and apply a person-centred approach to nursing care, demonstrating shared assessment, planning, decision making and goal setting when working with adults, their families, communities, and populations of all ages;
- Effectively assess a person's capacity to make decisions about their own care and to give or withhold consent;
- Understand and apply the principles and processes for making reasonable adjustments and best interest decisions someone does not have capacity;
- Demonstrate and apply knowledge of human development from conception to death; knowledge of body systems and homoeostasis, human anatomy and physiology, biology, genomics, pharmacology, and social and behavioural sciences when undertaking full and accurate person-centred nursing assessments to develop appropriate care plans;
- Demonstrate and apply knowledge of all commonly encountered mental, physical, behavioural, and cognitive health conditions, medication usage and treatments when undertaking full and accurate assessments of nursing care needs and when developing, prioritising, and reviewing person-centred care plans;
- Demonstrate the knowledge, skills, and ability to act as a role model for others in providing evidence-based nursing care to meet people's needs related to nutrition, hydration, and elimination;
- Recognise and assess people at risk of harm and the situations that may put them at risk, ensuring prompt action is taken to safeguard those who are vulnerable.

(Adapted from NMC, 2018a)

Consent, Mental Capacity and Confidentiality

In accordance with the NMC *Code* (2018b), a person must give informed consent before any actions (including treatment, investigations, or care) are provided. Informed consent means that, as nurses, we need to be able to provide people with all the relevant accurate and truthful information in a way that they can understand to help them make an 'informed decision' about their care. A person has the right to refuse or withdraw consent at any time and as a nurse we must always act in their best interests (NMC, 2018b). However, occasionally this might mean that we must respect and support a person's right to refuse care and treatment if they have the mental capacity to make that decision. Having mental capacity means having the ability to make your own decisions. The Mental Capacity Act 2005 (www.legislation.gov.uk/ukpga/2005/9/contents) aims to protect vulnerable adults who are not able to make decisions for themselves. In 2019 in England, Wales and Northern Ireland, this act was further amended to encompass the concept of the Deprivation of Liberty Safeguards (DoLS) with an overall revised approach resulting in the current Liberty Protection Safeguards (LiPS).

Furthermore, any information obtained within a nursing assessment or that relates to any aspects of their care must remain confidential. As a nurse, or indeed any other healthcare professional, we owe a duty of confidentiality to all those in our care. Information about a person can only be shared with their permission or when their safety or that of others overrides the need for confidentiality (NMC, 2018b).

Activity 3.1

You can find out more by reading the documents outlined below:

Consent in England and Wales: www.rcn.org.uk/clinical-topics/consent

Consent in Northern Ireland: www.rcn.org.uk/clinical-topics/Consent/Consent-in-Northern-Ireland

Consent in Scotland: www.rcn.org.uk/clinical-topics/Consent/Consent-in-Scotland

The Mental Capacity Act (2005) and Mental Capacity (Amendment) Act (2019) Available at: www.legislation.gov.uk/ukpga/2005/9/contents and www.legislation.gov.uk/ukpga/2019/18/contents (last accessed 21 July 2022).

Mental Capacity Act (Northern Ireland) (2016) and Mental Capacity Amendment (Northern Ireland) (2019) Available at: www.legislation.gov.uk/nia/2016/18/contents and www.legislation.gov.uk/ukpga/2019/18/contents (last accessed 21 July 2022).

Scottish Government (2000) Adults with Incapacity (Scotland) Act (Short Guide). Available at: www.gov.scot/policies/social-care/adults-with-incapacity/ (last accessed 21 July 2022).

NHS England (2019) *Confidentiality Policy*. Available at: www.england.nhs.uk/publication/confidentiality-policy/ (last accessed 21 July 2022).

Liberty Protection Safeguards: Available at: www.gov.uk/government/publications/liberty-protection-safeguards-factsheets/liberty-protection-safeguards-what-they-are. (last accessed 26 August 2022).

Care Planning

Care planning is a highly skilled process. Applying a systematic approach to care planning is a way of encouraging us to think clearly about what we do for people receiving care and why we do certain things rather than carrying out nursing tasks in a ritualistic fashion. It also provides us with opportunities to plan, implement and evaluate care effectively, considering all the factors that can impact on health. The nursing process was first conceived by Orlando (1961) as a cyclical way of focusing on person-centred nursing problems, setting agreed measurable and realistic goals intended to improve health. The modern-day process ASPIRE (Barrett et al., 2012) includes the following:

- *Assessment*: finding out what person can or cannot do;
- *Systematic diagnosis*: making a nursing diagnosis – identifying the health and nursing care needs of an individual;
- *Plan*: in discussion with the person concerned, coming to an agreement about how their identified health and nursing needs can be met, setting mutually agreed goals;
- *Implement*: delivering evidence-based nursing interventions;
- *Recheck*: considering if the interventions selected are helping to meet the agreed goals;
- *Evaluate*: measuring and carefully documenting whether agreed interventions and approaches have been successful.

Following the evaluation of our nursing interventions, the cycle begins again with a reassessment and evaluation of the effectiveness of any care undertaken in close collaboration with the person concerned. The cycle ensures that their needs are constantly re-evaluated using the latest evidence-based care. Yet, according to Toney-Butler and Thayer (2022), some nurses lack the necessary knowledge and experience to be able to apply this process in practice. High nurse–patient ratios and a lack of required resources are cited as contributory factors.

Nursing Assessment

The assessment of an individual's needs and their care requirements involves the systematic and continuous collection of data; sorting, analysing, and organising that data; and the documentation and communication of the data collected (Toney-Butler and Unison-Pace, 2021). This can be achieved with the use of nursing models. For example, the Roper Logan and Tierney model (Roper et al., 2000) encompasses 12 activities of daily living (ADLs) (Figure 3.1). ADLs are the fundamental activities required by an individual to manage basic physical needs. This framework or model can help us to structure a holistic assessment of their needs.

The ADL model is applicable to all individuals, irrespective of the disease or problems they are experiencing. Using it allows us to gain valuable information relating to the level of help that may be required for them to be able to enact day-to-day activities. However, care must

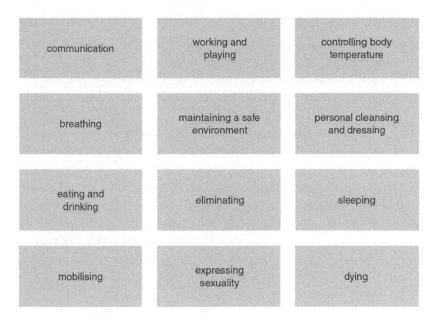

Figure 3.1   Activities of daily living (ADL)

be taken to ensure that the 'list' of ADLs is not merely used as a checklist. Instead, it should be incorporated within a person-centred approach to care planning, which involves the nurse and person concerned setting short and long-term goals for the actual and potential problems identified. However, although using a systematic nursing process and the ADL framework is useful, as you work your way through this chapter you will no doubt begin to recognise that one assessment tool will not always fit every situation; you may sometimes need to 'mix and match' additional tools and frameworks to ensure that the best approach is adopted, so that you can provide good-quality, holistic nursing care. For example, the Instrumental Activities of Daily Living (IADL) scale (Lawton and Brody, 1969) was developed to assess more complex activities associated with independent living. According to Mlinac and Feng (2016), these activities are more sensitive to early cognitive decline because IADL function is usually lost before ADL capability. Gold (2012) suggests that assessing cognitive and functional capabilities in these areas helps to evaluate the impact of cognitive impairment in adults. Activities include:

- Ability to use the telephone or mail;
- Shopping and food preparation;
- House cleaning and home maintenance: personal laundry and performing domestic tasks to keep the living space tidy;
- Managing transportation: either driving or arranging other means of transport;
- Managing medications: being responsible for ensuring medication is taken correctly;
- Managing finances: paying bills or keeping track of income and expenditure.

- Will these models/frameworks successfully capture information that is needed?
- What other nursing models might be more suitable depending on the care setting?
- What models or frameworks are used to underpin nursing assessments in **your** workplace setting?

It is important to remember that some people may not be able to fully address all the above because of physical and/or mental illness or disability. For example, depression or anxiety can have a significant impact on a person's ability to self-care.

According to the World Health Organization (2022), 1 in every 8 people (970 million) live with a mental disorder; anxiety and depressive disorders being the most common.

Depression is described by Taylor and Ashelsford (2008: 49) as a 'medical condition involving changes in mood, appetite, sleep, thoughts and psychomotor activity' and can be a reaction to life events such as physical illness, bereavement, or problems with relationships or finances (Hardy, 2013). Three key symptoms include persistent sadness or low mood, loss of interest or pleasure, and fatigue or low energy, but may also include other associated symptoms, for example disturbed sleep, poor concentration or indecisiveness, low self-confidence, poor or increased appetite, suicidal thoughts or acts, agitation or slowing of movements, and guilt or self-blame.

Alternatively, anxiety can present as restlessness and irritability, excessive fear, worry or panic, difficulty in concentration or withdrawal and making threats or demands. Thus, as an adult nurse you will need to be alert for signs of depression, anxiety, or other mental health disorders, and engage in accurate assessment as part of a therapeutic relationship with those in your care.

Activity 3.2

Access and read the WHO Mental Disorder Factsheet available at: www.who.int/news-room/fact-sheets/detail/mental-disorders?

- Consider how each of these disorders might affect a person's ability to self-care or engage with health-care services.
- Identify how a person's mental health needs are assessed in your own workplace.

Ruth

Ruth, a frail 77-year-old, is admitted to hospital accompanied by a relative, although normally lives alone. On admission, Ruth appears confused.

Initially, as Ruth appears confused, you would need to assess the capacity for Ruth to make decisions about care provision and to give or withhold consent. You would need to understand and apply the principles and processes for making reasonable adjustments and best interest decisions if you determine that Ruth lacks mental capacity. If Ruth has mental capacity, you would seek consent for treatment. You would offer constant reassurance and provide ongoing information about what was happening. At the earliest opportunity, you would take a full nursing history using a systematic approach, for example using the ADL and IADL frameworks outlined earlier as a guide.

- What other evidence-based frameworks or tools might help you in this process?
- What initial observations would you carry out?

We have already determined that Ruth will need a mental capacity assessment. Other additional assessments might include:

- A pressure injury risk assessment;
- A falls risk assessment (FRAT);
- A nutritional assessment;
- A depression and anxiety assessment.

Making Reasonable Adjustments

It is more than 15 years since the MENCAP report (2007), *Death by Indifference*, relayed the stories of the avoidable deaths of six people with learning disabilities and raised concern about hospital care for people with learning disabilities. This includes the sad case of 43-year-old Martin with a severe learning disability who was admitted to hospital following a stroke. Martin could not speak or swallow so speech and language therapists advised that eating or drinking activities should not be attempted and that alternative feeding methods should be used. Apart from intravenous fluids, no other attempts were made to provide nutrition and after having no food for the 26 days spent in hospital, Martin died.

The inadequacies in care that contributed to the 6 deaths were attributed to a lack of concern for individual disabilities.

Common areas of concern include poor communication, poor partnership working and coordination, poor relationships with families and carers, a failure to follow routine procedures, poor management, and a lack of advocacy (Parliamentary and Health Service Ombudsman, 2009). Unfortunately, persistent issues remain. In 2017, NHS England reported delays in treatment, gaps in service provision, organisational dysfunction, and neglect or abuse adversely affecting the health of people with learning disabilities. More recently, a report by White et al. (2022) suggested that although there are some examples of good practice, people with learning disabilities continue to receive poor standards of care and have a shorter life expectancy (with 6 out 10 dying before age 65, compared to 1 out of 10 for people from the general population). Those with epilepsy and from minority ethnic backgrounds were also more likely to die younger. Their findings also indicate a general lack of awareness amongst staff and a lack of experience working with people with a learning disability.

Sean

37-year-old Sean has moderate learning disabilities and lives at home with both parents who are designated main carers, although the family has some help from outside agencies. Sean has been admitted to a surgical ward for exploratory surgery to investigate a potential cancer diagnosis.

Make some suggestions about what 'reasonable adjustments' you might make to accommodate Sean's needs.

The above case scenario encourages you to consider how Sean and his family might cope with Sean's acute admission to hospital and how you might make reasonable adjustments to improve the provision of care. You probably decided that an assessment of Sean's needs would be appropriate to apply your general knowledge to this specific and unique situation.

Public Health England (2018) declare that individuals regardless of their age, gender or label should receive care that is based on their unique needs, that is appropriate in its design and effective in its delivery, outlining core principles that should be used to inform professional practice. This should include adopting a 'capabilities approach,' focusing on what Sean **can** do rather than cannot and includes a mental capacity assessment. According to Phillips (2012), other significant considerations would include assessing the effect on Sean of being in hospital. Hospitalisation is stressful for anyone but particularly for people with learning disabilities (Doyle et al., 2016). As previously illustrated, hospital routines often fail to cater for the needs of people with learning disabilities and staff tend to lack knowledge and experience of dealing with such individuals (Phillips, 2012; NHS England, 2017; White et al., 2022). Reasonable adjustments may be needed to comply with the legal requirements of the Equality Act 2010 (see www.legislation.gov.uk/ukpga/2010/15/contents). Public Health England (2018) suggests that making reasonable adjustments involves making changes to services to ensure all people can access (e.g., changes to building access, policies and procedures and staff training). It also requires possession of knowledge about the health vulnerabilities that are specific to people with learning disabilities, coupled with an assessment of that individual's communication abilities, views and preferences (Thomas and Atkinson, 2011). The Confidential Enquiry into Premature Deaths of People with Learning Disabilities (CIPOLD; Heslop et al., 2013) suggests the following reasonable adjustments to services:

- A mental capacity assessment each time a decision needs to be made, applied on the basis that sometimes individuals can make some decisions about their care but not at other times;

- Annual health checks to monitor health and detect health problems early on;
- Summary care records to ensure ease of finding and consulting information;
- Health action plans: these documents contain an outline of the individual's health and illness history, health problems and treatments;
- Informed decision making: knowledge and appropriate use of the Mental Capacity Act 2005 to ensure that an individual makes their own decisions as far as possible, or decisions that are made on the individual's behalf are in that person's best interests;
- Learning disability liaison nurses: Morton-Nance (2015) suggests that these professionals use their expertise to coordinate care and provide advice and are best placed to support care within the acute setting.

The potential role of Sean's parents is also another consideration. With Sean's permission, for example, how might they be encouraged to continue to help and support Sean during his hospital stay?

Activity 3.3

Access the Public Health England (2018) guidance *Learning Disabilities: Applying All Our Health* via the following website:

- www.gov.uk/government/publications/learning-disability-applying-all-our-heal th/learning-disabilities-applying-all-our-health

Make a list of any actions/interventions that should be adopted in your own current and future workplace settings.

Activities of daily living

Breathing

Breathing is fundamental to life. It provides the cells in our body with oxygen and helps us to expel waste products. Without oxygen, our cells and tissues would begin to die after a few minutes. Where there is reduced oxygen intake (i.e., because of injury or disease), there is a risk of a person developing hypoxia (low oxygen levels in the tissues or cells) or hypoxemia (low oxygen levels in the blood). The main causes of breathlessness are chronic lung diseases, such as chronic obstructive pulmonary disease (COPD), emphysema and chronic bronchitis which cause breathing difficulties characterised by the restriction of airflow. These can have a significant impact on a person's ability to undertake normal daily activities because exercise capacity can be reduced, which often results in worsening health status and physical inactivity (van Helvoort et al., 2016).

Daniel

65-year-old Daniel is living with COPD and is admitted to hospital with a chest infection, accompanied by another family member. Daniel is breathless and finding it difficult to hold a conversation.

What knowledge and skills would you need to have to undertake a respiratory assessment?

The ability to undertake a full respiratory assessment requires a good understanding of the anatomy and physiology of the respiratory system. It might be obvious from looking at Daniel that he is unwell. He may look warm and sweaty or pale and clammy. You would of course speak to him and offer constant reassurance. You would want to seek consent to treatment and keep him informed of what was happening throughout. You could initially make Daniel comfortable, repositioning and supporting him with pillows if it helps with his breathing to sit upright and administer any initial treatment as prescribed. As Daniel is quite breathless, with permission you could try to gain as much information as possible from the accompanying relative before consulting with Daniel again once he is well enough to contribute.

In accordance with your own levels of competence, you would measure, record, and interpret (i.e., recognise healthy ranges and clinically significant low/high readings) all baseline observations (i.e., respiration rate, pulse oximetry, peak flow, blood pressure, pulse, temperature, blood glucose levels) to detect signs and symptoms of physical ill health. You would undertake a whole-body systems assessment, focusing initially on his respiratory problems (which should include chest auscultation and interpretation of the findings), but then also a full assessment of Daniel's circulatory, neurological, musculoskeletal, and cardiovascular systems, recording and reporting your findings accurately. You would undertake venepuncture, cannulation and blood sampling, interpreting normal and common abnormal blood profiles and venous blood gases. If Daniel has a productive cough, you would collect and observe his sputum, sending a sample to the laboratory for further analysis if needed. You might also take a urine sample to screen for abnormalities (e.g., leucocytes, blood, glucose, etc.). At the earliest opportunity (e.g., once Daniel is more able) you would take a full nursing history using a systematic approach (e.g., using the ADL framework and/or other suitable assessment tools as a guide).

In accordance with the nursing process, you would assess the need for care interventions that would be agreed with Daniel and provided in accordance with current evidence-based guidelines and care pathways (NICE, 2018). You would closely monitor Daniel's progress, amending the plan of care in response to progress and his wishes.

Other related clinical skills required for entry to the nursing register (NMC, 2018a) include

- Responding to restlessness and agitation using appropriate interventions;
- Managing airway and respiratory processes and equipment;
- Managing inhalation, humidifier, and nebuliser devices;
- Managing the administration of oxygen using a range of routes and best practice approaches.

Nutrition and Hydration

To keep healthy, warm, and active, we need energy. The importance of good nutrition and hydration cannot be over-emphasised. Malnutrition is both a cause and an effect of ill health (NICE, 2012a). According to Manz and Wentz (2005), even mild dehydration can have a negative impact on health. Therefore, ensuring that the nutrition and hydration needs of individuals are met is an important part of the nurse's role.

However, to be able to undertake a thorough nutritional assessment, a sound knowledge base is needed. This knowledge should comprise of a good understanding of related anatomy and physiology of the gastrointestinal system, the normal processes involved in the acquisition and assimilation of nutrients, the factors that can influence nutrition, and the effects of malnutrition on health and healing, for example. To manage a person's nutritional needs effectively, a baseline assessment must first be undertaken, and this should then be reviewed regularly. Once an assessment has been completed, problems can be identified and a plan of care developed, implemented, and evaluated.

- What factors might impact on a person's ability to eat and drink?

The NICE quality standard for nutritional support in adults recommends that 'people in care settings are screened for the risk of malnutrition using a validated screening tool' (NICE, 2012a: 7). This suggests that all individuals, irrespective of setting, should be screened. As an adult nurse you will undertake many of these assessments, often as part of the initial assessment or hospital admission process. It is therefore important that you understand the assessment tools you are using to ensure an accurate and appropriate outcome for each person. One commonly used tool is the Malnutrition Universal Screening Tool or MUST (BAPEN, 2011). This is used in many health care organisations across the UK and comprises five simple steps that identify whether a person is at low, medium, or high risk of malnutrition. The overall score is determined by body mass index (BMI), which will require you to measure the person's weight and height measurements; an assessment of unplanned weight loss in the past three to six months and how acutely ill the person is in terms of poor nutritional intake for more than five days. Those individuals identified as low risk should have repeat screening – the regularity of this is determined by local protocol and is often influenced by where the person is being cared for (e.g., annual screening is recommended for individuals over 75 living in their own homes). Those at medium risk should be observed, which involves documentation of their dietary intake for three days, with action taken after that. Those at high risk should be treated unless this is of no benefit to the individual and includes referral to a dietician. In a simple way, the MUST tool identifies level of risk and suggests basic actions to take.

Activity 3.4

Access a copy of the Malnutrition Universal Screening Tool (MUST) (BAPEN, 2011) and familiarise yourself with it.

- Do you think this provides an adequate assessment of nutritional status?
- What other tools are available?

It needs to be acknowledged (as with all screening tools) that they are meant to be used as a guide only, together with your own knowledge and professional judgement. Following on from the assessment, regular monitoring should be undertaken. This may be because of the person being identified as medium risk or on the recommendation of the dietician and may involve the use of a food diary or fluid balance monitoring.

It is the nurse's role to ensure that individuals receive adequate nutrition and hydration. As some people may be unable to feed themselves, this requires assisting them to eat and drink. Care may need to be taken with some individuals due to swallowing difficulties, and advice from professionals such as the speech and language therapist about issues such as thickness of fluids will need to be adhered to. The nurse's role in health promotion and nutrition is vital here. To provide advice and support about a person's diet, you will need to be knowledgeable yourself. Of course, the dietician can provide additional in-depth information, but it is beneficial to have some knowledge and awareness of what a healthy diet is, the impact of nutritional deficiencies, and some of the diet restrictions involved in certain conditions (e.g., diabetes mellitus). Some individuals will be unable to take nutrition orally. In such circumstances, NICE (2006) provides guidance in relation to enteral and parenteral nutrition. As nurses we need to ensure that those who cannot take food orally (e.g., due to a swallowing impairment after a stroke or if unconscious) are adequately fed and hydrated.

Documentation (as with other aspects of nursing) is also vital in relation to fluid and nutritional management. Records of the administration of enteral and parenteral nutrition and intravenous fluids should be made, so that accurate calculations can be made about progress. This will include keeping accurate records of fluid balance (i.e., intake and output), regularly documenting assessment findings such as subsequent MUST scores, recording a person's BMI, keeping food diaries, and noting any changes and amendments to their care plan.

Other related clinical skills required for entry to the register (NMC, 2018a) include

- Assisting with feeding and drinking and using appropriate feeding and drinking aids;
- Recording fluid intake and output, and identifying, responding to, and managing dehydration or fluid retention;
- Managing nausea and vomiting;
- Inserting, managing and removal of oral/nasal/gastric tubes;
- Managing artificial nutrition and hydration using oral, enteral, and parenteral routes;
- Managing the administration of intravenous (IV) fluids;
- Managing fluid and nutritional infusion pumps and devices.

Elimination: Bladder and Bowel Health

Bladder and bowel elimination are essential to maintain health. The urinary and gastrointestinal systems provide the ability to eliminate most of the body's waste products, maintaining the body's homoeostasis and ensuring effective excretion of toxins. However, an individual's ability to effectively eliminate waste products can be affected by various physical, psychological, sociocultural and/or environmental factors, or surgery. To be able to undertake a thorough assessment of elimination needs, you will need to have a good understanding of related anatomy and physiology of the gastrointestinal and urinary systems. Bowel and bladder problems can also affect fluid and electrolyte balance, hydration, and nutrition.

When seeking a detailed elimination history, you will need to approach the subject sensitively, acknowledging the intimate nature of nursing interventions and ensuring that the person's privacy and dignity are always respected. Health issues faced by some individuals can include constipation, faecal impaction or diarrhoea, and urinary and faecal incontinence. It is important to identify any specific problems and toileting needs, accurately assessing not only the person's capacity for independence and self-care but also determining the need for support and intervention (e.g., assisting with toileting or assessing elimination patterns to identify and respond to potential issues appropriately).

Other related clinical skills required for entry to the register (NMC, 2018a) include

- Collecting and observing urine, stool, and vomit specimens, undertaking routine analysis and interpreting findings;
- Selecting and using appropriate continence products;
- Inserting, managing, and removing catheters for all genders, and assisting with self-catheterisation when required;
- Managing bladder drainage;
- Administering enemas and suppositories, and undertaking rectal examination and manual evacuation when appropriate;
- Undertaking stoma care and identifying and using appropriate products and approaches.

Assisting with Personal Care

When considering best practice approaches for meeting the needs for care and support with hygiene and the maintenance of skin integrity, again it is important accurately to assess a person's capacity for independence and self-care before agreeing appropriate interventions. This would include assessing needs for help with washing, bathing, shaving and dressing, oral, dental, eye and nail care; identifying and managing any skin conditions (e.g., irritations, rashes or wounds and sores) and taking into account when onward referral to other members of the multidisciplinary team (MDT) is appropriate (e.g., dentist, podiatrist, tissue viability nurse). The Essence of Care benchmarks (DH, 2010a) state that personal hygiene is 'the physical act of cleansing the body to ensure that the hair, nails, ears, eyes, nose and skin are maintained in an optimum condition'. It also includes mouth hygiene, which is the effective removal of plaque and debris to ensure that the structures and tissues of the mouth are kept in a healthy condition. As an adult nurse you may encounter many individuals who have pre-existing periodontal disease made worse by their current health status (Table 3.1).

Table 3.1 At-risk groups: individuals with pre-existing periodontal disease that is often exacerbated by current health status

Dementia	Individuals receiving oxygen therapy or head and neck radiation
Frail elderly	Ventilated individuals
Learning disabilities	Immunocompromised individuals
Palliative care	People with poor mobility
Chemotherapy	Individuals who have suffered a stroke
Delirium	Individuals with physical disabilities
Mental health issues	

Activity 3.5

Identify a care-dependent adult who might need assistance with their oral health.

- How often do they receive oral care?
- What equipment is used?
- How does this compare with hospital policy in your area?

Skin Integrity

You may be familiar with a criticism that the modern graduate nurse is 'too posh to wash.' This rests with the idea that delivering personal care can be an unpleasant, repetitive, and mundane task that involves physical demanding work. However, personal care is an essential nursing responsibility that contributes to the comfort, safety, wellbeing, and dignity of the individual. It also provides an opportunity to assess a person's activity levels and gain valuable insights into the appearance of the skin, hair, nails, and mucous membranes that may be present in healthy and diseased states. The term 'skin integrity' refers to the skin being a sound and complete structure in unimpaired condition. As we age subcutaneous fat is diminished and the skin becomes thinner, drier, and less elastic. Sebaceous and sweat gland activity is reduced, as is capillary blood flow. The cumulative effect of the ageing process is that skin becomes significantly more vulnerable to damage and there are delays in wound healing. Skin conditions, xerostomia (dryness), fissures (cracks) and pruritus (itching) are common in elderly people but often go unrecognised and untreated (Cowdell and Garrett, 2014). Alterations in the colour, moisture, temperature, texture, mobility and turgor of skin, and the presence of skin lesions can alert the nurse to an underlying pathology. Only when you have assessed and documented the condition of a person's skin can you then formulate an appropriate care plan to maintain skin integrity.

There are several acute and chronic wounds that will breach the integrity of the skin. Three will briefly be considered here:

1 Pressure injuries;
2 Leg ulcers;
3 Surgical wounds.

Pressure injuries

A pressure injury is defined as 'localised damage to the skin and/or underlying soft tissue usually over a bony prominence or related to a medical or other device which occurs as a result of intense and/or prolonged pressure or pressure in combination with shear' (National Pressure Injury Advisory

Panel, 2016). The most common anatomical sites are the sacrum and the heels. Severity varies from erythema to full-thickness skin loss, and incidence increases in elderly people. Although seen as largely preventable, between April 2015 and March 2016 there were 24,674 newly acquired pressure injuries reported, costing the NHS more than £3.8 million a day (Stephenson and Fletcher, 2020). Risk factors include:

- Significantly limited mobility (e.g., Individuals with a spinal cord injury);
- Significant loss of sensation;
- History of a previous or current pressure injury;
- Nutritional deficiency;
- The inability of an individual to reposition themselves;
- Significant cognitive impairment.

A pressure injury risk assessment should be included for all individuals admitted to secondary care, care homes or receiving NHS care in other settings within six hours of admission. They should be reassessed after a surgical or interventional procedure, or after a change in their care environment following a transfer (NICE, 2015). There are available risk assessment tools that alert practitioners to the most common risk factors that predispose individuals to pressure injury development (Moore and Cowman, 2014). Completing a risk assessment allows the nurse to protect a person's skin integrity through careful moving and handling techniques, regular repositioning, the use of pressure-redistributing devices, and the need for nutritional supplements and hydration.

Fatima

Fatima is an 82-year-old admitted from the Accident and Emergency department having fallen six hours ago sustaining a fractured left neck of femur. Fatima is normally independent and in good health but is currently bedbound. You estimate that Fatima has a below-average BMI, dry skin and suffers occasionally from stress incontinence.

Complete a risk assessment using the approved tool in your current placement. What measures would you put in place to prevent pressure damage?

Leg ulcers

Venous leg ulcers are a form of chronic wound characterised by skin loss below the knee on the leg or foot that remains unhealed after four weeks. They can affect one in 500 people in the UK and cost the NHS up to £400 million a year (Stanton et al., 2016). The incidence of leg ulcers rises with age and can take longer to heal in people from lower socioeconomic groups (Scottish Intercollegiate Guidelines Network or SIGN, 2010). Venous leg ulcers are caused by sustained venous hypertension that is exacerbated by obesity, immobility, a history of varicose veins and deep vein thrombosis. Individuals with leg ulcers endure numerous bio-psychosocial problems, which include pain, odour, sepsis, absence from work, loss of independence and social isolation. Care provision often takes place in community settings, in their own home or in a specialist leg ulcer clinic. Such individuals may be admitted to hospital if experiencing secondary sepsis. Local wound care and graduated compression therapy that improves microcirculation is the cornerstone of leg ulcer management (O'Meara et al., 2012). However, it is reported that many individuals cannot tolerate, compression therapy.

- What are the reasons why someone might not tolerate compression therapy?
- As an adult nurse, what things would you consider when managing this situation?

Surgical wounds

The aim of postoperative wound care is to allow the wound to heal rapidly without complications, and with the best functional and aesthetic results. Due to the natural mass of microorganisms in the environment, it is not possible to achieve sterility in a typical healthcare setting. However, the principles of asepsis – to remove viable pathogenic microorganisms at the time of a high-risk procedure – is a more achievable aim and helps to protect an individual's portal of entry. Aseptic Non-Touch Technique (ANTT) has garnered approval throughout the world as being a specific type of standardised principles, practices and procedures that ensure only uncontaminated equipment, referred to as 'key parts,' comes into contact with susceptible areas, called 'key sites' during clinical procedures (Association for Safe Aseptic Practice (ASAP), 2019).

Key components of Aseptic Non-Touch Technique to reduce cross infection are:

- ANTT Risk assessment (e.g., determining whether Surgical ANTT or Standard ANTT approach is required);
- Environmental Management (e.g., environmental risks removed or avoided, and work areas cleaned and/or disinfected);
- Decontamination and Protection (e.g., hand cleansing and use of personal protective equipment);
- Aseptic Field Selection and Management (e.g., critical, or micro-critical aseptic fields);
- Non-touch technique (e.g., desirable, or essential).

Broadly, the risks of surgical wound infection can be separated into the preoperative period, the intraoperative period and postoperative period. A recent review (Harris et al., 2018) suggested that where possible the following 12 key risk factors should be identified and addressed in the preoperative period:

1   Obesity;
2   Malnutrition;
3   Smoking;

4   Hypertension and coronary artery disease;
5   Pre-existing body site infection;
6   Diabetes mellitus (poor glycaemic control);
7   Size and virulence of the microbial inocula;
8   General health and co-morbid disease processes, including medications that affect integrity of an individual's host defences;
9   Alcohol or substance use;
10 Physical activity and mobility limitations;
11 Previous complications with anaesthetic and surgeries;
12 Advanced age.

Activity 3.6

Access the National Institute for Health and Care Excellence (2019) *Surgical Site Infections: Prevention and Treatment* (updated 2020) guidelines via the website below:

www.nice.org.uk/guidance/ng125/resources/surgical-site-infections-prevention-and-treatment-pdf-66141660564421

Identify actions needed to reduce the risk of surgical site infections.

Important components of the intraoperative risks (during surgery) can include length of the procedure, whether it is 'clean' or 'contaminated,' the methods used, how well peripheral perfusion is maintained, whether it is an elective or emergency procedure, and the presence of an implant. Delayed healing can take place in the postoperative period through dehiscence (i.e., the wound breaking open) and infection. As an adult nurse, you should look for the following signs when you undertake a postoperative wound review: fever, haematoma, seroma, separation of wound edges and purulent discharge from the wound. NICE (2019) have also made several recommendations for postoperative wound management, and this includes keeping wounds clean and debriding non-viable tissue. If wound infection is suspected, a specimen should be taken, and empirical antibiotic therapy commenced based on the suspected pathogen. Once the pathogen and sensitivity have been identified the antibiotic should be tailored as required.

Mobility

The ability for individuals to move around safely is important to prevent complications associated with inactivity or long-term bedrest (e.g., deep vein thrombosis, pressure ulcers/bed sores, constipation, loss of muscle strength and confidence). Any loss of mobility, even for a fleeting period, can have an untoward impact on a person's independence and health (Ness and Murray, 2009). To be able to undertake a thorough assessment of mobility issues a nurse will need to have a good understanding of related anatomy and physiology of the musculoskeletal and nervous system.

• What are the factors that can impact on an individual's ability to mobilise?

Your nursing assessment would need to determine whether someone has any medical condition that might impact on their ability to mobilise safely (e.g., muscle weakness, poor vision or balance, low blood pressure or anxiety related to the risk of falling). You would need to assess any mobility restrictions or limitations on how far they could walk. You would also need to establish whether they needed any walking aids (e.g., a walking stick or Zimmer frame) or other specialist equipment to move around.

Although mobilisation can help people regain or maintain function and reduce complications, unsafe or reduced mobilisation increases the risk of falls. Growdon et al. (2017) highlight the tensions faced by healthcare practitioners when considering the need to promote mobility while also preventing falls. Indeed, Kneafsey et al. (2013) point out that nurses will often focus on keeping people safe to prevent problems, rather than focusing on a rehabilitation goal. However, Growden et al. (2017) argue that promoting mobility may help to prevent injury sustained by falls, and therefore they question the customary practice of immobilising individuals for the sake of fall prevention. In consideration of these issues, required and agreed interventions should be aimed at maximising mobility and independence while also maintaining a person's safety; for example, encouraging them to move around as much as possible, referring to a physiotherapist to help agree a personalised mobility plan, providing required walking aids and teaching gentle exercises and techniques to move from bed to chair or wheelchair.

Activity 3.7

Download a copy of the current NICE (2013) Guidelines for Falls Risk Assessment www.nice.org.uk/guidance/cg161/evidence/falls-full-guidance-190033741

Compare these with local guidelines and fall risk assessment policies that you have in your own placement setting. Are there any similarities or differences?

Other related clinical skills required for entry to the register (NMC, 2018a) include

- Using appropriate safety techniques and devices;
- Using a range of contemporary moving and handling techniques and mobility aids;
- Using appropriate moving and handling equipment to support people with impaired mobility.

Resting and Sleeping

Sleep plays a vital role in our physical health. According to the National Heart, Lung, and Blood Institute (NHLBI, 2011), sleep has a restorative function and helps to protect not only our health but also our quality of life and safety. Ongoing sleep deficiency can be linked to an increased risk of heart disease, kidney disease, high blood pressure, diabetes, and stroke (NHLBI, 2011). Assessing and meeting the needs for care and support with rest, sleep and comfort involve making enquiries about the quality and duration of rest and sleep, identifying, and addressing any factors that might adversely impact on this (e.g., noise, other disturbance, anxiety, depression, pain, etc.).

Activity 3.8

Access and review the following:

Dubose, J. and Hadi, K. (2016) 'Improving inpatient environments to support patient sleep', *International Journal for Quality in Health Care*, 28(5), 540-53.

Irish, L.A, Kline, C.E, Gunn, H.E., Buysse, D.J. and Hall, M.H. (2015) 'The role of sleep hygiene in promoting public health: a review of empirical evidence', *Sleep Med Rev.* 2015 August; 22: 23-36.

Consider what actions you could take to help promote an individual's rest and sleep in your own placement area?

Infection Prevention and Control

Healthcare Associated Infection (HCAI), also referred to as 'nosocomial' or 'hospital' infection, is an infection occurring in someone during the process of care in a hospital or other healthcare facility which was not present or incubating at the time of admission. It is associated with significant morbidity and mortality (particularly if caused by multi-drug-resistant bacteria), protracted hospital stays and increased healthcare costs (Loveday et al., 2014). The COVID-19 pandemic reminds us of the intractable nature of HCAI. In the first 6 months of the pandemic up to 1 in 6 Sars-Cov-2 infections were attributed to hospital transmission. At the same time, there was an increase in central line-associated blood stream infections (CLABSI), catheter-associated urinary tract infections (CAUTI), and methicillin-resistant *Staphylococcus aureus* (MRSA) bacteraemia (Baker, 2022).

It is a legal requirement for registered providers of health and social care in England to comply with a code of practice that makes explicit the way they develop and maintain high levels of infection prevention (Health and Social Care Act, 2008). There are comprehensive evidence-based guidelines produced by EPIC (Loveday et al., 2014) and NICE (2016), which underpin the Code of Practice, and these are complemented by the NMC's standards (NMC, 2018a), outlined below. These form the basis of this short section on infection prevention and control.

Meeting needs for care and support with the prevention and management of infection include:

- Observing, assessing, and responding rapidly to potential infection risks using best practice guidelines;
- Using standard precautions protocols;
- Safely decontaminating equipment and environment;
- Safely using and disposing of waste, laundry, and sharps;
- Using appropriate personal protection equipment including gloves and masks;
- Using evidence-based hand-washing techniques;
- Implementing isolation procedures;
- Using effective aseptic, non-touch techniques;
- Safely assessing and managing invasive medical devices and lines.

Risk assessment and the cycle of infection

Contemporary acute healthcare settings can be understood as places where large numbers of sick people with weakened immune systems are placed close together. As a result of their pre-existing morbidities this often means an increase in invasive treatments that bypass the body's natural defences. To exacerbate this, these treatments are often undertaken by busy staff, in environments of diminished resources. To observe, assess and respond rapidly to potential infection risks, the adult nurse needs to have some understanding of the interplay of the host, pathogen, healthcare workers and healthcare organisations that can result in HCAI. The 'chain of infection' (Figure 3.2) is a well-established framework that captures the epidemiology of HCAI by taking what is known about the nature of microorganisms and describing how they can spread from one person to another. In short, a pathogenic microorganism must be present, and transmission will occur when it leaves its reservoir, or its common resting place, through a portal of exit; it is then conveyed by some mode of transmission, and enters a susceptible host through a

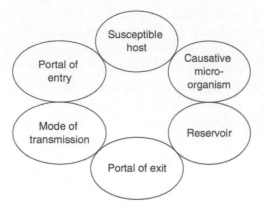

Figure 3.2   The six links within a chain of infection

portal of entry to cause an infection (Centers for Disease Control and Prevention or CDC, 2012). Many of the key principles of infection, prevention and control are based on targeting, and then breaking, the separate 'links' of the chain.

Infectious agent

Microorganisms (often referred to as pathogens) that are responsible for HCAI are classified as bacteria, viruses, or fungi. Gastrointestinal viruses such as norovirus, respiratory viruses, such as influenza, and fungal infections that cause oral thrush can all be problematic in healthcare settings. However, it is bacteria that are largely responsible for the incidence of HCAI (Khan et al., 2017). Paradoxically, bacteria also form an essential part of a human's microbiota and up to 1000 varied species can be found colonising the upper respiratory tract, bowel, skin, and female reproductive tract. Under normal circumstances this is part of a normal synergistic host–microbe relationship because bacteria aid digestion, produce essential vitamins and can create a microbial antagonism, whereby more benign species take up the space and nutrients that are required by more aggressive pathogens. However, when these bacteria grow beyond their normal range, as often seen in people with suppressed immune systems, or begin to populate 'sterile' areas, often through medical devices, they may become more invasive. As a nurse you cannot remove all bacteria, but you can appreciate the conditions that allow them to thrive and how they create abnormal colonisations that result in infection.

Standard precautions

Standard precautions (Table 3.2) refer to a cocktail of infection control practices that aim to minimise, and where possible eliminate, the risk of transmission of infectious agents from their natural reservoirs to a susceptible individual. They are called standard because they offer a basic

Table 3.2 Standard precautions

Hand hygiene
Personal protective clothing
Safe handling of sharps
Cleaning and decontamination of equipment and the environment
The handling and disposal of healthcare waste
The handling and disposal of linen
The management of blood and body fluid spillages

level of care that should be used by all staff, in all care settings, at all times, for all people regardless of their perceived or confirmed infectious status. Standard precautions particularly target the portal of exit and the mode of transmission as a nurse may become contaminated because they come into contact with a person's excretions, secretions, and skin scales.

Understanding the routes of transmission of infection helps to plan strategies to prevent cross-infection. There are four main routes as follows:

1 **Contact**: this is the most frequent mode of transmission and can be through direct physical contact with a person or indirect though contact with equipment or the environment (e.g., methicillin-resistant *Staphylococcus aureus* [MRSA]);
2 **Airborne**: through inhalation of light aerosol droplets that remain airborne for an extended period and are breathed in (e.g., pulmonary tuberculosis, chickenpox);
3 **Faecal–oral**: hand-to-mouth transmission typically seen in enteric infections (e.g., *Campylobacter* spp., *Clostridium difficile*);
4 **Blood and body fluids**: this includes vertical transmission (mother to baby) or horizontal transmission (sharing needles, unprotected sex, e.g., HIV, hepatitis B and C).

Bacteria grow best when there is an ample supply of nutrients and water, an optimum pH, temperature, and oxygen requirements. For these reasons, the exact role that the environment may play in cross-infection can be difficult to quantify. What is known is that the fabric of a building, its furnishings and the medical equipment used on people do become contaminated with hazardous substances. When these are then handled, they can be passed on to a susceptible host. Decontamination is a generic term that refers to the removal of contaminants by a process of cleaning, disinfection, or sterilisation. The precise method used will depend on the level of risk. So, a surgical instrument entering a sterile body cavity would need to be sterilised to remove all microorganisms and their spores, whereas a blood pressure cuff that comes into contact with intact skin could be cleaned to remove contaminants to a safe level. In some cases, a piece of equipment may not withstand a decontamination method and would be deemed a single-use item. Manufacturers of medical devices are legally obliged to provide information on how their devices should be decontaminated and this must be followed. If the instructions appear inappropriate or incomplete this should be reported to the Medicine and Health products Regulatory Agency (MHRA) as an adverse incident (MHRA, 2015).

A coroner reported a case of cross-infection caused by poor decontamination of laryngoscope handles and their blades (MHRA, 2015).

- How do you think this equipment should have been decontaminated?
- How do you think it was decontaminated?
- What are the possible reasons for the variations?
- What risks does this pose to the nurse and an individual in their care?

Hand Hygiene

Hand-mediated cross-infection is seen as a major contributing factor in the acquisition and spread of HCAI (Loveday et al., 2014). In 2009 the World Health Organization (WHO) developed the five moments of hand hygiene and this has been adopted throughout NHS policies:

1   Before touching a person;
2   Before clean/aseptic procedure;
3   After body fluid exposure risk;
4   After touching a person;
5   After touching a person's surroundings.

This was an attempt to identify the key moments when hand hygiene should be performed and place them within a framework that was easy to learn, logical and applicable to a wide range of settings. Moreover, it could be woven into the natural workflow of care (WHO, 2009).

Activity 3.9

Next time you are in a practice setting, observe your colleagues performing hand hygiene.

- Did you think compliance would be the same across all five moments?
- Were you right?
- Can you explain the differences between moments?
- Now read page 86 of the WHO hand hygiene guidelines. Available at: https://www.who.int/publications/i/item/9789241597906

As the requirement for hand hygiene increases, the technique required to systematically remove all transient bacteria from the hand may deteriorate. Posters that demonstrate an approved technique are often present in clinical environments. As well as identifying a good technique, posters will show the parts that are frequently missed: the thumbs and finger pads. These can be a useful aide memoire to the nurse. Broadly speaking, there are three products that can be used to decontaminate hands: antiseptic solutions which are rarely necessary outside the confines of a high-risk environment or procedure; soap and water, which should be used when hands are visibly soiled, potentially contaminated with body fluids, or when caring for people with vomiting or diarrhoeal illness; and alcohol-based hand-rub which is the preferred product after direct person contact with hands that are not visibly soiled (WHO, 2009). The frequent use of some hand hygiene products may cause damage to the skin and alter normal hand flora. The increased colonisation of pathogenic microorganisms and reductions in hand hygiene seen in nurses with damaged skin can increase the risk of cross-infection. Damaged skin and sore hands should be reported to the occupational health department.

Personal Protective Equipment

Personal protective equipment (PPE) is equipment 'that is intended to be worn or held by a person to protect them from risks to their health and safety while at work' (NICE, 2012b: 25). Common examples include gloves, aprons, and eye and face protection. PPE fulfils two functions – to protect the nurse and to protect those being cared for. In making decisions about PPE the nurse will need to undertake a risk assessment. Primarily, this involves asking three questions:

What is the risk of contamination to the nurse?

What is the risk of transmission of microorganisms to another person?

What is the suitability of the equipment for the proposed use?

Plastic aprons and gloves are the most used pieces of PPE. Although the evidence is unclear on whether a nurse's uniform plays a significant part in cross-infection they do become heavily contaminated during clinical care. Plastic aprons offer some protection, as well protecting clothing from the splashing effects of blood or body fluids (DH, 2010b). Similarly, gloves can provide a physical protective barrier that protects the nurse's hands when they come into contact with body fluids. There are different types of gloves (e.g., sterile or non-sterile, latex, vinyl, and nitrile). It is important that you are aware of the gloves available within a clinical setting. You can then assess the task, take note of any allergies that may be present, for example to latex, before selecting the correct product. Aprons and gloves protect those being cared for by preventing the nurse from becoming a portal of exit if their hands and clothing become contaminated when performing routine clinical care. Masks, goggles, and visors tend to focus more on protecting the nurse. Facial protection guards the mucous membranes of the eyes, nose, and mouth from aerosol-generating procedures, such as sputum induction, suctioning and bronchoscopy, or from splash, spray or splatter of blood and body fluids from a poorly controlled haemorrhage.

It is important that you wear the appropriate PPE when coming into contact with contaminated waste, linen, or spills of body fluids. These can all be contaminated with hazardous microorganisms, and need to be handled, disposed of, or managed in a safe manner. You should be aware of the colour-coded system for the disposal of clinical waste and know how to locate water-soluble alginate plastic bags to remove soiled linen. Spills of high-risk body fluids should be removed as soon as possible. This may involve pre-treatment using hypochlorite granules. All healthcare facilities will have a policy on this. As an adult nurse you will frequently come into contact with sharp objects when performing procedures such as injections. Between 1997 and 2018 Public Health England received 8765 reports where healthcare workers (HCWS) experienced significant exposure to Bloodborne Viruses (Public Health England, 2020). Not only do these injuries constitute a major threat to healthcare workers' psychophysical wellbeing, but the true number is likely to be significantly higher because needlestick injuries are notoriously underreported.

Aseptic Non-touch Technique

Due to the natural mass of microorganisms in the environment it is not possible to achieve sterility in a typical healthcare setting. However, the principles of asepsis – to remove viable pathogenic microorganisms at the time of a high-risk procedure – is a more achievable aim and helps to protect a person's portal of entry. Aseptic non-touch technique has garnered approval throughout the NHS as a set of standardised practices and procedures to ensure that only uncontaminated equipment, referred to as 'key parts' or sterile fluids, come into contact with susceptible areas, called 'key sites,' during clinical procedures (Rowley et al., 2010). As stated earlier in the chapter, the key components of aseptic non-touch technique are:

- Always wash hands effectively;
- Non-touch technique is always used to protect key parts;
- Touch non-key parts with confidence;
- Take appropriate infective precautions.

Healthcare organisations that have standardised aseptic technique with aseptic non-touch technique report improved compliance with the core components of aseptic technique and associated reductions in the incidence of HCAI (Clare and Rowley, 2018). Aseptic non-touch technique is particularly targeted at the maintenance of susceptible body sites because the presence of intravenous catheters, urethral catheters, mechanical ventilation, and surgical wounds exponentially increases the risk of HCAI. They do this by undermining a person's anatomical barriers to infection, allowing bacteria to create abnormal colonisations and resistant biofilms that attach to medical devices. The standard precautions that have been already outlined, (e.g., aseptic non-touch technique, hand hygiene, the use of PPE and a clean, managed environment) help to manage risk. Nevertheless, medical devices are frequently implicated in both local and systemic infections. To be able to observe, assess and respond rapidly to these challenges, nurses need to maximise the opportunities available to them. For example, there are risk assessment tools such as the visual infusion phlebitis (VIP) chart (Jackson, 1999) which allows a daily assessment of a vulnerable site, identifying early complications of phlebitis and prompt timely removal. Another idea that is gaining approval within infection prevention and control is the notion of empowerment. According to McGuckin (2016), people want to be empowered and contribute to their own health, but to do this they need the nurse to communicate information to them in a way that they can understand and be convinced that this knowledge will give them a shared responsibility in their health.

- What opportunities have you seen where empowerment would help both the person being cared for and the nurse to prevent and control HCAI?

Isolation

Isolation is another practice that seeks to address several links within the chain of infection. Broadly, there are two types of isolation: *source isolation* (barrier nursing) where the person being cared for is the source of the infection and *protective isolation* (reverse barrier nursing) where the person being cared for requires protection, for example if they are immunocompromised. Source isolation is more commonly encountered, and it has become a mainstay in the management of multi-drug-resistant organisms such as MRSA and enteric infections such as *Clostridium difficile*. Source isolation is best carried out in a single room that has en-suite facilities and a handwashing basin. When demand for single rooms outstrips supply, individuals with the same infection can sometimes be placed in the same area, and this is called cohort nursing. There are times when demand outstrips supply and tough decisions must be made about allocation of resources. This is where you would use your knowledge of the cycle of infection and perform a risk assessment. So, for example, if you had two individuals – one with MRSA and one with *Clostridium difficile* – who would you allocate a single room to? At this point you may require further information. If you discovered the MRSA was in a wound that was covered with an occlusive dressing, but the *Clostridium difficile* infection was associated with explosive diarrhoea, do you now have enough information to make a confident decision? It is important to note that, from a psychological point of view, it is the infectious microorganism that is being isolated and not the person. There is some evidence to suggest that people who are isolated are more likely to exhibit symptoms of depression, develop pressure ulcers, suffer falls, and have longer lengths of stay (Chittick et al., 2016). Moreover, nurses have been shown to have fewer direct interactions with and perform fewer examinations on isolated individuals. It is important not to forget the human face of infection prevention and control.

Compliance

Despite a compelling evidence base to support the use of standard precautions, they are sometimes seen as basic, repetitive, and small scale. Moreover, the rewards for performing them in a systematic way are not always obvious. There might be times when you witness poor practice. Several studies have demonstrated that healthcare workers are not always compliant with the five moments of hand hygiene. When they do wash their hands, it may not be for the 10–15 seconds of vigorous rubbing recommended in the guidelines. Some may have a habitual preference for soap and water, despite campaigns that encourage the greater use of alcohol hand rub (AHR). AHR has been found to be quicker, more effective, and kinder to hands. At times healthcare workers may don gloves when there is no contact with blood or body fluids but continue to wear them when they have become contaminated. They may place themselves at unnecessary risk by not adorning facial protection (even when they should) overfilling sharps containers and re-sheathing needles. Documentation might not always be complete and those individuals receiving care are often passive in their contribution to preventing HCAI. This is merely to state the challenges that the adult nurse faces in today's busy contemporary healthcare. There are enormous opportunities as well. Compliance may not be perfect but there has been a cultural change in the way the NHS manages HCAI. Cases of MRSA and *Clostridium difficile* infection have fallen significantly, and these are testament to the excellent care that is taking place. Each NHS organisation will employ an infection control team and nurses play a vital role in infection prevention and control.

Activity 3.10

Find out who the infection control nurse is for your area.

Arrange a meeting to discuss the contribution you can make to preventing infection in vulnerable people.

Related clinical skills required for entry to the register (NMC, 2018a) include

- Safely decontaminate equipment and the environment;
- Safely assess and manage invasive medical devices and lines.

Developing Your Clinical Skills

The NMC (2018a) requires registered nurses to be proficient in a range of technical and non-technical procedures and list an extensive range of clinical skills that the adult nurse is expected to perform as part of their sphere of practice. However, clinical skills should not be viewed as task related, nor should skills be performed without critical thought. They should be seen as a vital part of caring for a person and not in isolation. Indeed, the NMC (2018a) stresses that all nursing procedures should be carried out as part of holistic person-centred care. Furthermore, as a registrant you will always need to ensure that you do no harm to those in your care. Performing a clinical skill for which you do not have the appropriate education and recent experience may have a negative impact on the person's experience and the safety of their care.

Simulation-based Learning

Some would argue that the most valuable learning experiences take place in practice. However, Dewey (1933) suggests experience is only the raw material for learning. Therefore, it is how you utilise the learning experience and what you do with it that matters. Simulated learning can take place in a clinical skills laboratory, in a classroom, in the clinical area away from direct care environments or online. High-fidelity simulation is defined by Rehmann et al. (1995: 2) as 'as much realism as possible', and virtual-reality technology offers the chance to experiment and practise clinical skills and procedures, providing opportunities for individualised learning, repeated exposure, and mistakes to be made without anyone coming to harm (Lewis et al., 2012). Technology can be used to expose a learner to scenarios that they might not encounter in clinical practice to help bridge the gap between theory and practice. Activities may focus on cognitive (critical thinking), affective (feelings, attitudes) and psychomotor skills, offering the prospect of reflection and feedback within a safe and supportive environment (Yuan et al., 2012; Cooper, 2015; Sundeler et al., 2015; Wighus and Bjork, 2018). Recognising the value of simulated learning, the NMC (2023) has acknowledged this method as an acceptable way to learn clinical skills.

Activity 3.11

In each of your placement areas, you should be thinking about opportunities for developing your clinical skills and considering which clinical skills you need to develop.

- Set yourself three learning objectives for each skill you need to develop;
- Take part in learning the clinical skill;
- Reflect on your learning in your portfolio. Have you met your learning objectives? If not what else can you do to meet your learning needs?

Chapter Summary

It is crucial that nurses can deliver person-centred, evidence-based nursing care in a sensitive and compassionate manner. Systematic approaches to nursing care and the use of assessment frameworks and models offer us processes by which we can work closely with people to plan individualised care pathways and guide the delivery of high-quality person-centred nursing care. However, to be able to do so, our decisions need to be informed and underpinned by a proficient level of knowledge and understanding of the associated anatomy, physiology and pathophysiology, an understanding of the need to protect safety and an ability to integrate theory, simulation, and practice.

Further Reading

Cook, N., Shepherd, A. and Boore, J. (2020) *Essentials of Anatomy and Physiology for Nursing Practice*, 2nd edn. London: Sage.

Delves-Yates, C. (2022) *Essentials of Nursing Practice*, 3rd edn. London: Sage.

Lister, S., Hofland, J. and Grafton, H. (2020) *The Royal Marsden Manual of Clinical Procedures*, 10th edn. Chichester: Wiley.

Holland, K. and Jenkins, J. (2019) *Applying the Roper–Logan–Tierney Model in Practice*, 3rd edn. Edinburgh: Elsevier.

Moore, T. (2017) 'Observations and monitoring'. In T. Moore and S. Cunningham (eds), *Clinical Skills for Nursing Practice*. Oxon: Routledge, Chapter 7.

Pellatt, G.C. (2007) 'Clinical skills: bed making and patient positioning', *British Journal of Nursing*, Mar 8-21; 16(5): 302–5. doi: 10.12968/bjon.2007.16.5.23010. PMID: 17505378.

Wilson, B, Woollands, A. and Barrett, D (2019) *Care Planning: A Guide for Nurses*, 3rd edn. New York: Routledge.

References

Association for Safe Aseptic Practice (2019) *Aseptic non-touch technique (ANTT): a practice framework for clinical practice*. Available at: www.antt.org/antt-practice-framework.html. (last accessed 21 July 2022).

Baker, M.A., Sands, K.E., Huang, S.S., Kleinman, K., Septimus, E.J., Neha Varma, N., Blanchard, J., Poland, R.E., Coady, M.H., Yokoe, D.S., Fraker, S., Froman, A., Moody, J., Goldin, L., Isaacs, A., Kleja, K., Korwek, K.M., Stelling, J., Clark, A., Platt, R. and Perlin, J.B. (2022) 'The impact of Coronavirus disease 2019 (COVID-19) on healthcare-associated infections', *Clin Infect Dis*. May 30; 74 (10): 1748–54.

Barrett, D., Wilson, B. and Woollands, A. (2012) *Care Planning: A Guide for Nurses*, 2nd edn. Harlow: Pearson.

British Association for Parental and Enteral Nutrition (2011) *Malnutrition Universal Screening Tool*. London: BAPEN. Available at: www.bapen.org.uk/pdfs/must/must-full.pdf. (last accessed 27 July 2022).

Centers for Disease Control and Prevention (2012) *Principles of Epidemiology in Public Health Practice*, 3rd edn. *An Introduction to Applied Epidemiology and Biostatistics*. Available at: www.cdc.gov/ophss/csels/dsepd/ss1978/lesson1/section10.html (last accessed 25 July 2022).

Chittick, P., Koppisetty, S., Lombardo, L., Vadhavana, A., Solanki, A., Cumming, K., Agboto, V., Karl, C. and Band, J. (2016) 'Assessing patient and caregiver understanding of and satisfaction with the use of contact isolation', *American Journal of Infection Control*, 44: 657–60.

Clare, S. and Rowley, S. (2018) 'Implementing the Aseptic Non-Touch Technique (ANTT®) clinical practice framework for aseptic technique: a pragmatic evaluation using a mixed methods approach in two London hospitals', *Journal of Infection Prevention*, 19: 6–15.

Cooper, S. (2015) 'Simulation versus lecture? Measuring educational impact: considerations for best practice,' *Evidence Based Nursing*, 19(2). Available at: http://dx.doi.org/10.1136/eb-2015-102221. (last accessed 25 July 2022).

Cowdell, F. and Garrett, D. (2014) 'Older people and skin: challenging perceptions', *British Journal of Nursing*, 23(12): S4–S8.

Department of Health (2010a) *Essence of Care Benchmarks for Personal Hygiene*. London: DH.

Department of Health (2010b) *Uniforms and Workwear: Guidance of Uniforms and Workwear Policies for NHS Employers*. London: DH.

Dewey, J. (1933) *How We Think: A Restatement of Reflective Thinking to the Educative Process*. Boston, MA: Heath.

Doyle, C., Byrne, K., Fleming, S., Griffiths, C., Horan, P. and Keenan, P.M. (2016) 'Enhancing the experience of people with intellectual disabilities who access health care', *Learning Disability Practice*, 19(6): 19.

Gold, D.A. (2012) 'An examination of instrumental activities of daily living assessment in older adults and mild cognitive impairment', *Journal of Clinical and Experimental Neuropsychology*, 34(1): 11–34.

Growdon, M.E., Shorr, R.I. and Inouye, S.K. (2017) 'The tension between promoting mobility and preventing falls in the hospital', *JAMA Internal Medicine*, 177(6): 759–60.

Hardy, S. (2013) 'Prevention and management of depression in primary care', *Nursing Standard*, 27(26): 51–6.

Harris, C., Kuhnke, J. and Haley, J. (2018) *Best Practice Recommendations for the Prevention and Management of Surgical Wound Complications*. Available at: www.woundscanada.ca/docman/public/health-care-... Best practice recommendations for the prevention and management of skin tears.... /public/555-bpr-prevention-and-management-of-surgical-wound-complications-v2/file. (last accessed 25 July 2022).

Health and Social Care Act (2008) *Code of Practice on the Prevention and Control of Infections and Related Guidance*. London: Department of Health and Social Care.

Heslop, P., Blair, P., Fleming, P., Hoghton, M., Marriott, A. and Russ, L. (2013) *Confidential Inquiry into Premature Deaths of People with Learning Disabilities (CIPOLD)*. Bristol: Norah Fry Research Centre, University of Bristol. Available at: www.bristol.ac.uk/cipold. (last accessed 25 July 2022).

Jackson, A. (1999) *IV Therapy and Care*. Rotherham General Hospital NHS Trust.

Khan, H., Kanwal Baig, F. and Mehboob, R. (2017) 'Nosocomial infections: epidemiology, prevention, control and surveillance', *Asian Pacific Journal of Tropical Biomedicine*, 7(5): 478–82.

Kneafsey, R., Clifford, C. and Greenfield, S. (2013) 'What is the nursing team involvement in maintaining and promoting the mobility of older adults in hospital? A grounded theory study,' *International Journal of Nursing Studies*, 50: 1617–29.

Lawton, M.P. and Brody, E.M. (1969) 'Assessment of older people: self-maintaining and instrumental activities of daily living', *Gerontologist*, 9: 179–86.

Lewis, R., Stachan, A. and McKenzie Smith, M. (2012) 'Is high fidelity the most effective method for the development of non-technical skills in nursing? A review of the current evidence,' *Open Nursing Journal*, 6: 82–9.

Loveday, H., Wilson, J., Pratt, R., Golsorkhi, M., Tingle, A., Bak, A., Browne, J., Prieto, J. and Wilcox, M. (2014) 'Epic3: national evidence-based guidelines for preventing healthcare-associated infections in NHS hospitals in England', *Journal of Hospital Infection*, 86(Suppl 1): S1–S70.

Manz, F. and Wentz, A. (2005) 'The importance of good hydration for the prevention of chronic diseases', *Nutrition Review*, 63(6 Pt 2): S2–S5.

McGuckin, M. (2016) 'Patient and healthcare worker empowerment'. In P. Elliot, J. Storr and A. Jeanes (eds), *Infection Prevention and Control: Perceptions and Perspectives*. Boca Raton, FL: CRC Press, pp. 175–88.

Medicines and Healthcare products Regulatory Agency (2015) *Managing Medical Devices*. London: MHRA.

MENCAP (2007) *Death by Indifference: Following up the Treat me Right! Report*. London: MENCAP. Available at: www.mencap.org.uk/sites/default/files/2016-06/DBIreport.pdf. (last accessed 25 July 2022).

Mlinac, M.E. and Feng, M.C. (2016) 'Assessment of activities of daily living, self-care and independence', *Archives of Clinical Neuropsychology*, 31, 506–16.

Moore, Z. and Cowman, S. (2014) 'Risk assessment tools for the prevention of pressure ulcers', *Cochrane Database Systematic Reviews*, 5(2): CD006471.

Morton-Nance, S. (2015) 'Unique role of learning disability liaison nurses', *Learning Disability Practice*, 18(7): 30–4.

National Heart, Lung, and Blood Institute (2011) *Your Guide to Healthy Sleep*. Bethesda, MD: NHLBI.

National Institute for Health and Care Excellence (2006) *Nutritional Support for Adults: Oral Nutritional Support, Enteral Tube Feeding and Parenteral Nutrition*. Available at: www.nice.org.uk/Guidance/cg32. Updated Aug 2017. (last accessed 25 July 2022).

National Institute for Health and Care Excellence (2012a) *Nutrition Support in Adults (Quality Standard)*. Available at: www.nice.org.uk/guidance/qs24/resources/nutrition-support-in-adults-pdf-2098545777349. (last accessed 25 July 2022).

National Institute for Health and Care Excellence (2012b) *Healthcare-associated Infections: Prevention and Control in Primary and Community Care*. London: NICE.

National Institute for Health and Care Excellence (2015) *Pressure Ulcers (Quality Standard)*. London: NICE.

National Institute for Health and Care Excellence (2016) *Healthcare-associated Infections (Quality Standard)*. London: NICE.

National Institute for Health and Care Excellence (2018) *Managing Exacerbations of COPD (Care Pathway)*. London: NICE. Available at: https://pathways.nice.org.uk/pathways/chronic-obstructive-pulmonary-disease. (last accessed 25 July 2022).

National Institute for Health and Care Excellence (2019) *Surgical Site Infections: Prevention and Treatment* (updated 2020). London: NICE.

National Pressure Injury Advisory Panel (2016) *Pressure Injury and Stages.* Available at: https://cdn.ymaws.com/npiap.com/resource/resmgr/NPIAP-Staging-Poster.pdf. (last accessed 21 July 2022).

Ness, V. and Murray, J. (2009) 'Mobilising'. In C. Doherty and J. McCallum (eds), *Foundation Clinical Nursing Skills.* Oxford: Oxford University Press, pp. 379–421.

NHS England (2017) *The Learning Disabilities Mortality Review (LeDeR Programme) Annual Report,* December 2017. Bristol: Norah Fry Centre for Disability Studies.

Nursing and Midwifery Council (2023) *Future Nurse: Standards of Proficiency for Registered Nurses.* London: NMC.

Nursing and Midwifery Council (2018b) *The Code: Professional Standards of Practice and Behaviour for Nurses and Midwives.* Available at: www.nmc.org.uk/globalassets/sitedocuments/nmc-publications/nmc-code.pdf (last accessed 22 August 2022).

O'Meara, S., Cullum, N., Nelson, E., et al. (2012) 'Compression for venous leg ulcers', *Cochrane Database of Systematic Reviews,* 11: CD000265.

Orlando, I.J. (1961) *The Dynamic Nurse–Patient Relationship: Function, Process, and Principles.* New York: G.P. Putmans & Sons. [Reprinted, 1990, New York: National League for Nursing.]

Parliamentary and Health Service Ombudsman (2009) *Six Lives: The Provision of Public Services to People with Learning Disabilities.* Available at: www.gov.uk/government/publications/report. (last accessed 25 July 2022).

Phillips, L. (2012) 'Improving care for people with learning disabilities in hospital', *Nursing Standard,* 26(23): 42–58.

Public Health England (2018) *Learning Disabilities: applying ALL Our Health.* Available at: www.gov.uk/government/publications/learning-disability-applying-all-our-health. (last accessed 21 July 2022).

Public Health England (2020) *Eye of the Needle Report: Surveillance of Significant Occupational Exposures to Bloodborne Viruses in Healthcare Workers in the United Kingdom – update on seroconversions.* London: Public Health England.

Rehmann, A., Mitman, R. and Reynolds, M. (1995) *A Handbook of Flight Simulation Fidelity Requirements for Human Factors Research.* Defense Technical Information Center. Technical report DOT/FAA/CT-TN95/46.

Roper, N., Logan, W.W. and Tierney, A.J. (2000) *The Roper–Logan–Tierney Model of Nursing: Based on Activities of Living.* London: Churchill-Livingstone.

Rowley, S., Clare, S., Macqueen, S. and Molyneux, R. (2010) 'ANTT v2: an updated practice framework for aseptic technique', *British Journal of Nursing,* 19(5): S5–S11.

Scottish Intercollegiate Guidelines Network (2010) *Management of Chronic Venous Leg Ulcers.* Edinburgh: SIGN. Available at: www.sign.ac.uk/our-guidelines/management-of-chronic-venous-leg-ulcers/. (last accessed 25 July 2022).

Stanton, J., Hickman, A., Rouncivell, D., Collins, C. and Gray, D. (2016) 'Promoting patient concordance to support rapid leg ulcer healing', *Journal of Community Nursing,* 30(6): 28–35.

Stephenson, J. and Fletcher, J. (2020) *NHS England/ Improvement National Pressure Ulcer Prevalence and Quality of Care Audit – Cohorts 1 and 2 National Stop the Pressure Programme Audit report.* NHS England. Available at: https://huddersfield.app.box.com/s/mgl1c3bspfed9i3hdthtyxsgd2tqpr56. (last accessed 25 July 2022).

Sundeler, A., Pettersson, A. and Burglund, M. (2015) 'Undergraduate nursing students' experiences when examining nursing skills in clinical simulation laboratories with high-fidelity patient simulators: a phenomenological research study', *Nurse Education Today,* 35: 1257–61.

Taylor, V. and Ashelsford, S. (2008) 'Understanding depression in palliative and end of life care', *Nursing Standard,* 23(12): 48–57.

Thomas, B. and Atkinson, D. (2011) 'Improving health outcomes for people with learning disabilities', *Nursing Standard*, 26(6): 33–6.

Toney-Butler, T.J. and Thayer, J.M. (2022) *Nursing Process*. In: StatPearls [Internet]. Treasure Island (FL): StatPearls Publishing. Available at: www.ncbi.nlm.nih.gov/books/NBK499937/. (last accessed 25 July 2022).

Toney-Butler, T.J. and Unison-Pace, W.J. (2021) *Nursing Admission Assessment and Examination*. In: StatPearls [Internet]. Treasure Island (FL): StatPearls Publishing. Available at: www.ncbi.nlm.nih.gov/books/NBK493211/. (last accessed 25 July 2022).

van Helvoort, H.A., Willems, L.M., Dekhuijzen, R., van Hees, H. and Heijdra, Y.F. (2016) 'Respiratory constraints during activities in daily life and the impact on health status in patients with early-stage COPD: a cross-sectional study', *NPJ Primary Care Respiratory Medicine*, 26: 16054.

White, A., Sheehan, R., Ding, J., Roberts, C., Magill, N., Keagan-Bull, R., Carter, B., Ruane, M., Xiang, X., Chauhan, U., Tuffrey-Wijne, I. and Strydom, A. (2022) *Learning from Lives and Deaths – People with a learning disability and autistic people (LeDeR) report for 2021*, Autism and learning disability partnership, King's College, London.

Wighus, M. and Bjork, I.T. (2018) 'An educational intervention to enhance clinical skills learning: experiences of nursing students and teachers', *Nurse Education in Practice*, 29: 143–9.

World Health Organization (2009) *WHO Guidelines on Hand Hygiene in Health Care*. Geneva: WHO.

World Health Organization (2022) *Mental Disorders*. Available at: www.who.int/news-room/fact-sheets/detail/mental-disorders. (last accessed 25 July 2022).

Yuan, H., Williams, B. and Fang, J. (2012) 'The contribution of high-fidelity simulation to nursing students' confidence and competence', *International Nursing Review*, 59: 26–33.

4

INTERPROFESSIONAL AND MULTIDISCIPLINARY TEAM WORKING

Jean Rogers and Sarah Booth

Chapter objectives

- Define the terms multidisciplinary and interprofessional working;
- Reflect upon and identify the factors that contribute to the development of partnerships and team working, considering how you can develop these skills;
- Identify and reflect upon factors that can prevent collaborative partnerships and team working;
- Explore strategies for overcoming the barriers to interprofessional working and consider how you can develop these skills;
- Explore the benefits of effective team working in the provision of safe and effective healthcare and consider how you can apply these within a contemporary healthcare setting.

So far, the previous chapters have focused on the knowledge and skills required to be an adult nurse as well as the concept of safe and effective person-centred care. However, often good health care cannot be provided or achieved by one individual- it takes a team of health and social care professionals to deliver truly effective, person-centred care. The aims of this chapter are to explore how interprofessional and multidisciplinary working can positively impact the health needs of individuals and identify factors that contribute to the development of collaborative working partnerships.

Related Nursing and Midwifery Council (NMC) Proficiencies for Registered Nurses

The overarching requirement of the NMC is that all nurses must be able to play an active and equal role in the interdisciplinary team, collaborating and communicating effectively with a range of colleagues. They must work effectively across professional and agency boundaries, actively involving and respecting the contribution of others to ensure the provision of integrated person-centred care. They must know when and how to communicate with and refer to other professionals and agencies to respect the choices of service users and others, promoting shared decision making to deliver positive outcomes and coordinating smooth, effective transition within and between services and agencies (NMC, 2018a).

━━━━━ TO ACHIEVE ENTRY TO THE NMC REGISTER

YOU MUST BE ABLE TO ━━━━━

- Demonstrate an understanding of the roles, responsibilities, and scope of practice of all members of the nursing and interdisciplinary team, and know how to make best use of the contributions of others involved in providing care;
- Understand and apply the principles of partnership, collaboration, and interagency working across all relevant sectors;
- Demonstrate the knowledge and confidence to contribute effectively and proactively within an interdisciplinary team;
- Demonstrate the ability to write accurate, clear, and timely records and documentation;
- Effectively and responsibly use a range of digital technologies to access, input, analyse and apply information and data within teams and between agencies;
- Confidently and clearly share and present verbal, digital and written reports or information and instructions with individuals and groups when delegating or handing over responsibility for care;
- Demonstrate knowledge of when and how to refer people safely to other professionals or services for clinical intervention or support.

(Adapted from NMC, 2018a)

Throughout this chapter we will use real examples and case studies so that you can gain a wider perspective of interprofessional and multidisciplinary working. However, before exploring interprofessional and multidisciplinary work in more detail, it would be useful to consider what each term means.

- What do the terms 'multidisciplinary' and 'interprofessional' working mean to you?

Multidisciplinary working describes the mechanism by which holistic care is ensured and a seamless service delivered across the boundaries of primary, secondary, and tertiary care (Hastie et al., 2016). However, it is about the task and not necessarily the collective working process, so it does not imply collaboration. There are some distinct advantages and disadvantages to multidisciplinary working (Table 4.1).

Alternatively, Pollard et al. (2014: 13) define *interprofessional* working as:

'the process whereby members of different professions and/or agencies work with each other and patients/service users, to provide integrated health and/or social care for the latter's benefit'.

This is supported by NHS England (2014: 12) who advise that working together enables professional teams to 'explore problems outside of normal boundaries and reach solutions based on a new understanding of complex situations'. Similarly, there are also some clear advantages and disadvantages to interprofessional working, which will be discussed later in the chapter.

Table 4.1 Advantages and disadvantages of multidisciplinary working

Advantages	Disadvantages
Individuals receive better all-round care.	Different professions work together but keep their defined role (working in their silos).
All plans can be discussed so that all pros and cons can be considered.	Takes more time to come to conclusions.
More likely to provide comprehensive care and less likely that anything is missed.	Information not always shared properly.
Team members aware of progress in case anyone becomes ill.	Communication can be a challenge.
Better use of resources.	Professional rivalry and mistrust.
Reduces the number of people to whom recipients of care need to relate.	

Jovanović et al. (2020) believe the prefix 'multi' indicates the involvement of personnel from different professions and does not imply collaboration, whereas 'inter' implies collaboration. Therefore, it is sensible to define collaboration.

- What does the term 'collaboration' mean to you?

Wei et al. (2020) define collaboration as working together to achieve something that no profession could achieve alone. When working collaboratively, knowledge and expertise are brought together to facilitate decision making, which is undertaken jointly with shared viewpoints from several professions, for the benefit of those receiving care. The terms 'interprofessional' and 'multidisciplinary' are often used interchangeably and thus, for the purposes of this chapter, we will be using the term 'interprofessional working.'

Interprofessional team working is a key objective in any contemporary health and social care setting and working interprofessionally is seen by all professional bodies as essential for promoting effective care. However, it is not a new concept because team working has been an integral part of healthcare from the 1960s onwards (Baldwin, 1993). Before this, staff from various disciplines worked in distinct professional teams (silos) and had no concrete knowledge of what each other's roles entailed. This required multiple duplication of documentation, which often resulted in those receiving care being repeatedly asked for the same details. Care delivery was also fragmented. Ongoing developments in approaches to service delivery has resulted in elevated levels of specialisation. Babiker et al. (2014) maintain that this meant it was not possible for any one professional to have the knowledge and skills to respond appropriately, particularly where the complex needs of communities or individuals are required.

- What do you think are the key strengths of interprofessional working?

One of the key strengths of interprofessional working is that the combined expertise of a range of health professionals is used to deliver seamless, comprehensive care to individuals. The World Health Organization (2010) suggests that interprofessional collaboration is an essential component of satisfactory service delivery. Mayo and Woolley (2016) argue that the quality of service received is dependent on how effectively different professions work together. This is supported by Jovanović et al. (2020) who believe that the modernisation of healthcare delivery has initiated a move towards the collaborative delivery of care and that effective teamwork links to more positive care outcomes. The UK healthcare provision has changed radically and rapidly in the last decade, and this is reflected in political and policy decisions at all levels; regionally, nationally, and internationally (Department of Health, 2021). Due to the unprecedented pressures faced, the NHS has had to adapt and evolve their systems to meet these new challenges. As a result, we have seen collaboration in health and social care increase at an unimaginable scale and pace (Department of Health, 2021).

Activity 4.1

What recent changes are you aware of that have impacted on the delivery of health and social care services? Make a list of these.

Now access one of the following websites below and identify the relevant government health policy documents that highlight the changing context in which healthcare is delivered in your area:

England: www.gov.uk/government/organisations/department-of-health
Scotland: www.scotland.gov.uk
Northern Ireland: www.dhsspsni.gov.uk
Wales: www.wales.gov.uk

In England, several documents highlight the changing context in which healthcare is delivered. These include the *Health and Social Care Act* (DH, 2012) (see www.legislation.gov.uk/ukpga/2012/7/contents/enacted), *Willis Commission Report* (2012), *The Care Act* (2014) (see www.legislation.gov.uk/ukpga/2014/23/contents/enacted), the *Health and Social Care (safety and quality) Act* (DH, 2015), *The Berwick Report* (DH, 2013), *The NHS Long Term Plan* (DH, 2019), *Build Back Better: Our Plan for Health and Social Care* (DH, 2022a) and *Coronavirus: Lessons Learned to Date* (DH, 2022b). These documents emphasise the increasingly busy environment in which care delivery takes place; the constantly changing staff population; the growing use of technology; the increasing acuity of recipients of care; an ageing population and the move to more community-based services with limited resource availability. It is expected that these changes will continue and there is now, more than ever, a realisation of the importance of holistic person-centred care and a wider recognition that true collaborative working requires all team members to work closely together (Wei et al., 2020). Morley and Cashell (2017) also maintain that the active contribution of recipients of care to the decision-making process will make working together truly collaborative with UK governments promoting the principle of working in partnership. There are some excellent examples where health and social care teams have been able to work effectively and collaboratively together. For example, *'Discharge to Assess'*, a new integrated person-centred approach model, was introduced to ensure the safe and timely discharge of individuals from an acute setting to a community setting, whilst acknowledging the need for assessment of health *and* social care needs (GMCA, 2017). Other examples include health and social care professionals working together in intermediate care settings addressing the complex needs of those receiving care by combining expertise, perspectives, and resources; forming a common goal to restore, maintain and improve care outcomes.

Reflect on the teams you have previously worked within.

- Has your experience been a positive or a negative one?
- Why do you think this might be?

Over the last decade considerable progress has been made towards creating environments where interprofessional working can thrive and be a positive experience, but in some practice areas this is not so easy to achieve and has been implemented on less than robust evidence (Lalani et al., 2020). There have been numerous examples where difficult interprofessional working has been reported. Rawlinson et al. (2021) suggest that this is because some professionals are not convinced of the benefits for those receiving care; some care providers perceive it as a loss of continuous and holistic care, a loss of professional identity or of their own jobs' attributes.

You may recall in Chapter 1 we highlighted that until late in the twentieth century, some groups predominantly male occupations (e.g., medicine), were identified as professions with distinct characteristics of completing a course of education to at least graduate level, having autonomy and self-regulation, and remaining free from managerial control. Alternatively, other predominantly female occupations (e.g., nursing and midwifery) were seen as semi-professions, who in contrast received 'training' and were regulated and overseen by other occupational groups (Traynor, 2013). However, today, nursing is seen as a profession with qualified nurses (and other professionals) having the autonomy and authority to work independently (The King's Fund, 2020).

Healthcare Provision in A Prison Setting

A large prison sends individuals with medical problems for scans to the local hospital. Only one person at a time can attend for security reasons and must be accompanied by a member of prison staff at a cost of £250 a visit. Therefore, waiting times for these individuals are significant. There are also further problems in that those in need of a scan must be handcuffed, resulting in a high failure rate for scans (for security reasons the individual receiving care is not told in advance the day or time of the scan). This often means that they are not prepared properly, for example having eaten when they should not have done so. In response to the issues identified above, the prison service and local Clinical Commissioning Group (CCG) developed a more collaborative approach to meet healthcare needs. The local CCG commissioned a GP-led ultrasound team who visit the prison once a week, working with and alongside the prison healthcare team, scanning seven or eight individuals at any one time. This has the potential to save money, improve efficiency and provide dignity for those receiving care.

The above scenario provides a good example of how money can be saved in the NHS. However, it is not just about saving money, but also utilising precious resources more efficiently and effectively, to achieve a better standard of care for individuals and their families. This may require greater involvement and collaboration between the private sector and charities, as well as healthcare providers. The public have also become much more knowledgeable through the increase in technology and education, making knowledge more accessible. However, sometimes that knowledge is incorrect or limited and does not provide the full picture. It can then be much more challenging to negotiate and compromise with members of the public. This has influenced policy, creating turbulence where policy is formulated to achieve political goals, address systemic failings, and produce rapid-fire responses to public disillusionment (Buzelli et al., 2022). Healthcare professionals working within these environments are often left to make sense of new ways of working and demands, i.e., what they do and how they should go about it.

List the reasons why people may lose faith in the NHS.

- What effect do you think this might have on the healthcare professionals working within this service?

Across the UK poor interprofessional collaboration has been identified as a contributing factor in numerous high-profile cases with poor outcomes, for example, Mid Staffordshire NHS Foundation Trust (2013), Morecambe Bay (Kirkup, 2015), Liverpool Community Trust (Kirkup, 2018) and Shrewsbury and Telford NHS Foundation Trust (Ockenden Report, 2020). Following such criticisms, people lose faith in the NHS because they are concerned with carelessness in services, long waits, and poor communication. For health professionals this can cause disillusionment within the profession and lower morale. There are assumptions that interprofessional working will prevent such tragedies as well as poor practice; however, as yet there is no real research or evidence to support this assumption. This is due to the complex nature of the research, the funding available and the collaboration needed across practice and higher education institutions (HEIs) (Hammond and Morgan, 2022).

- There are some advantages to interprofessional working. What do you think these are?

The advantages to interprofessional working include:

- Enhancing personal and professional confidence;
- Promoting mutual understanding of all professionals and their roles;
- Promoting interprofessional communication and breaking down barriers to communication;
- Recognising and respecting each professional role and their contribution to care provision;
- Contributing to job satisfaction: working together in harmony makes working life much better;
- Sharing information and knowledge to provide improved decision making about person-centred care;
- Problem sharing: as the adage goes 'a problem shared is a problem halved.' Just talking through care delivery issues with another professional colleague can sometimes help to provide the solution to a problem.

Sanjit

Sanjit was admitted to hospital after a stroke resulting in left-hand side weakness and speech difficulties. Once medically stable, Sanjit was transferred to a Discharge Assessment Unit for further multidisciplinary assessment, prior to discharge home. The multidisciplinary team which included an occupational therapist, physiotherapist, and members of the nursing team worked closely with the community specialist teams (e.g., moving and handling team, speech and language therapy and social workers), to ensure a smooth discharge home with a full package of care. However, the physiotherapist was concerned that Sanjit's family would not be able to manage. Therefore, a joint home assessment was also carried out with all staff involved, to ensure the appropriate equipment was in place. Family members living at home were trained to use the equipment as required.

Referring to the above scenario:

- What do you think went well?
- What could have been improved and how?

This scenario displays good interprofessional working, although this could have been improved further by including Sanjit and his family in the discussions. Service users and carers can offer a unique perspective on how a particular illness or disease affects them or their loved ones. It is therefore essential that interprofessional teams ensure that those receiving care and their carers, are fully consulted, involved in decision-making processes about care provision and that their contribution to care planning, implementation and evaluation is meaningful.

Over the last decade healthcare policy in the UK and Scotland has been centred on empowerment, with service users/carers being at the centre of decisions made around their care (DoH, 2019). One example is that of individuals with dementia who come into hospital with their own passport of care. In this case, the multidisciplinary team members who have been working with the person with dementia clearly identify what they have been doing and what works or does not work for that person. The individual receiving care and their important others are also able to input their thoughts, feelings and needs. This then allows staff to work towards getting the individual home in optimal health.

Team Working

Working in health and social care settings usually involves some aspect of team working. Effective teamwork does not just happen when a team of people work together – in fact, teamwork could be poor in a group of people working together or could be effective. The Royal College of Physicians (2017: 3) define teamwork as:

> 'a small number of people with complementary skills who are committed to a common purpose, performance goals and approach for which they hold each other mutually accountable'.

James (2021) agrees, though he advises that teamwork also requires more than just communication and mutual goals. He states that effective teamwork requires a collaborative mindset and a recognition of the value of the team model and a commitment to building effective relationships.

Within health and social care settings, teamwork is vital in delivering high-quality care. The best outcomes are achieved when professionals work and learn together as well as engaging in audits and generating innovative ways of moving the practice and service forward.

Consider your current or recentplacement and the teams you have worked in:

- Did the teams work well together or not?
- Why do you think this was the case?
- Try to identify all the potential barriers to effective team working. How do you think these might be overcome?

There are some key factors required to encourage teamwork (Babiker et al., 2014) including the following:

- *Personal commitment*: this comes from individuals who are committed to the success of the team and requires that the leader of the team allows members to ask questions. In teams where this occurs, all members will have an idea about what best practice is and are not expected to go beyond their level of competence unsupported. An individual's weaknesses are minimised and their strengths maximised, thereby releasing their true potential.
- *A common goal or vision*: all teams need to develop a common goal or vision. When teams are working towards a common goal they are committed and this inspires team members to learn and gain confidence. In fact, within a healthcare team there may need to be two visions – one for the team and one for the organisation.
- *Clarity of roles*: team members need to be clear about their various roles within a team because this will maintain their motivation. It is also important that they are clear about the roles of the other team members. In today's environment, we are increasingly working with members from different organisations and professional groups. It is thought that this understanding encourages a team approach to care needs assessment, where information and knowledge are shared to enable improved decision making about care provision (Hammond and Morgan, 2022). This will also encourage mutual trust and respect within teams.
- *Communication*: effective communication between team members is crucial for safe care provision. It encourages joint problem solving and the provision of excellent interprofessional person-centred care. The team should adopt two-way information giving rather than unidirectional pathways; thus, ensuring that information is shared with the whole team.
- *Support*: the best teams work most effectively where there is a framework to support interprofessional working, although Green and Johnson (2015) believe the degree of support can be variable.

Activity 4.2

Consult the views of current members of the team in which you are working.

• What do they think are the advantages and disadvantages of team working?

There are some clear advantages to team working in a healthcare setting (Royal College of Physicians, 2017; Rosen et al., 2018). In the activity above, your colleagues may have identified some or all of these:

• *Improvements in the quality-of-care provision*: when the team communicates effectively and works together as a unit, the quality of care increases. They have a clear commitment to excellence of care. This increases coordination, especially in complex cases.
• *Improvements in safe care provision*: if teamwork is effective the person in receipt of care can become an active partner. They are listened to, monitored and the procedures implemented are based on their feedback. This has the potential to reduce medication errors and unnecessary procedures, thereby creating a safer care environment.
• *Improvements in staff satisfaction*: teams that work efficiently and effectively brainstorm and problem solve together. The workload tends to be distributed more evenly and stress is reduced.
• *Improvements in communication*: because the team members regularly interact with each other they can contribute to the decision making in the team, thus making their shared goals and visions achievable.
• *Improved knowledge of each person's role*: a team working well together will learn about each person's role and limitations. This strengthens relationships and builds unity in the team.
• *Enhanced reflection*: efficient and effective teams regularly reflect on how they work together and how effective they are being.
• *More innovative approach to work*: a team that works well together can potentially be more innovative in their outlook. There is verbal and practical support for innovative ideas, thus moving the team forward.
• *Improved problem solving*: an effective team bounces ideas off each other. Each person offers their unique perspective on a problem and produces the best solution.
• *Enhanced skills*: no one person is the same as another and so teams need to use each person's unique skills to improve one another and be more productive in the future.

Disadvantages of team working

As you can see, there are many advantages to team working that are often talked about, but there are some disadvantages here too (Sims et al., 2014; Wei et al., 2020) including the following:

- *Unequal participation*: sometimes some members of the team will sit back and let others do most of the work. This can have an adverse effect by causing resentment, which can then cause conflict and affect morale.
- *Members who are not team players*: some people do not function well as part of a team and prefer to work alone. They can be excellent workers in the right situation but have difficulty fitting into a team, thus causing dissatisfaction and disharmony.
- *A lack of constructive conflict*: once a team works well together members may become reluctant to argue or dispute a point. If all conflict is avoided resentment can build up and team members can become lazy and apathetic, thus stifling creativity.
- *Traditions and professional cultures*: for some this can cause split loyalties between the team and their own discipline. Some team members may be reluctant to accept suggestions from other professions and become very defensive, particularly if they are used to assuming sole responsibility.
- *Personality clashes*: not all people can get on all the time and personality clashes can occur. These can then cause unwanted conflict in a team and even split the team.

You will no doubt have come across some of the barriers identified above in some of your practice learning environments. How do you think these could be overcome? Before reading on, note down your ideas.

Barriers to effective team working

While acknowledging that there are some real advantages to interprofessional working, we must also admit that there are some real barriers. Rawlinson et al. (2021) maintain that not acknowledging barriers to interprofessional working is a cause of failure and therefore advise that it is crucial to recognise all the obstacles encountered. Some of the common barriers to interprofessional working might include the following:

- Suspicion of the motives behind collaboration e.g., is it about improving care or is there a different agenda?
- A lack of confidence in one's own professional knowledge base for fear of being wrong, e.g., a newly qualified nurse might not challenge a more senior practitioner because of fears they may be wrong and do not want to appear as if they are not sure what they are talking about.
- Traditional professional cultures, e.g., joint working is difficult where there are perceived status differences between occupational groups. Some practitioners view this as a threat to their professional status, autonomy and control when asked to participate in more democratic decision making.

- Mistrust of other professions due to a lack of knowledge leading to stereotyping.
- Lack of training and preparation to work in teams.
- Lack of shared values, visions, and principles.
- Lack of investment on an individual, professional, and organisational level.

Overcoming the barriers

Barriers can be overcome with time and patience and by undertaking the following:

- *Choosing the right members of the team*: although this is not always possible in a healthcare setting, as far as it is practicable this should be done. Some team players may have to move to another area if they cannot work collaboratively in the team.
- *Team building*: allow time for team members to get to know each other and each person's role and unique contribution to the team. This allows team members to develop respect for each other.
- *Developing an atmosphere of trust and respect in the team members*: this takes time and effort, and actions speak louder than words.
- *Ensuring clarity of team goals*: members of the team need to understand the team's common goal and vision. These should include specific and measurable outcomes.
- *Encouraging a supportive environment*: make sure that all members are aware how their action or inaction might impact on those in their care and other team members.
- *Encouraging debate and constructive challenges*: this can help the team to keep improving and producing their own ideas. Mechanisms need to be developed to review goals and roles over time.

Practice Learning Models

Over recent years, a range of models have developed to help meet the need for increased learning opportunities within practice settings, whilst maintaining the required quality of educational support (NHS Employers, 2022a). These new models can also provide excellent opportunities to promote interprofessional learning as an important part of the overall practice learning experience. The Nursing and Midwifery Council's (NMC) *Standards for Student Supervision and Assessment* (NMC, 2019a), move away from a traditional mentoring model, to one that separates out the supervisor and assessor roles. The standards advise that students can be supervised by either an NMC registered nurse, midwife, nursing associate or any other registered health and social care professional. The NMC (2019b) therefore advise that learning experiences should also have an interdisciplinary and interprofessional learning focus, which includes learning with and from other healthcare professions where relevant. These models use a coaching approach whereby students are directly involved in hands-on care delivery and are empowered to take a greater level of responsibility for their own self-directed learning. Students from different year groups work together as a team, supported by a practice-based educator who uses a coaching approach to encourage them to explain their practice and identify their own learning needs. They are also encouraged to work alongside other healthcare students and staff to promote collaborative learning and enhance person-centred care. Collaborative learning in practice (CLiP) is the most commonly used coaching model (NHS Employers, 2022b). This model encourages a 'whole team approach' to learning, giving students more exposure to a range of different clinical areas and professionals, providing them with a much more realistic view of care delivery and pathways (NHS Employers, 2022b).

Activity 4.3

- What different practice learning models have you experienced?
- How might these models help you to develop your team-working skills?

Skills that could be achieved by applying a coaching model include:

- *Gaining a greater understanding of other professional roles;*
- *Developing effective collaborative working skills to enhance care;*
- *Development of practice assessment skills;*
- *Development of negotiation and delegation skills;*
- *Development of reflection skills;*
- *Development of leadership and management skills.*

Reflect on the above list of skills with your practice supervisors and assessors. Do you feel your practice learning experiences have helped you to develop any of these skills? What else would help you to develop these skills further?

Team integration

Wherever you are working, it is essential that you try to integrate into the team as soon as possible. There are many challenges and opportunities in healthcare today. You will need to plan and identify your learning needs before you enter the practice learning environment and, once there, it is a good idea to let your assessor/practice supervisor know what these are.

As a student (or even as a newly qualified nurse moving into another area of practice), consider how you might integrate into a new team.

- Who will be the members of the team?
- What could you do to enhance your integration into the team?

Here are some suggestions:

1   Do a little detective work and find out about the team you are joining before you get there. This might involve visiting the organisation's website or calling the practice learning area to ask them a little about themselves. If possible you are near try to arrange to pop in for a short visit. This can often make a good first impression, although consideration should always be given to the demands on staff, particularly in a busy environment.
2   Once you are in a practice learning setting, find out who the key members of the multi-professional team are and arrange to spend time with them, in collaboration with your assessor or practice supervisor. Identifying key members of the team can help you identify relevant learning opportunities.
3   Be proactive rather than reactive and try to take responsibility for your own learning needs where appropriate, rather than always waiting to be directed by your supervisor. This will help make a good impression and may also help you to meet your own personal learning needs.
4   Know what you want to learn about the specialism and the team before you meet with your practice supervisor/assessor. So long as this plan meets your specified learning outcomes, the team should help you achieve these.
5   Demonstrate a willingness to work as part of the team in all aspects of care planning and delivery.
6   Ask questions. Learn as much as you can about all the professionals working to provide holistic person-centred care. Do not be afraid to ask any member of the team what they contribute to the overall package of care (no question is a silly question!).

The Importance of Record Keeping and Teamwork

There is no denying that record keeping is crucial in healthcare and each member of a team has personal responsibility and accountability for good record keeping, including students (NMC, 2018b).

Record keeping is one of the most basic clinical tools that we can use to ensure that individuals receive the best possible care. This helps us communicate with each other and is essential for ensuring that an individual's assessed needs are met in a timely and efficient manner.

The principles of good record keeping apply to all types of records (e.g., electronic, hand-held, or written), with the electronic record becoming more popular. The essential ability for healthcare professionals to be able to communicate effectively also demands that systems are developed that will allow this collaboration. Mayo and Woolley (2016) suggest that the related technology is the easy bit. What is much harder is navigating the legal framework around data sharing. This is where clinicians need to have a satisfactory level of knowledge and understanding of local and national policies to allow them to safely share medical information without fear of legal repercussions.

- What can you do to ensure that you are involved in effective record-keeping processes?

It is important that you are involved in all aspects of record keeping. You will need to discuss with your assessor/supervisor the best ways you can do this within your placement. However, your record keeping should clearly differentiate between facts, opinion, and judgements.

The way in which record keeping is undertaken is set out by the employer and in the past each discipline within a multi-professional team would have maintained their own separate records. However, with an ever-increasing focus on improving the quality of care, one of the main components of clinical governance is the use of high-quality systems to effectively monitor care for clinical record keeping and the collection of relevant information (NHS England, 2021). This has led to many employers looking towards integrating record keeping for all disciplines. The NMC (2023) supports the use of the same documentation within agreed protocols by all members of the team providing care, because this can enhance collaborative working. The advantages of having one document for a care recipient's notes are:

- Improved communication;
- Reduction in the duplication of information;
- Reduction in the recording of irrelevant data;
- Maintaining the continuity of a person's care journey;
- Encouraging deeper discussion about an individual and their care.

Electronic record keeping has now become more prevalent, as national programmes for the use of information, communication technology and electronic record keeping are introduced throughout the UK. Electronic records that are complete, integrated, and legible offer added value because they can be accessed from multiple sites and used to generate risk alerts and prompts, indicating that added information is available (Pullen and Loudon, 2006). This approach can sometimes cause issues for learners in the practice area because they need to be able to obtain a password to access the systems. However, paper records are not yet obsolete and the principles of good record keeping must be adhered to regardless of how records are held.

Confidentiality

Confidentiality is as crucial in record keeping as it is in all aspects of healthcare and is identified in Article 8 of the European Convention on Human Rights (European Court of Human

Rights, 1990). It is not acceptable for any member of staff to discuss an individual or their care outside the clinical setting (e.g., in public where they could be overheard or on social media), or to leave records unattended where they could be seen. People need to be assured and have confidence in all staff that their data is protected. All of this is covered by the Data Protection Act 2018 (see www.gov.uk/data-protection) which governs the processing of information that can identify individuals. This is covered by legislation from common law and statute law. Common law refers to decisions made by a court of law; statute law is passed in parliament. Under these laws every individual can expect that any information given to a healthcare practitioner (including students) will be used only for the purpose given. It also encompasses a person's right to control access to their health information. Therefore, if a relative were to ask for information on an individual, that person would have to be consulted. In fact, confidentiality requirements also continue after the death of a person.

Consider how a person's confidentiality can be breached.

- How might this occur?
- What would you do if you suspected that there had been a breach in confidentiality?

If you believe there has been a breach of confidentiality you must raise your concerns with someone in authority. A risk or breach of confidentiality may be a result of individual behaviour or organisational systems or procedures. *The Code* (NMC, 2018b: 14) is clear on this and states: *'Act without delay if you believe that there is a risk to patient safety or public protection'*. We all have a professional duty to take action to ensure that the people in our care are protected and failing to take such action could amount to professional misconduct. There are, however, certain circumstances where records can be disclosed.

Disclosure

In all circumstances, if possible, individuals should be consulted and access to their records given with consent. They need to know why and with whom the information is being shared and give their consent freely. The only time that information about a person can be shared without consent is if it is in the 'public interest.' This includes the detection and prevention of serious crime and to prevent abuse or serious harm to others. As healthcare professionals we need to be aware that disclosures of this nature must be justified to the courts and the NMC, so clear and accurate decision trails and documentation, need to be kept. Contrary to widely held belief, the police do not have an automatic right to access an individual's health records and must obtain a warrant to do so. However, if a person is at risk of serious harm, then it is acceptable but must be discussed with your management team and/or your union or NMC and the individual's consent should also be sought.

Record keeping in healthcare is a potential minefield. Therefore, you need to ensure that you abide by *The Code* (NMC, 2018b) and the local policies of the organisation within which you are working.

Interprofessional Education

The high-profile cases already mentioned previously highlight the need not only to move towards collaborative team working, but also to review professional education and training in the UK, with a view to making this interprofessional, as well as driving the interprofessional agenda within health and social care organisations (Van Diggele et al., 2020).

At this point it is judicious to define and explore the concept of interprofessional education further. The World Health Organization (WHO) Framework for Action on Interprofessional Education and Collaborative Practice (2010: 13) defines interprofessional education (IPE) as 'when two or more individuals from different professions within health and social care engage in learning from and about each other to enable effective collaboration and improve health outcomes'. In the past, nurses, doctors, and allied health professionals (AHPs) were educated separately with no real opportunities for learning together. Therefore, cohesive team working in everyday practice did not always occur. However, as a profession we are now much more forward-thinking and across healthcare settings there is an increasing reliance on teams from a variety of specialties (e.g., nursing, physician specialties, physical therapy, social work) to provide care (Mayo and Woolley, 2016). Therefore, the necessity for a more cohesive cross-professions approach to education is becoming more prevalent (Hammond and Morgan, 2022).

The context of healthcare policy and the nature of healthcare itself, have both had a major influence on educational developments in relation to interprofessional teaching and learning. The WHO began to promote IPE and, following their lead, some countries developed organisations that were dedicated to IPE. At the forefront in the UK is the Centre for the Advancement of Interprofessional Education (CAIPE, 2007). Numerous other drivers include relevant professional bodies: the Nursing and Midwifery Council (NMC, 2018a; 2018b; 2018c; 2018d), the Health Professionals Council (HPC, 2017) and the General Medical Council (GMC, 2015). This has resulted in IPE beginning to be provided globally by universities as part of a student's prequalification for graduate practice (Mishoe et al., 2018).

IPE should take place as early as possible within professional development programmes, to help break down the artificial walls that separate professional groups, reinforcing silo working (Lairamore et al., 2018; Berger-Estililita et al., 2020). It is recommended that interprofessional curricula be implemented where students from all disciplines can meet and collaborate before they enter practice settings, so that they can build the basic values of working in interprofessional teams. The WHO (1988) argues that if healthcare professionals are taught together and learn to collaborate throughout their student years, there is much more chance that they will work together in their professional lives. Khullar (2015) advocates that this will ensure practitioners are equipped with effective team-working skills to enhance care delivery. This is supported by Herrman et al. (2015), who believe that the face-to-face interaction of different professionals should help to prevent stereotyping and inform and challenge outdated beliefs. Although this is the ideal, it is not always possible in practice and can prove difficult to achieve logistically.

Role-emerging placements

'Role-emerging placements' are currently being used by some allied health profession programmes to support practice learning provision. For example, the College of Occupational Therapists (RCOT, 2006) describes 'role-emerging placements' occurring at a site where there is no current occupational role established. Learners are supported by 'on-site' supervisors. They are also supported and assessed by a 'long-arm' educator who is a qualified Occupational Therapist (OT), who may be working in a different local organisation. The OT long-arm educator meets regularly with the learner (either face-to-face or online) to support and guide their practice. They also liaise closely with the on-site supervisors to assess the learner's progress during the learning process.

A Role-emerging Placement

A small charity drop-in centre acts as a role-emerging learning environment for occupational therapy (OT) students. Two members of staff at the charity are registered nurses who have extensive experience of supporting learning in a practice setting and are allocated to the role of 'on-site' supervisors. The drop-in centre provides crucial support for vulnerable adults within a deprived area and includes the following services: a foodbank, signposting service, mental health support, access to computers, other weekly activities to support people's mental health and wellbeing (e.g., 'knit and natter,' craft sessions and a wellbeing group). The charity works in close partnership with the local council, housing services and other local mental health support organisations. This learning environment provides an excellent opportunity for interprofessional and interagency working. At the end of the experience, learners realise that one individual discipline does not necessarily have the means and resources to meet the complex needs of individuals and their families. Working at the charity provides an excellent experience and example of the importance of reaching out and linking in with other services and professions, which is vital to ensure an all-encompassing supportive plan of care can be made to meet service user needs.

Activity 4.4

1 How do you think the example practice learning experience highlighted above could benefit other healthcare students?
2 Why is it important to work closely with other disciplines or agencies to meet the needs of individuals and their families?
3 What local charities and services are you aware of which it might be useful to work collaboratively with to help meet the needs of those in your care?

Reflecting upon your current and any previous practice learning environments, identify all the potential/actual opportunities available to you for interprofessional learning:

1 Have these been arranged by your employment organisation or your educational provider?
2 Is there potential for you to be able to arrange individualised/bespoke/informal IPE for yourself (i.e., bespoke experience days with other professionals)?

Write down/make a list of all the potential opportunities available to you. Discuss the practicalities and possibilities of these with your practice assessor/supervisor.

You can often find creative ways for IPE to occur throughout your career so that you can continuously develop the skills you will need to work with other professions. Although IPE does take place in practice on a day-to-day basis, Rees et al. (2018) explore how learners and staff may have a different understanding of this and therefore IPE may not always be easily recognised or acknowledged by staff; if it does occur, it is usually very sporadic and ad hoc, with a lack of planning for specific experiences and a reliance on opportunistic experiences. Rudawska (2017) agrees and believes that even if staff do value the importance of IPE, they choose to prioritise profession-specific skills.

It is important here that we differentiate IPE from 'shared learning' (e.g., where professionals sit in the same lecture theatre). Recognising that some key skills all health professionals use could be taught together (e.g., communications skills such as listening, gathering information, and building a rapport with those in receipt of care) would help learners challenge discriminatory statements about other professions (Reeves et al., 2016). IPE should, however, also include the opportunity to collaborate, discuss and learn about each other with the aim being to improve care provision. The aims of IPE are to enhance the sharing of skills and knowledge across healthcare professions, which in turn allows for a better understanding of each other, sharing values and respecting each other's role. If this can be established, then the quality and safety of care provision can be optimised. We have already seen in the high-profile cases identified earlier how poor healthcare team working and communication can have a negative impact on care outcomes.

IPE can work well if all professions can work together to make this happen in both practice and academic settings (Mayo and Woolley, 2016; Hammond and Morgan, 2022).

IPE

A community occupational therapist (OT) attends an 'Interprofessional Learning (IPL) Champions' Forum' (a forum that has been developed to enable IPL champions from all disciplines to meet and learn together). Another member of the group (a podiatrist) shares information about some new drop-in sessions that they are holding in their area and is surprised that the OT was unaware of these as the information had already been distributed on flyers to all the clinics. However, the OT is based in another building that had not been included in the distribution. In addition, due to the hectic pace of NHS work, flyers and distribution information is often missed. The IPL Forum allows time for the podiatrist and OT to liaise and learn more about each other's services and remit, and the specific changes that are being implemented locally to improve care. The OT immediately starts to refer individuals to the drop-in, which leads to much more timely treatment being provided for those in their care. The podiatrist also becomes much more aware of the necessity for effective communication and the need to ensure that all appropriate colleagues are aware of any new services.

Over recent years, the need for IPE and collaborative learning has been recognised as being more important than ever (Singh and Matthews, 2021). Park (2022) agrees, advising that IPE presents a conduit, aligning professional requirements with professional strategies and workplace demands, thereby bridging the liminal space between practice and theory, though delivery can be complex. For example, online conversion of IPE can be challenging, presenting barriers to some, and widening participation to others. Look at further examples of IPE approaches below:

Case examples

1 A virtual ward is developed at one hospital to facilitate students from various disciplines to learn together. It is designed collaboratively as an innovative way of enabling different professions to work together in teams and develop their communication skills, learning about each person's role and responsibilities while caring for people.

2 A Higher Education Institution (HEI) uses simulation scenarios (SIM) to encourage learners from different professions to work together in problem solving complex care issues. This is undertaken in the SIM suite where everyone can work together in a safe environment and make mistakes without causing any harm to care recipients. It involves recreating real-life events so that learners can experience that event through use of a high-fidelity environment, thereby gaining new skills, knowledge, and attitudes. This can be extended further by scenarios being enacted in the clinical areas at random and with no prior notice.

3 An IPL forum founded in partnership with a mental health trust and the local council brings together key staff interested in education and learning where they can work towards integrated learning in practice. This involves having IPE champions at all levels in the

organisation to help promote IPE in practice. A person-centred approach is promoted, and the IPL forum advocates the importance of partnership working with all practitioners involved in care delivery.

4   An organisation has an online preceptorship programme which brings different professions together via an online platform, allowing staff to learn together and share examples of good practice during the first year of their new roles.

In some areas HEIs have yet to pursue IPE fully, due to the organisational complexities involved. In the past some have argued that there has been a lack of research as to the effectiveness of IPE, suggesting that the cost, amount of labour required, lack of support and timetabling difficulties have helped to fuel this reluctance (Van Dieggele et al., 2020). For example, even simple differences such as terms, length and different assignment requirements can often cause a problem and make it logistically difficult to achieve. However, in the UK evidence has grown for its implementation (Choudhury et al., 2020).

Health Education England (HEE) have recognised the need for extra support for learning in practice and developed the role of the practice education facilitator (PEF). This has now been extended, with a realisation that developing a sustainable growth in allied health professions' workforce is vital to delivering ambitions of the NHS long term plan (DoH, 2019). Scotland also focused on practice education in their paper The Healthcare Quality Strategy for NHS Scotland (Morrison, 2010), and have extended this by developing the Quality Standards for Practice (NHS Quality Improvement in Scotland, 2020). Wales has also developed a similar role (RCN (Royal College of Nursing) Wales, 2016). Although initially slow to develop (Wright and Lindqvist, 2008), the role has been instrumental in the practice setting for supporting and managing practice-based multi-professional learning. As the PEF role has developed and the need for IPE has become more widely recognised, the role of the PEF has now expanded to assist and support assessors/supervisors and students across all disciplines. Indeed, most healthcare organisations have embraced the notion of IPE and developed structures to support it.

It has also been recognised that, as well as the need to work interprofessionally with other healthcare professionals within one area or organisation, there is also a broad consensus about the importance of working across both acute and community settings. This includes working collaboratively with a wider range of NHS, private and voluntary organisations to meet future complex care needs. *The NHS Long Term Plan* (DoH, 2019) and *Build Back Better: Our Plan for Health and Social Care* (DoH, 2022a) continues to describe a future that will see the NHS dissolving the classic divide between GPs (General Practitioner), hospital care and health and social care. Instead, the NHS will form primary care networks which will empower those receiving care to take more control over their own treatment plans. The review also calls for a radical upgrade in prevention and public health, recognising the crucial role that healthcare students can play within this important agenda. The increasing need for all healthcare students to gain valuable public health experience, together with the new models of integrated working across both health and social care services, has led to new opportunities for increased interprofessional working experiences for pre-registration students which could also play a crucial role in their public health exposure.

IPE Case Study: Promoting Public Health

Public health experiences within practice learning environments are often ad hoc and dependent on the mindset of the practice assessors/supervisors. One organisation was keen to develop a new initiative that would strengthen, promote, and formalise the public health experience for learners, providing them with a deeper understanding of the wider issues involved when caring holistically for individuals and their families. They developed an annual 'Public Health Conference' for healthcare learners in collaboration with two local HEIs and a private healthcare organisation. The conference provided a more formalised opportunity for attendees from a range of professions to learn together about local public health services and explore their role in promoting health and signposting services to those in their care. This enabled the learners to see public health in action and helped them link theory to real-life practice.

- What opportunities do you think public health might bring in relation to IPL for healthcare learners?
- How do you think your own public health experience could be strengthened and formalised?
- When providing holistic care what do you think the wider issues might be in relation to public health?
- Do you think it is important for learners from different professions to learn together?
- What do you think the key learning might be for those attending this conference?
- How do you think this conference might improve the care provided to individuals?

IPE advantages and challenges

There are some key advantages to IPE including:

- Understanding the theoretical principles of team working and collaboration early in a student's career;
- Understanding all the roles involved in the service-user experience;
- An ability to communicate appropriately and understand the language of different healthcare professionals;
- An understanding of the professional responsibilities, values, and accountability of healthcare professionals in meeting the needs of individuals;
- Being able to work effectively in an interprofessional team;
- Understanding how different professions make decisions about care provision;
- Understanding how IPE produces better teamwork, which in turn improves care delivery;
- Removal of the fear of other professions;
- The ability to challenge professionals to ensure quality care provision.

There are also some challenges, including:

- Difficulty in mapping the curricula for different professions;
- Recognising that there needs to be a commitment from all stakeholders to effective planning of IPE;
- Recognising that time and opportunity need to be given for professions to address differences;
- Allowing for coordination and resourcing difficulties because learning in small groups is often labour-intensive and costly;
- A lack of evaluation of the IPE that has already been implemented; rigorous and robust evaluation is essential;
- A lack of preparation and support for the IPE teachers;
- A lack of student involvement in planning the IPE; Freeth et al. (2005) maintain students should be actively involved in steering their IPE.

Looking into the future of the healthcare service, Schot et al. (2020) believe that we must change the way we educate professionals and change the milieu in which they work. Silo working and training cannot continue, and the development of an integrated, interprofessional, multi-dimensional workforce is critical. For all of this to happen, teamwork is also crucial.

Chapter Summary

Interprofessional working and learning are not new concepts; however, it is obvious that they are essential to the future of healthcare and adult nursing. Indeed, the NMC (2018d) are clear that nursing students should be given opportunities and chances to learn with other professionals and as far as is possible with learners from other professions. However, for this to occur, all professions need to show a commitment to learning and working together to provide the best high-quality person-centred care. This often involves breaking down traditional boundaries and barriers and working flexibly. It also requires clear leadership and a commitment to ongoing collaborative education, all of which should help to build sustainable relationships with mutual understanding, respect and communication which occur through influencing and negotiating. This involves breaking down hierarchical structures and taking a leap of faith and commitment to work proactively for true collaboration.

The key challenges have been identified here and the commitment to work through these challenges and develop effective policies is apparent (Park, 2022). For adult nurses, teamwork is key and therefore every opportunity should be taken during your programme to join in all teamwork activities.

Further Reading

Day, J. (2013) *Interprofessional Working. An Essential Guide for Health and Social Care Professionals*. Hampshire: Cengage Learning.

Department of Health (2021) *Integration and Innovation: working together to improve health and social care for all*. Available at: www.gov.uk/government/publications/working-together-to-improve-health-and-social-care-for-all/integration-and-innovation-working-together-to-improve-health-and-social-care-for-all-html-version (last accessed 17 February 2023).

James, T. (2021) *Teamwork as a Core Value in Health Care*. Harvard Medical School. Available at: https://postgraduateeducation.hms.harvard.edu/trends-medicine/teamwork-core-value-health-care (last accessed 25 January 2023).

McLaney, E., Morassaei, S., Hughes, L., Davies, R., Campbell, M. and Di Prospero, L. (2022) 'A framework for interprofessional team collaboration in a hospital setting: advancing team competencies and behaviours', *Healthcare Management Forum*, 35(2): 112–17.

Thistlethwaite, J.E. (2012) *Values-Based Interprofessional Collaborative Practice. Working Together in Health Care*. Cambridge: Cambridge University Press.

References

Babiker, A., El Husseini, M., Nemri, A.A., Frayh, A,A., Juryyan A.N., O Faki, M., Assiri, A., Al Saadi, M., Shaikh, F. and Al Zamil, F. (2014) 'Health care professional development: working as a team to improve patient care', *Sudanese Journal of Paediatrics*, 14(2): 9–16.

Baldwin, D. (1993) *Development of Health Professionals to Maximise Health Provider Resources in Rural Areas. National Rural Health Association HRSA Contract*. Washington, DC: Bureau of Health Professions.

Berger-Estilita, J., Chiang, H., Stricker, D., Fuchs, A., Greif, R. and McAleer, S. (2020) *Attitudes of Medical Students Towards Interprofessional Education: A mixed methods study*. Available at: https://doi.org/10.1371/journal.pone.0240835 (last accessed 4 February 2023).

Buzelli, L., Cameron, G. and Gardner, T. (2022) *Public Perceptions of the NHS: and social care performance, policy, and expectations*. Available at: www.health.org.uk/publications/long-reads/public-perceptions-performance-policy-and-expectations (last accessed 30 January 2023).

Centre for the Advancement of Interprofessional Education (2007) *Creating an Interprofessional Workforce: An Education and Training Framework for Health and Social Care*. London: CAIPE (supported by the Department of Health).

Choudhury, R.I., us Salam, M.A., Mathur, J. and Choudhury, S.R. (2020) 'How interprofessional education could benefit the future of healthcare – medical students' perspective', *BMC Med Educ* 20, 242. Available at: https://doi.org/10.1186/s12909-020-02170-w (last accessed 17 February 2023).

College of Occupational Therapists (2006) *Developing the Occupational Therapy Profession: Providing new work-based learning opportunities for students*. London: COT.

Data Protection Act (2018) Data Protection Act 2018. [online] Legislation.gov.uk. Available at: www.legislation.gov.uk/ukpga/2018/12/pdfs/ukpga_20180012_en.pdf (last accessed 12 July 2022).

Department of Health (2012) *Health and Social Care Act*. London. DH. Available at: www.legislation. gov.uk/ukpga/2012/7/contents/enacted (last accessed 1 January 2023).

Department of Health (2013) *Berwick Report into Patient Safety*. London: DH.

Department of Health (2015) *Health and Social Care (Safety and Quality) Act 2015*. London: DH.

Department of Health (2019) *The NHS Long Term Plan*. London: DH. Available at: www.england. nhs.uk/long-term-plan/ (last accessed 17 February 2023).

Department of Health (2021) *Integration and Innovation: Working together to improve health and social care for all*. Available at: www.gov.uk/government/publications/working-together-to-improve-health-and-social-care-for-all/integration-and-innovation-working-together-to-improve-health-and-social-care-for-all-html-version (last accessed 17 February 2023).

Department of Health (2022a) *Build Back Better: Our Plan for Health and Social Care*. London: DH.

Department of Health (2022b) *Coronavirus: Lessons learned to date. (Sixth Report of the Health and Social Care Committee and Third Report of the Science and Technology Committee of Session 2021–22)*. London: DH.

European Court of Human Rights (1990) *Article 8 of the European Convention on Human Rights*. Available at: www.echr.coe.int/documents/convention_eng.pdf (last accessed 1 January 2023).

Freeth, D., Hammick, M., Reeves, S., Koppel, I. and Barr, H. (2005) *Effective Interprofessional Education: Development, Delivery and Evaluation*. Oxford: Blackwell.

General Medical Council (2015) *Promoting Excellence: Standards for Medical Education and Training*. Manchester: GMC.

GMCA (2017) *Discharge to Assess – Standards for Greater Manchester*. Manchester: GMCA.

Green, B.N. and Johnson, C.D. (2015) 'Interprofessional collaboration in research, education, and clinical practice: working together for a better future', *Journal of Chiropractic Education*. 29(1): 1–10. doi: 10.7899/JCE-14-36 (last accessed 27 July 2022).

Hammond, K.M. and Morgan, C.J. (2022) 'Development of interprofessional healthcare teamworking skills: mapping students' process of learning', *Journal of Interprofessional Care*, 36(4): 589–98.

Hastie, C.R., Fahy, K.M., Parratt, J.A. and Grace, S. (2016) 'Midwifery students' experience of teamwork projects involving mark-related peer feedback', *Women and Birth*, 29(3): 252–9.

Health Professionals Council (2017) *Standards in Education and Training*. London: HPC.

Herrman, G., Woermann, U. and Schelgel, C. (2015) 'Interprofessional education in anatomy: learning together in medical and nursing training', *Anatomical Sciences Education*, Jul-. Aug; 8(4): 324–30.

James, T. (2021) *Teamwork as a Core Value in Health Care*. Harvard Medical School. Available at: https://postgraduateeducation.hms.harvard.edu/trends-medicine/teamwork-core-value-health-care (last accessed 25 January 2023).

Jovanović, S., Maja Stanković, M., Kilibarda, T., Trgovčević, S. and Ivanović, S. (2020) *The terminology used to describe teamwork in the health care system: A literature review*. UDC. Available at: https://scindeks-clanci.ceon.rs/data/pdf/0365-4478/2020/0365-44782004013J.pdf (last accessed 16 February 2023).

Khullar, D. (2015) 'Doctors and nurses not learning together'. https://archive.nytimes.com/well.blogs.nytimes.com/2015/04/30/doctors-and-nurses-not-learning-together/ (last ast accessed 4 February 2023).

Kirkup, B. (2015) *The Report of the Morecambe Bay Investigation*. London: The Stationery Office, William Lea Group.

Kirkup, B. (2018) *Report of the Liverpool Community Health Independent Review*. Available at: www.england.nhs.uk/2018/02/independent-review-liverpool-community-health-nhs-trust-published/ (last accessed 1 January 2023).

Lairamore, C., Morris, D., Schichtl, R., George-Paschal, L., Martens, A., Maragakis, A., Garnica, M., Jones, B., Grantham, M. and Bruenger, A. (2018) 'Impact of team composition on student perceptions of interprofessional teamwork: a 6-year cohort study', *Journal of Interprofessional Care*, 32(2): 143–50.

Lalani, M., Bussu, S. and Marshall, M. (2020) 'Understanding integrated care at the frontline using organisational learning theory: a participatory evaluation of multi-professional teams in East London', *Social Science and Medicine*, 2020 Oct; 262:113254. doi: 10.1016/j.socscimed.2020.113254. Epub 2020 Jul 31. PMID: 32768774.

Mayo, A.T. and Woolley, A.W. (2016) 'Teamwork in health care: maximizing collective intelligence via inclusive collaboration and open communication', *AMA Journal of Ethics*, September 18(9): 933–40.

Mid Staffordshire NHS Foundation Trust (2013) *Report of the Mid Staffordshire NHS Foundation Trust Public Inquiry: Executive Summary*. London: HMSO.

Mishoe, S.C., Tufts, K.A., Blando, J.D. and Hoch, J.M. (2018) 'Health professions students' attitudes toward teamwork before and after an interprofessional education co-curricular experience', *Journal of Research in Interprofessional Practice and Education*, 8(1): 1–16.

Morley, L. and Cashell, A. (2017) 'Collaboration in healthcare', *Journal of Medical Imaging and Radiation Sciences*, 48(2): 207–16.

Morrison, C. (2010) *The Healthcare Quality Strategy for NHS Scotland*. The Scottish Government. Available at: www.gov.scot/publications/healthcare-quality-strategy-nhsscotland/ (last accessed 206th June 2023).

NHS Employers (2022a) *Expanding Placement Capacity*. NHS Employers. Available at: www.nhsemployers.org/articles/expanding-placement-capacity. (last accessed 16 February 2023).

NHS Employers (2022b) *Clinical Placement Supervision Models*. Available at: www.nhsemployers.org/articles/clinical-placement-supervision-models (last accessed 17 February 2023).

NHS England (2014) *MDT Development – Working toward an effective multidisciplinary/multiagency team*. Available at: www.england.nhs.uk/wp-content/uploads/2015/01/mdt-dev-guid-flat-fin.pdf (last accessed 17 February 2023).

NHS England (2021) *Records Management Code of Practice 2021*. Available at: https://transform.england.nhs.uk/media/documents/NHSX_Records_Management_CoP_V7.pdf (last accessed 1 February 2023).

NHS Quality Improvement in Scotland (2020) *Quality Standards for Practice Learning (QSPL)*. NHS Education for Scotland.

Nursing and Midwifery Council (2018a) *Future Nurse: Standards of Proficiency for Registered Nurses*. London: NMC.

Nursing and Midwifery Council (2018b) *The Code: Professional Practice and Behaviour Standards of Nurses and Midwives*. London: NMC.

Nursing and Midwifery Council (2018c) *Fitness to practise outcomes*: April to September 2018. London: NMC.

Nursing and Midwifery Council (2018d) *Future nurse: Standards of proficiency for registered nurses*. London: NMC

Nursing and Midwifery Council (2019a) *Part 2: Standards for Student Supervision and Assessment*. London: NMC.

NMC (2019b) *Different Learning Opportunities*. Available at: www.nmc.org.uk/supporting-information-on-standards-for-student-supervision-and-assessment/learning-environments-and-experiences/types-of-learning-experiences/different-learning-opportunities/ (last accessed 16 February 2023).

Nursing and Midwifery Council (2023) Part 1: *Standards Framework for Nursing and Midwifery Education*. London: NMC.

Ockenden, D. (2020) *Ockenden Report: The emerging findings and recommendations from the independent review of maternity services at Shrewsbury and Telford Hospital NHS Trust*. London: Department of Health.

Park, V. (2022) Moving interprofessional education to a virtual platform (comment), *British Journal of Nursing*, 10 March 2022. Available at: www.britishjournalofnursing.com/content/comment/moving-interprofessional-education-to-a-virtual-platform/ (last accessed 12 July 2022).

Pollard, K.C., Sellman, D. and Thomas, J. (2014) 'The need for interprofessional working'. In J. Thomas, K.C. Pollard, and D. Sellman (eds), *Interprofessional Working in Health and Social Care, Professional Perspectives*, 2nd edn. Basingstoke: Palgrave Macmillan, Chapter 1.

Pullen, I. and Loudon, J. (2006) 'Improving standards in clinical record keeping', *Advances in Psychiatric Treatment*, 12: 280–6.

Rawlinson, C., Carron, T., Cohidon, C., Arditi, C., Hong, Q.N., Pluye, P., Peytremann-Bridevaux I. and Gilles, I. (2021) 'An overview of reviews on interprofessional collaboration in primary care: barriers and facilitators', *International Journal of Integrated Care*, Jun, 21(2): 32. (last accessed 1 February 2023).

RCN Wales (2016) *Future of Nurse Education in Wales: Education Strategy*, RCN Wales leadership summit, Cardiff.

Rees, C.E., Crampton, P., Kent, F., Brown, T., Hood, K., Leech, M., Newton, J., Storr, M. and Williams, B. (2018) 'Understanding students' and clinicians' experiences of informal interprofessional workplace learning: an Australian qualitative study', *BMJ Open* 2018; 8. https://bmjopen.bmj.com/content/bmjopen/8/4/e021238.full.pdf (last accessed 5 February 2023).

Reeves, S., Fletcher, S., Barr, H., Birch, I., Boet, S., Davies, N., McFadyen, A., Rivera, J. and Kitto, S. (2016) 'A BEME systematic review of the effects of interprofessional education: *BEME Guide No. 39*', *Medical Teacher*. Jul; 38(7): 656–68. doi: 10.3109/0142159X.2016.1173663. Epub 2016 May 5. PMID: 27146438.

Rosen, M.A., DiazGranados, D., Dietz, A.S., Benishek, L.E., Thompson, D., Pronovost, P.J. and Weaver, S.J. (2018) 'Teamwork in healthcare: key discoveries enabling safer, high-quality care', *American Psychologist*, 73(4): 433–50.

Royal College of Physicians (2017) *Improving teams in healthcare Resource 1. Building effective teams*. Available at: www.rcplondon.ac.uk/projects/outputs/improving-teams-healthcare-resource-1-building-effective-teams (last accessed 25 January 2023).

Rudawska, A. (2017) 'Students' team project experiences and their attitudes to teamwork', *Journal of Management and Business Administration*, 25(1): 78–97.

Schot, E., Tummers, L. and Noordegraaf, M. (2020) 'Working on working together. A systematic review on how healthcare professionals contribute to interprofessional collaboration', *Journal of Interprofessional Care*, 34(3): 332–42.

Sims, S., Hewitt, G. and Harris, R. (2014) 'Evidence of collaboration, pooling of resources, learning and role blurring in interprofessional healthcare teams: a realistic synthesis', *Journal of Interprofessional Care*, 25(1): 20–5.

Singh, J. and Matthews, B. (2021) 'Facilitating interprofessional education in an online environment during the COVID-19 pandemic: A mixed method study', *Healthcare (Basel)*. May 11; 9(5): 567. doi: 10.3390/healthcare9050567. PMID: 34065009; PMCID: PMC8151389.

The King's Fund (2020) *The King's Fund History of Nursing* (online). Available at: https://my.visme.co/view/q6jz4wre-the-king-s-fund-nursing-exhibition-2020. (last accessed 7 July 2022).

Traynor, M. (2013) *Nursing in Context. Policy, Politics, Profession*. London: Palgrave Macmillan.

Van Diggele, C., Roberts, C., Burgess, A. and Mellis, C. (2020) 'Interprofessional education: tips for design and implementation', *BMC Medical Education* 20: 455. Available at: https://doi.org/10.1186/s12909-020-02286-z (last accessed 12 July 2022).

Wei, H., Corbett, R.W., Ray, J. and Wei, T.L. (2020) 'A culture of caring: the essence of healthcare interprofessional collaboration', *Journal of Interprofessional Care*, 34(3): 324–31.

Willis Commission (2012) *Quality with Compassion: The Future of Nurse Education*. London: Royal College of Nursing.

World Health Organization (1988) *Learning Together to Work Together for Health*. Geneva: WHO.

World Health Organization (2010) *Framework for Action on Interprofessional Education and Collaborative Practice*. Geneva: WHO.

Wright, A. and Lindqvist, S. (2008) 'The development, outline, and evaluation of the second level of an interprofessional learning programme: listening to the students', *Journal of Interprofessional Care*, 22(5): 475–87.

5

DIGITAL LITERACY

Dawn Dowding and Siobhan O'Connor

Chapter objectives

- Critically evaluate the role of digital health technology to support evidence-based decision making, care quality and safety of care in professional nursing practice;
- Understand how to maintain professional values (including data and information governance, privacy, security, and professional conduct) when using digital technologies;
- Recognise the importance of digital data, including data standards, clinical coding, nursing terminologies and how data is captured and used to support nursing practice;
- Understand the role of digital technologies in communicating with people and colleagues, and monitoring and supporting people to manage their own health;
- Evaluate the use of data and digital technologies to support evidence-based decision making, care quality, and patient safety;
- Recognise how digital health technologies can be utilised in public health.

This chapter will consider the role of digital technologies in healthcare, and how their implementation and use can support professional nursing practice. It will discuss the factors you need to be aware of when using digital technology and the skills you need to practice as a nurse in a digitally enabled healthcare environment.

Related Nursing and Midwifery Council (NMC) Proficiencies for Registered Nurses

The overarching requirement of the Nursing and Midwifery Council (NMC) is that nurses play a key role in providing, leading and coordinating care that is compassionate, evidence based and person-centred. They should always act professionally, communicate effectively, delivering safe and effective nursing care. Nurses work across interdisciplinary teams, collaborating and communicating effectively with a range of colleagues (NMC, 2018a).

━━━━━━━━ **TO ACHIEVE ENTRY TO THE NMC REGISTER**

YOU MUST BE ABLE TO ━━━━━━━━━━

- Demonstrate the numeracy, literacy, digital and technological skills required to meet the needs of people in your care to ensure safe and effective nursing practice;
- Demonstrate the ability to keep complete, clear, accurate and timely records;
- Provide information in accessible ways to help people understand and make decisions about their health, life choices, illness and care;
- Effectively and responsibly use a range of digital technologies to access, input, share, and apply information and data within teams and between agencies.

(Adapted from NMC, 2018)

The use of digital technology is becoming increasingly widespread in health and social care organisations. Hence, it is vital that nurses are aware of the benefits, limitations and risks associated with using digital technology, to ensure that people receive the best available care and are not disadvantaged in any way. In England, the NHS Long Term Plan (NHS, 2019) sets out ambitions by the UK Government that by 2024 all NHS organisations should be using digital rather than paper records, and that people will be increasingly cared for and supported at home using remote monitoring and digital tools. It is assumed that digitally enabled care will improve the effectiveness and efficiency of healthcare provision as it can be used to:

- Improve person-centred care and empower people to access care at their convenience. This includes increasing an individual's involvement in their own care;
- Provide quality care through enhanced monitoring and data that can inform personalised care pathways;
- Expand the knowledge base for both nurses and the people they care for by making personal health-related information easily accessible;
- Remove the time needed to read through paper notes;
- Reduce errors and improve care safety by improved communication of information and efficient handover systems.

Before exploring the role and potential implications of the use of digital technologies in healthcare, it is useful to examine what we mean by digitally enabled nursing practice. Iyawa et al. (2016: 246) define digital health as:

> 'an improvement in the way healthcare provision is conceived and delivered by healthcare providers through the use of information and communication technologies to monitor and improve the wellbeing and health of patients (sic) and to empower patients (sic) in the management of their health and that of their families'.

Digitally enabled nursing practice refers to nurses' use of digital technologies to support nursing practice and education. There are an increasing number of different types of technology being introduced into the healthcare sector. A summary of some of the most common technologies reported in the nursing literature can be found in Table 5.1.

Table 5.1   Types of digital health technology (adapted from Booth et al., 2021)

Digital Technology	Description
Artificial intelligence (AI) / Big data	Use of statistical techniques to develop algorithms (sets of rules) to analyse large data sets (big data). Typically used to make predictions or classifications based on the data.
Assisted living devices	Sensors and devices to monitor physiological, behavioural, and environmental aspects in a person's home or other setting.
Automation technologies (e.g., robotics, drones)	Machines able to carry out a complex series of actions automatically - examples in healthcare include robots used in hospital to deliver medications/laboratory specimens.
Clinical decision support systems (CDSS)	Computerised systems that integrate evidence with characteristics of individual patients to provide guidance and support to decision making (see Chapter 8).
Electronic health records (EHRs)	A digital/electronic version of a person's paper health/medical record.
Gaming technologies	Use of gaming platforms where a user controls a virtual avatar that can interact in simulated environments.
Mobile health (mHealth)	Use of mobile communication technologies such as smartphones and tablet computers, as well as wearable devices such as smart watches.
Telehealth/telemedicine	Healthcare services delivered remotely through a variety of communication technologies.
Personalised/precision health	Use of information obtained from a variety of sources that can be used to tailor interventions to an individual's unique characteristics and behaviours.
Social media and online information (Internet)	Digital technology that enables the instant generation and sharing of information through virtual communities and networks.
Virtual and augmented reality	Augmented reality technologies combine elements from a digital world with real world components. Virtual reality is a computer-generated simulation of the real world.

Professional values and the use of digital technology

The widespread use of digital technologies, such as smartphones, and the increasing inter-activity of communities using social media means there can be a blurring between per-sonal and professional lives. For example, posting unprofessional material online, such as negative remarks about a person you are caring (or have cared) for, peers, or your work environment, that includes profanity, prejudicial language or breaching a per-son's privacy could all lead to being dismissed from your nursing programme (Booth, 2015; Westrick, 2016; De Gagne et al., 2019). It is important that you remember what your responsibilities are as a member of the nursing profession (as discussed in Chapter 1). This includes being aware of how you behave and share information in the virtual world, as the NMC *Code* (NMC, 2018b) applies equally to your online presence as your 'real-world' behaviours.

Activity 5.1

Read the NMC guidance on using social media responsibly (social-media-guidance.pdf nmc.org.uk)
　　Make a note of all the actions you may need to take to make sure you act responsibly online.

The obligation to be digitally professional also extends to how you access, use and share infor-mation. The use of electronic health records (EHR) is becoming more common across health and social care organisations. Whilst the use of digital technologies means that it is often much easier to share information with others than if you have a paper record, it does not mean that you should do so. The principles you adhere to for confidentiality and security of information apply in a digital environment as well as a paper-based one. There are laws surrounding how you manage and use information or data, based on the European Union General Data Protec-tion Regulation (GDPR) (https://gdpr.eu/) and the UK Data Protection Act 2018 (www.gov.uk/data-protection). This sets out the legal framework around which you both manage and share information with others who are involved in a person's care. There are some basic principles that you should adhere to, which are identified in the legislation as follows:
　　Information should be:

- Used fairly, lawfully, and transparently;
- Used for explicit purposes;
- Used in a way that is adequate, relevant, and limited to only what is necessary;
- Accurate and where necessary kept up to date;
- Kept for no longer than is necessary;
- Handled in a way that ensures appropriate security, including protection against unlawful or unauthorised processing, loss, destruction, or damage.

So, what does this mean for you as a student and as a registrant? First, in a digital world you should not be sharing logins or passwords with others, as this means that any information recorded in a digital record is not accurately linked to the individual providing the care. You should have your own separate login and password to any digital system you are being asked to use in practice settings. This is important for digital security; you need to make sure that everyone who accesses a system has the appropriate clearance to do so. Also, make sure that you only ever access an individual's clinical notes with good reason and if you are uncertain if you should be sharing information with others, ask for advice. This is particularly relevant if you use a smartphone or mobile device in a practice setting, as accessing such technology while with a person in your care may seem unprofessional (Mostaghimi et al., 2017). The Royal College of Nursing (2016) has a statement on the use of personal mobile devices that you may find useful.

The Role of Data in Nursing

Data is the information that we collect as nurses, often as part of clinical care. It could be related to an individual's clinical status, individual characteristics, or treatments they are receiving. Data has been defined as 'discrete entities that are described objectively without interpretation' (Ronquillo et al., 2016: E2). To turn data into something useful for care it needs to be interpreted, organised or structured, and then used and applied to particular care situations. This transition of data into something that can be used for practice (wisdom) has been identified as the Data, Information, Knowledge, Wisdom framework (Ronquillo et al., 2016). Digital technologies (which are only one source of information we need in nursing) can collect data, but it is through the interaction with the users of that data (e.g., nurses and other healthcare professionals) that it is transformed into knowledge used to inform clinical decision making and care (see Chapter 8) and (Figure 5.1).

The way we collect and use data in nursing is important, as it is used to help organise and coordinate care, improving communication between healthcare professionals and care organisations, to support care decision making, for quality improvement/audit purposes, and to provide valuable insights and evidence for the care nurses provide.

Activity 5.2

Watch this video where Tim James discusses digital innovations and his use of data in clinical practice: www.youtube.com/watch?v=yzx34K2mYrE

What do you think the benefits are of using data and digital in nursing practice?

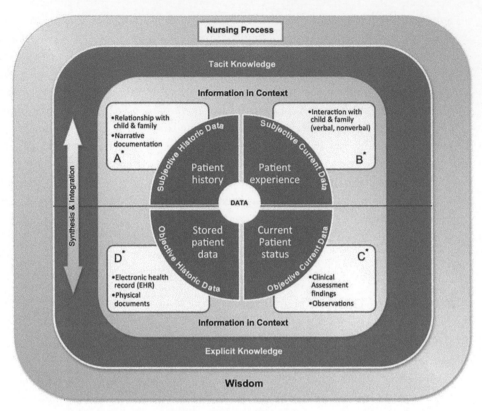

Figure 5.1   The Data Information Knowledge Wisdom framework applied to nursing

Nursing languages and terminology

To ensure that data is collected in the same way across organisations, we have a set of data standards. In the UK, we have an independent organisation, the Professional Record Standards Body (PRSB) (https://theprsb.org/), which produces standards for how care is recorded or documented in a care record. This is built on a system of codes, which are ways of classifying and categorising elements of an individual's care and treatment. These codes are often used to calculate the cost of a person's care but may also be used to provide details on the quality of care provided and feed into national datasets about care provision.

There are several ways of coding information or data, often known as 'ontologies' or terminologies. Standardised nursing terminologies or languages are a way of systematically grouping and defining terms used when nurses assess, manage and care for people, including definitions that represent that knowledge. There is no one standardised terminology in nursing due to the complexities of nursing practice, such as the variety of settings nurses work in and the diversity of care groups and problems that people may have which require many distinct types of care. However, most terminologies group nursing activity according to nursing assessments (diagnoses), evidence-based interventions, and outcomes. Using nursing terminologies to code and classify what nurses do means it is possible to explore and identify the evidence base for nursing practice, as well as enhancing the ability to share information between organisations (Schwirian, 2013).

Table 5.2 provides an overview of different nursing terminology systems, some of which have been developed specifically for distinct types of care settings (e.g., the Omaha system was developed for community nursing) (Fennelly et al., 2021). The majority have been developed in the USA, with the exception being the International Classification for Nursing Practice (ICNP). Some of the terminologies are linked (mapped) to standardised medical terms and clinical codes used in EHR systems (often known as reference systems). In the UK, clinical coding is mapped to a reference terminology known as SNOMED.

Table 5.2 Summary of common nursing terminologies (adapted from Schwirian, 2013)

Terminology	Details
Clinical Care Classification (CCC)	Research-based terminology designed to be computerised and applicable to all care settings. Includes nursing diagnoses, interventions, and outcomes.
Omaha System	Research-based terminology originating in community and home care and designed to be computerised. Has evolved to be applicable in a variety of nursing care settings. Has an assessment, intervention, and outcomes component.
Nursing Intervention Classification (NIC)	Research-based standardised classification of interventions performed by nurses. Includes 554 interventions grouped into 30 classes and 7 domains. Continually updated and mapped to SNOMED.
Nursing Outcomes Classification (NOC)	Outcomes of care that are responsive to nursing interventions. Developed for all settings and patient populations. Includes 490 outcomes grouped into 32 classes and 7 domains. Mapped to SNOMED.
NANDA International (Nursing Diagnoses, Definitions and Classification)	Classification of nursing judgements (diagnoses) made by nurses providing care. Diagnoses used as the basis for selecting appropriate interventions and outcomes.
International Classification for Nursing Practice (ICNP)	Standardised vocabulary and classification of nursing phenomena, interventions and outcomes for both paper and electronic records. Is mapped to SNOMED.

If you use a digital system such as an EHR to record an individual's care, and you are asked to complete a series of assessments or identify care interventions you have provided (often using a tick box), you are providing data that is probably linked to a nursing terminology or language in the digital system. This type of data is called 'structured' data, and when it is collected and classi-fied in this way, it means it can easily be identified, retrieved, and used again for other purposes. For example, if you record that a person has a stage 2 pressure injury in an electronic record, this information can be used to identify the appropriate care they need, can be communicated easily to other individuals (as you can find it easily), as well as being used by your care organisa-tion to monitor the quality of care being delivered. It is for this reason that it is important to understand how and why data is recorded in a particular way in digital systems, which may be different to the way you might record it in a paper record.

Data quality

Data quality is an important aspect of digital technology to make sure information is robust and safe to use in decision making. Data quality has several key dimensions including: 1) accuracy, 2) completeness, 3) uniqueness, 4) consistency, 5) timeliness, and 6) validity (Figure 5.2).

All these aspects of data quality are important in nursing, both in paper and digital records. Digital technologies such as EHRs (electronic health records) can improve aspects of data quality by replacing hand-written paper records with digital information that is legible and easier to understand (Weiskopf and Weng, 2013). However, data can still be of inferior quality even if it is in an EHR (e.g., the information may have been entered incorrectly into the record). It is also important to remember that data quality can diminish over time as the lives of those we care for change and historical data (clinical and administrative) that we hold about them may no longer be accurate. Therefore, it is important as a nurse to apply clinical judgement when using digital information to inform decision making and care.

Digital Technology and Nursing Care

There are a range of digital technologies used by nurses across all areas of health and social care to support their practice.

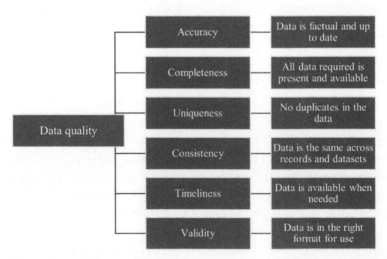

Figure 5.2   Dimensions of data quality

Clinical decision support

As discussed in Chapter 8, clinical decision support systems (CDSS) are used as a way of helping clinicians with different elements of their judgement and decision making in clinical practice settings. Whilst decision support tools can be paper based, they are increasingly being inte-grated into digital technology systems. There are several types of decision support systems, all of which are designed to target different elements or parts of a decision process and/or help clinicians prevent common decision errors (due to the use of heuristics in decision making for example – see Chapter 8). In general, computerised CDSS can be categorised into two main types of approaches to using data/information collected from digital systems and transform this into knowledge and guidance for decision making (Figure 5.3). Knowledge-based CDSS uses rules (known as IF-THEN statements) to link different bits of information/data to produce an action or outcome. The rules used to direct the decision support could come from research evidence, expert consensus, or the person receiving care (Sutton et al., 2020). Non-knowledge-based CDSS are built on analytical approaches such as artificial intelligence or machine learning, where sta-tistical models take clinical data, and look for patterns across those in receipt of care to produce predictions or insights into the likely outcome or correct action to take in a specific situation (O'Connor et al., 2022).

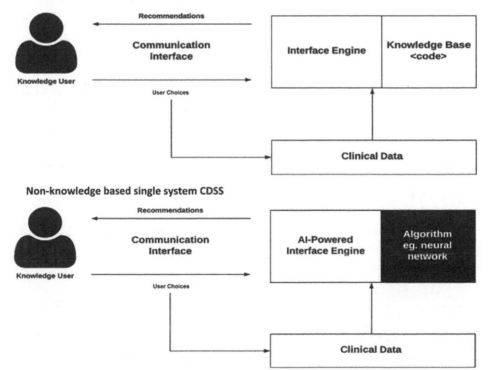

Figure 5.3 Knowledge-based, and non-knowledge-based CDSS (Sutton et al., 2020)

Both knowledge-based and non-knowledge-based CDSS use data stored digitally (often from EHR systems) to inform the decision guidance that they give to clinicians.

There are several examples of computerised CDSS that have been developed in nursing. A systematic review of computerised CDSS that has been developed and evaluated in the nursing, midwifery and allied health professions identified 35 studies (Mebrahtu et al., 2021). CDSS has been developed for a range of several types of clinical area and decisions, including triage prioritisation, pain assessment and management, supporting glycaemic control in intensive care settings, the management of cancer symptoms, risk assessment, falls and pressure injury prevention, and oral anticoagulant control (Mebrahtu et al., 2021). The review suggests that using CDSS can improve care processes (such as adherence to care guidelines) and healthcare outcomes (such as better glycaemic control).

Telehealth and telemedicine

Telehealth is a way for people to receive healthcare services remotely through various information and communication technologies, e.g., using remote monitoring of symptoms in a person's home can help identify early exacerbations of disease. This can improve clinical outcomes for individuals at home who are living with chronic conditions such as diabetes, asthma, stroke, and mental illness, among others (Snoswell et al., 2021). There are several devices that can be used at home to measure blood pressure, heart rate, weight, and other physiological signs. These devices can be connected or send data to a telehealth system which transmits these data from a person's home to clinicians in hospital, general practice, or community settings to support decision making and care delivery. This regular monitoring can help identify if someone is having problems at home and enable the clinician to provide further assessment and care if needed. Telehealth can be used in a range of settings including a person's own home, with older adults in care homes or other residential facilities, and people in prisons to facilitate the remote delivery of care (Groom et al., 2021).

Activity 5.3

Watch the Royal College of Nursing (RCN) YouTube video from Morag Hearty who is a nurse that helps to run a telehealth programme in Lanarkshire, Scotland (6:27 minutes): www.youtube.com/watch?v=GF2G8BPsKmg

What do you think are the benefits of using telehealth to support nursing care?

Telehealth is often combined with telemedicine which is remote peer-to-peer digital consultations between people and clinicians. This is sometimes referred to as a 'virtual ward' as clinicians can check in with the people they care for every day over videoconferencing technologies to see how they are managing their illness at home (Figure 5.4).

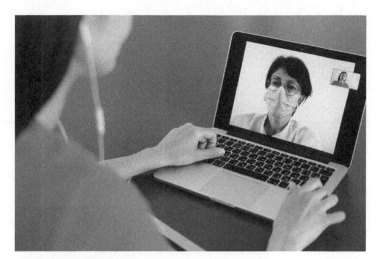

Figure 5.4   A tele-consultation between a healthcare professional and their client

Supporting and promoting health

Digital technologies can also be used to monitor health and disease, and support and promote health (see Chapter 11). For example, data (information) collected in hospital settings about people diagnosed and treated with cancer is automatically sent to a national cancer registry. Each country of the UK has its own cancer registry; in England, this organisation is called the National Cancer Registration and Analysis Service (NCRAS). The NCRAS collects electronic information on over 300,000 cases of cancer every year. This digital dataset is then analysed to understand the incidence and prevalence of cancer in England and how individuals are diagnosed and treated as well as their care outcomes. This population level digital information can then be used to plan and improve cancer care services around the country as well as facilitate clinical research to find better ways of diagnosing, treating and supporting people with cancer and their families. For example, clinical nurse specialists (CNS) can use statistics from the NRCAS to improve cancer care by providing targeted genetic counselling to individuals with a strong family history of cancer who may be at risk of developing this disease (Barr et al., 2018).

Digital technologies are often used as a way of supporting and promoting health. Look at the case example of Mary and answer the questions afterwards about this in Activity 5.4.

Mary

A group of cardiovascular nurse specialists in an NHS Trust run a virtual programme targeting behaviours such as smoking, obesity and lack of exercise that increase the risk of cardiovascular events. Mary, one of the group participants, is 55 years old, with high blood pressure and is overweight. All group participants receive a home blood pressure monitor, a Fitbit watch, and a tape measure to track their health over 12 weeks. Video group sessions with participants are run twice a month with a nurse who provides individualised coaching consultations so that they can discuss their progress, needs and goals they want to achieve. With this support, Mary was able to achieve weight reduction and reach the target blood pressure over the 12-week digital health programme.

Activity 5.4

- Can you make a list of the things that you think may have helped the digital health programme be successful for participants such as the one highlighted above?
- What sort of things would nurses need to be aware of if they wanted to introduce this type of digital service into professional practice?

In the scenario above, nurses introduce a range of technologies to support people to manage their health at home. This includes a standard medical device such as a home blood pressure machine, a wearable device (i.e., Fitbit), and video consultations. The digital health programme combines these technologies with regular peer support and professional support from a nurse who specialises in cardiovascular health which leads to better outcomes for participants.

Social media platforms are another digital tool being increasingly used to support and promote health in the general population. For example, social networking platforms such as Facebook and Twitter are being used to tailor and target multimedia content (e.g., videos, images or photographs, visualisations, and text) for groups of people with specific diseases/conditions. Anti-smoking campaigns have been designed and rolled out on social media such as YouTube and Instagram to encourage young people to quit smoking and discourage the use of cigarettes. Targeted reminders can be sent via notifications that pop up on a person's smartphone and can be combined with messaging applications like *WhatsApp* to communicate with closed groups of people. These digital forms of health promotion have been shown to improve smoking-related outcomes such as greater abstinence, reduction in relapses, and increases in attempts to quit smoking (Naslund et al., 2017). Moderated online discussions such as Twitter chats are also being used by public health agencies to engage people in two-way communication to educate them about a range of issues from responsible drinking to road safety.

Digital tools are also increasingly being used to support preventative health by encouraging diet and lifestyles changes and some infectious diseases which can be halted through vaccination programmes. Many nurses are actively involved in national vaccination programmes including Measles, Mumps, Rubella (MMR), the Human Papillomavirus (HPV), and coronavirus disease (COVID-19). Technology is critical in supporting the roll out of vaccination programmes in the community so that the public can receive reminders via their smartphone to encourage them to participate, arrange a vaccine appointment online or through their mobile device, and get confirmation of attendance (Mbunge et al., 2021). There is also some evidence to suggest that digital tools can help increase vaccination rates among different populations (Diaz et al., 2022).

Person-Facing Technology

There are many types of technologies that individuals can use to monitor and manage their own physical and mental health and that the public can utilise for self-care. Telehealth and telemedicine were discussed earlier in this chapter, other tools include mobile devices and mobile applications (apps) as well as wearable technologies. Mobile health has been defined as

> 'medical and public health practice supported by mobile devices, such as mobile phones, patient monitoring devices, personal digital assistants (PDAs), and other wireless devices'. (World Health Organization, 2011)

These digital tools can help individuals collect their own health data via an app on their smartphone which can process the information and provide recommendations and guidance on a regular basis on how to stay healthy. Healthcare providers can send reminders to individuals via text messages, email or video messages to their mobile phone reminding them to take medication, get exercise, and eat a healthy diet. For example, a nursing quality improvement initiative created a mobile health messaging service for new mothers and sent them regular text or email video reminders over 60 days explaining how to put their infant baby to sleep correctly in the supine position to try to reduce the risk of sudden infant death syndrome (Moon et al., 2017).

Other examples of person-facing technology include gaming platforms, where users can interact with each other in simulated virtual environments or follow a digital avatar who talks them through different activities such as exercises or brain training games to improve aspects of physical and mental health (Fleming et al., 2016). This is sometimes referred to as a *serious game* where a commercial gaming platform is used for purposes other than pure entertainment. Sometimes games can be accessed via mobile devices and mobile heath apps are increasingly using features from computer gaming (a process called gamification) such as running competitions between users and receiving digital rewards to engage individuals and keep them using the app on a regular basis.

Activity 5.5

Watch this YouTube video from Dr Emma Stanmore, a rheumatology nurse and member of the nursing faculty at the University of Manchester, UK who talks about her research developing and testing a video gaming platform called MIRA with older adults to help reduce falls and frailty (3:49 minutes): www.youtube.com/watch?v=-vOOwkcOuGQ

What do you think the benefits might be of using MIRA with older adults compared to more traditional fall prevention interventions?

Millions of people receiving care and their families also use the Internet every day to access health information and digital services from healthcare providers that are accessible online. A common digital mental health service that is offered by the NHS is computerised Cognitive Behavioural Therapy (CBT). See the following case scenario for an example of this.

Case scenario

NHS Cumbria, Northumberland, Tyne and Wear provide a platform called SilverCloud (www.cntw.nhs.uk/services/first-step/what-does-first-step-offer/ccbt/) to individuals who can access online psychological therapy that can help them with anxiety, depression, phobias and stress. The benefit of this approach is that it is flexible, so they can select the date and time that suits them, and it is also very convenient as they can access this digital service from the comfort of their own home and there are no waiting lists as it is available immediately. Some people prefer this ease of access and the privacy it offers, while others prefer to go to face-to-face CBT sessions with a healthcare practitioner.

Other benefits that individuals receiving care and family carers can get from accessing the Internet and being online is the social support that they can receive through various social media platforms. Many groups and organisations have Facebook, Twitter, Instagram, YouTube and other social media accounts that can be followed, which they use to share the latest advice and guidance on how to manage various aspects of an illness or new and emerging treatments. Research suggests that individuals and carers can benefit from emotional and technical support by participating in online communities on social media (Gavrila et al., 2019). Patients-LikeMe (www.patientslikeme.com) is an extremely popular social networking platform that is exclusively for those who can benefit from sharing knowledge of real-world experiences of healthcare services and how to manage an illness at home.

Other digital devices and tools that are increasingly being introduced to monitor and support a person's health at home or in other residential settings such as care homes, include sensors and robots. This can include sensors on doors, kitchen equipment (e.g., smart kettles or smart fridges), and mats or other furnishings that may indicate someone is moving around their house, and digital heating systems that can measure the room temperature to make sure it is not too hot or too cold. Some pilots of these technologies, often called 'smart homes', with older adults have demonstrated that using a range of connected devices at home could help identify when they are having problems such as mobility and alert a family carer or healthcare provider who can offer support (Marikyan et al., 2019).

Robots are also being developed and tested with a range of people to see if they can improve their physical and mental health. For example, care homes are trialing the use of robopets with residents to see if they can improve aspects of wellbeing such as loneliness, depression and quality of life (Abbott et al., 2019). PARO the seal is one type of robopet that has been used with people with dementia to determine if interacting with the robot has a positive therapeutic effect on their biological and psychosocial outcomes. Other types of robotics are being created to support nurses in their work, with numerous kinds of exoskeletons developed to support upper and lower limb movements. These can be used by nurses when transferring people in and out of bed or mobilising them in the bathroom (e.g., showering or toileting) to minimise any back pain they experience and support the safe transfer of individuals (O'Connor, 2021).

Technology for Teaching and Learning

Other novel technologies include virtual and augmented forms of reality. Virtual reality (VR) is defined as

> 'the use of interactive simulations created with computer hardware and software to present users with opportunities to engage in environments that appear and feel similar to real-world objects and events'. (Weiss et al., 2006: 183)

Augmented reality (AR) is slightly different where objects in the real world are enhanced by using computer-generated visual, audio, or haptic information that is overlaid or interwoven with a real environment using a range of digital tools. They are increasingly being used in healthcare as a method of simulation education to teach healthcare practitioners new clinical knowledge and skills. Traditional approaches to simulation education such as using mannequins or human actors in a simulation laboratory are not always feasible or affordable ways to deliver education. Therefore, some universities and health services are starting to use VR and AR to train nurses and other professionals, as immersive 3D simulations can enable in-depth visualisations of human anatomy resulting in greater technical proficiency, skills acquisition, and improved performance (Gasteiger et al., 2022). These technologies are also being used to educate individuals and help them learn how to manage disease symptoms and other problems at home (van der Kruk et al., 2022).

The Future of Digital Health

The nature of digital health technologies is that they are rapidly advancing, so it is difficult to identify precisely what innovations will be developed in the future. However, there are some areas where advances in science and technology will begin to impact on nursing care. One example is Artificial Intelligence (AI) which is the term given to advanced computational or statistical techniques that are combined in different ways to create predictive software algorithms which are applied to health datasets. Nurses are starting to use AI techniques in several ways to improve the prediction of care outcomes which can inform clinical decision making and care delivery (O'Connor et al., 2022). For instance, in one example nurses analysed an existing dataset using a few machine learning techniques to help predict falls among community dwelling older adults (Yang et al., 2021). This AI-based approach could be developed as a digital tool for nurses to help them to quickly identify those individuals at risk of falling and intervene early by introducing strategies to minimise falls.

Another example is precision health (also known as 'personalised' medicine or genomic health) which is an approach to tailoring treatments for people based on their unique genetic makeup, lifestyle and environment. At present, most medical treatments are generic in nature and designed to suit the 'average' person, which might not work for everyone (Calzone et al., 2018). Some genomic services already exist such as prenatal screening and new-born screening (i.e., blood spot test or heel prick) to identify diseases such as sickle cell disease, cystic fibrosis and congenital hypothyroidism, among others. In the future, it is likely that more genomic services will emerge to screen people who might be at risk of developing certain diseases. AI is becoming important in advancing precision health as genomic sequencing requires the analyses of large amount of complex health data and machine learning techniques can facilitate this (Xu et al., 2019). Pharmacogenetics is an emerging area within precision health where an individual's genome can be analysed to identify the safest, most effective drug for them. This could improve how well drugs works for individuals and reduce the side effects they can experience.

Limitations of Digital Health

Although technologies can help improve many areas of nursing practice, every piece of technology (hardware and software) has its limitations, and these can cause problems for nurses in their day-to-day practice, and people at home. It is important to understand the potential impacts of digital technologies in more detail, as their introduction may lead to unintended consequences. For example, if nurses find a particular technology difficult to use, they may experience more burnout and the outcome for those they care for is worse (Kutney-Lee et al., 2019).

Data quality

Although digital data in a computer system like an EHR or a CDSS can be better quality than hand-written notes, as the information is legible, this does not guarantee that the data quality is perfect. Sometimes data can be entered into the wrong electronic healthcare record, or it can be put in the wrong part of a record, or it might not be entered into an EHR in a timely manner if staff are busy, which can affect the accuracy of digital information (Feder, 2017). Hence, you should always use your clinical judgement as well as taking on board digital information and any guidance provided by technology in practice. Information on the Internet can also vary hugely in terms of its quality which can impact on people's understanding of health. Social media contains lots of information (e.g., text, images, audio and video) on many healthcare topics and some of this can be 'fake news' or misinformation that is deliberately created and posted by certain people and organisations for their own economic or political reasons. For example, there is a belief that childhood vaccinations are linked to autism which is not based on decent quality scientific evidence, although this misinformation may have influenced some parents not to vaccinate their children against certain diseases (Merchant and Asch, 2018).

Cost

Another limitation of technology is the cost of purchasing and installing hardware and software in a hospital, care home, or a person's own home. Computer equipment also needs to be maintained by specialist information technology (IT) staff on an ongoing basis. A national roll-out of electronic health records and other computing systems in NHS England, called the National Programme for Information Technology (NPfIT), over a decade ago, was estimated to cost in the region of £12 billion (Slight et al., 2014). Technology also needs to be upgraded or replaced if it is broken or out of date, which can add to the expense. This means that the cost of implementing digital health solutions needs to be balanced with the benefits technology can bring for nurses, other health professionals, and NHS management and the people who access healthcare.

Interoperability (data sharing)

Interoperability or data sharing is another limitation of digital health. Some technologies may not be able to share digital data with each other as they use different hardware and software that cannot communicate and exchange data. This can cause problems in health and care systems when we try and bring together healthcare data that is collected in various parts of a hospital such as medical wards, surgery and theatre, critical care, the emergency department, radiology, or across different care organisations (Lehne et al., 2019). The impact of interoperability for nurses is in the inability to share data between professional groups working across acute, primary, and community/social care settings. Poor levels of interoperability also affect individuals receiving care, as they often must repeat their health information regularly to separate groups of professionals which can slow down the coordination and delivery of their care.

Usability

A further limitation with some technology is its usability. Certain software and hardware can be easy to use but some of it can be more difficult to use which can affect how often and how well nurses and those they care for use technology. If a computer system such as an EHR is easy to log into and navigate around, then nurses will be able to quickly enter and find information that they need to inform clinical decision making and care delivery. Some key usability issues with IT in nursing and their impact are listed in Table 5.3. There are other practical usability issues with

Table 5.3 Usability issues with information technology in nursing and their impact (Staggers et al., 2018)

Themes	Categories	Sample Quotes
Usability pain points	Health IT Design	'EHRs are not designed to support nurses' professional practice or the way they think about their work.'
	Fit to workflow	'Vendors must understand the different workflows and information required in different settings, different speciality areas and levels of nursing.'
	Excessive documentation and handoffs	'Nurses are documenting requirements for other departments versus concentrating on what they need to provide good nursing care.'
	Interoperability	'Integration is needed with non-EHR health IT, such as smart pumps, point of care devices, BCMA, and other bar-coded devices that might avoid the nurse having to be the data copier. Current information is siloed in separate systems.'
	Lack of information to support the process of care	'The data nurses are able to retrieve often does not support the processes of care.'
Importance of the issues	Significance	'Issues are across all sites, patient populations, and health IT vendors.'
	Impacts	'Usability problems are fundamentally changing the way nurses practise.'
	Threats to patient safety	'Health IT creates patient safety issues, work-arounds, sentinel events.'
The Responsibility Gap	No win for nurses	'Everyone complains about these issues but other team members have a seat at the table. The perception seems to be that nurses will just use what they are given.'
	Contractual issues and nondisclosure clauses	'By not sharing information and applying a nondisclosure, the same incidents keep happening.'
	Training and education	'Tendency to shy away from training due to the impression that we shouldn't need a lot of training for technology.'
	Resources	'Must understand nursing role today. Outline information needs at each point. Holistic approach to understand tasks nurses are doing.'
Acting on usability issues	Solutions	'One thing to approve is to assign ownership to someone. Make them own it.'
	Usability methods	'Building awareness to create bridges between nursing and other disciplines like human factors engineers creates opportunities for exploration and better design.'
	Voice of nursing	'Nursing needs a digital strategy. Leaders need more knowledge about informatics.'
	We need a new vision	'(Health IT visions) need to be centred around the scope of practice for all disciplines for interprofessional team-based care.'

technology as the battery life in some devices can be short and they need to be charged regularly. Connectivity can also be a challenge if the device needs to access the Internet to send or receive data. Broadband or Wi-Fi can be slow or non-existent in some rural and urban areas which can affect nurses, other healthcare professionals, as well as individuals and their families.

Digital literacy and the digital divide

Digital literacy is the ability to use technologies including the use of specific devices/tools (such as a computer or smartphone) as well as the software/interfaces associated with them (Kuek and Hakkennes, 2019). People with limited digital knowledge and skills can become excluded from using digital health services and prevented from accessing useful health information and resources online. This is referred to as digital inequality or the 'digital divide,' which can be exacerbated for people who live in rural/remote regions and in urban areas where there is poor Internet access. It is also an issue for people in lower socio-economic groups as technology such as smartphones and Internet access can be expensive to purchase for those on low incomes or unemployed (Robinson et al., 2015). As nurses we need to be aware of our own digital literacy capabilities and improve these to ensure we can use EHRs, CDSS and other technologies to facilitate care provision. We also need to be cognisant of people's digital literacy and support them to improve their digital knowledge and skills, so they can use different technologies to help manage their illness at home and provide self-care.

Accountability, autonomy and burnout

Some additional risks associated with digital health are concerns among some nurses and other healthcare professionals that technology will be used to replace them or supersede their clinical decision making, leading to a loss of accountability and autonomy. There are also reports of healthcare professionals, including nurses experiencing burnout when using electronic health records. This is related to the amount of digital health data and documentation required in some countries, and certain EHR systems not designed to fit clinical workflows. This can cause usability issues for staff that can be frustrating and add to the busy workload they already have, which can lead to higher rates of stress and burnout among healthcare professionals over time (Kroth et al., 2019).

What Can You Do To Develop Your Digital Skills?

Digital health education

Nurses need good digital knowledge and skills throughout their careers whether they are working as a staff nurse in a hospital or community setting, or a nurse manager or nurse director overseeing nursing services in acute or primary care. There are many ways to develop your digital skills as a nurse. Some may choose to take postgraduate education courses or PhD qualifications while working as a nurse. Many universities run level 7 programmes on health informatics (digital health) and programmes that are specific to nurses may include a course on digital health. If interested in doing clinical research, either full-time or part-time, others might choose to complete a PhD where research methods are explored, followed by completing a focused research project on a digital health area in the NHS over a period of 3 to 4 years, while supported by a supervisory team.

NHS England have also set up their own NHS Digital Academy (https://digital-transformation. hee.nhs.uk/learning-and-development/digital-academy) to provide education and training for all clinicians (including nurses) on different topics in digital health such as the ones covered in this book chapter. You can also join professional associations such as the Faculty for Clinical Informatics (https://facultyofclinicalinformatics.org.uk/) in the UK to improve your digital skills further, as they run workshops and seminars on different topics in clinical informatics. International professional associations such as the International Medical Informatics Association (https://imia-medinfo.org/wp/) and the American Nursing Informatics Association (www.ania.org/) may also be useful to join and attend their conferences and other events to learn more about the world of digital nursing and digital health. Many nursing research conferences, such as the annual one run by the Royal College of Nursing in the UK, have presentations from nurses on digital health projects in the NHS and other settings. This can be another good way to learn about what is happening with technology in healthcare and nursing to improve your digital knowledge and skills.

Chapter Summary

This chapter has provided you with an introduction to the role of digital technologies in supporting nursing practice. It has highlighted the issues that you need to be aware of as a student and registered nurse when using digital technology in your practice, as well as providing an overview of the wide range of technologies that are being used across health and care settings. It has also provided you with insights into both the benefits and limitations of using technology in your practice, and highlighted the importance of being aware of these issues when using technology. The nature of technology development means that there will be a number of innovations you may come across in your clinical practice that have not been mentioned in this chapter. Make sure that you are always aware of both the pitfalls and promise of technology for supporting practice, and make sure that you use your clinical judgement when you need to.

Further Reading

Booth, R.G., Strudwick, G., McBride, S., O'Connor, S. and López, A.L.S. (2021). How the nursing profession should adapt for a digital future. *BMJ, 373:n1190.* https://doi.org/10.1136/bmj.n1190.

Coiera, E. (2015) *Guide to Health Informatics*, 3rd edn. Boca Raton, FL: CRC Press.

Nelson, R. and Staggers, N. (2018) (eds) *Health Informatics: An interprofessional approach*, 2nd edn. St. Louis, Missouri: Elsevier.

Acronyms

Acronym	Description
AI	Artificial Intelligence
BCMA	Bar Code Medication Administration
CBT	Cognitive Behavioural Therapy
CCC	Clinical Care Classification
CDSS	Clinical Decision Support System
CNS	Clinical Nurse Specialist
COVID-19	Coronavirus
EHR	Electronic Health Record
GDPR	General Data Protection Regulation
HPV	Human Papillomavirus
ICT	Information and Communication Technologies
ICNP	International Classification for Nursing Practice
IT	Information Technology
MMR	Measles, Mumps, Rubella
NANDA	Nursing Diagnoses, Definitions and Classification
NCRAS	National Cancer Registration and Analysis Service
NHS	National Health Service
NIC	Nursing Intervention Classification
NMC	Nursing and Midwifery Council
NOC	Nursing Outcomes Classification
NPfIT	National Programme for Information Technology
PDA	Personal Digital Assistant
PRSB	Professional Record Standards Body
RCN	Royal College of Nursing
SNOMED	Systematized Nomenclature of Medicine
UK	United Kingdom
VR	Virtual Reality
WHO	World Health Organization

References

Abbott, R., Orr, N., McGill, P., Whear, R., Bethel, A., Garside, R., Stein, K. and Thompson-Coon, J. 2019. 'How do "robopets" impact the health and well-being of residents in care homes? A systematic review of qualitative and quantitative evidence'. *International Journal of Older People Nursing*, 14(3): p. e12239. https://doi.org/10.1111/opn.12239

Barr, J.A., Tsai, L.P., Welch, A., Faradz, S.M., Lane-Krebs, K., Howie, V. and Hilman, W., (2018) 'Current practice for genetic counselling by nurses: an integrative review', *International Journal of Nursing Practice*, 24(2): e12629.

Booth, R.G. (2015) 'Happiness, stress, a bit of vulgarity, and lots of discursive conversation: a pilot study examining nursing students' tweets about nursing education posted to twitter', *Nurse Education Today*, 35(2): 322–7.

Booth, R.G., Strudwick, G., McBride, S., O'Connor, S. and Lopez, A.L.S. (2021) 'How the nursing profession should adapt for a digital future,' *BMJ*, 373: p. n1190.

Calzone, K.A., Kirk, M., Tonkin, E., Badzek, L., Benjamin, C. and Middleton, A. (2018). 'The global landscape of nursing and genomics. *Journal of Nursing Scholarship*, 50(3): 249–56. https://doi.org/10.1111/jnu.12380

De Gagne, J.C., Hall, K., Conklin, J.L., Yamane, S.S., Roth, N.W., Chang, J., & Kim, S.S. (2019). Uncovering cyberincivility among nurses and nursing students on Twitter: A data mining study. *International journal of nursing studies*, 89: 24–31. https://doi.org/10.1016/j.ijnurstu.2018.09.009

Diaz, D., Chacko, S., Sperling, A., Fleck, E., Louh, I., Trepp, R., & Ye, S. (2022). Assessment of Digital and Community-Based Outreach Interventions to Encourage COVID-19 Vaccination Uptake in an Underserved Community. *JAMA Network Open*, 5(6): e2217875-e2217875. https://doi.org/10.1001/jamanetworkopen.2022.17875

Feder, S.L. (2017) 'Data quality in electronic health records research: quality domains and assessment methods', *Western Journal of Nursing Research*, 40(5): 753–66.

Fennelly, O., Grogan, L., Reed, A. and Hardiker, N.R. (2021) 'Use of standardized terminologies in clinical practice: a scoping review', *International Journal of Medicine Informatics*, 149: 104431.

Fleming, T.M., Bavin, L., Stasiak, K., Hermansson-Webb, E., Merry, S.N., Cheek, C., & Hetrick, S. (2017). Serious games and gamification for mental health: current status and promising directions. *Frontiers in psychiatry*, 7: 215. https://doi.org/10.3389/fpsyt.2016.00215

Gasteiger, N., van der Veer, S.N., Wilson, P. and Dowding, D. (2022) 'How, for whom, and in which contexts or conditions augmented and virtual reality training works in upskilling health care workers: realist synthesis', *JMIR Serious Games*, 10(1): e31644.

Gavrila, V., Garrity, A., Hirschfeld, E., Edwards, B., & Lee, J.M. (2019). Peer support through a diabetes social media community. *Journal of diabetes science and technology*, 13(3): 493–497.

Groom, L.L., McCarthy, M.M., Stimpfel, A.W. and Brody, A.A. (2021) 'Telemedicine and telehealth in nursing homes: an integrative review', *Journal of the American Medical Directors Association*, 22(9): 1784–1801.e7.

Iyawa, G.E., Herselman, M. and Botha, A. (2016) 'Digital health innovation ecosystems: from systematic literature review to conceptual framework', *Procedia Computer Science*, 100: 244–52.

Kroth, P.J., Morioka-Douglas, N., Veres, S., Babbott, S., Poplau, S., Qeadan, F., Parshall, C., Corrigan, K. and Linzer, M. 2019. 'Association of electronic health record design and use factors with clinician stress and burnout'. *JAMA network open*, 2(8): pp.e199609-e199609 *https://doi.org/10.1001/jamanetworkopen.2019.9609*

Kuek, A. and Hakkennes, S. (2019) 'Healthcare staff digital literacy levels and their attitudes towards information systems', *Health Informatics Journal*, 26(1): 592–612.

Kutney-Lee, A., Sloane, D.M., Bowles, K.H., Burns, L.R., & Aiken, L.H. (2019). Electronic health record adoption and nurse reports of usability and quality of care: the role of work environment. *Applied clinical informatics*, 10(01): 129–139. https://doi.org/10.1055/s-0039-1678551

Lehne, M., Sass, J., Essenwanger, A., Schepers, J., & Thun, S. (2019). Why digital medicine depends on interoperability. *NPJ digital medicine*, 2(1): 79. https://doi.org/10.1038/s41746-019-0158-1

Marikyan, D., Papagiannidis, S. and Alamanos, E. (2019) 'A systematic review of the smart home literature: a user perspective', *Technological Forecasting and Social Change*, 138: 139–54.

Mbunge, E., Dzinamarira, T., Fashoto, S.G. and Batani, J. (2021) 'Emerging technologies and Covid-19 digital vaccination certificates and passports', *Public Health in Practice*, 2: 100136.

Mebrahtu, T.F., Skyrme, S., Randell, R., Keenan, A.M., Bloor, K., Yang, H., Andre, D., Ledward, A., King, H. and Thompson, C. (2021) 'Effects of computerised clinical decision support systems (CDSS) on nursing and allied health professional performance and patient outcomes: a systematic review of experimental and observational studies'. *BMJ open*, 11(12): p.e053886

Merchant, R.M. and Asch, D.A. (2018) 'Protecting the value of medical science in the age of social media and "fake news"', *JAMA*, 320(23): 2415–16. DOI: 10.1001/jama.2018.18416

Moon, R.Y., Hauck, F.R., Colson, E.R., Kellams, A.L., Geller, N.L., Heeren, T., Kerr, S.M., Drake, E.E., Tanabe, K., McClain, M. and Corwin, M.J. 2017. 'The effect of nursing quality improvement and mobile health interventions on infant sleep practices: a randomized clinical trial'. *JAMA*, 318(4): 351–9.

Mebrahtu, T.F., Skyrme, S., Randell, R., Keenan, A.M., Bloor, K., Yang, H., Andre, D., Ledward, A., King, H. and Thompson, C. 2021. 'Effects of computerised clinical decision support systems (CDSS) on nursing and allied health professional performance and patient outcomes: a systematic review of experimental and observational studies'. *BMJ open*, 11(12): p.e053886

Mostaghimi, A., Olszewski, A.E., Bell, S.K., Roberts, D.H., & Crotty, B.H. (2017). Erosion of digital professionalism during medical students' core clinical clerkships. *JMIR Medical Education*, 3(1): e6879.

Naslund, J.A., Kim, S.J., Aschbrenner, K.A., McCulloch, L.J., Brunette, M.F., Dallery, J., Bartels, S.J. and Marsch, L.A. (2017) 'Systematic review of social media interventions for smoking cessation'. *Addictive Behaviors*, 73: 81–93

NHS (2019) *The NHS Long Term Plan*. [Online]. Available at: www.longtermplan.nhs.uk/ (last accessed 13 October 2022).

NMC (2018a) *Future Nurse: Standards of Proficiency for Registered Nurses*. London: Nursing and Midwifery Council. Available at: www.nmc.org.uk/standards/standards-for-nurses/standards-of-proficiency-for-registered-nurses/ (Online). (last accessed 13 October 2022).

Nursing and Midwifery Council (2018b) *The Code* (Online). Available at: www.nmc.org.uk/globalassets/sitedocuments/nmc-publications/nmc-code.pdf (last accessed 1 January 2023).

O'Connor, S. (2021) 'Exoskeletons in nursing and healthcare: a bionic future', *Clinical Nursing Research*, 30(8): 1123–6.

O'Connor, S., Yan, Y., Thilo, F.J., Felzmann, H., Dowding, D. and Lee, J.J. (2023) 'Artificial intelligence in nursing and midwifery: a systematic review'. *Journal of Clinical Nursing* 32 (13–14): 2951–2968. https://doi.org/10.1111/jocn.16478

Robinson, L., Cotten, S.R., Ono, H., Quan-Haase, A., Mesch, G., Chen, W., Schulz, J., Hale, T.M. and Stern, M.J. (2015) 'Digital inequalities and why they matter'. *Information, Communication & Society*, 18(5): pp.569–82.

Ronquillo, C., Currie, L.M. and Rodney, P. (2016) 'The evolution of data-information-knowledge-wisdom in nursing informatics', *Advances in Nursing Science*, 39(1): E1–18.

Royal College of Nursing (2016) *RCN Position Statement: Nursing staff using personal mobile phones for work purposes.* Available at: www.rcn.org.uk/-/media/royal-college-of-nursing/documents/publications/2016/november/005705.pdf?la=en. (last accessed 1 January 2023).

Schwirian, P.M. (2013) 'Informatics and the future of nursing: harnessing the power of standardized nursing terminology', *Bulletin of the American Society for Information Science and Technology*, 39(5): 20–4.

Slight, S.P., Quinn, C., Avery, A.J., Bates, D.W. and Sheikh, A. (2014) 'A qualitative study identifying the cost categories associated with electronic health record implementation in the UK'. *Journal of the American Medical Informatics Association, 21(e2)*, e226–e231

Snoswell, C.L., Chelberg, G., De Guzman, K.R., Haydon, H.H., Thomas, E.E., Caffery, L.J, and Smith, A.C. (2021) 'The clinical effectiveness of telehealth: a systematic review of meta-analyses from 2010 to 2019'. *Journal of Telemedicine and Telecare, 1357633X211022907*

Staggers, N., Elias, B.L., Makar, E. and Alexander, G.L. (2018) 'The imperative of solving nurses' usability problems with health information technology', *JONA: The Journal of Nursing Administration*, 48(4).

Sutton, R.T., Pincock, D., Baumgart, D.C., Sadowski, D.C., Fedorak, R.N., & Kroeker, K.I. (2020). An overview of clinical decision support systems: benefits, risks, and strategies for success. *NPJ digital medicine*, 3(1): 17.

van der Kruk, S.R., Zielinski, R., MacDougall, H., Hughes-Barton, D., & Gunn, K.M. (2022). 'Virtual reality as a patient education tool in healthcare: a scoping review'. *Patient Education and Counseling*

Weiskopf, N.G. and Weng, C. (2013) 'Methods and dimensions of electronic health record data quality assessment: enabling reuse for clinical research', *Journal of the American Medical Informatics Association*, 20(1): 144–51.

Weiss, R., Kizony, R., Feintuch, U. and Katz, N. (2006) 'Virtual reality in neurorehabilitation'. In L. Cohen, F. Gage, S. Clark, and P. Duncan (eds), *Textbook of Neural Repair and Rehabilitation.* Cambridge, UK: Cambridge University Press, pp. 182–97.

Westrick, S.J. (2016) 'Nursing students' use of electronic and social media: law, ethics, and e-professionalism', *Nursing Education Perspectives*, 37(1).

World Health Organization (2011) *Mhealth: New horizons for health through mobile technologies: Based on the findings of the second global survey on ehealth.* [Online]. Available at: https://apps.who.int/iris/handle/10665/44607 (online). (last accessed 13 October 2022).

Xu, J., Yang, P., Xue, S., Sharma, B., Sanchez-Martin, M., Wang, F., Beaty, K.A., Dehan, E. and Parikh, B. 2019 'Translating cancer genomics into precision medicine with artificial intelligence: applications, challenges and future perspectives'. *Human Genetics*, 138(2): pp.109–124.

Yang, R., Plasek, J.M., Cummins, M.R. and Sward, K.A. (2021) 'Predicting falls among community-dwelling older adults: a demonstration of applied machine learning', *CIN: Computers, Informatics, Nursing*, 39(5).

6

MEDICINES MANAGEMENT

Laura Green, Morgan Evans and Brendan Garry

Chapter objectives

- Identify the role of registered nurses in medicine management;
- Describe the processes and the associated skills required for safe and effective medicine management;
- Understand some of the legal and ethical issues relating to medicine management;
- Identify factors that may increase the risk of medication errors;
- Demonstrate an awareness of some recent developments of the registered nurse's role in relation to medicine management;
- Understand why good pharmacological knowledge is needed for safe and effective care.

Medicine management is a core responsibility for the registered nurse, requiring competent decision making and risk management. It is an activity that often evokes concern for nurses on account of the high risk nature of managing medicines. However, it is also a rewarding aspect of the role in which nurses can play a key part not only in the management of conditions and symptoms, but in education and advocacy for those receiving care as well as their carers.

Related Nursing and Midwifery Council (NMC) Proficiencies for Registered Nurses

The overarching requirements of the NMC are that all nurses must understand the principles of safe and effective administration and optimisation of medicines in accordance with local and national policies and demonstrate proficiency and accuracy when calculating dosages of prescribed medicines. They must be able to apply knowledge of pharmacology to the care of people, demonstrating the ability to progress to a prescribing qualification following registration (NMC, 2018a).

━━━━━━━━ **TO ACHIEVE ENTRY TO THE NMC REGISTER**

YOU MUST BE ABLE TO ━━━━━━━━

- Carry out initial and continued assessments of people receiving care and their ability to self-administer their own medications;
- Understand the principles of safe, effective administration and optimisation of medicines in accordance with local and national policies and demonstrate proficiency and accuracy when calculating dosages of prescribed medicines;
- Demonstrate the numeracy, literacy, digital and technological skills required to meet the needs of people in your care to ensure safe and effective nursing practice;
- Demonstrate knowledge of pharmacology and the ability to recognise the effects of medicines, allergies, drug sensitivities, side effects, contraindications, incompatibilities, adverse reactions and prescribing errors, and the impact of polypharmacy and over-the-counter medication usage;
- Demonstrate knowledge of how prescriptions can be generated, the role of generic, unlicensed, and off-label prescribing, and an understanding of the potential risks associated with these approaches to prescribing;
- Recognise the various procedural routes under which medicines can be prescribed, supplied, dispensed and administered, and the laws, policies, regulations and guidance that underpin them;
- Use the principles of safe remote prescribing and directions to administer medicines;
- Undertake accurate checks, including transcription and titration, of any direction to supply or administer a medicinal product;
- Demonstrate an understanding of how to identify, report and critically reflect on near misses, critical incidents, major incidents, and serious adverse events to learn from them and influence their future practice;
- Exercise professional accountability in ensuring the safe administration of medicines to those receiving care.

(Adapted from NMC, 2018a)

Medicines management has been defined by the UK's Medicines and Healthcare Products Regulatory Agency as

> the cost effective and safe use of medicines to ensure patients get the maximum benefit from the medicines they need, while at the same time minimising potential harm.
> (National Institute for Clinical Excellence, 2015b)

Medicine management involves understanding the kinds of systems, contexts and behaviours that may influence how medicines are used, both by prescribers and by recipients. The nurse plays a key role in optimising the use of medicines. The goal of medicine management is to help people to improve their health outcomes, ensure they take medications correctly and avoid the risks of unnecessary medicines such as polypharmacy. It can also help us to achieve sustainability goals; wasted medications has a serious environmental and economic impact. In this chapter, we explore how medicines management can maximise safety and effectiveness of prescribed treatments, how nurses can engage collaboratively in related processes and how ultimately this can contribute to optimal healthcare.

For nurses, guidance and clinical support for medicines management can be found in the RCN/GPhC joint document relating to prescribing and administration of medicines (Royal Pharmaceutical Society, 2020). In terms of professional responsibilities around administration, the NMC no longer provide specific guidance on medicines management as this has been encompassed within the overarching guidelines provided by the General Pharmacological Council (Royal Pharmaceutical Society, 2019). Additionally, in hospital settings there will be specific policies and procedures governing medicine management. These may relate to the use of a person's own medicines, Patient Group Directives (which enable registered nurses to administer commonly used drugs without a specific prescription, such as paracetamol), and particular requirements for the management of controlled drugs.

For nurses working in a community setting, the importance of educating people in receipt of care is a high priority because individuals themselves or their carers usually take responsibility for administration. Nurses have a key role in supporting concordance, and this involves ensuring that the person and/or their relatives understand the reasons for the medication being prescribed and the possible consequences of not taking the medication as directed. A person's ability to open containers and to remember when to take their medication may need to be assessed and monitored. Advice should also be provided about storing medicines correctly and securely, for example kept out of the reach of children and other vulnerable groups. It is also important to monitor the effects and identify side effects or problems experienced by those receiving medications in the community.

Complex packages of care for residents are often in place in many care homes in the community. The need to improve the management of medicines for vulnerable residents was identified in The Care Home Use of Medicines Study (Barber et al., 2009). There are now seventeen recommendations aimed at improving practice in the NICE guideline on Drug Allergy Diagnosis and Management (NICE, 2014) which sits alongside the standard for Managing Medicines in Care Homes (National Institute for Clinical Excellence, 2015a).

A Medicine's 'Journey'

To understand the role of the nurse in medicine management it can be useful to have an over-view of the journey taken by medicines from the point of manufacture to the point of use or disposal. Table 6.1 below summarises this.

Table 6.1   A medicine's journey

Stage	Definition
Manufacture and marketing	Ensuring that medicines are manufactured legitimately and safely, and that advertising complies with ABPI standards.
Procurement	Ensuring medicines are purchased from a legitimate source.
Selection	Ensuring legal processes are adhered to for medicines, particularly prescription-only medicines.
Dispensing	Ensuring that medicines are dispensed correctly.
Sale or supply	Medicines that are available over the counter either as over-the-counter medicines or in pharmacies, pharmacy-only medicines. The supply of medicines is medicines that are supplied to someone in a pre-dispensed form, for example over labelled medicines, and are given to a person directly by the clinician.
Personal use	How a person engages in medicine management e.g., self-administration and adherence.
Disposal	Safe disposal of medicines that have not been used or have been partially used.

The Medicine Management Process

Medicine management incorporates nursing assessment, knowledge of a person's individual care plan, medicine administration and monitoring. In the next section, we will look at each of these stages in greater depth to explore the nurses' role.

1. Nursing assessment

A key component to a holistic nursing assessment is an accurate record of current and recent drug history. This may be obtained directly from the person receiving treatment, from their medical record, or from caregivers and other members of the multidisciplinary team. It is vital that this record includes not only what is prescribed but how it is taken. It should include formulation, dose, frequency, and times. Any allergies must be documented. It should also be noted if someone takes any medications over the counter, as well as any herbal remedies or recreational drugs.

Demi

Demi a 38-year-old who experiences migraine headaches and depression, has recently been diagnosed with pre-menstrual dysphoria disorder and has been commenced on a daily dose of fluoxetine. Demi reports feelings of despondency and thinks nothing has changed since starting fluoxetine other than some unpleasant side effects. A friend has suggested taking St John's Wort as it is a safe and effective herbal remedy for depression that has been used for hundreds of years. Demi asks you what you think about this.

Activity 6.1

How would you respond to Demi's query?
Who might you approach for help or advice?
Where might you look for additional information?

In your answer to the above question, you may well have referred to the British National Formulary (BNF). As the UK's primary resource for prescribing professionals, this contains a wealth of information about medications, including the recommended dose ranges, indications and contraindications, and interactions. It also addresses issues to consider in specific situations such as when prescribing or administering a drug to a person with renal or hepatic impairment, or who is pregnant or breastfeeding.

Although it is primarily a resource for prescribers, it is invaluable for nurses as a means of orientating oneself to drugs that may be in use in a particular clinical setting. Using the BNF would inform you that there is a known interaction between fluoxetine and St John's Wort, in which there is a risk of serotonin syndrome. Both St John's Wort and fluoxetine act to inhibit the re-uptake of serotonin from the presynaptic space, with the effect that serotonin will exert its pharmacological action for longer and help to address some of the symptoms of depression. However, when taken together there is risk of a rare but serious syndrome known as serotonin syndrome which can lead to life-threatening hypertension and neurological disturbances.

When assessing a person-particularly one who is new to the clinical setting – it is vital to include a comprehensive drugs history as part of the overall assessment. Not only is this a valuable way to establish rapport and give important insights into their general health beyond the presenting condition, the way in which a person shares their medical history can indicate their preferences and concerns.

Kris

You are admitting Kris to the ward following a fall at home and enquire what regular medications have been taken. Kris presents you with a piece of paper and reads out the list. It includes antihypertensives, diuretics and sleeping tablets. On further questioning, Kris admits to sometimes avoiding taking diuretics because of a fear of wetting the bed and doubling up on medications if forgotten. Kris's lifelong partner died last year of a stroke and Kris is worried about having a stroke so makes sure to never forget to take the blood pressure tablet. Kris appears tearful and stressed, and continuously asks whether it will still be possible to live at home.

Activity 6.2

What insight does this brief encounter give to you about Kris' potential nursing needs around medicine management?

Reflecting on Kris' concerns, several issues appear to have arisen in relation to what might have initially seemed a simple or straightforward question. Discussing the prescribed diuretic has led to Kris sharing a range of concerns, from bereavement to anxiety about potential loss of independence and fear about future health. These are all valuable insights for the nurse in the development of a therapeutic relationship.

2. Care planning

It is essential that nurses involved in medication administration are aware of the needs of individuals receiving medication. Prescribed medication will be a part of an overall treatment plan but the specifics of the plan may vary from person to person. For example, someone with diabetes who is taking insulin will need assessing for clinical stability which may involve testing their blood glucose level prior to administration. The timing of the insulin will need to consider their usual pattern of eating. Each individual is likely to have a slightly different target blood sugar level. Further, an assessment will need to be made regarding the availability and safe storage of their insulin as well as the injection sites. Any concerns or deviations from the plan must be communicated to the clinician in charge of their diabetes management regimen.

Allergies

Drug allergies are a specific type of adverse drug reaction and make up 5–10% of all adverse drug reactions (Warrington et al., 2018). Drug allergies occur due to an immune response to a drug – hence they are described as 'immunologically mediated hypersensitivity reactions'. Drug allergies will present clinically in a variety of ways according to the precise immunological mechanism that is activated by a drug. The Gell and Coomb (Dispenza, 2019) classification system describes these mechanisms and if understood can be used to help recognise drug reactions.

1   Type I reactions are mediated by immunoglobulin E (IgE), occur minutes to hours after drug administration and present as anaphylaxis, urticaria, bronchospasm or angioedema.
2   Type II reactions are cytotoxic and mediated by Immunoglobulin (Ig) M (IgM) or Immunoglobulin G (IgG). These reactions can occur within a variable time frame but will result in lysis of drug-coated blood cells, thus causing haemolytic anaemia and/or thrombocytopaenia.
3   Type III reactions occur due to the deposition of drug-antibody immune complexes within the tissue which causes vasculitis, rashes, fever, arthralgia and/or serum sickness. This will occur 1–3 weeks after drug administration.
4   Type IV reactions are delayed type hypersensitivity reactions that occur due to T cell activation. T cell activation causes the release of pro-inflammatory mediators 2–7 days after drug administration which results in contact dermatitis, Steven-Johnson syndrome, or AGEP (acute generalised exanthematous pustulosis).

Nurses must not only be able to recognise drug allergies, but they must also fulfil their role in the prevention of drug allergies and in educating those receiving treatment. Each year there are around 62,000 annual hospital admissions of individuals experiencing serious allergic reactions to drugs.

Between 2005–2013 there were 18,079 incidents reported to the National Reporting and Learning System involving the prescription or administration of a drug to someone with a known drug allergy to that specific drug/drug class. This included 13,071 near misses, 4980 other harms, 19 severe harms and 6 deaths (National Institute for Clinical Excellence, 2014). To reduce the frequency of these incidents, there is a structured process of documentation that must be observed following a suspected drug allergy. This includes documentation of the generic and brand name of the drug suspected to have caused the reaction, the strength of the drug formulation, the date and time of reaction, the time elapsed between drug administration and reaction, and a detailed description of the reaction.

In terms of educating individuals receiving medication there must be a discussion with that person (or their family/carers) regarding their drug allergy and written structured information must be provided to them. They also must be advised to inform all health professionals about their allergy when asked about their medication history. Since 2007, patients in NHS hospitals in the UK with a known drug allergy have been issued with red wristbands. However, if a person does not have a red wristband never assume that they have no allergies – questioning those individuals about drug allergies should always be a basic standard within nursing practice.

3. Administration

When administering a medication from a prescription the following items must be established:

1   Name of the medication
2   Dose and route of administration
3   Time
4   Prescriber's signature (and role if non-medical)
5   Start date

The prescription should be legible if handwritten, and any doubts should be referred to the prescriber. Prior to administration, the expiry date of the medication should be checked. All medicines come with the manufacturer's guidance as to the correct way to store them safely. Exposure to light or heat may interfere with the therapeutic properties of medications.

A core set of principles for avoiding errors when administering medications is to consider the five 'rights':

1   Right person
2   Right drug
3   Right dose
4   Right time
5   Right route

The use of electronic prescribing and medicines administration (EPMA) systems can help to reduce risk but do not ameliorate it entirely. A study by Slight et al. (2019) found that although EPMAs can reduce certain errors (such as dose or allergy identification), they do not impact on broader aspects of medicines management such as appropriate monitoring and follow-up, and that errors such as wrong selection of drug from drop-down menus can occur.

Drugs Calculations

Numeracy skills are a fundamental component of medicine management. This may mean calculating the number of tablets to make up a particular dose, the rate of infusion of an intravenous fluid, or a dose calculation based on a titration regimen. Miscalculations are a common cause of nursing medication errors: unit measurement such as micrograms and milligrams may be misunderstood, calculation errors that lead to wrong doses, or using the wrong equipment to measure dosages.

Drugs calculations are often a source of worry for students and universities will have a specific focus on numeracy as part of the pre-registration programme.

Building confidence in drug calculations

The following steps, adapted from the RCN's PEACE framework (RCN, 2023) can be helpful:

PLAN: Consider what your task is, including any person-specific factors.

ESTIMATE: Looking at the drug prescription and the available strengths. Can you make a rough guess at how many tablets or what volume will be required? This can help to identify if your calculation appears significantly different to what you are expecting.

APPROACH: If this is a complex calculation, do you need to find a quiet place to work it out? Do you need to double check your estimation with a colleague?

CALCULATE: The following formula is used whether you are administering liquid medicines or tablets:

$$\frac{\text{what you want}}{\text{what you've got}} \times \text{what it's in} = \text{dose}$$

For example, if you are asked to give 75mg amitriptyline and you have a packet of 25mg tablets, your calculation would look like this:

$$\frac{75}{25} \times 1 \text{tablet} = 3 \text{tablets}$$

Now let us try a calculation with a liquid medication.

Activity 6.3

You are asked to administer 5mg of liquid haloperidol. The oral liquid comes in a solution of 2mg/ml. What volume do you need to give to obtain the required dose?

Use the formula above to try and work this out.

Evaluate

Does your answer look correct? You can check this by repeating the formula calculation. Do you need to monitor the recipient to check their response to the medicine? For example, if you have administered analgesia, how will you follow up to see how effective it has been?

Routes of Administration

The most common route of administration of medications is oral, in the form of tablets, capsules, liquids or suspensions. However, medicines are frequently administered via alternative routes for several reasons. This may be because the medication cannot be absorbed via the gastrointestinal tract (e.g., insulin, would be digested by gastric enzymes and therefore must be administered subcutaneously) or because of personal factors, such as an inability to swallow medicine devices.

As an adult nurse, you will need to have sufficient knowledge to administer medications via several routes and the skills to ensure the safe use of any devices. These include pots, spoons and syringes for oral medications, syringes and needles for parenteral administration (injections), and oxygen masks and nebulisers for inhalation.

Mina

Mina has recently completed a cycle of chemotherapy for advanced cancer and is now being cared for at home but is experiencing problems with nausea and vomiting. Mina informs you that ondansetron (an antiemetic) was prescribed by the hospital to be taken at mealtimes, but is currently unable to keep anything down - even the tablets. Mina is also finding it difficult to take the prescribed oral modified-release morphine tablets, which are supposed to be taken twice a day.

Activity 6.4

What advice could you give Mina about the timing of the prescribed medication?
What might be an alternative option if the problems with nausea and vomiting do not resolve?
What other routes of administration can you think of for medications?
For each of the above routes, are there any specific individual considerations you would need to consider?

There are several devices for administering medications via various routes. In the above example, you might have suggested that Mina requires the antiemetic to be given via a different route, such as a subcutaneous injection. This would have potentially resolved the issues with not absorbing the antiemetic, and improved nausea and vomiting symptoms. However, there are times when a person requires multiple injections, or else a means of administration of medication that provides a steady plasma level of drug rather than peaks or troughs. This is often the case in palliative care (see Chapter 16), and is the primary reason that syringe drivers, or continuous subcutaneous infusion (CSCI) are used.

In the acute setting intravenous infusions are often used for administration of fluids, blood products or medications directly into a person's vein. The fluid is administered via a cannula that has been inserted into a small peripheral vein. Cannulas may come in several forms, varying both in the gauge (width) of the lumen and the number of connectors. Smaller gauge cannulas tend to be used for children and infants or those who are difficult to cannulate and are used for low-viscosity fluids such as normal saline. Wider gauge cannulas are used for products that are more viscous- such as blood or platelets- to enable flow at the required rate. Individuals receiving intensive care or who are receiving longer term intravenous medicines or fluids may have a more permanent cannula in situ, such as a peripherally inserted central catheter (PICC) line. When caring for a person on intravenous medication, you must ensure that you have received the appropriate training and that the device has been recently serviced. All devices should display a label showing the due date of the next service.

Table 6.2 Safety checklist

The medication	What has been prescribed? What is the dose? Do you know the side effects to watch out for? Is the medication in date and is the vial intact?
The individual receiving medication	Has consent been given? Have name and date of birth been checked? Check again for allergies.
Aspects of IV medication	Use aseptic no-touch technique for all IV procedures, check for signs of swelling, redness or pain at the cannula insertion site. What volume of diluent (if any) should be used? Is this to be given as a bolus or an infusion? If infusion, what rate?

Prior to administering any intravenous medication, the following checklist is a useful memory aid for maintaining safety:

Finally, some individuals who are unable to swallow might have a percutaneous endoscopic gastronomy or radiologically inserted gastronomy tube (PEG or RIG), which enables administration of liquid or suspensions of medicine via a tube directly into the stomach. The NEWT guidelines (Smyth, 2015) provide evidence-based support on administering medicines to those with enteral feeding tubes or swallowing difficulties, including data on the safety of crushing tablets or opening capsules in the cases of certain medications. For example, tablets should never be crushed unless there is clear safety data on their efficacy. Enteric-coated medications should never be crushed. If a person is unable to swallow these, the prescriber must be consulted to issue a more appropriate formulation.

Monitoring

The nursing role does not end with the administration of a drug. It is vital that the person receiving medication is monitored for any signs of adverse effects or side effects, as well as the efficacy of the drug, where appropriate. For example, administering post-operative analgesia according to a prescription chart must be accompanied with some evaluation of how effectively pain has been managed. In some cases, adjustments to prescriptions will need to be made. For example, an individual might experience unacceptable side effects (e.g., drowsiness), or their pain may not yet be well controlled. Other means of recording response to medication might include physiological observations such as blood pressure, pulse, or respiratory rate. Administration of insulin will require monitoring of blood glucose levels in accordance with the individual's care plan.

It is important to familiarise yourself with common side effects of medications you are involved with administering. Many drugs have side effects that are not related to their therapeutic effect. Side effects can impact on concordance to prescriptions, but in some cases effective communication and concurrent prescribing of other medications to counter the side effects can ameliorate potential non-concordance.

Tarik

Tarik is seen by a GP (General Practitioner) after sustaining a cut to the right hand. After attending the minor injuries unit where the wound was cleaned and dressed, a course of flucloxacillin for cellulitis is prescribed. On follow-up with you a few days later, you find out that Tarik decided to stop taking the antibiotic after three days due to experiencing side effects of diarrhoea and deciding that the cellulitis was better anyway.

Activity 6.5

What would you advise Tarik?
Write some brief notes which explain the difference between a side effect and an adverse drug reaction.

Adverse Drug Reactions

An adverse drug reaction (ADR) is a response to a medicinal product which is noxious and unintended. Response in this context means that a causal relationship between a medicinal product and an adverse event is at least a reasonable possibility. Adverse reactions may arise from use of the product within or outside the terms of the marketing authorisation or from occupational exposure. Conditions of use outside the marketing authorisation include off-label use, overdose, misuse, abuse, and medication errors. The reaction may be a known side effect of the drug, or it may be new and previously unrecognised. (Medicines and Healthcare products Regulatory Agency, 2020)

Adverse drug reactions (ADRs) continue to produce an increasing public health issue due to increases in life expectancy, co-morbidities, polypharmacy and the development of new drugs (De Angelis et al., 2016). Failed monitoring and management of ADRs leads to unplanned hospital admissions (ADRs cause 5–8% of unplanned admissions in the UK), increased morbidity and mortality and an increased financial burden on the NHS (4–6% of bed occupancy and an annual cost of £1 billion–£2.5 billion in the UK) (Jordan et al., 2016). It is not only the major life threatening ADRs that can cause significant impact. Minor problems can also cause significant discomfort for people and require a significant cascade of medical intervention to remedy, all reducing a person's quality of life. Due to the variety of reactions and the varying severity of reactions that can occur, the following classification system exists for ADRs and labels them:

Type A-E (Medicines and Healthcare products Regulatory Agency, 2020):

a   **Type A** – 'augmented' reactions which are dose dependent and due to a drug's normal pharmacological activity being exaggerated e.g., bleeding when taking warfarin. Also includes when the reaction that occurs is not linked to the pharmacological action of the drug e.g., dry mouth when taking tricyclic depressants/nephrotoxicity when taking aminoglycosides.

b   **Type B** – 'bizarre' reactions that are not expected based on the pharmacological activity of the drug e.g., urticaria or anaphylaxis when taking penicillin.

c   **Type C** – 'continuing' reactions that persist over time e.g., hypothalamic-pituitary-adrenal axis suppression by corticosteroids.

d   **Type D** – 'delayed' reactions develop after a period of time since commencing treatment e.g., tardive dyskinesia after taking antipsychotic medication.

e   **Type E** – 'end of use' reactions that are associated with ending treatment e.g., insomnia after stopping benzodiazepines.

Fifty per cent of ADRs are preventable (De Angelis et al., 2016) and 50% occur in the first five days following admission (Jordan et al., 2016). Due to the nature of their job, nurses are in a prime position to identify ADRs. If a person experiences an ADR, nurses can and should take the following steps:

1   Record this ADR in the person's notes.
2   Inform the prescriber of the ADR.
3   Inform the Yellow Card Scheme immediately.
4   Inform the person that they can independently report this ADR to the Yellow Card Scheme.

Reporting ADRs to the Yellow Card Scheme inputs the event to a database of 'potential causal relationships' between drugs and adverse drug reactions. This data is then used to determine whether the reported drug reaction combinations are likely to be true drug reactions. This allows the latest information regarding adverse reactions to be published and for guidelines to change around administration, usage, or accessibility (Medicines and Healthcare products Regulatory Agency, 2020). Clinical trials alone may fail to truly assess the safety and side effect profile of medications when administered to those individuals already susceptible to ADRs. Therefore, pharmacovigilance is required in everyday practice to ensure the safety of drugs is ever improving (Gabe et al., 2011). Consequently, under reporting of ADRs provides significant problems for pharmacovigilance (De Angelis et al., 2016). Under reporting can occur due to inadequate identification of non-life threatening ADRs, uncertainty of which/if any medication is attributable for the reaction, and difficult pathways to report ADRs (Jordan et al., 2016). Nurses need to be able to identify ADRs amongst those individuals in their care. The methods to identify an ADR include:

a   *Listening* to an individual receiving medication and/or family members/carers and the symptoms that may have developed since commencing a new medication – this may reveal adverse reactions that are apparent;
b   As not all reactions will be apparent, *looking* for changes in observations or baseline laboratory results is often required.

Other ways to increase the rate of ADR reporting, specifically by nurses, include increasing nurses' knowledge of pharmacology and the definition of ADRs to help gain confidence in reporting, reporting all ADRs (not only the novel reactions) and reporting all ADRs immediately (De Angelis et al., 2016). However, to reduce morbidity and mortality of ADRs at the origin, good monitoring and management by nurses is required. This includes increased awareness of risk factors those receiving medicines may possess that lead to increased susceptibility to ADRs (e.g., atopy, polypharmacy, renal/hepatic/cardiac disease, increasing age), taking a good drug history (including all OTC medications, prescribed medications, herbal products, and doses), and increased case-study based teaching (Jordan et al., 2016). Reducing rates of ADRs and increasing ADR reporting is not just a role for nurses. Instead, these objectives require multidisciplinary collaboration and widespread organisational changes to increase pharmacovigilance by all healthcare professions.

Medicine Errors

There are around 237 million medication errors in England every year (NHS England and NHS Improvement, 2019) of which 66 million are thought to be clinically significant. Errors can take place at any of the stages of the medication process, from prescribing through to dispensing, administering, and monitoring. They are different from adverse drug effects which are physiological responses to the medicine itself. At the core of medicine errors are human and system factors.

Rebecca

Rebecca (a registered nurse) has just commenced the drug round before becoming aware that there are several 'buzzers' sounding. The other staff on the ward include a registered nurse from a nursing agency, three healthcare support workers and a student.

Rebecca arrives at bed 3 where Gerald is awaiting an antibiotic. Rebecca checks Gerald's wristband against the drug chart to confirm identity and opens the trolley. Rebecca cannot see any ciprofloxacin capsules so returns to the stock cupboard to check availability. However, Rebecca then realises that the drug chart is still at the end of Gerald's bed but manages to find clarithromycin and adds it to the trolley. The next day Rebecca is contacted by her manager after another nurse undertaking the morning drug round discovers that there is no ciprofloxacin in the trolley but there is a box of clarithromycin with a capsule missing and deduces that this has been adminstered in error. Thankfully Gerald experiences no adverse effects from this error. Rebecca is distraught and despite support from the manager, takes time out from work for stress-related illness.

Activity 6.6

What human factors do you think might contribute to this error?

If you were Rebecca what would help you to learn from this experience?

What support do you think you would need?

Incident reporting

If a medication error takes place it is vital that it is reported promptly to minimise the potential impact of the error. The nurse has a duty of candour, as outlined by *The Code* (Nursing and Midwifery Council, 2018b). Openness and honesty are fundamental professional and moral qualities. Failure to act on discovery of a medication error can not only lead to significant harm for the individual receiving the medication but also to serious sanctions for the nurse.

Root cause analysis is an investigatory tool that is often used when an incident such as a medication error occurs. Using a systematic approach, the aim is to identify what factors (root causes) led to the medication error. This is an important process aimed at improving safety and is explained further in Chapter 9.

Polypharmacy

The term polypharmacy describes the concurrent use of at least five medications (Aggarwal et al., 2020) or simply a person taking more drugs than are clinically indicated (Barnett, 2022). In England, 8.4 million people are prescribed five or more medications regularly, and 20% of hospital admissions in the over-65s are from adverse drug effects (Department of Health and Social Care, 2021). Polypharmacy and overprescribing may occur due to medication being used first-line where lifestyle modifications could be alternatively suggested, a lack of prescription reviews being completed leaving people with medications they no longer require or inappropriate medication being prescribed for a person that worsens other comorbidities (Department of Health and Social Care, 2021). Healthcare outcomes are negatively affected by polypharmacy. Consequences of polypharmacy include adverse drug reactions from drug–drug interactions and drug–disease interactions, falls leading to fractures, renal failure, reduction in physical function, increase frailty, lower cognitive function, and increased hospital admissions (Wastesson et al., 2018). There is also increased risk of non-adherence to treatment and increased costs to the NHS (Pasina et al., 2014). Nurses therefore, must be aware of the impact of polypharmacy when working in any healthcare setting, especially when working with older people.

Unfortunately, polypharmacy is set to increase in future years. In England, one quarter of people over 60 have two or more chronic conditions, and with an ageing population (between 2013 and 2050 the global number of people aged over 60 is set to increase from 841 million to 2 billion) (Aggarwal et al., 2020), this will increase the burden of polypharmacy on the population and on the NHS. With 30–50% of medications prescribed for chronic conditions not being taken as intended, an ageing population with an increasing level of polypharmacy could have grave financial and clinical consequences. Additionally, the number of investigations and tests in UK primary care increases by 8.5% annually, producing more diagnoses and more prescriptions (O'Sullivan et al., 2018). Therefore, practitioners must focus on actively trying to avoid polypharmacy by prescribing fewer than five medications per day and on person-focused deprescribing which involves considering an individual's wishes, co-morbidities, lifestyle (Barnett, 2022). Nurses can facilitate this by identifying those taking multiple medications, organising a medication review with the prescriber or a pharmacist and discussing with people how they are coping with taking their medications (Royal Pharmaceutical Society, 2022).

Antimicrobial Stewardship

Nurses must recognise the concepts of infection prevention and control, particularly in relation to antimicrobial resistance and antimicrobial stewardship (Laging et al., 2015). Antimicrobial stewardship means using evidence-based decisions to reduce unfavourable consequences of antimicrobial therapy and promote the best possible health outcomes for individuals. The inappropriate use of antimicrobials has a host of consequences such as worse health outcomes, increased recovery times, treatment failure, toxicity, and antimicrobial resistance. With inappropriate use of antimicrobials ranging between 20 to 45% in high-income countries (Kirby et al., 2020), antimicrobial resistance is fast becoming one of the largest threats to health for all countries with widespread global consequences for morbidity and mortality (Gotterson et al., 2021).

Previously, the roles that doctors and pharmacists play in antimicrobial stewardship have been the focus for advancement in the field; however, nurses can and should have significant impact on the management of antimicrobial therapy. A nurse's role in antimicrobial therapy includes monitoring and assessment of individuals, administering prescribed antimicrobials and person-centred education. Given that nurses will regularly monitor and detect changes to a person's condition, there is good potential for nurses to guide the choice of antimicrobials and the dose and duration of treatment.

Concepts for nurses to focus on in practice to maintain antimicrobial stewardship include:

1   Act as an advocate for individuals (e.g., helping them to receive the right treatment promptly).
2   Have a good knowledge of antimicrobials (e.g., their mechanism of action and which bacterial strains are sensitive to them).
3   Be aware of and implement trust antimicrobial stewardship policies.
4   Collaborate with other health professionals to come to best decisions for those we care for.
5   Ensure correct techniques and trust protocols are adhered to when collecting cultures.
6   Obtain and document a person's allergies to antimicrobials prior to prescribing decisions being made.
7   Ensure correct disposal of antimicrobials.
8   Fastidiously follow trust infection control protocols.

Controlled Drugs

In accordance with current guidelines (National Institute for Health and Care Excellence, 2016), controlled drugs (CDs) such as strong opioids must be kept in locked cupboards within institutional settings that can only be accessed by a registered nurse. The registered nurse in charge of a shift is responsible for the safe storage and use of CDs, although specific tasks such as administration may be delegated to another registered nurse. They are similarly responsible for requisitioning, using a specific CD book and detailing the name of the hospital and ward, date, drug name, form and strength, total quantity required in dosage units (e.g., number of tablets, ampoules, or millilitres), and signature alongside the printed name of the nurse in charge or delegated nurse. The same information should be recorded on receipt of the ordered medications.

Where a CD must be administered it is a requirement that two people are present, one of whom must be a suitably qualified registered nurse. The second person may be another nurse, a student nurse, or a doctor. In some exceptional instances it is possible for a single nurse to administer the medication, for example in a community setting where there is only one nurse. There will be local operating procedures to guide you if this is the case.

When administering CDs, the process to follow is the same as for other medications, with the following additional safeguards:

1. Stock must be reconciled with the record in the CD book after removing the required quantity. At the bedside, both practitioners independently check the recipient's details, confirm the absence of allergies, and the details of drug, dose, and volume.
2. The name and dose of the drugs given must be documented, as well as the volume of bolus or infusion, the diluent used, the drug expiry date and the route of administration.
3. The CD register should then be updated with the correct details, finally logging the remaining balance in stock.
4. Where only a part of an ampoule is used, the registered nurse should document the amount administered as well as the amount discarded, and this should be witnessed and signed by a second registrant.

Ethical Considerations

As in all areas of nursing practice, it is of utmost importance to uphold core ethical principles when engaged in person-centred care. But what does this mean in relation to medicine management? In this section, we consider some issues that a nurse may encounter and offer some guidance as to how to navigate the terrain in an ethical and compassionate way.

Concordance, adherence, or compliance?

Supporting an individual to manage their condition with medication is much more than a mechanical task. The relationship between a recipient of care and their healthcare team is key in promoting concordance in line with the principles of person-centred care. Individuals are sometimes described as being 'non-compliant' with their treatment if they do not take it as prescribed but this implies a level of paternalism that is at odds with current healthcare philosophy. Involving the individual concerned as a partner in care is essential, particularly in areas such as medicine management.

Some people hold views about their disease or condition and about the treatments they take. For over twenty years, healthcare professionals have been encouraged not to use the word 'compliance' when talking about people and their treatments, and yet still it is a frequently heard term. However, it implies a relationship of inequality between healthcare professionals where a person is a passive recipient of care, and in which they have been instructed to take their treatment.

A further term, 'adherence,' can also be used in clinical practice. This describes the extent to which a person is taking their medication as it has been prescribed. It is always worth checking to see if someone is taking their medicine as prescribed. They may be adjusting the dose or timings, or there may be some other reason that influences adherence. Some examples of factors affecting adherence are poor manual dexterity, making it difficult to open blister packs, and cognitive impairment.

Concordance is a more recent concept in medicines management and describes the development of a relationship in which individuals and prescribers agree about the purpose of the treatment, the specifics of the prescription (Dickinson et al., 1999) and agree mutual goals of care. Within a concordance model, the individual concerned is at liberty to decline or moderate the treatment plan and the healthcare professional should respect this (Aronson, 2007).

Nurses play a significant role in enhancing medication adherence and promoting concordance in all clinical settings. Certain groups of the population are particularly in need of this additional support. For example, many older people have multiple conditions and may be taking many medications. When they are discharged from hospital they are at considerable risk of non-adherence. This may be because of issues obtaining supplies of medications, confusion about doses or timings, or taking too much medication because of combining discharge medications with stocks in the home. This can lead to problems of poor management of their condition and in some cases necessitate further hospital admission. Nurses are well placed to support such individuals both prior to discharge and afterwards at home. A systematic review of interventions to support adherence (Verloo et al., 2017) identified 14 studies reporting on nurse interventions, such as written fact sheets and medicine schedules, telephone and electronic reminders, comprehensive medicines assessments at community nurse home visits and electronic pill dispensers. There is some evidence that these interventions enhance medicine adherence, although the quality of the research is impaired by a lack of 'blinding,' (e.g., the process used in research by which study participants and carers, care providers, data collectors and data analysts are kept unaware of group assignment) as well as challenges in how to assess adherence.

Jakub

Jakub has recently moved to a care home following increasing concerns about safety at home and has several regular medications that are prescribed for various conditions including diabetes, hypertension, and depression. You are asked to administer Jakub's tablets in the morning, but when you arrive, Jakub does not want to take medication and wants to go back to sleep.

Activity 6.7

- What would you do?
- What factors would you need to consider?
- Who else would you involve?

This is a common scenario faced by nurses. Initially, you would try to ascertain Jakub's reasons for not wanting to take the prescribed medication. For example, is Jakub particularly unsettled following the recent move to a care home? Does Jakub resent being told when to take the medications rather than having control? Does Jakub's mood indicate a concern that might be contributing to a lack of motivation?

If someone expresses a wish not to take medication as prescribed, the next step would be to assess their mental capacity. Remember that people can make decisions that might not be in line with what is recommended if they are able to demonstrate mental capacity in accordance with the *Mental Capacity Act* (Department of Health, 2005). It might be appropriate to go through their medications individually to confirm their wish not to take them. Some will be more important than others in maintaining health and a conversation with a pharmacist or doctor could help to prioritise medicines or to discontinue those that are considered non-essential. Reducing tablet burden might help here.

If after undertaking all these steps, a person still declines their medicines and has capacity to do so, it is essential that this decision is recorded in their notes and on the prescription chart. There will be a local policy that explains the process to follow in the event of a person refusing to take their medications.

People with impaired capacity

People with dementia are often prescribed multiple medications, primarily to manage other conditions associated with older age such as pain. Managing medicines can be particularly complex for those with dementia and their caregivers. There are risks of harm through polypharmacy, under or over estimating symptoms, or non-adherence to treatment regimens. As dementia progresses, the ability to independently plan and organise one's own medications will be affected, leading to increasing reliance on caregivers. At such times, it can be helpful to explore what resources are available to them. For example, are there caregivers with regular contact who could support the person with obtaining, storing and taking their medicines? The use of visual aids or personal reminders can help to maintain a person's autonomy around medicines management.

Sometimes, those with cognitive impairment and/or behavioural concerns may refuse to take their medications. In such instances, it may become necessary to explore other avenues of administration such as covert administration.

Covert administration

Covert administration of medication refers to giving drugs to people who actively refuse their medications and who are considered to lack mental capacity in relation to that decision (Department of Health, 2005). This may only be done within the remit of an agreed management plan. Where it is deemed necessary, covert administration must take place within the context of legal and best practice professional frameworks. Healthcare institutions should have policies covering covert administration (Care Quality Commission, 2022).

It should only be considered where a person is actively refusing their medicine *and* they are deemed not to have capacity to understand the consequences of their refusal (as determined by the *Mental Capacity Act*), and that the medicine is deemed essential to the person's health and wellbeing.

Medicines may be concealed in food or drink or administered through a feeding tube where a person does not consent. In all cases, covert administration should be a last resort. There are professional, clinical, and ethical issues associated with this practice. Not least, it undermines an individual's autonomy and risks breaking the trusted relationship with the healthcare professional. Further, it can impact on enjoyment of food, particularly if the person feels under pressure to eat because of the medication concealed within the meal. Food and eating practices are sources of health, opportunities to exercise autonomy, ways to create valuable experiences (e.g., pleasure, cultural connections), ways to express/reinforce identity and ways of reinforcing/building connections with others. Eating is also a relational practice, one that entails significant vulnerability to and dependency on others (Pickering, 2020).

Pharmacokinetics and Pharmacodynamics

As you progress through your nursing career you will be exposed to a vast variety of medications. Your involvement in medicines management requires that you understand the key principles of pharmacokinetics and pharmacodynamics in order that you appreciate the requirements of certain medication conditions and how drugs are prescribed.

Pharmacokinetics refers to how the body deals with a drug once it has been administered – or put simply, what the body does to the drug. This covers the (1) *absorption*, (2) *distribution*, (3) *metabolism* and (4) *excretion* of the drug. These four stages describe (1) how the drug enters the body, (2) how it moves around the body, (3) how it changes in the body and (4) how it leaves the body.

Drugs are absorbed in various ways depending on the route of administration, and in some cases, this can affect the actual amount of active drug that enters the plasma. For example, intravenous morphine enters the bloodstream directly, and so all of it is available to exert its analgesic effect. However, when taken orally morphine undergoes *first-pass metabolism*, which means that a proportion of it (approximately 50%) is metabolised before it enters the blood. For this reason, dose adjustments need to be made when converting an oral to an intravenous dose of morphine and vice versa. If a drug is taken orally, it is absorbed via the small intestine and transported via the blood to the liver. This is known as first-pass metabolism. Metabolism turns the drug into the usable form, in which state it can be transported around the body. Distribution of a drug describes the transfer of a drug from one part of the body to another. Once a drug has undergone first-pass metabolism and is in its active state in the systemic circulation, it can travel to its site of action. This relies on transport processes and is concerned with how the drug accumulates at the site of action. It is influenced by several factors, including albumin levels in the drugs (for drugs that are protein-bound), levels of hydration, as well as by the presence of other drugs with which they may interact. Excretion is different from elimination. Excretion refers to the loss of chemically unchanged drug, whereas elimination refers to the loss of drug from the site of action. Thus, excretion refers to inactive products of metabolism leaving the body. Elimination refers to the removal of a medication from the body, such as might result from metabolism in the liver.

Activity 6.8

Case Scenario

Mohammed

Mohammed has chronic renal failure, dementia and severe osteoarthritis which is causing pain and interrupting sleep. One of Mohammed's family members comments that they have had excellent pain relief from ibuprofen for arthritis and suggests this might be helpful.

Refer to the information on ibuprofen in the British National Formulary at https://bnf.nice.org.uk/ Do you think ibuprofen would be a good option for pain management of Mohammed's arthritis?

Pharmacodynamics refers to the study of a drug's molecular and physiological effects in the body. In general, drugs act on the body to bring about the desired effect. Put simply, this can be seen as what the drug does to the body. Drugs that act on receptors may either have an agonist or an antagonist effect, as in the examples below. Some drugs have a partial agonist–antagonist effect.

Some drugs act by replacing or substituting a substance such as ferrous sulphate for iron-deficiency anaemia. Others may inhibit enzymes from working. Non-steroidal anti-inflammatories

Table 6.3   Drugs that act on receptors

Mechanism	Description of action	Example
Agonist	Chemical that activates a receptor to produce a response.	*Morphine* – activates opioid receptors to produce analgesic response.
Antagonist	Chemical that blocks the action at a receptor.	*Ranitidine* – blocks release of hydrochloric acid in response to gastrin.
Blocker	Chemical that occupies an electrolyte channel to prevent the transportation of certain electrolytes.	*Nifedipine* – blocks calcium channels to prevent constriction of blood vessels, thus treating high blood pressure.
Inhibitor	Chemical that inhibits neurotransmitters.	*Ondansetron*, an antiemetic, inhibits the neurotransmitter serotonin, which is implicated in the chemoreceptor trigger zone in the brain.
Cytotoxic	Chemical that destroys cells.	Chemotherapy acts by interfering with the cell cycle or with key cell signalling pathways in order to disrupt cell division.
Antimicrobial	Antibiotics, antifungal and antivirus drugs target the organism causing the infection.	*Nystatin* acts by increasing the permeability of the cell wall of certain yeasts so that they die, enabling treatment of oral and oesophageal thrush.

such as naproxen and ibuprofen are examples of these, and they act by preventing the production of prostaglandins by inhibiting an enzyme known as cyclo-oxygenase. In this way, they reduce inflammation (Adams et al., 2020). Pharmacodynamics also provides us with insight into the ways in which some drugs interact with one another. For example, simultaneous administration of a non-steroidal anti-inflammatory such as ibuprofen, and aspirin can increase the risk of gastric bleeding as they have an antagonistic effect on one another.

Sustainability

It has been estimated that £300 million of NHS prescribed medications are wasted every year. There are various kinds of pharmacological waste. Non-adherence is one example. Additionally, non-preventable waste occurs when a person dies or their treatment is adjusted meaning that their current medications are no longer needed. Preventable waste results from people stockpiling medications, or when items are dispensed from repeat prescriptions even when no longer required or surplus to requirements.

Nurses play a vital role in minimising waste through supporting people to take medicines as prescribed and identify any concerns or issues. It is also vital that communication between services is efficient, and patients are prescribed appropriate quantities for their needs. A 'one-size-fits-all' approach will not be appropriate here.

Medicine-related incidents are a significant concern for the healthcare service. In March 2017, the WHO (World Health Organization) launched its global safety challenge to reduce avoidable medication-related harms by 50% in the next five years.

Non-Medical Prescribing

Prescribing medication was at one time the sole remit of a medical professional. However, since 1992 changes in legislation enabled certain nurses to prescribe from an Extended Nurse Formulary (Cope et al., 2016). This role continued to develop and expand, leading to the development of Supplementary Prescribing in which nurses could prescribe specific medications for specific conditions within a supervisory partnership with a medical professional. Since 2006, there has been a rapid expansion in non-medical prescribing in the UK, with nurses and other allied health professionals undertaking additional training to be annotated with their professional regulatory bodies as independent prescribers. It is increasingly recognised that nurse independent prescribing can offer a safe and effective alternative to physician prescribing in certain circumstances. Nurse Independent Prescribers (formerly known as Extended Formulary Nurse Prescribers) can prescribe any medication for any condition, providing this activity falls within their level of professional experience and competence.

To be considered for acceptance onto a Prescribing Programme a nurse must demonstrate the required skills, knowledge and experience required to undertake the programme. It is no longer the case that this equates to a set period in clinical practice, because under the Future Nurse Proficiencies (NMC, 2018a) there is an expectation that newly qualified nurses will possess higher levels of skills that are relevant to prescribing, such as clinical assessment and diagnostics.

Chapter Summary

This chapter has provided an overview of the responsibilities of a nurse when it comes to safe administration of medications, considering the four key components of the medicines management process. It is recommended that this chapter is used as a guide to further study, and that when you are in clinical practice you make sure that you familiarise yourself with the most commonly prescribed drugs in that area. As well as knowledge of the individual and their care plan, understanding the indications for the drug, as well as how it is administered, absorbed and acts will be a valuable skill as you develop in your role. Medications management is often a source of anxiety for nurses, but with proper care and diligence it can be a significantly rewarding area of practicce. Understanding the key principles in this chapter will help you to become a safe, conscientious, and ethical professional nurse.

Further Reading

Adams, M., Holland, L. and Urban, C. (2020) *Pharmacology for Nurses: A Pathophysiologic Approach.* Upper Saddle River: Pearson.

British National Formulary (BNF) *Key information on the selection, prescribing, dispensing and administration of medicines.* Available at: https://bnf.nice.org.uk/

NHS England and NHS Improvement (2019) *The NHS Patient Safety Strategy: Safer culture, safer systems, safer patients.* Available at: www.england.nhs.uk/patient-safety/the-nhs-patient-safety-strategy/ (last accessed 1 January 2023).

NHS Wales (Website) *Medicines Management.* Available at: www.wales.nhs.uk/medicinesmanagement

Royal Pharmaceutical Society (2019) *Professional Guidance on the Administration of Medicines in Healthcare Settings.* London: RPS.

References

Adams, M., Holland, L. and Urban, C. (2020) *Pharmacology for Nurses: A Pathophysiologic Approach,* Upper Saddle River: Pearson.

Aggarwal, P., Woolford, S.J. and Patel, H.P. (2020) 'Multi-morbidity and polypharmacy in older people: challenges and opportunities for clinical practice', *Geriatrics (Basel),* 5.

Aronson, J.K. (2007) 'Compliance, concordance, adherence', *Br J Clin Pharmacol,* 63: 383–4.

Barber, N.D., Alldred, D.P., Raynor, D.K., Dickinson, R., Garfield, S., Jesson, B., Lim, R., Savage, I., Standage, C., Buckle, P., Carpenter, J., Franklin, B., Woloshynowych, M. and Zermansky, A.G. (2009) 'Care homes' use of medicines study: prevalence, causes and potential harm of medication errors in care homes for older people', *Quality and Safety in Health Care,* 18: 341–6.

Barnett, N. (2022) *Understanding polypharmacy, overprescribing and deprescribing* [Online]. Specialist Pharmacy Service. Available at: www.sps.nhs.uk/articles/understanding-polypharmacy-overprescribing-and-deprescribing/ (last accessed 1 January 2023).

Cope, L.C., Abuzour, A.S. and Tully, M.P. (2016) 'Nonmedical prescribing: where are we now?' *Therapeutic Advances in Drug Safety,* 7: 165–72.

Care Quality Commission (2022) *Covert Administration of Medication* [Online]. Available at: www.cqc.org.uk/guidance-providers/adult-social-care/covert-administration-medicines (last Accessed 5 August 2022).

De Angelis, A., Aolaceci, S., Giusti, A., Vellone, E. and Alvaro, R. (2016) 'Factors that condition the spontaneous reporting of adverse drug reactions among nurses: an integrative review', *Journal of Nursing Management,* 24: 151–63.

Department of Health (2005). *Mental Capacity Act.* London: HMSO.

Department of Health and Social Care (2021) *Good for you, good for us, good for everybody: A plan to reduce overprescribing to make patient care better and safer, support the NHS, and reduce carbon emissions.* Available at: https://assets.publishing.service.gov.uk/government/uploads/system/uploads/attachment_data/file/1019475/good-for-you-good-for-us-good-for-everybody.pdf (last accessed 1 January 2023).

Dickinson, D., Wilkie, P. and Harris, M. (1999) 'Concordance is not compliance', *British Medical Journal*, 319: 787.

Dispenza, M.C. (2019) 'Classification of hypersensitivity reactions', *Allergy Asthma Proceedings Journal*, 40: 470–3.

Gabe, M.E., Davies, G.A., Murphy, F., Davies, M., Johnstone, L. and Jordan S. (2011) 'Adverse drug reactions: treatment burdens and nurse-led medication monitoring', *Journal of Nursing Management*, 19: 377–92.

Gotterson, F., Buising, K. and Manias, E. (2021) 'Nurse role and contribution to antimicrobial stewardship: an integrative review', *International Journal of Nursing Studies*, 117: 103787.

Jordan, S., Vaismoradi, M. and Griffiths, P. (2016) 'Adverse drug reactions, nursing and policy: a narrative review', *Annals of Nursing Research & Practice*, 3: 1050.

Kirby, E., Broom, A., Overton, K., Kenny, K., Post, J.J. and Broom, J. (2020) 'Reconsidering the nursing role in antimicrobial stewardship: a multisite qualitative interview study', *BMJ Open*, 10: e042321.

Laging, B., Ford, R., Bauer, M. and Nay, R. (2015) 'A meta-synthesis of factors influencing nursing home staff decisions to transfer residents to hospital', *Journal of Advanced Nursing*, 71: 2224–36.

Medicines and Healthcare products Regulatory Agency (2020) *Yellow Card: Guidance on Adverse Drug Reactions*. Available at: https://assets.publishing.service.gov.uk/government/uploads/system/uploads/attachment_data/file/949130/Guidance_on_adverse_drug_reactions.pdf (last accessed 1 January 2023).

National Institute for Clinical Excellence (2014) *Drug Allergy: Diagnosis and management* [Online]. Available at www.nice.org.uk/guidance/cg183. (last accessed 1 January 2023).

National Institute for Clinical Excellence (2015a) *Medicines Management in Care Homes: Quality standard [QS85]*. Available at: www.nice.org.uk/guidance/qs85. (last accessed 1 January 2023).

National Institute for Clinical Excellence (2015b) *Medicines Optimisation: The safe and effective use of medicines to enable the best possible outcomes*. Available at: www.nice.org.uk/guidance/ng5. (last accessed 1 January 2023).

National Institute for Clinical Excellence (2016) Controlled Drugs: safe use and management NICE Guidelines [NG46]. Available at https://www.nice.org.uk/guidance/ng46 (last accessed 21 Jun 2023).

NHS England and NHS Improvement (2019) *The NHS Patient Safety Strategy: Safer culture, safer systems, safer patients*. Available at: www.england.nhs.uk/patient-safety/the-nhs-patient-safety-strategy/ (last accessed 1 January 2023).

Nursing and Midwifery Council (2018a) *Future Nurse: Standards of proficiency for registered nurses*. Available at: www.nmc.org.uk/globalassets/sitedocuments/standards-of-proficiency/nurses/future-nurse-proficiencies.pdf (last accessed 1 January 2023).

Nursing and Midwifery Council (2018b) *The Code: Professional Practice and Behaviour Standards of Nurses and Midwives*. London: NMC.

O'Sullivan, J.W., Stevens, S., Hobbs, F.D.R., Salisbury, C., Little, P., Goldacre, B., Bankhead, C., Aronson, J.K., Perera, R. and Heneghan, C. (2018) 'Temporal trends in use of tests in UK primary care, 2000-15: retrospective analysis of 250 million tests', *BMJ*, 363: k4666.

Pasina, L., Brucato, A.L., Falcone, C., Cucchi, E., Bresciani, A., Sottocorno, M., Taddei, G.C., Casati, M., Franchi, C., Djade, C.D. and Nobili, A. (2014) 'Medication non-adherence among elderly patients newly discharged and receiving polypharmacy', *Drugs Aging*, 31: 283–9.

Pickering, N.J. (2020) 'Covert medication and patient identity: placing the ethical analysis in a worldwide context', *Journal of Medical Ethics*, 0:1–4. Available at: https://jme.bmj.com/content/medethics/early/2020/12/16/medethics-2020-106695.full.pdf (last accessed 1 January 2023).

Royal College of Nursing (2023) Learning Resources. Available at: https://www.rcn.org.uk/Professional-Development/Learning-Resources (last accessed 21 Jun 2023).

Royal Pharmaceutical Society (2019) *Professional Standards on the Administration of Medicines in Healthcare Settings*. Available at: www.rpharms.com/Portals/0/RPS%20document%20library/Open%20access/Professional%20standards/SSHM%20and%20Admin/Admin%20of%20Meds%20prof%20guidance.pdf?ver=2019-01-23-145026-567 (last accessed 5 August 2022).

Royal Pharmaceutical Society (2020) *Professional Guidance on the Safe and Secure Handling of Medications*. Royal Pharmacological Society. Available at: www.rpharms.com/recognition/setting-professional-standards/safe-and-secure-handling-of-medicines/professional-guidance-on-the-safe-and-secure-handling-of-medicines (last accessed 5 August 2022).

Royal Pharmaceutical Society (2022) *Polypharmacy: Getting our medicines right* [Online]. Available at: www.rpharms.com/recognition/setting-professional-standards/polypharmacy-getting-our-medicines-right (last accessed 28 August 2022).

Slight, S.P., Tolley, C.L., Bates, D.W., Fraser, R., Bigirumurame, T., Kasim, A., Balaskonis, K., Narrie, S., Heed, A., Orav, E.J. and Watson, N.W. (2019) 'Medication errors and adverse drug events in a UK hospital during the optimisation of electronic prescriptions: a prospective observational study', *The Lancet Digital Health,* 1: e403-e412.

Smyth, J. (2015) *The NEWT Guidelines*. Wrexham: Betsi Cadwaladr University Local Health Board (Eastern Division).

Verloo, H., Chiolero, A., Kiszio, B., Kampel, T. and Santschi, V. (2017) 'Nurse interventions to improve medication adherence among discharged older adults: a systematic review', *Age Ageing,* 46: 747–54.

Warrington, R., Silviu-Dan, F. and Wong, T. (2018) 'Drug allergy', *Allergy, Asthma & Clinical Immunology*, 14: 60.

Wastesson, J.W., Morlin, L., Tan, E.C.K. and Johnell, K. (2018) 'An update on the clinical consequences of polypharmacy in older adults: a narrative review', *Expert Opinion on Drug Safety,* 17: 1185–96.

7

EVIDENCE-BASED PRACTICE AND THE IMPORTANCE OF RESEARCH

Ann Wakefield

Chapter objectives

- Explore the origins of evidence-based practice, define the term, and examine why it is important in contemporary healthcare;
- Develop the 'right' clinical question following identification of a problem;
- Search and retrieve evidence;
- Identify and appraise different types of evidence;
- Consider how to utilise and apply evidence-based practice within healthcare;
- Evaluate the impact of using evidence in clinical practice, outlining the barriers to and enablers of implementation.

This chapter will explore the origins of evidence-based practice, define the term 'evidence-based practice,' and explore how to go about searching, critiquing, and synthesising literature. We will then consider how to implement evidence-based principles into clinical practice by examining strategies that can be employed to encourage nurses to use evidence as part of their everyday work. Hence, we will investigate some of the barriers to nurses using evidence-based principles and explore how these might be overcome. The aim of this chapter is to help you nurture your ability to appraise evidence critically and make informed decisions about the care you administer. We also intend to support the development of critical appraisal skills so you can decide if the evidence available is based on robust research principles.

Related Nursing and Midwifery Council (NMC) Proficiencies for Registered Nurses

The overarching requirements of the NMC are that all nurses must act in the best interests of people, putting them first and providing person-centred, evidence-based, safe and compassionate nursing care. Nurses should always act professionally and use their knowledge and experience to make evidence-based decisions about care. Registered nurses need to continually reflect on their practice and keep abreast of new and emerging developments in nursing, health, and care (NMC, 2018a).

——————— TO ACHIEVE ENTRY TO THE NMC REGISTER

YOU MUST BE ABLE TO ———————

- Demonstrate an understanding of research methods, ethics, and governance to critically analyse, safely use, share, and apply research findings to promote and inform best nursing practice;
- Demonstrate the knowledge, skills, and ability to think critically when applying evidence and drawing on experience to make evidence-informed decisions in all situations;
- Safely demonstrate evidence-based practice in all skills and procedures;
- Demonstrate the ability to accurately process all information gathered during the assessment process to identify needs for individualised nursing care, and develop person-centred, evidence-based plans for nursing interventions with agreed goals;
- Understand how the quality and effectiveness of nursing care can be evaluated in practice and demonstrate how to use service delivery evaluation and audit findings to bring about continuous improvement.

(Adapted from NMC, 2018a)

The Origins and Purpose of Evidence-based Practice

Florence Nightingale is the first 'nurse' to have used evidence to improve healthcare outcomes in the 1850s. Following her experience in the Crimean War, Nightingale was asked to oversee the management of the barrack hospital in Scutari, Turkey, known for its unsanitary conditions. It was there Nightingale critically examined how the environment influenced health and healthcare outcomes. Hence, Nightingale utilised statistics to help generate the evidence needed to fully understand and predict morbidity and mortality rates amongst those receiving nursing care (Nightingale, 1992; Aravind and Chung, 2010; Mackey and Bassendowski, 2017).

Contemporary evidence-based practice has its origins in evidence-based medicine, which emerged in the early 1970s. Cochrane, a UK epidemiologist, found that people were not getting the care they needed so undertook a randomised controlled trial to compare usual care with care based on evidence. Not only did those receiving evidence-based care achieve better outcomes, the care they received was also better (Mackey and Bassendowski, 2017).

Conversely, modern evidence-based nursing only started to manifest from the 1990s onwards. Evidence-based nursing practice is a decision-making process used to optimise healthcare outcomes, improve clinical practice, and ensure accountability in nursing (Canadian Nurses Association, 2018). Consequently, evidence-based practice encourages nurses to assess the available research evidence, clinical guidelines and other information sources based on high-quality findings to apply the results found to their clinical practice (American Academy of Medical and Surgical Nurses Association, 2017).

What is evidence-based practice and why is it important?

Evidence-based practice has been defined as

> 'the conscientious, explicit, and judicious use of theory-derived, research-based information in making decisions about care delivery to individuals or groups of patients by considering an individual's needs and preferences'. (Ingersoll, 2000: 152)

As indicated in Figure 7.1, evidence-based practice is a way for nursing and nurses to minimise the theory-to-practice gap. Hence, evidence-based practice constitutes a problem-solving approach to

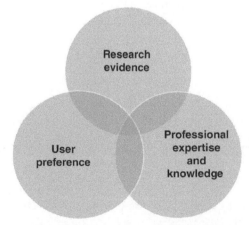

Figure 7.1   The relationship between theory and practice can be achieved when practicing from an evidence base

'clinical decision-making that incorporates a search of the best available literature and latest evidence, clinical expertise and assessment, and patient preference values within a context of caring'. (International Council of Nurses, 2012: 6)

The use of research has steadily increased since the 1990s, thereby improving both health and healthcare services, turning evidence into everyday practice. Thus, by incorporating evidence into practice uncertainties can be minimised when engaging in clinical decision making. Hence, nurses can now choose from a series of alternatives rather than basing their practice on tradition.

Go back to the International Council of Nurses' definition of evidence-based practice and note down why you think each of the elements has been listed. Best available literature, clinical expertise and assessment, together with an individual's own preferences and values are important components of evidence-based practice.

Identifying Distinct Types of Evidence

The knowledge you need to gain greater understanding about what you are doing as nurses and why, is generated from three key sources (Table 7.1):

1   Empirical research;
2   Clinical expertise;
3   An individual's own values.

Table 7.1   Potential sources of evidence

Type of Evidence	Examples of the evidence†sources	Generated by
Empirical research	Qualitative Quantitative Mixed methods	Empirical research Curiosity Questioning practice Critical thinking Reflection
Clinical expertise	Expert opinion Clinical guidelines	Research Trial and error Formal learning Conferences Reflection
Person-centred values	Individual preferences Attitudes Beliefs Choice	Action research Questioning Listening to individuals Communication

Empirical research

The 'gold standard' form of empirical research is the randomised controlled trial – this form of research is employed in quantitative research studies when the researcher wants to evaluate the effectiveness of an intervention.

Randomised controlled trials (RCTs) are part of the positivist, deductive paradigm. In other words, the researcher uses logical reasoning to understand and make sense of their findings. If conducted correctly, RCTs help to minimise bias because the results are not prejudiced by any direct involvement from the researcher. For example, if the RCT is double blinded (e.g., neither the researcher nor the participant knows who is receiving what intervention), nothing should occur by chance and any change should normally occur only because of the intervention. Therefore, RCTs are akin to experiments, and for this reason they are considered to have greater significance in terms of their position on the evidence hierarchy than other forms of evidence, as outlined below. Experimental designs without randomisation, such as cohort, case-control or case report-based studies are still part of the quantitative paradigm but constitute lower levels of scientific evidence. For more details about the hierarchy of evidence, see Ingham-Broomfield (2016) in 'Further reading' at the end of the chapter.

Nevertheless, not all research questions can be answered through positivist, deductive or what is often referred to as quantitative research strategies. Healthcare is not straightforward; rather it is embedded within personal, environmental, cultural, and social dimensions. Consequently, quantitative approaches are not appropriate when exploring such elements of the person or their environment. For this reason, interpretative approaches are needed to explore how knowledge is socially constructed by an individual or group of individuals. Thus, qualitative research explores people's experiences or feelings to generate understanding and meaning of their world, in a bid to uncover how people engage in interactions with others and how they make decisions, or how and why they live their lives in the manner chosen.

Qualitative researchers are therefore interested in gaining insight into the complexities of human behaviour rather than establishing cause and effect. The types of research approach used to generate this form of evidence might include ethnography, grounded theory, naturalistic enquiry, phenomenology, case study and a general, qualitative, descriptive design. Hence, rather than experimental, survey, or questionnaire-based data used in quantitative studies, data collection in qualitative research is likely to incorporate individual face-to-face (including online video-based) interviews, telephone interviews, focus groups, diary recordings, oral histories and/or observations. Hierarchies for qualitative evidence are less well used, although study rigour remains an important consideration. For more details about the qualitative hierarchy of evidence, see Daly et al. (2007) and, for more details about rigour in qualitative research, see Forero et al. (2018) in 'Further reading' at the end of the chapter.

Activity 7.1

Challenge yourself by reading more about qualitative research and thinking about how this might be conducted. Read the suggested texts within the further reading section about case studies, ethnography, general descriptive qualitative designs, grounded theory, naturalistic enquiry, or phenomenology. Compare these with the texts on randomised controlled trials and survey research, and write down what you think the advantages and disadvantages of using each type of research might include. You might also like to find your own reading materials to see if you can use databases effectively and if you can source your own robust materials.

Increasingly, studies that draw on more than one methodological approach are becoming more prolific as the complexities of human behaviour impact various aspects of healthcare. An example of this might include an individual's concordance with treatment. For example, it is no use producing the best-ever cancer drug that will kill off all the cancer cells, only for a person to disagree with treatment plan because the side effects are unbearable. For this reason, many drug trials based on RCTs now include a qualitative element, whereby researchers interview people about their experiences of taking the drug and the impact of any side effects. This type of research is called the mixed method approach, which some would argue, enables researchers to gain a complete picture of the phenomenon in question (Brannen, 2005). Others however, would argue that such research only amplifies the weaknesses of both approaches (Tariq and Woodman, 2013).

Activity 7.2

What do you think are the values of mixed methods research? Have a look at what others have had to say about this form of research and then write down the reasons why mixed methods is a useful strategy to employ.

Creswell, J.W. and Clark, V.L.P. (2007) *Designing and Conducting Mixed Methods Research*. Wiley online library.

Korstjens, I. and Moser, A. (2022) 'Series: practical guidance to qualitative research. Part 6: longitudinal qualitative and mixed-methods approaches for longitudinal and complex health themes in primary care research', *European Journal of General Practice*, 28(1): 118-24.

Schoonenboom, J. and Johnson, R.B. (2017) 'Wie man ein Mixed Methods-Forschungs-Design konstruiert' (How to construct a mixed methods research design), *KZfSS Kölner Zeitschrift für Soziologie und Sozialpsychologie*, 69(2): 107-31. Available at: https://link.springer.com/article/10.1007/s11577-017-0454-1

Timans, R., Wouters, P. and Heilbron, J. (2019) 'Mixed methods research: what It Is and what It could be', *Theory and Society*, 48(2): 193-216. Available at: https://link.springer.com/article/10.1007/s11186-019-09345-53

Now write a list of all the possible limitations of mixed methods research based on what you have read and your own thoughts.

Clinical expertise

Clinical expertise can be based on research; however, it is often based on clinicians' observations of many cases and comparisons of different individual outcomes. This accumulated wealth of knowledge, based on non-research-based evidence, also needs to be considered when engaging in and implementing evidence-based practice. Such evidence might be sourced from or informed by case studies, conferences or discussion papers, and government reports. Consequently, Sackett et al. (1996) argue the clinician's 'proficiency and judgement' gained from university, continuing education and clinical practice experience should be taken into consideration when making care decisions. However, clinical expertise, although important, cannot be used as the sole basis for 'informing evidence-based practice' or clinical decision making. (The latter is elaborated on in Chapter 8.)

Individual values

The values and preferences of an individual can be defined as: 'The collection of goals, expectations, predispositions, and beliefs individuals have for certain decisions and their potential outcomes' (Guyatt et al., 2015: 12). It is those who use health services that benefit from care delivered by professionals who can interpret research findings, understand an individual's unique circumstances, and then working with that individual, construct a plan of care in their best interests, however the recipient of care defines it. Hence, without the incorporation of clinical expertise and individual preferences, best evidence could be used indiscriminately, so a person may choose not to 'adhere' to a treatment plan, or the treatment may not be the most appropriate intervention for that individual, and therefore be ineffective. However, had the clinician consulted the individual to establish their values and preferences, the treatment may not have been considered in the first place and an alternative intervention selected instead. See Figure 7.2 to see the potential relationship between evidence, clinical expertise and individual preference and the impact these three components may have on improving healthcare outcomes.

Hierarchy of Evidence

The evidence hierarchy is a form of ranking based on how robust (i.e., accurate and non-biased) a study may be. Hence, the evidence hierarchy can be considered as a pyramid with systematic reviews and other types of review, focusing on empirical research, sitting at the top of the hierarchy whilst other forms of evidence are located further down the hierarchy, depending on how reliable, valid, credible, and trustworthy the data emerging from such evidence sources may be considered, as illustrated in Figure 7.3. However, before continuing we would like to draw your attention to the difference in systematic reviews, meta-analyses, and meta-synthesis, so you know what each of these terms refers to.

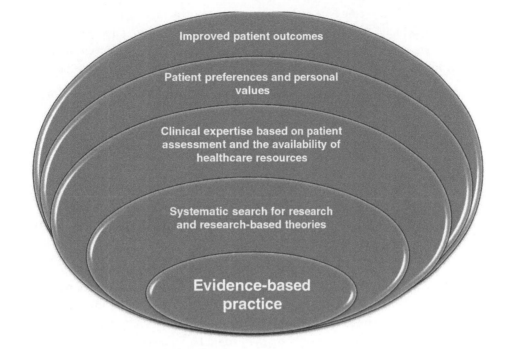

Figure 7.2   The relationship between evidence-based practice, clinical expertise, individual preferences, and the potential to improve healthcare outcomes

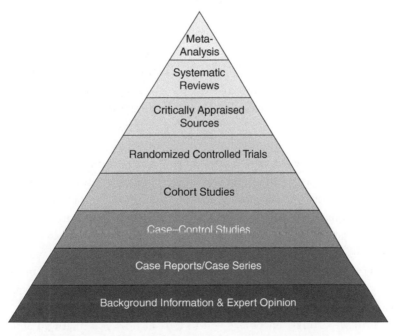

Figure 7.3   Hierarchy of evidence. (Adapted from Porzsolt et al., 2003.
© 2001–2017, The Board of Regents of the University of Wisconsin System)

Systematic review is a specific type of literature review to generate a synthesis of the available literature. The Cochrane Collaboration has produced a handbook to guide people in how to undertake a systematic review of interventions, edited by Higgins and Green (2022), which outlines key features of all systematic review methodologies. A systematic review has:

- Clearly stated objectives underpinned by a set of predefined eligibility criteria to help you decide which studies to include in the review;
- An explicit, reproducible methodology;
- A systematic search that attempts to identify all studies that would meet predefined eligibility criteria;
- An assessment of the validity of the findings of the included studies (e.g., through the assessment of risk of bias);
- A systematic presentation, and synthesis, of the characteristics and findings that have been drawn from the included studies to highlight a set of conclusions and recommendations for future reference and development.

Meta-analysis is the use of statistical methods to combine and summarise the results generated by two or more or even a series of independent studies (Glass, 1976). By combining data generated from relevant studies focusing on the same issue, meta-analyses can provide a more accurate estimate of the effects of healthcare than could be achieved if you drew on data from an individual study. Hence, by combining data from a variety of related studies you can increase the statistical power of the data generated as part of a collective, rendering it more robust (Higgins and Green, 2022). For more information on statistical power, see Porter (2018) in 'Further reading'.

Meta-synthesis is an intentional and comprehensive approach to analysing data drawn from several qualitative studies. Meta-synthesis allows researchers to identify a specific research question, search, select, appraise, summarise and combine the evidence from qualitative studies to then address the identified research question. This process uses rigorous qualitative methods to synthesise existing qualitative studies to construct greater meaning through an interpretative process. For more information on meta-synthesis see Erwin et al. (2011) in 'Further reading'.

As you can see from Figure 7.3, the hierarchy of evidence encompasses quantitative methods. Therefore, the hierarchy as presented would imply qualitative research is less valuable than quantitative forms of research. However, as we have already pointed out in the section related to mixed methods, qualitative research can play a vital role in healthcare by helping us to better understand the people we are dealing with daily. As a result, we need to exercise a degree of caution when considering what research evidence to draw on, particularly when searching the databases for evidence on which to base clinical practice. If we focus on only one type of study, we are unlikely to gain a complete understanding of the topic or the phenomenon we want to examine to administer the best possible care.

For this reason we strongly encourage you to look at how you might go about generating robust evidence on which to base your practice.

Activity 7.3

Reflect on the concept that all three components of evidence-based practice are equal; namely, research, clinical expertise, and an individual's personal preferences. Compare this notion with the ideas presented in the evidence hierarchy. Does the hierarchy imply the research element has greater import over the other two? Should this be the case? Why do you think that? Write your ideas down and share them with your peers.

Steps Involved in Evidence-based Practice

Evidence-based practice comprises six interrelated steps which incorporate the examination and application of robust research within clinical practice as outlined below and in Table 7.2.

Table 7.2 Evidence-based practice in six steps

Assessing an individual	Frequently when assessing an individual, questions might arise where you want to answer why or how something happens, works (or not), or something has simply piqued your interest such that you want to find out more.
Asking the (right) question	When asking a question, it needs to be well constructed so it addresses what you are interested in finding out.
Acquiring the evidence	Here it is vital you gain access to the best and most appropriate resources such as the most appropriate databases or documents to help you conduct a thorough search and generate the evidence you need to appraise, or establish how robust that information might be.
Appraising the evidence	To ensure the evidence you have found is appropriate you need to consider whether it is valid (i.e., sound or credible) and applicable (i.e., can be used or transferred into tangible clinical practice).
Applying the evidence	Evidence needs to be incorporated into clinical practice by combining it with your own or the team's clinical expertise and aligning it with an individual's personal preferences.
Evaluating the impact of evidence in practice	Evaluating the impact of evidence-based practice could involve you undertaking more research to find out how successful the change in practice has been; hence, a new question is generated and the process recommences.

Developing the 'right' clinical question after identification of a problem

As you engage in clinical practice questions will constantly arise, given you should be curious about the world you encounter and those you nurse. Consequently, you need to ask yourself how things can be improved or why something happens or does not work. Alternatively, you might ask what would happen if things had been done differently. The type of question asked will dictate which research approach you adopt to answer it. For example, if you wanted to ask descriptive, comparative, or relationship-based questions you would need to use a quantitative approach to generate the answers. Alternatively, if you wanted to ask exploratory, predictive, or interpretive questions then you would adopt qualitative approaches to your data gathering. Table 7.3 gives a brief overview of what aspect each type of question addresses.

Consequently, how you frame your question is a key element of evidence-based practice, as we will explore in the next section.

Table 7.3   Types of research question

	Type of question	Definition of what each type of question addresses
Quantitative questions	Descriptive	This type of question is used to describe something such as why a particular dressing is used to heal a wound.
	Comparative	This type of question is used to explore the difference between two concepts or variables, e.g., why one dressing is used in preference to a different form of wound dressing or why one drug is better than another.
	Relationship based	This type of question looks at how one variable influences another, e.g., how might rest and/or elevation of a limb assist in healing a leg ulcer.
Qualitative questions	Exploratory	Although similar in nature to the descriptive questions outlined above, exploratory questions are used in qualitative work to try to gain greater understanding about the topic of interest. For example, you might explore why some individuals do not adhere to their medication regimen. Or what forms of care a person might want to receive if they had a choice and why that might be.
	Predictive	This type of question tries to predict why a person would take a particular course of action.
	Interpretive	This type of question tries to gather feedback about a particular issue or topic and as such might seek to make sense of events such as why and/or how nurses organise their work in the way they do. Alternatively, such questions might attempt to establish how acceptable a particular form of treatment is and why that might be.

Asking the right question

To find the most relevant, robust, and reliable evidence it is essential to ask the **right** clinical question, which is grounded in practice.

Questions can be developed in a variety of ways:

- Undertaking or reviewing the research literature;
- Questioning your own or others' clinical expertise and practice;
- Reviewing a person's experiences and examining service-user feedback.

To help you develop your question you need to ensure it meets the following five criteria, namely the question should be:

1 Clinically relevant;
2 Contemporary;
3 Clear and simple;
4 Consistent with the needs of individuals, carers, or service;
5 Manageable.

Let us use a sample question to look at how best to ask the right question in more detail. If we take the following question:

> What impact does case management have on health-related quality of life and satisfaction for cancer survivors?

You could frame the above as either a quantitative or a qualitative question depending on what focus you want to adopt. However, when engaging in evidence-based practice it is usual to adopt a formal framework or structure to help you focus your question and generate key terms. One of the frameworks you can use is referred to as the PICO (Springett and Campbell, 2006) or PICo framework (Joanna Briggs Institute, 2014).

PICO stands for:

P **patient, problem,** or **p**opulation
I **i**ntervention
C **c**omparator or **c**ontrol
O **o**utcome

whereas PICo stands for:

P **p**opulation
I area of **i**nterest
Co **c**ontext

Let us have a look at how you can use both frameworks to address the question identified (Table 7.4).

> What impact does case management have on health-related quality of life and patient satisfaction for cancer survivors?

Table 7.4 Quantitative question broken down using the PICO framework

Element of the framework	Clinical question
P	Cancer survivors
I	Case management
C	Impact on health-related quality of life
O	Patient satisfaction

Now let us see what happens if you apply the same question to the PICo framework (Table 7.5).

Table 7.5 Qualitative question broken down using the PICo framework

Element of the framework	Clinical question
P	Cancer survivors
I	Case management
Co	Impact on patient satisfaction and health-related quality of life

Searching the evidence

If you are going to be successful when searching and retrieving the required evidence, you must be able to identify what literature has been written previously about the topic. However to retrieve robust evidence about a particular topic, you must first generate a comprehensive set of search terms to enter into the database(s) to identify what data is available related to your chosen topic. You need to start by formulating a comprehensive set of alternative words or terms that best capture or describe the main concepts you have identified in your question.

In Tables 7.6 and 7.7 we have identified each element of the PICO/PICo framework that corresponds to our question, and then applied the appropriate element of our question to the corresponding element of the PICO/PICo seen under the 'Clinical question' heading. Next, we have identified alternative terms that correspond with the original question under the 'Potential search terms' heading. By adopting this approach, we can enter as many terms as possible that reflect what we want to explore in the database(s), to be certain we are accessing all the possible research that has been published to date. The reason we need to identify alternative search terms is because researchers do not always use universal words or expressions to describe a particular phenomenon; so, by looking for as many relevant key words as possible we can ensure we capture all the relevant papers that have been published related to the topic.

So far, we have talked only about the PICO/PICo framework. However, there are other equally appropriate frameworks you can use to generate key words and organise your search effectively, depending on what the focus of your search is. These frameworks include the following: SPIDER (Cooke et al., 2012), SPICE (Booth, 2006), ECLIPS(E) (Wildridge and Bell, 2002) and BeHEMoTH

Table 7.6 Generating key words using the PICO framework

Element of the framework	Clinical question	Potential search terms
P	Cancer survivors	Cancer survivors or people with cancer.
I	Case management	Case management or case management model of care or case management model.
C	Impact on health-related quality of life	Impact or effect or influence or outcome or result or consequence. Health-related quality of life (HRQoL) or quality of life (QoL).
O	Patient satisfaction	Patient satisfaction or patients' experiences or patients' perceptions or patient attitudes.

Table 7.7 Generating key words using the PICo framework

Element of the framework	Clinical question	Potential search terms
P	Cancer survivors	Cancer survivors or cancer patients.
I	Case management	Case management or case management model of care or case management model.
Co	Impact on patient satisfaction and health-related quality of life	Impact or effect or influence or outcome or result or consequence. Health-related quality of life (HRQoL) or quality of life (QoL). Patient satisfaction or patients' experiences or patients' perceptions or patient attitudes.

(Booth and Carroll, 2015). Although we have not discussed each framework in detail here, there are dedicated texts linked to each of these alternative frameworks outlined in the references at the end of the chapter.

Activity 7.4

What is the value of using other frameworks to structure a question to define precisely what you want to find out? Reflect on the value of using more detailed frameworks and the additional complexities this may generate. Discuss with your peers the pros and cons of limiting searches depending on what you are searching the literature for.

Try to generate a question for yourself that reflects what you want to look at in practice and apply it to one of the frameworks listed.

Acquiring and retrieving the evidence

Once you have generated your search question you need to use a database, or preferably several databases, to access the most relevant articles (sometimes referred to as papers or hits) so you can review them and establish if they are relevant to your research or are appropriate sources of evidence on which to base your practice. The articles accessed need to be based on sound sources of evidence, so you need to look for research-based evidence in what are termed academic databases because these will enable you to access peer-reviewed journal papers, which should be your main sources of evidence to draw upon and generate your review.

Academic databases

An academic database is a computer program that has been instructed to collate information in an organised manner after your search criteria have been entered into the search box. Academic databases enable you to access peer-reviewed journal articles, conference proceedings, newspaper articles, government and legal reports, patents, and books efficiently.

In effect, a database can be compared with a sophisticated electronic filing system (Oracle Cloud Infrastructure, 2022). However, there are many databases to choose from and you will need to decide which are the most appropriate to help you to access the type of information you think you require. Table 7.8 lists some of the databases relevant to nursing and healthcare. However, if you are going to generate the most comprehensive search possible you will usually need to access more than one database.

Table 7.8   Examples of database information related to nursing and healthcare

Database	Type(s) of information held in the database
AgeLine	Ageing, economics, public health and policy
ASSIA (Applied Social Sciences Index and Abstracts)	Health, social services, psychology, sociology, economics, politics, race relations and education
British Nursing Index (BNI)	UK nursing and midwifery
CINAHL (Cumulative Index to Nursing and Allied Health Literature)	Nursing and allied health
The Cochrane Library	Systematic reviews and meta-analyses of high-quality medical research
DARE (Database of Abstracts of Reviews of Effects)	Systematic reviews
DOAJ (Directory of Open Access Journals)	Open access scientific and scholarly journals
EMB Evidence-Based Medicine Reviews	Best evidence about medical decision making
Embase Biomedical Database	Biological and pharmacological data
Health Technology Assessment Database	Health technology assessments worldwide
Medline	Medicine, dentistry and nursing-related topics
PsycINFO	Behavioural sciences and mental health
PubMed	Health, medicine, nursing, audiology and biology

Reproduced with the permission of *Nursing Standard*.

Activity 7.5

Using Table 7.9 as a template, list what you think might be the advantages and disadvantages of using each of the databases listed, to help you choose the most appropriate database for your task.

Inclusion and exclusion criteria

Once a clear set of search terms has been developed you next need to develop a set of clear and robust inclusion and exclusion criteria, so if we return to our question:

Table 7.9 Advantages and disadvantages of using different databases

Name of database	Advantages	Disadvantages
ASSIA		
CINHAL		
Cochrane library		
EMBASE		
MEDLINE		
PsycINFO		
PubMED		

> What impact does case management have on health-related quality of life and
> service-user satisfaction for cancer survivors?

We might set the following inclusion criteria, in other words, when we have found our papers and start to review them, they must address the following issues, namely the paper must:

- Focus on cancer survivorship:
  - and be related to any form of cancer;
  - associated with individuals from any age group or gender;
- Focus on individuals who have been exposed to case management processes as part of their cancer management plan;
- Address issues concerned with health-related quality of life;
- Address the impact of case management on the person with cancer and their quality of life.

We can also add in additional limiters to focus the papers we review even further; this might include the following, namely the papers must be:

- Published in the English language only;
- Published in the last 10 years only;
- Based only on empirical research;
- Available in full text only.

The exclusion criteria will be all those features that fall outside the inclusion criteria; for example, papers related to cancer that do not address survivorship, case management or health-related quality of life, and fall outside the additional limiters set.

However, you need to be aware that placing limiters on the type of text you uncover means you could potentially miss papers or other sources of evidence that are important to your search. Nevertheless, if you are undertaking the search process for an undergraduate dissertation or review of a particular topic, placing limiters on the types of text you uncover will make the process more manageable. In contrast, if you were undertaking a systematic review, then full text limiters would not be appropriate because you would need to access as many of the papers that had been written as possible to gain a holistic view of the topic.

Boolean operators

An additional way to refine your search is to use Boolean operators to identify the logical relationship(s) between terms. To retrieve the most relevant information you need to link key concepts or keywords together; you can do this with the use of the terms OR, AND, NOT. These terms are the most used; however, another abbreviation you can include is ADJ, which looks for terms that are near to or like the term you want (see Table 7.10 below). For more details see also EBSCO help searching with Boolean operators in 'Useful websites'.

Table 7.10 Using Boolean operators

Boolean operator	Use	Example
OR	Either one term or another is present	Depression OR Mood disorders
AND	Both key words are present	Depression AND Anxiety
ADJ	Finds near or adjacent terms	Childhood ADJ Trauma
NOT	To specify a term that should not be present	Books NOT Internet

Truncations

A further way in which you can improve your search is to use what are called truncations; these are symbols used to represent different types of endings for the same word. For example, if you are searching for something related to nurses or nursing, rather than entering both terms into the database you could use a truncation sign; this is usually represented by the dollar sign ($), although some databases use other signs such as (#). If we go back to our nurse example, if we enter nurs$ into the database it will pull up all variations of the word, including nurse, nurses, nursing, nursery. As you can see, if we want to look only at papers related to nursing, using the truncation symbol will pull up papers not related to the topic, in this case nursery, consequently truncations need to be used with caution. Although truncations can help you capture multiple variants of a term, allowing you to broaden your search, they can make it too broad by adding in unwanted or inappropriate terms. Please move to after paragraph below (wildcards).

Wildcards

A further tool you can use is the wildcard symbol, which allows you to search for words that mean the same but are spelt differently, e.g., behavior and behaviour; by inserting the wildcard symbol into the search term section you can ensure you capture all variations of the term you are looking for. Wildcards can be used in two ways: first as a substitute for one letter (#), e.g., analy#e to find analyse and analyze, and second, as an additional letter (?), e.g., behavio?r to find behavior and behaviour.

Activity 7.6

Try entering a term relating to a question you might want to ask then identify what difference it makes to the number and quality of hits you generate when you use the wildcard and/or truncation tools.

Medical subject headings: 'MeSH' headings

The final tool you can use to help you search the databases is the thesaurus or MeSH terms function. Databases have different sorts of tools to help you find alternative terms or words to broaden your search and are present in most, if not all, databases (Jones and Smyth, 2004; Hek and Moule, 2006).

MeSH, or 'medical subject headings' to give it its full title, comprises a list of over 27,000 terms that precisely describe the content of medical documents (e.g., journal articles). The MeSH vocabulary is a distinctive feature of the Medline database produced by the National Library of Medicine (NLM). The NLM indexers examine articles and other publication types and assign specific MeSH headings to a paper that most appropriately describes what it is about to help you identify more precisely the most suitable papers you need for your search.

Consequently, MeSH headings make searching the evidence more relevant. For example, if you were to enter the word 'aids' into a keyword search in Medline, you would retrieve all articles where the word 'aids' is used; this would include terms such as AIDS, hearing aids and clinical aids as an example. However, if you were to undertake a MeSH search it would map the word 'aids' to the term 'acquired immune deficiency syndrome' (the MeSH heading) and limit the search to that medical condition. Hence, MeSH terms may make your searches more relevant because they allow you to focus your search by research topic.

Activity 7.7

Using the Medline database, enter a term you have used as part of your question into the search section; first, use a free text search and see what results you obtain. Now do the same thing, this time using the MeSH filter, and compare the two searches to see what has changed and whether the information you generate is more relevant to what you want to achieve.

Running a search of the databases

Bearing in mind all we have said so far you should now be ready to run your own search, so in the case of our original question we could enter the following terms into the database(s) to see what sorts of papers we can generate (Figure 7.4):

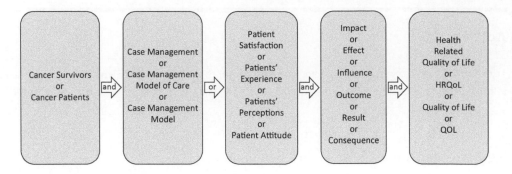

Figure 7.4   Search strategy

What impact does case management have on health-related quality of life and patient satisfaction for cancer survivors?

Activity 7.8

Enter the terms we have identified in Figure 7.4 into a database. We used CINHaL Plus; however, you might choose to use Medline or another accessible database. To narrow the search down further, we limited the texts to full texts published in English from 2012 to 2022. Then to narrow the search down further still, we limited the texts generated by stipulating the terms outlined had to appear in the exact major subject heading list and the papers had to have been published only in academic journals.

You might want to try different combinations of limiter to see what impact your actions have on the accuracy of your results and the number of hits (i.e., texts/papers) you generate.

Identifying and appraising the different types sof evidence/literature

Once the evidence has been retrieved you will need to make a decision about what evidence is the most relevant, reliable, robust, and appropriate to use to help you answer your clinical question. Assessing the evidence can be limited by a range of factors including time and database availability. Practical resources to support evidence-based practice are continually evolving and as health professionals we should always look at the highest level of evidence available.

The first part of appraising the evidence is to sift the papers you have located to identify the most appropriate and relevant evidence to answer your question. This involves a four-stage process as identified in Table 7.11.

Table 7.11 Literature-searching filters

Preliminary literature-filtering process
Title. Look at the title to decide whether it addresses the subject matter you are interested in.
Abstract. Read the abstract in full to compare its content with the topic and your inclusion and exclusion criteria to see if the article addresses these.
Full text. Read the full text to compare the content with the topic, purpose of the study, and your inclusion and exclusion criteria to see if the article meets all your requirements.
Type of article. In this final stage, you will need to decide if the article is what you want. For example, if you want to use only empirical research data in your review.

Adapted from Wakefield (2014).

It is often useful to critique papers as part of a team or with a second person to help to ensure you have drawn robust conclusions about the papers found and the strength of the evidence you have sourced. The more accurate your critique the more confident you can be of the accuracy, relevance, and applicability of your clinical decision to use the evidence you have sourced. However, if you are undertaking a review for an academic piece of work you are not able to critique the papers you have found as part of a group because you could be in danger of being accused of academic malpractice in the form of collusion, so how might you achieve a robust assessment and critique of the papers on your own? Write down your thoughts and discuss them with your peers.

Critiquing the literature

Once you have decided which papers you are going to keep you need to critique them to see if they document robust evidence on which to base your practice. The best way to do this is to use a critiquing tool; these tools can either be generic or specific. Generic checklists are not designed to appraise one particular type of research design (Moule et al., 2017). In contrast, there are several specific tools designed to critique different sorts of research; for example, the Critical Appraisal Skills Programme (CASP) has developed a series of checklists that can be freely downloaded from their website, addressing the following type of studies: systematic reviews, RCTs, qualitative studies, case–control studies and cohort studies, as well as economic evaluation, clinical prediction and diagnostic checklists. (See CASP online learning on how to critique RCTs within the useful websites section at the end of this chapter).

The Joanna Briggs Institute also produce checklists that can be downloaded addressing the following forms of study: case–control studies, case reports, case series, cohort studies, diagnostic test accuracy studies, economic evaluations, prevalence studies, quasi-experimental studies (non-randomised experimental studies), RCTs, systematic reviews, text and opinion papers, analytical cross-sectional studies, and qualitative research.

As you can see, there is considerable overlap between the types of tools produced by both organisations; however, neither provides tools that help you to appraise mixed methods studies critically. Hong et al. (2018) designed a tool specifically for mixed methods reviews called the mixed methods appraisal tool (MMAT). The checklist was developed as part of an international collaboration lead by McGill University to provide a quality appraisal tool for quantitative, qualitative, and mixed methods studies including systematic mixed studies reviews.

Activity 7.9

Choose two papers from your search and undertake a critique of both using an appropriate tool.

Applying the Evidence

Applying research-based evidence to your practice is the next step to implementing evidence-based nursing practice. However, before we discuss how you might try to apply evidence to practice, we are first going to explore some of the barriers to implementing evidence-based practice to help you generate innovative ways in which your peers and your clinical colleagues could be stimulated and motivated to consider making evidence-based practice an integral part of their everyday clinical practice.

Barriers to implementing evidence-based practices within the clinical context

Multiple barriers have been identified as prohibiting the incorporation of evidence into clinical practice (Grol and Wensing, 2004). The following list is not exhaustive, nevertheless it offers some insight into why evidence does not always get translated into practice:

- Lack of time;
- Lack of mentoring or training;
- Lack of skills;
- Lack of confidence;
- Lack of perceived value of evidence-based practice;
- Lack of access to the best evidence; and
- Lack of administrative support.

(Alatawi et al., 2020)

Lack of time

In the current healthcare climate there is often little time to read; hence, nurses frequently do not engage in reading to improve or change their practice. More importantly, trying to implement change on your own is of little value because change management needs to have an impetus behind it; therefore you need a cadre of like-minded individuals to support you in your endeavour (see chapter 10). Moreover, having one person do all the work is not realistic either because it is too much for one person to implement change or motivate others to engage in evidence-based practices, as opposed to those who base their practice on tradition and do not challenge practice.

Lack of mentoring or training

As with any other skill, the factors needing to be taken into consideration when implementing evidence-based practice also need to be learned. It is vital team members have some form of training in how to search for, critically appraise and synthesise the literature so evidence-based practitioners draw only on robust high-quality evidence. For this reason, you need to be aware of how to appraise research so you can be sure you chose the best evidence to take forward for implementation in practice.

Lack of skills

Many nurses do not have the skills to be able to critique the available evidence so they need to be taught these skills to become proficient in critically appraising the research they find to change practice in accordance with the latest evidence.

Lack of confidence

Some nurses have the skills yet doubt their abilities; so it is vital to encourage such individuals to contribute to any debate about practice and the sorts of changes you might want to invoke, considering everyone's views. It is important to have inclusive discussions at clinically based meetings and in practice areas, so that change becomes a negotiated process that everyone agrees to make the change happen.

Lack of perceived value of evidence-based practice

Sometimes nurses may perceive evidence-based practice as simply another fad needing to be implemented to keep managers or those receiving care happy. However, it is important to provide such individuals with convincing evidence to show them how and why evidence-based practice – as opposed to practice based on tradition or 'what we have always done' – is more robust and likely to bring about more positive care outcomes.

Lack of access to the best evidence

This element might be more difficult to overcome if there are strong firewalls in place to protect data and restrict access from rogue outside influences. Hence, it is vital strong links are made with either the local higher education institute or a relevant medical library site to facilitate access to databases and web-based resources. In this way access to the best available evidence can be better facilitated.

Lack of administrative support

Administrative support may not seem to be important. However, if you want to be able to access research papers and disseminate them among the team, having to spend time copying documents is not an effective use of clinical resources. You will need to negotiate with managers in your clinical area about how you might gain access to the necessary resources. Alternatively, if you have access to institutional logins to journals via an organisation, hospital, or educational institution you may be able to gain electronic access to your selected articles. Additional barriers to implemented evidence-based practice are referred to in Alatawi et al. (2020).

Utilising and Applying Evidence-based Practice within the Healthcare Environment

Knowing how to use and apply research-based evidence is now a vital part of the nursing role; this is clear from *The Code* (NMC, 2018b: 9) under the heading 'Practise effectively' whereby nurses are expected to:

> *'assess need and deliver or advise on treatment or give help ... on the basis of the best evidence available and best practice'.*
>
> (NMC, 2018b: 9, Clause 6: Practise effectively)

Consequently, in the final aspect of this chapter, we are going to explore how research-based evidence can be used in practice. For most of you reading this text, the type of evidence with which you will come into contact will be based on research undertaken by others because many of you will not have undertaken original research as part of your undergraduate programme. In view of this, we are going to explore how clinically based research can be championed by any individual working in a clinical area.

Using evidence in practice

There are many ways in which evidence can be used in practice; the following are some examples of how you can do this:

- Developing an information library;
- Ward-based research seminars;
- Journal clubs.

Developing an evidence-based information library for students and clinical staff

One of the ways you can help others to take note of research would be to formulate an evidence-based information library that could be located on an educational notice board in your clinical area. To generate your mini-library of evidence you need to locate and review a small number of contemporary, relevant and research-based papers about a topic relevant to the cases or people receiving care that you encounter.

Activity 7.10

Generate a mini library of papers and rationalise why you have:

1 Identified the papers you have included in your mini library;
2 Targeted journals from which to draw your papers;
3 Chosen specific limits to restrict the number of papers sourced;
4 Chosen to develop your mini library of up to 10 papers for one of the following groups:
   ○ Students;
   ○ Registered nurses;
   ○ Other members of the multi-disciplinary team, patients or service users;
   ○ Carers.

In addition, you also need to articulate how you know the papers you have sourced are high quality, robust, and based on sound research-based evidence.

Did you use the tools we suggested earlier in the chapter to help you decide which papers to choose or did you choose them based on the first 10 papers you found? Which approach is the most effective to use and why?

Write down your rationale and discuss this with your peers.

Ward-based research seminars

Research seminars offer an opportunity for small groups of staff to learn with and from each other about a particular topic or service-user group. Although these capture only a small number of people and may need to be run more than once to encompass a larger group, they are a useful way of stimulating conversations about research in a dedicated timeframe so individuals can stop and think about what they are doing as part of their practice and ask themselves why. You may decide to run such an event because this will help to consolidate your learning in practice and help you to understand better the research process and how evidence can be applied to practice. Engaging in such activities also stimulates discussion and questions practices that might be outdated or simply need to be refreshed.

Journal clubs

Integrating evidence-based practice awareness, critical thinking skills and critical evaluation of the current research literature and applying it to care provision activities can be facilitated best via the use of journal clubs (Lucia and Swanberg, 2018). Journal clubs are an extremely useful tool for encouraging dialogue with and between peers, reading about research and appraising its quality. Journal clubs have been shown to impact positively the development of evidence-based practice, knowledge, and skills (Eusuf and Shelton, 2022).

Activity 7.11

You have been asked by your manager to run a journal club for the staff in your workplace. How might you go about organising such an event? Write down your thoughts before moving on to the next section.

How to run a journal club

Although organising a journal club is not difficult, it is not just an excuse for a chat with your peers and colleagues. Hence, you need to give some serious thought to how you might go about arranging and running such an event. What follows is a brief outline of the considerations you need to consider as outlined below (Eusuf and Shelton, 2022):

Ten steps to success

Step 1: *Select a leader*
This person needs to be committed to the process because they need to review the paper or papers selected in detail prior to the session.

Step 2: *Create goals*
This aspect is vital because it cements what you want to achieve: a forum designed to help people learn how to critique research articles, or review evidence to support practice change.

Step 3: *Identify the audience*
This can be members of a team working in a specific clinical environment, people working in a specific department or specialty.

Step 4: *Select a time and place to meet*
This could be weekly, monthly, or quarterly and be based on site or take place via video conferencing tools such as Zoom/Teams.

Step 5: *Partner with your clinical library to select articles to review*
Connect with the clinical library to help select the most appropriate articles and provide additional training in relation to critiquing skills.

Step 6: *Create forms for summarising/analysing your articles*
Share these in advance of the meeting.

Step 7: *Market and promote your journal club*
Put up posters, send out email invitations or use institutional social media tools or intranet features.

Step 8: *Hold your first meeting*
Encourage and motivate participants to provide discussion and remember to invite a clinical librarian because this person may be able to help when you get stuck, so you do not shoulder all the responsibility of running the session on your own.

Step 9: *Evaluate your journal club*
At each session obtain feedback from participants; this can be verbal, or written via handouts, Padlet, online voting, QR code tools or online survey tools.

Step 10: *Adjust, if necessary*
Depending on your feedback, be prepared to make changes to the session format/content.

Evaluating the Impact of the Evidence in Practice

So far, we have discussed why evidence-based practice is an increasingly important part of contemporary nursing, given that it enables you to base your practice on the best available evidence, minimise risk and promote safe care provision. However, it is not appropriate to simply accept the evidence, implement best practice and continue with that practice recommendation. Instead, it is vital you evaluate whether the evidence is as robust as it claims to be, if improvements need to take place or ideas have been superseded. Additionally, it is important to undertake evaluation studies to ensure evidence is still relevant, or to engage in action research projects to see whether those in receipt of care feel the evidence-based practice is acceptable and fits with their personal values, preferences, and philosophies. In the concluding section of this chapter, we offer you a brief overview of how you might go about undertaking each type of study.

Evaluation and outcomes-based research

Evaluative research is undertaken to assess the worth or success of something (e.g., a programme, a policy, or a project. Evaluation-based research is an increasingly common form of applied social research). What distinguishes evaluation research from other types of research is its purpose; in other words, it is action oriented and often used to support or introduce a change in practice (Linsley, 2022).

In nursing the focus of evaluation research is often on care delivery. Therefore, outcomes will usually be determined by measuring the impact of an intervention, practice, or policy. Different approaches to undertaking evaluation research can be implemented depending on what is being evaluated and measured. These include goal-oriented approaches, which would be used to measure the extent to which an intervention has achieved specific goals or objectives. Economic evaluations are used to calculate the costs of resources and the benefits arising from these whereas utilisation-focused evaluations explore how every aspect of a project is used to determine the answers about a practice, policy, or intervention. Consequently, a variety of research methods can be used in evaluation research, including quantitative, qualitative, and mixed methods approaches. For more information on evaluation research, see Barlow (2004) in 'Further reading'.

Action research

Action research involves healthcare practitioners conducting a systematic investigation into their own practice and, consequently, it is seen as a 'hands-on' participatory approach to research. Action research is primarily focused towards improving practice; the purpose of undertaking the research is to bring about change in a specific context (Parkin, 2009). Action research is often seen as a cyclical process, beginning with the identification of a problem, planning actions, observing and finally reflecting on the outcomes. Nevertheless, the process still may not be completed at this point and may continue until a complete understanding of what is being investigated is fully understood or what is being investigated is achieved. Action research is therefore reliant on both participatory and collaborative working to generate change and new knowledge. In nursing, action research is often about improving standards and generating new knowledge, grounded in the reality of practice. For more information on participatory action research (PAR), see MacDonald (2012) in 'Further reading'.

Activity 7.12

What have you remembered? Test yourself.

Are you able to write a brief synopsis of what you have read without referring to the previous content?

For example, could you define what evidence-based practice encompasses? Could you formulate a robust search strategy? Can you remember how to identify the best evidence to answer a research question? Why might evidence not be implemented in practice?

Write your answers down and then go back over the content of the chapter to see how much you have remembered.

Chapter Summary

In this chapter we have discussed where evidence-based practice emerged from, what we mean by evidence-based practice and how to develop robust, clinically based questions. We have examined how you could search and retrieve the evidence effectively. Subsequently, we explored how you could appraise the evidence generated by quantitative, qualitative, and mixed methods research, as well as outlining the barriers to implementing evidence-based practice. In addition, we have demonstrated how you might go about utilising and applying evidence-based practice within healthcare environments. Finally, we explored how you might approach evaluating the impact of using evidence in clinical practice.

Useful Websites

CASP online learning on how to critique RCTs: https://critical-appraisal-skills-programme.teachable.com/

Centre for Evidence Based Medicine, Oxford: www.cebm.net

Centre for Reviews and Dissemination (University of York): www.york.ac.uk/crd/

EBSCO help searching with Boolean operators: https://www.ebsco.com/

EBSCO help using wildcards and truncations: https://connect.ebsco.com/s/share-video?language=en_US&vtui__mediaId=a1h5a000008bYCtAAM

Joanna Briggs Institute: https://jbi.global/

Mixed Methods Studies Appraisal Tool: http://mixedmethodsappraisaltoolpublic.pbworks.com (last accessed 2 June 2023).

Students4bestevidence: https://s4be.cochrane.org/

TRIP Medical database, Liberating the Literature: www.tripdatabase.com/

Further Reading

Barlow, A. (2004) 'Evaluation research: using comprehensive methods for improving healthcare practices', *Evidence-Based Midwifery*, 2(1): 4–8.

Claydon, L.S. (2015) 'Rigour in quantitative research', *Nursing Standard*, 29(47): 43–8.

Colorafi, K.J. and Evans, B. (2016) 'Qualitative descriptive methods in health science research', *HERD: Health Environments Research & Design Journal*, 9(4): 16–25.

Daly, J., Willis, K., Small, R., Green, J., Welch, N., Kealy, M. and Hughes, E. (2007) 'A hierarchy of evidence for assessing qualitative health research', *Journal of Clinical Epidemiology*, 60(1): 43–9.

Errasti-Ibarrondo, B., Jordán-Sierra, J.A., Díez-Del-Corral, M.P. and Arantzamendi, M. (2018) 'Conducting phenomenological research: rationalising the methods and rigour of the phenomenology of practice', *Journal of Advanced Nursing*, Jul; 74(7): 1723–34.

Erwin, E.J., Brotherson, M.J. and Summers, J.A. (2011) 'Understanding qualitative meta synthesis: issues and opportunities in early childhood intervention research', *Journal of Early Intervention*, 33(3): 186–200.

Forero, R., Nahidi, S., De Costa, J., Mohsin, M., Fitzgerald, G., Gibson, N., McCarthy, S. and Aboagye-Sarfo, P. (2018) 'Application of four-dimension criteria to assess rigour of qualitative research in emergency medicine', *BMC Health Services Research*, 18(1):1–11.

Hammersley, M. (2018) 'What is ethnography? Can it survive? Should it?' *Ethnography and Education*, 13(1): 1–17.

Harvey, M. and Land, L. (2017) *Research Methods for Nurse and Midwives. Theory and Practice*. London: Sage, Part 1, Chapters 4, 5 and 6.

Hensel, P. and Glinka, B. (2018) 'Grounded theory'. In M. Ciesielska and D. Jemielniak (eds), *Qualitative Methodologies in Organization Studies* (pp. 27–47). Cham, Switzerland: Palgrave Macmillan.

Ingham-Broomfield, R. (2016) 'A nurses' guide to the hierarchy of research designs and evidence', *Australian Journal of Advanced Nursing, The*, 33(3): 38–43.

MacDonald, C. (2012) 'Understanding participatory action research: a qualitative research methodology option', *Canadian Journal of Action Research*, 13(2): 34–50.

Mantzoukas, S. (2008) 'A review of evidence-based practice, nursing research and reflection: levelling the hierarchy', *Journal of Clinical Nursing*, 17(2): 214–23.

Mays, N. and Pope, C. (1995) 'Rigour and qualitative research', *British Medical Journal*, 311(6997): 109–12.

Perry III, L.G. and Perry, A. (2017) 'Facilitating student engagement research: a historical analogy for understanding and applying naturalistic inquiry', *Journal of Research Initiatives*, 3(1): 2.

Ponto, J. (2015) 'Understanding and evaluating survey research', *Journal of the Advanced Practitioner in Oncology*, 6(2): 168.

Porter, K.E. (2018) 'Statistical power in evaluations that investigate effects on multiple outcomes: a guide for researchers', *Journal of Research on Educational Effectiveness*, 11(2): 267–95.

Spieth, P.M., Kubasch, A.S., Penzlin, A.I., Illigens, B.M.W., Barlinn, K. and Siepmann, T. (2016) 'Randomized controlled trials–a matter of design', *Neuropsychiatric Disease and Treatment*, 12: 1341. doi:10.2147/NDT.S101938.

Thomas, E. and Magilvy, J.K. (2011) 'Qualitative rigor or research validity in qualitative research', *Journal for Specialists in Pediatric Nursing*, 16(2): 151–5.

Welch, C. (2018) 'Good qualitative research: opening up the debate'. In *Collaborative Research Design*. Singapore: Springer, pp. 401–12.

References

Alatawi, M., Aljuhani, E., Alsufiany, F., Aleid, K., Rawah, R., Aljanabi, S. and Banakhar, M. (2020) 'Barriers of implementing evidence-based practice in nursing profession: a literature review', *American Journal of Nursing Science*, 9(1): 35–42. Available at: www.sciencepublishinggroup.com/journal/paperinfo?journalid=152&doi=10.11648/j.ajns.20200901.16 (last accessed 14 June 2022).

American Academy of Medical and Surgical Nurses Association (2017) *What is Evidence Based Practice?* Available at: www.amsn.org/practice/evidence-based-practice (last accessed 23 June 2022).

Aravind, M. and Chung, K.C. (2010) 'Evidence-based medicine and hospital reform: tracing origins back to Florence Nightingale', *Plastic and Reconstructive Surgery*, 125(1): 403–9.

Booth, A. (2006) 'Clear and present questions: formulating questions for evidence-based practice', *Library Hi Tech*, 24(3): 355–68.

Booth, A. and Carroll, C. (2015) 'Systematic searching for theory to inform systematic reviews: is it feasible? Is it desirable?' *Health Information & Libraries Journal*, 32(3): 220–35.

Brannen, J. (2005) '*Mixed methods research: a discussion paper*'. NCRM methods review papers, *NCRM/005*. Available at: http://eprints.ncrm.ac.uk/89/1/MethodsReviewPaperNCRM-005.pdf (last accessed 23 June 2022).

Canadian Nurses Association (2018) *Evidence-Informed Decision-Making and Nursing Practice*. Available at: https://hl-prod-ca-oc-download.s3-ca-central-1.amazonaws.com/CNA/2f975e7e-4a40-45ca-863c-5ebf0a138d5e/UploadedImages/documents/Evidence_informed_Decision_making_and_Nursing_Practice_position_statement_Dec_2018.pdf (last accessed 23 June 2022).

Cooke, A., Smith, D. and Booth, A. (2012) 'Beyond PICO: the SPIDER tool for qualitative evidence synthesis', *Qualitative Health Research*, 22(10): 1435–43.

Eusuf, D. and Shelton, C. (2022) 'Establishing and sustaining an effective journal club', *BJA Education*, 22(2): 40_2. Available at: www.anesthesiologistpk.com/wp-content/uploads/2022/04/2022-Establishing-and-sustaining-an-effective-journal-club-BJA.pdf (last accessed 14 June 2022).

Glass, G.V. (1976) 'Primary, secondary, and meta-analysis of research', *Educational Researcher*, 5(10): 3–8.

Grol, R. and Wensing, M. (2004) What Drives Change? Barriers to and incentives for achieving evidence-based practice. *Medical Journal of Australia*, 180 (Suppl): S57.

Guyatt, G., Jaeschke, R. Wilson, M.C., Montori, V.M. and Richardson, W.S. (2015) What is evidence-based medicine In G. Guyatt, D. Rennie, M.O. Meade and D.J. Cook (eds), *Users' Guides to the Medical Literature: A Manual for Evidence-based Clinical Practice*, 3rd edn. New York McGraw-Hill education.

Hek, G. and Moule, P. (2006) *Making Sense of Research: An Introduction for Health and Social Care Practitioners*, 3rd edn. London: Sage.

Higgins, J.P.T. and Green, S. (eds) (2022) *Cochrane Handbook for Systematic Reviews of Interventions*, Version 6.3. London: The Cochrane Collaboration. Available at: https://training.cochrane.org/handbook/current (last accessed 22 June 2022).

Hong, Q.N., Pluye, P., Fàbregues, S., Bartlett, G., Boardman, F., Cargo, M., Dagenais, P., Gagnon, M.P., Griffiths, F., Nicolau, B. and O'Cathain, A. (2018) Mixed methods appraisal tool (MMAT), version 2018. *Registration of copyright, 1148552*(10). Available at: http://mixedmethodsappraisaltoolpublic.pbworks.com/w/file/fetch/146002140/MMAT_2018_criteria-manual_2018-08-08c.pdf (last accessed 4 July 2022).

Ingersoll, G.L. (2000) 'Evidence-based nursing: what it is and what it isn't', *Nursing Outlook*, 48(4): 151–2.

International Council of Nurses (2012) *Closing the Gap: From Evidence to Action*. Available at: www.nursingworld.org/~4aff6a/globalassets/practiceandpolicy/innovation–evidence/ind-kit-2012-for-nnas.pdf (last accessed 23 June 2022).

Joanna Briggs Institute (2014) *Reviewer's Manual*. Adelaide: Joanna Briggs Institute, University of Adelaide. Available at: https://nursing.lsuhsc.edu/JBI/docs/ReviewersManuals/Reviewers Manual.pdf (last accessed 23 June 2022).

Jones, L.V. and Smyth, R.L. (2004) 'How to perform a literature search', *Current Paediatrics*, 14(6): 482–8.

Linsley, P. (2022) 'Evaluation, Audit and Research'. In P. Linsley and R. Kane (eds), *Evidence-based Practice for Nurses and Allied Health Professionals*, 5th edn. London: Sage.

Lucia, V.C. and Swanberg, S.M. (2018) 'Utilizing journal club to facilitate critical thinking in pre-clinical medical students', *International Journal of Medical Education*, 9: 7–8.

Mackey, A. and Bassendowski, S. (2017) 'The history of evidence-based practice in nursing education and practice', *Journal of Professional Nursing*, 33(1): 51–5.

Moule, P., Aveyard, H. and Goodman, M. (2017) *Nursing Research: An Introduction*, 3rd edn. London: Sage, Chapters 5, 14, 15 and 21.

Nightingale, F. (1992) *Notes on Nursing: What It Is, and What It Is Not*. Philadelphia, PA: Lippincott Williams & Wilkins.

Nursing and Midwifery Council (2018a) *Future Nurse: Standards of Proficiency for Registered Nurses*. London: NMC.

Nursing and Midwifery Council (2018b) *The Code: Professional Standards of Practice and Behaviour for Nurses and Midwives*. London: NMC.

Oracle Cloud Infrastructure UK (2022) *What is a database?* Oracle. Available at: www.oracle.com/uk/database/what-is-database/ (last accessed 4 July 2022).

Parkin, P. (2009) *Managing Change in Healthcare: Using Action Research*. London: Sage.

Porzsolt, F., Ohletz, A., Thim, A., Gardner, D., Ruatti, H., Meier, H., Schlotz-Gorton, N. and Schrott, L. (2003) 'Evidence-based decision making: the six-step approach', *BMJ Evidence-Based Medicine*, 8(6): 165–6.

Sackett, D.L., Rosenberg, W.M.C., Mur Gray, J.A., Haynes, R.B. and Richardson, W.S. (1996) 'Evidence based medicine: what it is and what it isn't,' *British Medical Journal*, 312: 71–2.

Springett, K. and Campbell, J. (2006) 'An introductory guide to putting research into practice', *Defining the Research Question Podiatry Now*, 26–8. Available at: www.researchgate.net/publication/237406765_AN_INTRODUCTORY_GUIDE_TO_PUTTING_RESEARCH_INTO_PRACTICE_2_Defining_the_Research_Question/link/00b7d52a7b047bfcc4000000/download (last accessed 23 June 2022).

Tariq, S. and Woodman, J. (2013) 'Using mixed methods in health research', *JRSM Short Reports*, 4(6): 2042533313479197.

Wakefield, A. (2014) 'Searching and critiquing the research literature', *Nursing Standard*, 28(39): 49–57.

Wildridge, V. and Bell, L. (2002) 'How CLIP became ECLIPSE: a mnemonic to assist in searching for health policy/management information', *Health Information & Libraries Journal*, 19(2): 113–15.

8

CLINICAL DECISION MAKING

Dawn Dowding

Chapter objectives

- Critically review and discuss the relevance of clinical decision-making theory to practice;
- Identify relevant sources of information and knowledge that can be used to inform the decision-making process;
- Recognise the importance of sharing the decision-making process with service users, carers, families and other professionals;
- Identify key areas for personal development to improve your own decision-making and problem-solving abilities in practice.

This chapter considers the nature of judgement and decision making in professional nursing practice. It explores concepts such as uncertainty in healthcare practice and provides an overview of different theories related to judgement and decision making in healthcare contexts. The aim of the chapter is to give you understanding and insight into how you use knowledge (information) to inform the judgements and decisions you take in clinical practice. It will help you to appraise and critically evaluate your judgement and decision-making skills, as well as how to ensure individuals and their families (if required) are also involved in decisions about their care.

Related Nursing and Midwifery Council (NMC) Proficiencies for Registered Nurses

The overarching requirement of the NMC is that nurses play a key role in providing, leading and coordinating care, that is compassionate, evidence-based and person-centred. Nurses provide care for adults across a variety of settings, to people of all ages from different backgrounds, cultures and beliefs. They need to be skilled in caring for people with complex needs, in the context of a rapidly changing and evolving environment. As a registered nurse you will need to be able to work independently as well as part of a team and have the ability to think critically, apply knowledge and skills and provide expert, evidence-based nursing care (NMC, 2018).

TO ACHIEVE ENTRY TO THE NMC REGISTER
YOU MUST BE ABLE TO

- Demonstrate the knowledge, skills and ability to think critically when applying evidence and draw on experience to make evidence-informed decisions in all situations;
- Understand the need to base all decisions regarding care and interventions on a person's individual needs and preferences, recognising and addressing any personal and external factors that may unduly influence your decisions;
- Use a wide range of knowledge about individual biology, social and behavioural sciences to undertake accurate assessments of nursing care needs and developing prioritising and evaluating person-centred plans of care;
- Demonstrate the ability to accurately process all information gathered during the assessment process to identify needs for individualised nursing care and develop person-centred evidence-based plans for nursing interventions with agreed goals;
- Provide information in accessible ways to help people understand and make decisions about their health, life choices, illness and care;
- Work in partnership with people to encourage shared decision making to support individuals, their families, and carers to manage their own care when appropriate.

(Adapted from NMC, 2018)

In our day-to-day lives we are constantly making decisions. From the moment we wake up in the morning, to the time we go to bed, we are processing substantial amounts of information and using this to make choices about the things we do (or do not do). For example, we make decisions about what clothes to wear, what food to eat, how we spend our time. As a nurse, you will also be making decisions in your practice. What makes the decisions you take as a nurse different are the potential outcomes or consequences that are associated with your decision making. It is for that reason we will be focusing on how you use information (evidence or knowledge) to inform the eventual decisions you take about care provision and nursing practice interventions. Before we explore decision making in detail, complete Activity 8.1.

Activity 8.1

In Chapter 1 you were asked to consider 'Why did you become a nurse?' Ask yourself this again and reflect on the process you went through to make your decision.

- What information or factors did you consider?
- What were the alternatives that you thought about?
- Was there a key piece of information or factor that influenced your final choice?

Write down your answers.

Before we start to explore the process of judgement and decision making, it is helpful to provide a few definitions. First, it is useful to make a distinction between the concept of clinical judgement and that of a clinical decision. Dowie (1993: 9) defined a judgement as *'an assessment between alternatives'*. This definition has been expanded on by Chin-Yee and Upshur (2018) who suggest that the word *'judgement'* refers to the reasoning tasks we use to formulate diagnoses, treatment choices or prognosis. The phrase *'clinical'* refers to the context where this occurs – the world of healthcare practice (Chin-Yee and Upshur, 2018). In nursing, we often make judgements or assessments about a person's state, condition, and prediction of future events; for example, the assessment of risk of developing a pressure injury (Lamond, Crow et al., 1996; Cioffi, 2000). A decision is a *'choice between alternatives'* (Dowie, 1993: 9), and as before the 'clinical' refers to the context where choices or decisions are taken. Choices or decisions about treatment or interventions (plans of care) can be based on our assessment or evaluation (clinical judgement) of information about a person and their situation. Therefore, it is common to find that many authors combine the two concepts together into terms such as 'clinical decision making', 'clinical reasoning', 'clinical inference' or 'diagnostic reasoning' (Thompson and Dowding, 2009b).

Types of Judgements and Decisions

A significant amount of nursing practice consists of assessing individuals (making judgements) about their state or condition. For example, nurses assess pain, whether a person's condition is deteriorating, or their risk of falls, or developing pressure injuries. Nurses make numerous decisions, often based on their assessments or judgements. Thompson and Dowding (2009a) provide an overview of the different judgements and decisions nurses make in clinical practice, based on several different research studies (Table 8.1). Nurses have been recorded to make around 56 decisions every 8-hour shift (Karra et al., 2014) or every 30 seconds in a critical care unit (Bucknall, 2000). While there are differences in estimations of decision frequency (related to the way data were collected and decisions measured in the two studies), what is key is that nurses make a lot of decisions during their working shifts, and, consequently, how those decisions are taken, and the effect on care quality is important.

Table 8.1 Overview of nurse judgements and decisions (adapted from Thompson and Dowding, 2009a)

Type of Judgement	Definition	Example
Causal (diagnosis)	An individual's state or condition - identifies cause of signs/symptoms	Nurse assesses an individual and identifies cause of urinary incontinence
Descriptive	Description of a person's state/condition	Nurse assesses the individual's condition as stable
Evaluative	Identification of a qualitative difference in a person's state/condition	Nurse judges that the individual's condition has deteriorated
Predictive	Predicting what will happen to the person in the future	Individual is at risk of post-operative complications (based on information collected pre-operatively)
Type of Decision		
Intervention/ effectiveness	Choosing between interventions	Choosing a mattress for a frail elderly person
Targeting (Subcategory of intervention/ effectiveness decision)	Choosing individuals who will most benefit from a type of intervention	Deciding which individual(s) should get anti-embolism stockings
Timing	Choosing the best time to deploy an intervention	Choosing a time to commence asthma education for newly diagnosed individuals
Referral	Choosing a service to which a person may be referred for ongoing or specialist treatment	Choosing to refer a person with a leg ulcer for medical management rather than nursing management
Communication	Choosing ways of delivering information to and from individuals, family members and other healthcare professionals	Choosing how to approach cardiac rehabilitation following acute myocardial infarction for an elderly person who lives alone with her family nearby
Service delivery, organisation and management	Decisions related to the service configuration or processes of service delivery	Choosing how to organise handover so that communication is most effective

The concept of uncertainty is also key to understanding how we make judgements and decisions in nursing and healthcare contexts. This has been explained by Thompson and Dowding (2009c: 11) as:

> *Each decision they (nurses) make requires them to think about an uncertain future, in the present, using evidence that comes from a (more) certain past… everyone is unique, and no intervention ever leads with complete certainty to a given outcome.*

In other words, we are making judgements and decisions in situations where we may have incomplete information, where it is not clear what may be causing a person's signs, symptoms, or behaviour, and even if we think we know what action to take, the desired outcome we want may not be achieved. This makes the process of clinical judgement and decision making complex, and it is why it is important to understand if/how your reasoning and decision making can lead to different outcomes for adults in your care. Now complete Activity 8.2 below to see if you can identify the judgements/decisions you took in more detail.

Activity 8.2

Revisit your answers to the questions above – try to think about:

- How did the information you had influence the judgements and choices you made?
- How did you make your decision? Was it a process based on evaluating the information you had available, or did you use a discussion with others as a way of choosing what to do?
- So far – how would you evaluate your decision?

Why Do You Need to Understand the Judgement and Decision-Making Process?

As nurses, we are responsible and accountable for the decisions we take (NMC, 2018), which should, where possible, be based on the best evidence available to guide the decision process. It is important to understand the judgement and decision process because of the impact that individual decisions can have on the safety and quality of care that people receive, as well as the resources used by the health and care system to support that care.

Grace

Grace is 60 years-old and has just been admitted to the acute medical unit (AMU) with chest pain. The nurse looking after Grace has carried out an initial assessment focusing on pain and vital signs and has given Grace some pain medication. As Grace appears fit and well she tells her to call if needed but doesn't give any further information about the care or treatment. The nurse then leaves Grace to do something else. The medication given to Grace for pain causes dizziness resulting in Grace falling over and suffering a head injury when attempting to mobilise alone.

Activity 8.3

- What judgements and decisions did the nurse take when looking after Grace (use the typology in Table 8.1 to help you)?
- What do think could have been done differently to try and prevent Grace from falling?

In the previous scenario the nurse has made several judgements and decisions about Grace and the treatment provided. This includes judgements about what information to focus on as important for Grace's current status (e.g., assessing pain and vital signs – to make a judgement about level of pain and whether Grace is physiologically stable), and some assumptions about the level of function (e.g., fit and well). The nurse makes some decisions about interventions (e.g., giving pain medication – Grace appears to be able to manage without any real instruction), which lead, in this case, to a less than optimal outcome (e.g., Grace is dizzy when standing and is unaware about the potential side effects of the drug). As discussed in Chapter 9, how we as nurses manage risk and an individual's safety is a key part of nursing practice, and often incidents are a result of a number of factors, of which nurses' decision making may be one element. Understanding how we make judgements and decisions can therefore help to mitigate risk.

As well as individual harm, there are also issues related to the variation in the way nurses make decisions about care. For example, Gray et al. (2018) examined variation in the use of evidence-based treatments for individuals with complex wounds (such as pressure injuries and venous leg ulcers). They found that there was variation in the use of antimicrobial dressings (from 18% of dressings used in one area to 69% in another), variation in the use of compression therapy for venous ulcers (ranging from 70% to 98%), and variation in the use of pressure-relieving cushions/mattresses for people with a pressure injury (ranging from 27% to 64% of people having **no** cushion or mattress). There is little evidence that antimicrobial dressings are effective for promoting wound healing (Gray et al., 2018) and they often cost more than non-antimicrobial dressings. In comparison, compression therapy for venous leg ulcers and pressure-relieving mattresses for pressure injuries are evidence-based interventions, and their lack of use may not only compromise the quality of care but also cost the health service more (Gray et al., 2018).

Information and Evidence in Judgement and Decision Making

When we make judgements and decisions, we use information to inform the process. For example, if you are assessing an individual's pain or their home situation, you would collect data or information from various sources and use that information to inform your judgements and decisions. How you use information, including what information you use and where it comes from, is key to judgement and decision making in practice. This is particularly important with respect to using evidence as the basis for our decisions (see Chapter 8). We seek information to try to help reduce the uncertainty in a decision. To do that effectively, we need to access information that is useful and relevant, and available in a timely way. If crucial information is missing, this can lead to delays in decision making or decision errors.

Activity 8.4

Think about an example from a clinical setting where you were asked to carry out an assessment of an individual and/or write a care plan (or have witnessed another healthcare professional doing so). What information did you/they use to help you with the assessment process or care planning process? Where did your/their information come from?

In your response to the above activity, it is highly likely that the main types of information used were derived verbally (e.g., from asking the individual, their family or other colleagues), observation or drawing on own experience. Several studies have explored what information nurses use to inform their decisions. Ebenezer (2015) in a review of information behaviour found that nurses tend to use other colleagues or clinicians as their source of information, rather than seeking out information from more 'evidence-based' sources such as research literature. This is supported by a study in the USA, which observed nurses using professional colleagues and their own clinical experience to inform their decisions (Kouame and Hendren, 2022), even when other sources may be readily available. So, while nurses may have access to health information via the internet for example (Gilmour et al., 2016), in clinical practice settings they are often not used in practice. This is another reason why it is important to understand how you make judgements and decisions, to ensure that they are based on research evidence when it is appropriate to do so.

Overview of Theories of Decision Making

There are several different theories (explanations) that have been put forward to try and understand the judgement and decision-making process. In this chapter we will be focusing on 'descriptive theories,' which describe how individuals make judgements and decisions in practice environments. There are also several theories that focus on how decisions 'should' be taken (known as normative theories), and how we can 'improve' decision making (known as prescriptive theories). If you would like to read more about normative and prescriptive approaches a good introduction can be found in Thompson and Dowding (2009a). The basis for many theories of decision making is the information processing model of thinking.

Activity 8.5

This YouTube video (https://youtu.be/QwOBQsjCloO) gives you an overview of the principles of the information processing model.

After watching the video answer the following questions:

1   What is the difference between the three distinct types of memory?
2   How do you think that the distinct types of memory influence how you make decisions?

What the previous video clip highlights is the importance of how we pay attention to information, how we store it in our memory, and how we retrieve it. How we understand judgement and decision making relates to these basic cognitive (thinking) processes. If we fail to identify important information (cues) we will not retrieve the correct information from our memory to enable us to make an appropriate judgement or decision. Alternatively, ways in which our knowledge is stored or encoded in our long-term memory may affect what information we retrieve – and again impact on the decisions we take.

Hypothetico-deductive approach to reasoning

One of the first series of studies that explored how clinicians reason, was carried out by Elstein et al. (1978). They used simulations of different medical tasks or clinical situations to explore how physicians reached medical diagnoses. From this, they proposed a model of hypothetico-deductive reasoning (see Figure 8.1). A study by Tanner et al. (1987) found that nurses also use a hypothetico-deductive approach to carry out assessments of people described in different scenarios and decide on a management plan for the person.

What this model suggests is that clinicians go through stages to reach conclusions about their assessment or diagnosis of a person's condition or problem:

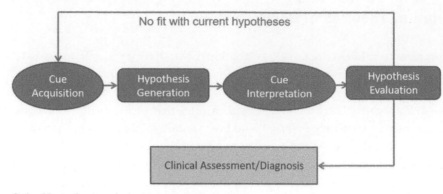

Figure 8.1 Hypothetico-deductive reasoning

- *Cue Acquisition*: first, individuals identify key pieces of information (or cues) from a situation or environment.
- *Hypothesis generation*: based on this information they generate possible explanations (hypotheses) for what the cause of those signs/symptoms may be (potential assessments).
- *Cue interpretation*: they then interpret the information/cues in the light of the hypotheses (e.g., so does the information they have 'match' with the potential assessments they are considering?).
- *Hypothesis evaluation*: if the information cues match a potential hypothesis, they reach a clinical assessment or diagnosis. If there is a mismatch between the information cues and potential hypotheses, the process starts again by collecting more information.

This reasoning process can be related to the process of decision making, where you have a variety of different options or alternative interventions, often chosen on the basis of your judgement/ assessment. Through exploring the evidence for the effectiveness of the different interventions (based on research evidence where it exists) as a decision maker you can then choose an optimal decision. Figure 8.2 gives an overview of this process based on the assessment and management of pain (Dowding et al., 2016).

Expertise and expert reasoning

Following on from the original research into hypothetico-deductive reasoning, other research-ers found that while individuals with little experience in an area (often referred to as novices) may use this approach, experts (more experienced individuals) often use different types of rea-soning. One of the most influential models of expert practice in nursing is that proposed by Benner (1984). Based on work by psychologists Dreyfus and Dreyfus (1980), Benner proposed a framework for how nurses develop expertise in clinical practice. The model proposes that when developing skills individuals pass through five levels (Figure 8.3):

Novice reasoning is characterised by using context-free rules to guide action. Because of nov-ices' limited experience in a situation, they are unable to identify when an exception to the

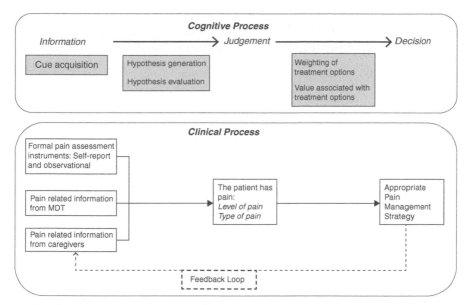

Figure 8.2 The hypothetico-deductive process for judgement and decision making (adapted from Dowding et al., 2016)

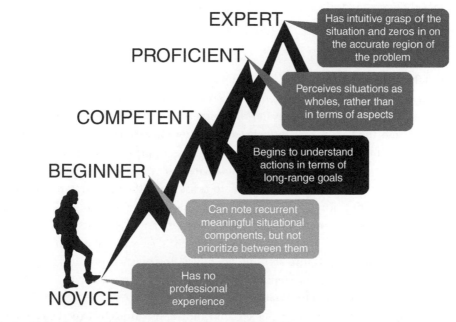

Figure 8.3 From novice to expert (Benner, 1982; 1984)

rule might be necessary. Advanced beginners can use some of their prior experience to use the rules to guide their actions but need help to identify priorities. Competent practitioners can assess situations more globally enabling them to identify what issues are important and what can be ignored. Proficient nurses see situations as 'wholes,' with experience they can identify typical events to expect in specific situations and plan in response to them. They are also able to identify when the 'normal' (what to expect) is absent. Experts can make decisions without using rules or guidelines to guide their actions, often described as having an 'intuitive grasp' of the situation (Benner, 1982). Carry out Activity 8.6 to explore how you match with Benner's framework.

Activity 8.6

Think back to a recent shift you completed in a clinical setting.

Consider your interaction(s) with a specific individual or their carer/relative where you know you made a difference (e.g., there was a positive change in the individual's response and their condition improved). Write down the events and describe in detail your responses during that interaction. Now have a short break before you read your description again.

- What happened during the interaction?
- How did you make the decisions that caused the difference in the person or their carer/family member?
- Are the thought processes/decision processes you used illustrated by any of the elements in Benner's novice to expert continuum (see Figure 8.3)?

Further research into the nature of expertise and expert practice also highlights how it varies according to the experience of the nurse involved. For example, Burger et al. (2010) explored how nurses they categorised as being advanced beginners, competent or expert prioritised an individual's care, and the factors that influenced changing plans of care during a work shift. They found that advanced beginners used a linear process to prioritise their work, focusing on tasks that needed to be completed. If they were interrupted, they struggled to reorganise their care, and relied on more experienced nurses to assist when they encountered unfamiliar situations. This is different to the approach used by competent nurses, who were much more adept at shifting priorities for care depending on the situation and were better able to manage care interruptions. Expert nurses were found to have a holistic view of the person, rather than focusing on care tasks, taking this into account when deciding on their prioritisation for care. In addition, expert nurses were more adept at anticipating future care needs whereas advanced beginner nurses tended to respond to situations or events.

The relationship between information perceived in clinical situations by experienced nurses, and how that enables them to retrieve strategies for decision making from their long-term memory is key to these differences in practice situations. Orique et al. (2019) found that nurses who had two or more years of experience working in medical or surgical units were more likely to identify individuals in a simulation task who demonstrated signs of clinical deterioration. This difference in the use of information was also found in a study by Hoffman et al. (2009), with expert nurses using more information to assess and manage people in critical care environments, and being more likely to be proactive in planning ahead for situations that might happen.

What these studies highlight is that with experience, nurses are more likely to be able to anticipate and identify where a person's conditions may change. This is what Cioffi (2012: 424) calls the '*deep smarts,*' the tacit knowledge that individuals have that they find hard to articulate (i.e., the intuition or 'just knowing' of expert practitioners). The issue with clinicians using this 'intuitive' approach to decision making is that, as it relies on the experience of the decision maker, it may be prone to errors or bias. It also makes it difficult to communicate the rationale for a decision to others, and whether decisions taken have been based on research evidence.

Heuristics and bias in judgement and decision making

Heuristics or bias are cognitive short cuts or 'rules of thumb' that we use to make judgements and decisions in complex situations. They are used when there is limited time to make a judgement or decision, and we are not aware of them as an approach to decision making. Heuristics are efficient and can save us a lot of time and cognitive (thinking) effort when making decisions. However, they can also lead to systematic errors or bias in our reasoning and decision making.

Activity 8.7

Look at the following scenarios and give a response to the question at the end of each one – try to write down your answer straight away.

Scenario 1

Imagine one of your relatives was diagnosed with a cancer that must be treated.
   Their choices are as follows:

- Surgery: Of 100 people having surgery, 50 live through the operation, and 40 are alive at the end of five years.
- Chemotherapy: Of 100 people having radiation therapy, all live through the treatment, and 20 are alive at the end of five years.

Question: Which treatment would you advise them to choose – surgery or chemotherapy?

Scenario 2

Bindie loves to listen to New Age music and faithfully reads her horoscope each day. In her spare time, she enjoys aromatherapy and attending a local spirituality group.

Question: Based on the description is Bindie more likely to be a schoolteacher or a holistic healer?

Scenario 3

Again, imagine one of your relatives was diagnosed with a cancer that must be treated. Their choices are now as follows:

- Surgery: Of 100 people having surgery, 50 die because of the operation and 10 of the 50 survivals die by the end of five years.
- Radiation therapy: Of 100 people having radiation therapy, none die during the treatment, and 80 die by the end of five years.

Question: Which treatment would you advise them to choose – surgery or radiation therapy?

For some of you reading this chapter your responses to the above scenarios would have used a heuristic approach to reasoning. Scenarios 1 and 3 are an example of a heuristic known as the *framing effect*. The decision choice in both scenarios is the same (e.g., the numbers for survival or death are the same for both surgery and chemotherapy/radiation) but one is framed in terms of survival and the other is framed in terms of deaths. How the problem is framed affects how risky individuals will be in their decision choice. Survival rates are regarded more positively as an opportunity, so decision makers are more likely to take risks and, in doing so, choose chemotherapy which has short-term benefits and long-term losses. If the decision is framed negatively in terms of death rates, then decision makers are more likely to be conservative and choose surgery. Have a think about the two scenarios – did you choose different options for each one?

The description in scenario 2 may trigger a response known as the *representativeness heuristic* where we estimate the likelihood of an event by comparing it to a model or 'prototype' in our memory. A prototype is the most relevant for a typical example of an object or event. This often leads to errors in judgement and decision making by overestimating the likelihood that something will happen. In this instance, you may have estimated that Bindie was a holistic healer because her characteristics fitted those of your prototype for holistic healers. Actually, there are more teachers than holistic healers in the population, so she is more likely to be a teacher.

The original research into heuristics and bias was conducted by Kahneman et al. (1982). There are several types of heuristic and bias that have been identified in medical decision making. A summary of some of the most frequently identified can be seen in Table 8.2.

A scoping review of heuristics and bias in nursing practice has been conducted by Thirsk et al. (2022). They separate out studies that explore *cognitive bias* (systematic errors in thinking) and *implicit bias* (automatic spontaneous stereotypes) confirming thoughts that lead to discrimination. Cognitive bias is associated with our thinking, but implicit bias is related to attitudes; both are out of our awareness of conscious thought (Thirsk et al., 2022). The review found 77 studies that explored biases focusing on nursing practice – they found 42 studies that explored aspects of implicit bias (such as effects of race, weight, gender, sexuality) and their

Table 8.2 Examples of heuristics and bias in medical decision making (adapted from Blumenthal-Barby and Krieger, 2014)

Heuristic/Bias	Definition	Example
Anchoring and adjustment heuristic	A clinician relies too heavily on specific data elements and then becomes set in his or her perception of the situation, failing to check for disconfirming evidence	In the example of Lewis Blackman, Acquaviva et al. (2013) suggest clinicians saw a healthy child who had experienced a successful surgical procedure even though subsequent data indicated their condition was deteriorating.
Availability heuristic	People assess the frequency of a class or the probability of an event by the ease with which instance or occurrences can be brought to mind (are available to recall)	After seeing several news reports about car thefts, you might make a judgement that vehicle theft is much more common than it really is in your area.
Confirmation bias	'The tendency to perceive more support of one's beliefs than actually exists in the evidence at hand'	One famous example is Andrew Wakefield's study that linked the MMR vaccine to autism. It was retracted from the *British Medical Journal* in 2010 after evidence that Wakefield manipulated and ignored much of his data. Wakefield's confirmation bias fuelled his desire to establish a link to regressive autism.
Loss/gain framing bias	Losses loom larger than corresponding gains	93% of PhD students registered early when a penalty fee for late registration was emphasised, with only 67% doing so when this was presented as a discount for earlier registration (Gächter et al., 2009).
Representativeness heuristic	'Probabilities are evaluated by the degree to which A is representative of B'	Nurses given a description of a person with symptoms of a stroke, either with or without the smell of alcohol on their breath. Of the nurses who read the scenario with the alcohol, 72.73% attributed the person's symptoms to inebriation – in the group that read the scenario without the alcohol 98.04% identified it as a physical illness(Brannon and Carson, 2003).

effects on practice situation such as pain management, care planning and triage. A total of 35 studies explored aspects of cognitive biases and heuristics, again focusing on areas of decision making such as identifying deterioration and ventilator weaning. The review highlights the implications that clinical judgements influenced by heuristics and bias have on individual outcomes, including receiving different pain medication, variation in triage decisions, escalations in calling a physician or a rapid response team (Thirsk et al., 2022) and in one example death (Acquaviva et al., 2013).

Dual process theory

Dual process theory is a theory of cognition (thinking) that suggests individuals use two different modes or ways of thinking depending on their expertise and the context of the decision situation.

System 1 thinking relies on heuristic processes and is characterised by automatic, quick, unconscious cognitive processing. It is the thinking process that underlies intuition (Thirsk et al., 2022). As already discussed, we often use heuristic reasoning as it is an efficient way of thinking, and whilst often correct can lead to some systematic errors in judgement.

System 2 thinking is slow, rational, conscious, and controlled, and requires more cognitive (thinking) energy (Thirsk et al., 2022). Because of this, most decisions that we take are made with System 1 thinking; we only engage System 2 thinking in specific circumstances (for example when we encounter something unusual).

We often move between System 1 and System 2 thinking depending on individual, contextual and social factors (Croskerry et al., 2013; Thirsk et al., 2022), and need to understand when our automatic, unconscious System 1 approach needs to be 'corrected' to minimise the risk of bias or errors with a more analytical and conscious System 2 approach.

See Figure 8.4 for an overview of System 1 and System 2 processing.

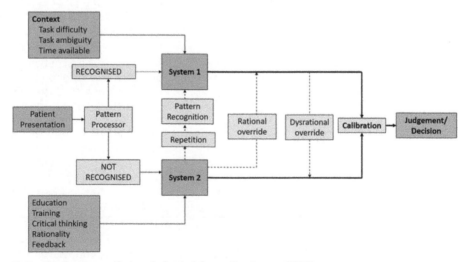

Figure 8.4 Dual process theory (adapted from Croskerry, 2009)

One approach to reducing the risk of judgement error or bias is the development of interventions known as cognitive debiasing (Croskerry et al., 2013a). For example, being aware of potential bias can stimulate individuals to change their approach to a decision situation (Croskerry et al., 2013a). To do this, a decision maker needs to be able to suppress automatic responses created intuitively, to override them and analyse the situation with different solutions to the decision situation. However, this can be challenging; by default, System 1 processing is unconscious and automatic, so it makes it difficult to address.

Croskerry et al. (2013b) identify strategies that can be used in the workplace to try and reduce the likelihood of errors in reasoning occurring. A summary of some of these can be seen in Table 8.3.

Table 8.3 Some strategies for overcoming bias in decision making (adapted from (Croskerry, Singhal et al., 2013b)

Strategy	Comment
Get more information	Heuristics and bias often occur as a result of too little information
Structure how you collect information	Forcing the systematic collection of information may enable you to identify less obvious signs/symptoms or a person's problems
Reflection on initial assessments	Deliberately analysing intuitive judgements to verify initial impressions
Slow down	Accuracy is affected when assessments/judgements are made too early and improves if you slow down the process
Group decision strategy	Seeking others' opinions when you are faced with complex situations can often help reduce bias
Decision support systems	Decision support systems are often designed to reduce errors in decision making

Activity 8.8

Return to your scenario in Activity 8.6, where you were thinking about expertise. Consider if any of the thought processes you identified could be considered as heuristic or biased (look at Table 8.2 to help you). Do you think there are any strategies you could use (for example the approaches in Table 8.3) that could reduce the risk of having biased approaches to decision making in the future?

Clinical decision support systems

Decision support systems or tools have been developed to try and support clinicians' decision making and reduce the likelihood of decision error or bias. Decision support tools integrate evidence (ideally from high-quality research) with the characteristics of the person being cared for to provide guidance and advice to support decision making during professional practice

(Dowding, 2008). Decision tools can provide information and advice to nurses in a variety of formats, including paper-based guidance, more structured approaches such as decision algorithms or using computerised systems. The key distinction between decision support systems, and systems that search for research evidence or information online, is that with decision support there is some form of integration with a person's own individual characteristics and the provision of advice/guidance to the decision maker.

If we relate this back to the simple judgement and decision process outlined in Figure 8.2, a decision support system may be designed to support one part of the decision process or several different elements of the process (Figure 8.5).

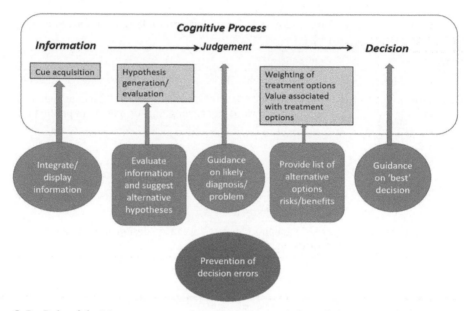

Figure 8.5 Role of decision support tools in the process of clinical decision making

For example, if you want to support the information gathering/cue acquisition phase of decision making, you may develop tools that assist with data integration or displaying information in a way that helps nurses process it more effectively. Many of the risk assessment tools you use in nursing practice are designed to help this part of the judgement and decision-making process, such as pressure injury risk assessment tools (Samuriwo and Dowding, 2014) or pain assessment tools (Dowding et al., 2016).

For hypothesis generation/evaluation, the tool may automate the process of information evaluation and suggest a variety of alternative hypotheses/diagnoses to the clinician. Some tools may also give guidance on what judgement is most likely (e.g., the probability of the person having a certain diagnosis/problem) based on the information provided. Alternative decision support tools may focus on helping with the decision process or helping clinicians/individuals in our care choose between different treatment options. This can include providing a list of alternative options and their risks and benefits and/or giving guidance on what would be the best decision/treatment option for a particular situation. The focus of many decision support tools is to try and promote more 'Type 2' or analytical thinking, with the overall aim of preventing diagnostic and decision errors (decision support systems are explored further in Chapter 5).

Involving People in Decisions: Shared Decision Making

The NHS Long Term Plan (NHS England, 2019) highlights a shift in care provision for nurses and other health care professionals, to deliver more 'person centred care' working alongside individuals and their families as partners in their care. This requires nurses to be able to engage people in decisions about their health and wellbeing, focusing on a process of shared decision making. Shared decision making is also the focus of a NICE guideline and should be part of routine communication with people about their care (NICE, 2021). Elwyn et al. (2017: 1) define shared decision making as:

'A process in which decisions are made in a collaborative way, where trustworthy information is provided in accessible formats about a set of options, typically in situations where the concerns, personal circumstances, and contexts of patients and their families play a major role in decisions'.

Adopting a shared decision-making approach is a collaborative process, where the person is an 'equal,' meaning that the role of the clinician is less patriarchal as in for example 'doctor knows best.' It also encourages the consideration and use of evidence from research, alongside the person's own views, experiences, and values to make a decision. In addition, it considers the extent to which a person wants involvement in the process. Involving someone in the process of decision making has been shown to increase influenza vaccination rates in adults (Sanftenberg et al., 2021), decrease the use of antibiotics when treating acute respiratory infections in primary care (Coronado-Vázquez et al., 2020) and improve an individual's knowledge about their condition (Saheb et al., 2017; Coronado-Vázquez et al., 2020).

Facilitating a more shared approach to decision making means you will need to concentrate on the way in which you talk to and share information with the person being cared for. Elwyn et al. (2017) propose the 'three-talk model' for consultations, which represents a formal process designed to help clinicians move someone from initial and potentially uninformed preferences to having informed preferences for different decision options to help them make a better quality decision. Key activities undertaken by the clinician include *Active listening* (paying close attention to what the person is saying and responding accurately) and *Deliberation* (the process by which you are thinking about options available and ensuring that they have been fully considered). The first phase of the three-talk model is that of '*Team Talk*,' where the focus is to encourage the clinician and person being cared for to work together to identify an optimal decision option. The second phase is that of '*Option Talk*,' where different alternatives are discussed, and the risks/benefits of each option are identified, and the options are compared. The third phase is *'Decision Talk*,' where a preference-based decision can be taken, as the individual receiving care now has informed preferences for the different options. It is important to note that the process may be iterative, and each phase informs the other.

One way you can present information or research evidence to people about the benefits or harms of different treatment options is by using a tool called a decision aid. Decision aids are different to decision support tools or systems; they are specifically designed to help people to make health and care decisions rather than supporting clinicians to make clinical decisions. They do vary in their content but normally contain information about:

- The benefits/harms of a treatment or intervention;
- Enough detail for an individual to make an evaluation about their choices;
- An exercise to help people identify what is most important to them (values clarification);
- Information from other people about their experiences, to provide insight into the different treatment options;
- A structured process to help people undertake a formal deliberation to identify the best option for them (Stacey et al., 2017).

There are a few different decision aids available for you and those you care for to help with common healthcare decisions. For example, NICE has published several decision aids that are linked to guidance documents (NICE, 2021) and the Ottowa Hospital Research Institute (2021) also has an online inventory of decision aids. A systematic review found that using decision aids increases knowledge, with individuals feeling better informed about the decisions they take, and accuracy of the risks associated with different treatment interventions (Stacey et al., 2017). To learn more about decision aids complete Activity 8.9.

Activity 8.9

Go to the NICE website for the decision aid for helping people with asthma discuss their options for inhaler devices (Patient decision aid: Inhalers for asthma (nice.org.uk)).

Imagine that you are someone who has just been diagnosed with asthma, and you are trying to decide what type of inhaler might be useful for you to help manage your condition. Work through the decision aid, and then decide the type of inhaler you think you might use in this situation.

- Did you find using the decision aid useful to help your thinking process?
- Reflect on how you might use decision aids like this to help you talk to people about their treatment interventions in the future.

What Can You Do to Help Your Decision-Making Skills?

Several things influence how nurses make clinical decisions, including experience and confidence, as well as external factors such as workload and time available to make decisions (Thompson et al., 2008; Nibbelink and Brewer, 2018). Table 8.3 has already highlighted some strategies that you can use to encourage a more systematic and analytical approach to decision making and 'debias' unconscious thought processes. In addition, Gillespie and Peterson (2009) propose the Situated Clinical Decision-Making Framework to help novice nurses reflect on the decisions they take in clinical practice and begin to develop the features of expert decision making. A schematic representation of the framework can be seen in Figure 8.6.

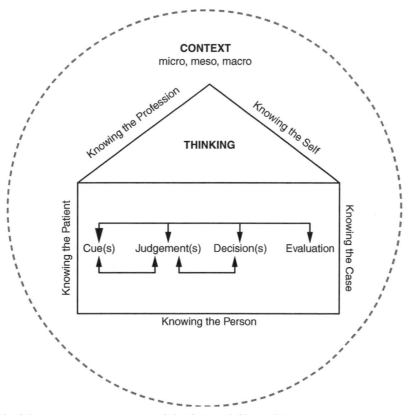

Figure 8.6 Schematic representation of the Situated Clinical Decision-Making Framework (Gillespie and Peterson, 2009)

The framework recognises the context where nurses work at *micro* (e.g., nurse and individual being cared for), *meso* (e.g., nursing unit or department) and *macro* (e.g., society, government, profession) levels. It identifies the foundational knowledge that informs nurses' clinical decision-making processes which include:

Knowing the profession: the ability to acknowledge and incorporate relevant principles, values, and standards of nursing and to use them to inform the decision-making process;

Knowing the self: the importance of being able to reflect on your own strengths and limitations, skills, experience, competence and learning needs, and to be willing to seek help and support if needed;

Knowing the case: the use of knowledge and understanding of related sciences (e.g., pathophysiology and typical patterns of health, disease and illness, patient responses, predicted outcomes) and the ability to apply this knowledge to the decision-making process;

Knowing the patient: focusing on a person's physiological state and being aware of the person's baseline data and the patterns within their individual physiological responses to treatment;

Knowing the person: builds on the concept of the therapeutic relationship and involves acknowledging that every person's experience of health and illness is unique, as is their capacity to be involved in the decision-making process.

Activity 8.10

Think of another situation where you were in clinical practice and had to assess and manage the clinical care of someone in your care. Reflect on this situation and answer the following questions related to the judgement/decision process you used:

1   Information cues – What observations did you make? What other information did you use to inform your judgements? What knowledge was it based on? Do you think you collected all the relevant information you needed to make an informed assessment? What would you do differently next time?

2   Judgements – What do you think was happening with this individual? What data/evidence supported this assessment? Did you need more information? Where would that come from? Was there anyone else you should/could involve or consult? What priority does the situation have?

3   Decision(s) – Different options could include should I wait and watch? Should I try something? Should I inform someone? Should I involve or consult someone else? How will I know if I made the best decision? What did I decide to do and why?

4   Evaluation of outcomes – Did the decision achieve what I wanted to happen? Should I make another decision? Should I collect more information? Whom should I involve or consult?

At the end of your reflection think about if or how you would manage the situation differently if you were faced with a similar individual again.

Chapter Summary

This chapter has focused on different theories that describe how nurses make judgements and decisions in clinical practice settings. It examined key concepts, including what clinical judgements and clinical decisions are, and how they are affected by the uncertainty that is part of healthcare practice. It has provided an overview of how clinical judgement and decision making varies depending on the experience of the person making decisions and how you can involve patients more in the decision process. All the strategies and concepts discussed in this chapter can help you to make effective, evidence-based (where appropriate) decisions in practice.

Further Reading

Benner, P.E. (1984) *From Novice to Expert: Excellence and power in clinical nursing practice*. Menlo Park, CA: Addison-Wesley.

Nibbelink, C.W. and Brewer, B.B. (2018) 'Decision-making in nursing practice: an integrative literature review', *Journal of Clinical Nursing*, 27(5–6): 917–28.

Thompson, C. and Dowding, D. (2009) *Essential Decision Making and Clinical Judgement for Nurses*. Edinburgh, Churchill Livingstone.

References

Acquaviva, K., Haskell, H. and Johnson, J. (2013) 'Human cognition and the dynamics of failure to rescue: the Lewis Blackman case', *Journal of Professional Nursing*, 29(2): 95–101.

Benner, P. (1982) 'From novice to expert', *The American Journal of Nursing*, 82(3): 402–7.

Benner, P.E. (1984) *From Novice to Expert: Excellence and power in clinical nursing practice*. Menlo Park, CA: Addison-Wesley.

Blumenthal-Barby, J.S. and Krieger, H. (2014) 'Cognitive biases and heuristics in medical decision making: a critical review using a systematic search strategy', *Medical Decision Making*, 35(4): 539–57.

Bucknall, T.K. (2000) 'Critical care nurses' decision-making activities in the natural clinical setting', *Journal of Clinical Nursing*, 9(1): 25–35.

Burger, J.L., Parker, K., Cason, L., Hauck, S., Kaetzel, D., Nan, C. and White, A. (2010) 'Responses to work complexity: the novice to expert effect', *Western Journal of Nursing Research*, 32(4): 497–510.

Chin-Yee, B. and Upshur, R. (2018) 'Clinical judgement in the era of big data and predictive analytics', *Journal of Evaluation in Clinical Practice*, 24(3): 638–45.

Cioffi, J. (2000) 'Recognition of patients who require emergency assistance: a descriptive study', *Heart & Lung*, 29(4): 262–8.

Cioffi, J.M. (2012) 'Loss of clinical nursing expertise: a discussion paper', *International Journal of Nursing Practice*, 18(5): 423–8.

Coronado-Vázquez, V., Canet-Fajas, C., Delgado-Marroquín, M.T., Magallón-Botaya, R., Romero-Martín, M. and Gómez-Salgado, J. (2020) 'Interventions to facilitate shared decision-making using decision aids with patients in Primary Health Care: a systematic review', *Medicine,* 99(32): e21389.

Croskerry, P. (2009) 'A universal model of diagnostic reasoning', *Academic Medicine,* 84(8): 1022–8.

Croskerry, P., Singhal, G. and Mamede, S. (2013a) 'Cognitive debiasing 1: origins of bias and theory of debiasing', *BMJ Quality and Safety,* 22(Suppl 2): ii58.

Croskerry, P., Singhal, G. and Mamede, S. (2013b) 'Cognitive debiasing 2: impediments to and strategies for change', *BMJ Quality and Safety,* 22(Suppl 2): ii65.

Dowding, D. (2008) 'Computerised decision support systems in nursing'. In N. A. Cullum, D. Ciliska, B. Haynes and S. Marks (eds), *Evidence-Based Nursing: An Introduction.* Oxford: Blackwell Pub/BMJ Journals/RCN Pub: 271–6.

Dowding, D., Lichtner, V., Allcock, N., Briggs, M., James, K., Keady, J., Lasrado, R., Sampson, E.L., Swarbrick, C. and José Closs, S. (2016) 'Using sense-making theory to aid understanding of the recognition, assessment and management of pain in patients with dementia in acute hospital settings', *International Journal of Nursing Studies,* 53: 152–62.

Dowie, J. (1993) 'Clinical decision analysis: background and introduction.' In H.A. Llewelyn (ed.), *Analysing How we Reach Clinical Decisions.* London: Royal College of Physicians: 7–26.

Dreyfus, S.E. and Dreyfus, H.L. (1980) *A Five-Stage Model of the Mental Activities Involved in Directed Skill Acquisition.* Berkeley, CA: Operations Research Center, University of California.

Ebenezer, C. (2015) 'Nurses' and midwives' information behaviour: a review of literature from 1998 to 2014', *New Library World,* 116(3/4): 155–72.

Elstein, A.S., Shulman, L.S. and Sprafka, S.A. (1978) *Medical Problem Solving: An analysis of clinical reasoning.* Cambridge, MA: Harvard University Press.

Elwyn, G., Durand, M.A., Song, J., Aarts, J., Barr, P.J., Berger, Z., Cochran, N., Frosch, D, Galasiński, D., Gulbrandsen, P., Han, P.K.J., Härter, M., Kinnersley, P., Lloyd, A., Mishra, M., Perestelo-Perez, L., Scholl, I., Tomori, K., Trevena, L., Witteman, H.O. and Van der Weijden, T. (2017) 'A three-talk model for shared decision making: multistage consultation process', *BMJ,* 359: j4891.

Gillespie, M. and Peterson, B.L. (2009) 'Helping novice nurses make effective clinical decisions: the situated clinical decision-making framework', *Nursing Education Perspectives,* 30(3): 164–70.

Gilmour, J., Strong, A., Chan, H., Hanna, S. and Huntington, A. (2016) 'Primary health-care nurses and Internet health information-seeking: access, barriers and quality checks', *International Journal of Nursing Practice,* 22(1): 53–60.

Gray, T.A., Rhodes, S., Atkinson, R.A., Rothwell, K., Wilson, P., Dumville, J.C. and Cullum, N.A. (2018) 'Opportunities for better value wound care: a multiservice, cross-sectional survey of complex wounds and their care in a UK community population', *BMJ Open,* 8(3): e019440.

Hoffman, K.A., Aitken, L.M. and Duffield, C. (2009) 'A comparison of novice and expert nurses' cue collection during clinical decision-making: verbal protocol analysis', *International Journal of Nursing Studies,* 46(10): 1335–44.

Kahneman, D., Slovic, P. and Tversky, A. (1982) *Judgment under Uncertainty: Heuristics and Biases.* Cambridge: Cambridge University Press.

Karra, V., Papathanassoglou, E.D., Lemonidou, C., Sourtzi, P. and M Giannakopoulou, M. (2014) 'Exploration and classification of intensive care nurses' clinical decisions: a Greek perspective', *Nursing in Critical Care,* 19(2): 87–97.

Kouame, G. and Hendren, S. (2022) 'Library tools at the nurses' station: exploring information-seeking behaviors and needs of nurses in a war veterans nursing home', *Journal of the Medical Library Association: JMLA*, 110(2): 159–65.

Lamond, D., Crow, R.A. and Chase, J. (1996) 'Judgements and processes in care decisions in acute medical and surgical wards', *Journal of Evaluation in Clinical Practice*, 2(3): 211–16.

NHS England (2019) *The NHS Long Term Plan*. NHS England.Available at: www.longtermplan.nhs.uk/ (last accessed 20 June 2023).

Nibbelink, C.W. and Brewer, B.B. (2018) 'Decision-making in nursing practice: an integrative literature review', *Journal of Clinical Nursing*, 27(5-6): 917–28.

NICE (2021) *Shared Decision Making* (NG197). London: National Institute for Health and Care Excellence.

NMC (2018) *Future Nurse: Standards of Proficiency for Registered Nurses*. London: Nursing and Midwifery Council.

Orique, S.B., Despins, L., Wakefield, B.J., Erdelez, S. and Vogelsmeier, A. (2019) 'Perception of clinical deterioration cues among medical-surgical nurses', *Journal of Advanced Nursing*, 75(11): 2627–37.

Ottawa Hospital Research Institute (2021) *A to Z Inventory – Patient Decision Aids*. Available at: https://decisionaid.ohri.ca/AZinvent.php. (last accessed 15 July 2022).

Saheb Kashaf, M., McGill, E.T. and Berger, Z.D. (2017) 'Shared decision-making and outcomes in type 2 diabetes: a systematic review and meta-analysis', *Patient Education and Counseling*, 100(12): 2159–71.

Samuriwo, R. and Dowding, D. (2014) 'Nurses' pressure ulcer related judgements and decisions in clinical practice: a systematic review', *International Journal of Nursing Studies*, 51(12): 1667–85.

Sanftenberg, L., Kuehne, F., Anraad, C., Jung-Sievers, C., Dreischulte, T. and Gensichen, J. (2021) 'Assessing the impact of shared decision-making processes on influenza vaccination rates in adult patients in outpatient care: a systematic review and meta-analysis', *Vaccine*, 39(2): 185–96.

Stacey, D., Légaré, F., Lewis, K., Barry, M.J., Bennett, C.L., Eden, K.B., Holmes-Rovner, M., Llewellyn-Thomas, H., Lyddiatt, A., Thomson, R. and et al. (2017) 'Decision aids for people facing health treatment or screening decisions', *Cochrane Database of Systematic Reviews*, (4).

Tanner, C., Padrick, K., Westfall, U. and Putzier, D. (1987) 'Diagnostic reasoning strategies of nurses and nursing students', *Nursing Research*, 36(6): 358–65.

Thirsk, L.M., Panchuk, J.T., Stahlke, S. and Hagtvedt, R. (2022) 'Cognitive and implicit biases in nurses' judgment and decision-making: a scoping review', *International Journal of Nursing Studies*, 133: 104284.

Thompson, C., Dalgleish, L., Bucknall, T., Estabrooks, C., Hutchinson, A.M., Fraser, K., de Vos, R., Binnekade, J., Barrett, G. and Saunders, J. (2008) 'The effects of time pressure and experience on nurses' risk assessment decisions: a signal detection analysis', *Nursing Research*, 57(5): 302–11.

Thompson, C. and Dowding, D. (2009a) *Essential Decision Making and Clinical Judgement for Nurses*. Edinburgh, Churchill Livingstone.

Thompson, C. and Dowding, D. (2009b) 'Introduction'. In C. Thompson and D. Dowding (eds), *Essential Decision Making and Clinical Judgement for Nurses*. Edinburgh: Churchill Livingstone: 1–9.

Thompson, C. and Dowding, D. (2009c) 'Uncertainty and Nursing'. In C. Thompson and D. Dowding (eds), *Essential Decision Making and Clinical Judgement for Nurses*. Edinburgh: Churchill Livingstone: 10–25.

9

LEADERSHIP AND MANAGEMENT

Dianne Burns

Chapter objectives

- Encourage consideration of your own identity as a leader and reflect upon the potential impact of personal resilience and emotional intelligence on your own leadership style and approaches;
- Critically explore various leadership and management philosophies, styles, skills, and approaches and consider the extent to which these can be adopted to make a positive impact on multi-professional care delivery;
- Explain the difference between 'risk aversion' and 'risk management' and apply effective strategies for risk assessment and management to provide a safe and healthy environment for service users, staff, and visitors.

So far in this book we have focused on the knowledge, understanding and skills required by a registered nurse to assess the needs of adults and deliver evidence-based care effectively in a variety of settings. Yet this is not enough; being able to manage the delivery of care, coordinate team activities, delegate care tasks and supervise the work of others is an essential part of every registered nurse's role and there is an increasing expectation that nurses will take on more leadership roles in the future (The King's Fund, 2011).

The aim of this chapter is to introduce you to a selection of leadership and management theories, models, styles, and approaches that can be applied within any contemporary healthcare setting. The activities in this chapter are designed to help you to reflect upon the importance of leadership and management skills, recognising areas for personal development to help you successfully lead healthcare teams in the future.

Related Nursing and Midwifery Council (NMC) Proficiencies for Registered Nurses

The overarching requirement of the NMC is that all nurses must provide leadership by acting as a role model for best practice in the delivery of nursing care. They are responsible for managing nursing care and are accountable for the appropriate delegation and supervision of care provided by others in the team, (including carers). They play an active and equal role in the interdisciplinary team, collaborating and communicating effectively with a range of colleagues. They assess risks to safety or experience and take appropriate action to manage those, putting the best interests, needs and preferences of people first (NMC, 2018a: 19).

▬▬▬▬▬ TO ACHIEVE ENTRY TO THE NMC REGISTER
YOU MUST BE ABLE TO ▬▬▬▬▬

- Demonstrate an understanding of how to make best use of the contributions of others involved in providing care;
- Exhibit leadership potential by demonstrating an ability to guide, support and motivate individuals, interacting confidently with other members of the care team;
- Understand the principles of effective leadership, management, group/organisational dynamics, and culture, applying these to team working and decision making to lead and manage the nursing care of a group of people safely and effectively;
- Demonstrate appropriate prioritisation, delegation, and assignment of care responsibilities to others involved in providing care;
- Apply an understanding of the differences between risk aversion and risk management and how to avoid compromising quality of care and health outcomes;
- Understand and apply the principles of health and safety legislation and regulations and maintain safe work and care environments;
- Demonstrate the ability to identify and manage risks and take proactive measures to improve the quality of care and services when needed;
- Demonstrate the ability to accurately undertake risk assessments in a range of care settings using a range of contemporary assessment and improvement tools;
- Understand the interrelationship of safe staffing levels, appropriate skills mix, safety, and quality of care, recognising the risks to public protection and quality of care, and escalating concerns appropriately;
- Demonstrate an understanding of how to identify, report and critically reflect on near misses, critical incidents, major incidents, and serious adverse events to learn from them and influence your future practice;
- Understand the principles and application of processes for performance management and how these apply to the nursing team;
- Demonstrate the ability to challenge and provide constructive feedback about care delivered by others in the team;

- Support others to identify and agree individual learning needs and provide encouragement in a way that helps them to reflect on and improve their practice;
- Demonstrate effective coordination and navigation skills through conflict, applying appropriate confrontation, negotiation, and de-escalation strategies.

(Adapted from NMC, 2018a)

The main purpose of leadership and management in healthcare settings is to maintain and improve care provision. This can be challenging when healthcare is constantly changing and there are a wide variety of competing factors to consider such as an ageing and increasingly culturally diverse population; continuous pharmacological, technological, and surgical advances, coupled with demands to meet government quality targets while also coping with rapid turnover; maintaining safety, managing risk, and containing rising costs in current financial climates. All of these are extraordinarily complex challenges. Added to this is evidence of serious deficiencies in care that have undermined public confidence and where leadership deficits have been clearly highlighted in previous chapters (Francis, 2013; Kirkup, 2015, 2018; Ockenden, 2022). Consequently, there are increasing calls for stronger leadership that not only positively influences the quality of care but also promotes a caring and compassionate culture (West, 2021). Clearly, healthcare organisations need strong, successful, and inclusive leaders and managers who can inspire and motivate others to achieve desired goals (The King's Fund, 2012, 2014; Rose, 2015; Messenger and Pollard, 2022).

So, what exactly are we talking about when we refer to 'management' and 'leadership' and what part, if any, do 'followers' play?

- What do the terms 'leadership,' 'management' and 'followership' mean to you?

Often leadership and management are viewed as being the same thing. However, some would argue that they are in fact distinct entities, albeit with some area of overlap. Most would agree that nurse managers and leaders are equally important and necessary to ensure that desired goals are successfully accomplished – although the focus of each of these roles may be different.

Management is mostly about processes. Huber (2010: 5) defines management as:

> *'the co-ordination of resources through planning, organising, co-ordinating, directing and controlling to accomplish specific institutional goals and objectives'.*

Put simply, managers focus on systems and structure. A manager's role is based upon authority and influence. Managers are usually formally appointed to a designated position although you could argue that the role of any qualified nurse involves some aspect of management, particularly when directing the work of junior staff or coordinating the delivery of care. Good management relies heavily on maintaining effective systems and involves ensuring that employees meet organisational goals and objectives; managers maintain stability (Huber, 2010). More specifically, expectations of a nurse manager's role include taking responsibility for the quality of a physical care environment, the standard of care delivery in relation to those who deliver care (the nursing team) and taking overall responsibility for those receiving care. This role often involves:

- Setting staffing levels and managing human resources (e.g., off-duty rotas, sickness and absence management and disciplinary procedures);
- Ensuring quality and maintaining safety (e.g., setting standards for care, data collection, audit, and service improvement);
- Coordinating care activities and supervising clinical care provision;
- Implementing new organisational policies and directives;
- Meeting government and organisational targets;
- Undertaking budgetary and resource management and control.

Nurse managers are also legally and professionally accountable for the decisions they make, having a *duty of care* to ensure the safety of service-users, visitors, and staff within their sphere of influence (Dimond, 2015). However, this does not detract from the fact that each healthcare worker is also personally accountable for the actions and omissions of their own practice (NMC, 2018b).

Leadership, on the other hand, is mostly about behaviour. It can be an informal role rather than an officially designated position and can occur spontaneously within any group. To influence others, leaders will often rely on their personal character and attitude to develop good interpersonal relationships. Described by Huber (2010: 4) as '*a complex and multi-dimensional process of influencing people to accomplish goals*', leaders focus primarily on people. Although leadership may be considered from a number of different perspectives, a widely accepted view is that it is an interactive event based on human relationships and can best be described as the ability to inspire confidence and encourage followers to follow, collaborating effectively in order to enthuse and motivate others to create and innovate (Kouzes and Posner, 2017). Moreover, leadership is necessary at all clinical levels and is not an activity reserved for those in positions of authority.

Leadership and followership behaviours are closely related because each of these affects the other. Being a follower is just as important as being a leader because without followers a leader would have no one to lead. Followership is also just as complex and multifaceted. Carsten et al. (2010) suggest that a follower's behaviour can be passive (e.g., obediently following direction with reduced responsibility taking), active (e.g., speaking up and making suggestions or verbalising ideas) or proactive (e.g., challenging the status quo for the good of the organisation). Chaleff (2009) suggests that the most effective followers are the ones who have initiative and can think for themselves. Therefore, competent and committed followers are an asset to be nurtured, developed, and valued by every aspiring leader. A leader should always understand the interests, ideas, attitudes and motivation of potential followers, and an ability and desire for their followers to release their potential.

In management, leadership and followership behaviours (Table 9.1), power is also intricately linked. According to Bass (1990), power is the underlying force for all social exchange. This falls into two broad categories – personal power or positional power (French and Raven, 1960) – each of which can be utilised to influence others. Although managers, leaders and followers all have different power bases they may use similar strategies (Table 9.1), skills and attributes to achieve their goals. Indeed, a leader, manager and follower may be the same person playing distinct roles at various times. Whichever role is adopted in any given circumstance, managers, leaders, and followers need to work together to improve the quality of care provision and the working environment.

Each of us will have preferred leadership, management or followership styles and behaviours, and it would be useful at this stage to reflect upon the type of leader or manager you are or want to be. Gaining a deeper understanding of your own preferences should help you identify areas for development to become a more effective manager, leader, and follower in the future.

The activities suggested below should help you identify your own preferences. It is more helpful to be honest with yourself rather than focusing on what you think is the right or wrong answer.

Table 9.1   Leaders, managers, and followers

Leaders	Managers	Followers
Informal role.	Formally designated role.	A member of an informal group/ formal team.
Personal power (Expert/ Referent) based on ability to influence.	Positional (Legitimate/Reward/ Coercive) power based on assigned position.	Information/Connection power based on ability and choice of whether to cooperate and collaborate effectively with leaders/managers.
Focus on people.	Focus on processes, systems and structure (achieving organisational objectives by planning, organising, supervising, negotiating, evaluating and integrating services).	Support managers, leaders and other team members. Contribute to creating a comfortable and safe working environment.
Influence, motivate, inspire and energise followers. Focus on the future. Visionary–they identify future goals and show the way forward. Innovate and create. An achieved position. Do the right thing. Do not need to be a good manager to be a good leader.	Direct and control followers, ensuring adherence to policies and procedures. Focus on the here and now? Responsible for maintaining quality and managing resources. Maximise output and productivity. An assigned position. Do things right. Need to be a good leader to be a good manager.	Follow the directions of managers. Cooperate and collaborate with leaders and managers. Focus on agreed tasks. A chosen position. Carry out agreed tasks. Good followers can be leaders, managers or neither!

Source: Adapted from Barr and Dowding (2012).

ACTIVITY 9.1

Use the leadership assessment instrument accessible via the weblink below to help you to define your current leadership view and approach:

> www.yumpu.com/en/document/read/63152643/conceptualizing-leadership-
> questionnaire

Take the time to reflect upon your preferences. Think back to your own positive and negative experiences of leadership and followership. How do you think your own experience has informed your views?

What are Management Theories?

Management theories attempt to describe the role and function of managers and how they engage with employees to achieve organisational goals. Developing a greater understanding of how to efficiently manage situations and people, we can achieve better outcomes while simultaneously maintaining or improving levels of productivity. There are many different management theories, and it is beyond the realms of this chapter to discuss all of these in any depth. What follows is a brief summary of management theory development.

Human relations theory promotes the idea that people want personal fulfilment, good social relationships and to be an accepted member of a group (Mayo, 1949). The main idea here is the belief that individuals cannot be coerced and forced to do things that they consider unreasonable – willing participants are needed.

Theory X and theory Y explore the motivation of workers and their attitude to work. Theory X individuals dislike work and need to be directed and controlled because they want security rather than responsibility. Theory Y individuals like work, are self-motivated and accept or seek responsibility (McGregor, 1960).

Contingency theory suggests that a manager's or leader's effectiveness is dependent on the match between a leaders/managers style and the setting or situation (Fiedler, 1967) and describes styles that are task or relationship motivated.

Situational theory argues that the effectiveness of a leader's/manager's style will be influenced by the situation itself and that as a basic principle managers/leaders will need to consider the situation alongside the competence and commitment of staff when making decisions. The essence of this approach suggests that leaders need to match their approach to follower readiness (Blanchard et al., 1993).

Systems theory suggests that to be effective, organisations need to consider a complex network of numerous factors and the interplay of structure, people, technology, and the environment (i.e., the provision of excellent care is dependent on the effective integration of effort across departments and disciplines). It is argued that changing one part of the system will affect the entire system because each system is a set of interrelated parts designed to achieve common goals (Senge, 1990). Some have seen this as a way of understanding management needs within healthcare settings (Goss, 2015).

Chaos theory draws on the emerging science of complexity to explain the unpredictable nature of organisations such as the NHS and the limitations associated with trying to organise a complex system into a 'manageable' state using rule-based frameworks (Tuffin, 2016).

What are Leadership Theories?

Leadership theories attempt to enhance our understanding of the desired characteristics and specific qualities, skills and approaches considered helpful in distinguishing a successful leader from a follower. By developing a greater appreciation of successful leadership approaches, we can use our influence as leaders to improve not only care provision but also the working environment for ourselves and others.

In general, leadership theories will vary according to:

- The emphasis placed on the personal characteristics of a leader;
- The effect of a leader on organisational functioning and culture;
- The emphasis placed on the leader and group behaviour (i.e., social interaction processes). (See Figure 9.1.)

'Great man'/trait theories are based on the belief that leaders possess exceptional qualities that influence the way a person leads (Bass, 1990). Numerous research studies have attempted to identify key traits and skills although there is still no complete agreement on the desired characteristics or skills. In one evidence-based review, West et al. (2015) suggest that desired leadership traits and skills include the following:

- High energy level and stress tolerance;
- Self-confidence;
- An internal locus of control (e.g., a belief that what happens around you is more under your control than the control of external forces);
- Emotional maturity (linked to the concept of emotional intelligence);
- Personal integrity;
- Socialised power motivation (i.e., use of power to achieve organisational objectives and to support the growth, development, and advancement of those they lead);
- Achievement orientation;
- Low need for affiliation.

However, critics argue that a trait approach fails to consider the influence of organisational culture and negates the part that social class, gender, and race inequalities play in the opportunity for leadership development.

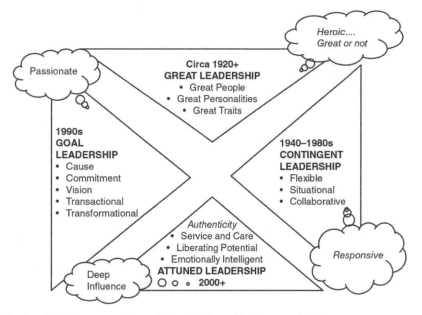

Figure 9.1 Leadership perspectives. (Adapted from Northouse, 2012)

Behavioural theories focus on the actions of effective leaders and how they behave (Hersey and Blanchard, 1988; Marquis and Huston, 2006). Indeed, the NHS Healthcare Leadership Model (NHS Leadership Academy, 2022) identifies what it believes to be the desired behaviours and attributes of leaders in healthcare – suggesting that both trait and behavioural theories still influence current thinking, and are often reflected as desired attributes within person specifications and job descriptions.

Contingency Theories A recognition of the more complex nature of the phenomenon of leadership resulted in the development of theories that examined leader characteristics and behaviour in the context of situational parameters. Contingency theories focus on the match between a leader's style and situational variables.

Situational theories attempt to explain how leaders adapt their leadership behaviours according to the situation. Fiedler (1967) concluded that no leadership style met the needs of every situation. Hersey and Blanchard (1988) suggest that different situations demand various leadership approaches and that leaders should adjust their leadership styles in accordance with the readiness of their followers.

Functional theories suggest that leadership effectiveness is dependent on the relationship between the leader and a group (Adair, 2009). They focus on how leadership supports the function of an organisation to carry out work and relates to a leader's source of power and influence over others (e.g., how various roles relate to the organisational functions to meet the needs of the organisation), task needs, needs of the team, needs of the individual and effects on group behaviours.

Activity 9.2

Access this short YouTube video clip, which provides a useful succinct overview of ten leadership theories: www.youtube.com/watch?v=XKUPDUDOBVo

Leadership and Management Styles

Leadership and management styles can be described as 'different combinations of tasks and relationship behaviours which are used to influence others to accomplish goals' (Huber, 2010: 6). Healthcare organisations are often overly complex, and the varied nature of the work involved along with the diverse nature of the workforce, has led to calls for the adoption of alternative approaches to the traditional top-down (autocratic) methods of leadership and management. Models of collaborative or shared/distributed leadership are now considered more appropriate within current healthcare settings (West et al., 2014; Messenger and Pollard, 2022). The NHS Leadership Academy (2022) suggest that effective leaders need to be able to work through others – supporting, motivating, and encouraging followers to achieve objectives, empowering them to use their skills effectively, recognising their achievements and thereby creating an engaged workforce. The demand for more honesty, openness and compassionate leadership within organisations is also growing. Ethical leadership encourages leaders and managers to take account of key ethical principles when making decisions to use their authority or influence for the common good (Ciulla, 2003). The authentic leadership approach (George, 2003) emphasises the importance of building honest relationships with followers by valuing their contributions and behaving ethically and transparently. Servant (Greenleaf, 1977) and spiritual leadership models emphasise the 'caring' principle (Northouse, 2012) in which leaders demonstrate care, compassion and are sensitive to the needs of others. Mindful leadership is considered an approach by which to improve personal and professional effectiveness and overall organisational productivity (Rowland, 2017), particularly when leading and managing change (we will explore this in a little more detail in Chapter 10). Emotionally intelligent (EI) leadership approaches (Goleman et al., 2013; Stein, 2017) focus primarily on how we can manage our own emotions to handle relationships with others effectively. West (2021) also highlights the concept of compassionate leadership, which draws on many of these previous ideas, arguing that leaders today should be seeking to 'develop cultures of compassion' in all workplace settings.

Looking closely at the literature around leadership and management styles it is possible to identify the similarities and how they overlap. Several commonly observed leadership and management styles are outlined in Table 9.2.

The evidence-based healthcare leadership model (NHS Leadership Academy, 2022) provides an outline of nine 'leadership dimensions', calling on future healthcare leaders to consider these when seeking to identify personal strengths and areas for development:

- Inspiring a shared purpose;
- Leading with care;
- Evaluating information;
- Connecting our service;
- Sharing the vision;
- Engaging the team;
- Holding to account;
- Developing capability;
- Influencing for results.

In summary, there are a range of styles of leadership. However, the most effective leaders are likely to be those who can recognise that one leadership style is not necessarily better than another. Historical leadership styles do not always meet the needs of today's workforce

Table 9.2 Leadership and management styles

Leadership Style	Advantages/Strengths	Disadvantages/Weaknesses
Laissez-faire Leaders exert minimal influence and take a 'hands-off' approach – leaving followers to decide upon the actions needed themselves.	Groups of fully autonomous and independent care providers working together can feel empowered to make decisions.	Can result in a lack of direction particularly where there is disharmony or a clash of work ethic values amongst team members.
Autocratic/Authoritarian/ Transactional Top-down approach (e.g., controlling, directing, goal/target setting). Use of recognition and reward incentives to influence motivation. Transactional leaders tend to focus more on tasks, dominating and making decisions without allowing for the views of others to be considered.	Can be very efficient in certain situations e.g., emergencies. Focuses upon the ability of leader/manager to monitor and correct subordinates.	Stifles creativity, fosters dependence, submissiveness and loss of individuality. Very little/limited collaboration and delegation. Shared values are not communicated. This can create discontent, hostility and even aggression amongst group members or followers.
Democratic Leaders work with and guide rather than direct followers. *Transformational* Based on the idea that leaders motivate others to perform by encouraging a shared vision and changing their perception of reality (e.g., shares the decision-making and planning processes as well as responsibility for their implementation).	Increased job satisfaction for followers. Followers feel more motivated to get involved, empowered.	Takes more time and effort to execute effectively.

and therefore, leadership has had to evolve to match a growing sense of democracy and independence in the workforce. The current complexity and philosophy of healthcare provision today also emphasise the need for effective leadership at all levels. To achieve optimum healthcare outcomes for service-users, enhance satisfaction and maintain healthy work environments you will need to be able to recognise a range of factors that influence your own chosen leadership style. You will have to adapt and adopt a range of leadership styles and approaches depending on the demands of the situation, remembering that leaders who perform well tend to be highly visible and thrive on collaboration and network building (Hardacre et al., 2011; The Kings Fund, 2012).

Developing Your Leadership Potential

As previously highlighted, self-awareness is considered an integral attribute of a good leader (Goleman et al., 2013). Goleman et al. (2013) and Stein (2017) argue that the way we manage ourselves is a central part of being an effective leader, suggesting that it is important to recognise that personal qualities such as self-awareness, self-confidence, self-control, self-knowledge, personal reflection, resilience, and determination, are the foundation of how we behave.

Activity 9.3

Access the short video clip below:

www.youtube.com/watch?v=Yosh5o64ujO

After you have viewed the clip consider how your own emotions influence your leadership practice. Try to think of some examples from your own workplace.

Now, click on the link below and complete the short quiz *'How emotionally intelligent are you*?' at www.mindtools.com/pages/article/ei-quiz.htm

How did you do? What areas (if any) do you need to work on (e.g., self-awareness, self-regulation, motivation, empathy, social skills)? What could you do to improve your scores in these areas? What could you do differently to embody an 'emotionally intelligent' leadership approach?

Whilst there are lots of ways we can support others as a leader it is also important to remember to be kind to ourselves too. Emotional, physical, and psychological stressors are prevalent within current healthcare environments and failure to acknowledge the detrimental impact of these on both leaders and followers can lead to stress, burn-out or mental health issues. Personal resilience is the most valuable resource for coping well during challenging times, enabling us to see things more clearly and solve problems more effectively. The American Psychological Association (2018) has discovered that several factors modify the negative effects of adverse life situations. Strong relationships at home and work that provide care and support, create trust, and offer encouragement and reassurance are critical to developing resiliency. Additional factors associated with resilience include the capacity to make realistic plans and carry them out, having self-confidence and a positive self-image, developing communication and problem-solving skills, and the capacity to manage strong feelings and impulses. Additionally, self-care activities that seek to support and nourish mind, body, and spirit such as meditation and mindfulness (Rowland, 2017; Behan, 2020), yoga (Cocchiara et al., 2019) or gentle exercise are also thought to be beneficial.

Table 9.3 below provides some suggestions on how you can enhance your leadership behaviour.

Table 9.3   Enhancing your leadership behaviour (Northouse, 2012)

Trait/Behaviour	Suggested activity
Intelligence	Keep well informed, by reading widely about topical issues.
Confidence	Develop a clear understanding of what is required. This will help you feel more confident when identifying and using future opportunities to take on leadership roles (e.g., leading a student discussion or speaking out in group work activities, volunteering, serving on committees and interest groups).
Charisma	You may or may not be a naturally charismatic or outgoing person. Nevertheless, by demonstrating that you are competent and can clearly articulate your goals, that you have strong values and high expectations, that you can encourage and show confidence in the ability of others – inspiring and exciting others with your ideas – will motivate others to follow.
Determination	Know where you are going and how you intend to get there. Show initiative, be persistent, proactive and persevere; give direction to others if needed.
Sociability	Make an effort to establish pleasant, social relationships. Try to be friendly and outgoing, courteous, tactful and diplomatic, kind, thoughtful and supportive to others in the group – make others feel included.
Integrity	Be open with others. Always act honestly and be loyal and dependable.

Similarly, the six pillars of character in Table 9.4 outline how you might exhibit an ethical leadership approach in practice (Northouse, 2012).

Being a member of an effective team means that you will often be required to shift between leadership and followership positions within the team depending on your expertise, level of contribution and the overall goal. Engaged followership is also crucial in determining successful outcomes. The *Five Dimensions of Courageous Followership* (Chaleff, 2009) outlined in Table 9.5 provide a useful framework when considering areas for developing your followership skills.

Table 9.4 The six pillars of character (Northouse, 2012)

Ethical principles	Six pillars of character - suggested behaviour
Veracity and fidelity	Trustworthiness: be open and honest, represent reality as fully and completely as possible. Keep promises. This also links to professional integrity (e.g., adhering to high moral values and professional standards) and confidentiality (e.g., in relation to personal or private matters).
Justice	Try to be non-judgemental: treat everyone equally and fairly; respect and value their views and ensure that you do not use followers as a means of meeting your objectives rather than their own. Encourage informed decision-making processes of the group based on a sound knowledge and understanding of issues. Use morally appropriate actions to achieve goals. Give credit to others when deserved.
Autonomy	Responsibility and freedom of choice: accept responsibility for the actions you take as a leader.
Non-maleficence	Care for others to avoid harm: caring leadership behaviour link to the notion of servant leadership and highlights the requirement to be attentive to the needs of others (e.g., establish goals that all parties can mutually agree to and assist others to develop emotional resilience).
Beneficence	Develop good citizenship by making decisions that promote the common good of 'doing the right thing'. Develop collegiality and share goals. Demonstrate compassion by listening deeply to others in order to try to understand things from their perspective (West, 2021). Focus on the needs of followers in order to help them become more autonomous and knowledgeable by mentoring/teaching and promoting team building.

Table 9.5 Five dimensions of courageous followership (Chaleff, 2009)

The courage to assume responsibility.	Know what you are expected to do and how you will achieve it. Take personal responsibility for completing (or not) any agreed tasks. Utilise effective communication skills to keep the leader and other team members fully informed.
The courage to serve.	Followers do not serve leaders. Rather, followers and leaders each serve a common purpose by supporting agreed decisions and shared values - creating a relationship of trust and support. Offer encouragement to the leader when necessary and help to communicate the leader's vision to others throughout the organisation. Cooperate and work energetically with others to achieve the agreed common goal. Provide timely and accurate feedback to the leader and other members of the group.
The courage to participate in transformation.	Make time and effort to consider what skills and attributes you will need to develop in order to transform the leader–follower relationship.
The courage to challenge.	This does not equate to being argumentative and unreceptive. However, good followers should not be afraid to constructively challenge the leader when necessary. Be courageous and voice your opinion when it really matters to challenge current thinking or leadership decisions that you believe are misguided or unethical. Providing accurate feedback on plans will help to ensure that the leader has the necessary information to make critical decisions.
The courage to take moral action.	Be honest and trustworthy. Demonstrate a 'courageous conscience'. You should always seek to carry yourself with integrity and self-respect. If you do not morally agree with a leader's approach or agenda then this is the time to stand up for what you believe is the right thing to do. Leaving the group/team or even whistle-blowing is one option that may need to be exercised rarely.

At this stage, you may want to take some time to stop and think about the difference you want to be able to make as a manager or leader. Consider the additional areas/skills/attributes you think you need to develop to make yourself a better leader/manager/follower in the following scenarios:

- An emergency (e.g., dealing with an individual who has collapsed);
- Implementing a new way of working.

Leading and Managing People

The provision of safe, high quality, compassionate care is an essential priority for any nurse. However, it is not possible to achieve this alone. In Chapter 4, we identified the skills required to be able to work effectively within teams and explored the facilitators and barriers of effective teamwork. When leading interprofessional teams nurses must be able to offer supportive and empowering leadership to others within their sphere of influence. This involves providing clarity, encouragement, support, and feedback so that others are not only able to practice safely but are empowered to innovate and introduce new and improved ways of working. Collaborative teamwork is an important contributor to the quality of healthcare provision. Research evidence suggests that good team leadership is a determinant of high-quality care and positive care outcomes (Wong et al., 2013; Sfantou et al., 2017). The leaders of today must acknowledge the need to work together with other professionals and support workers to deliver high-quality care across traditional boundaries as the complexity of care increases (Messenger and Pollard, 2022).

Delegating Responsibly

Every registered nurse needs to be able to coordinate work activities and delegate care to co-workers and other members of the team (NMC, 2018a). This requires a variety of skills such as the ability to communicate clearly and directly, provide instructions, explanations, support, guidance, and feedback. However, sometimes we may be reluctant to delegate to others either because we lack the confidence to do so or because we fear that the task will not be carried out properly. However, the most effective leaders and managers are those who can build a trusting and supportive culture where all members feel valued and will flourish irrespective of their role.

Delegation is the process by which you (the delegator) transfer authority and responsibility for completing a task to another competent person (the delegatee). You remain responsible for the overall outcome of the task and are accountable for your decision to delegate. However, the delegatee is responsible for their decisions and actions they take (NMC, 2020).

The Code (NMC, 2018b) sets out clear expectations that a registered nurse needs to meet when delegating care to others. It is important to remember that as a registered nurse you will remain legally and professionally accountable for the decision to delegate care and for the overall management of care delivery.

To ensure that you always delegate safely and effectively, you should always consider the context of the situation, rather than just focusing on the task alone. When delegating care to others you will need to consider (NMC, 2020):

- The stability of the person being cared for;
- The knowledge, skills, abilities and standards of proficiency of the delegatee and whether they are willing to accept responsibility for undertaking and completing the task;
- The complexity of the task being delegated and whether the delegatee has the authority (via national guidance, organisational policies, and protocols) to perform the task;
- The expected outcome of the delegated task;
- The availability of resources to meet those needs.

On occasion, the points highlighted here might be difficult to ascertain particularly if you are working in unfamiliar surroundings or with unfamiliar people. Therefore, you should check that the person you are delegating to fully understands what is required and expected of them. You should provide clear information and instruction (verbal, digital or written) direction and supervision where necessary Once the task has been completed, you should check that it has been carried out satisfactorily and offer appropriate constructive feedback, identifying areas for improvement if necessary. Delegating work to others can sometimes be difficult, particularly when staffing levels are low, or when the delegated task is considered unpleasant due to a fear of causing conflict (Hasson et al., 2013). Later in the chapter we will be exploring how such conflict can be dealt with appropriately.

Activity 9.4

Watch the following video clip produced by the Nursing and Midwifery Council (2020) which provides an overview of accountability and the responsibilities of all team members when delegating care to others: www.nmc.org.uk/standards/code/code-in-action/delegation/#

- What tasks might you consider delegating to others and in what situations?
- What strategies or skills could help you further develop your delegating abilities?

Obviously, the potential range of tasks you could delegate to someone else is considerable. However, following professional guidance frameworks can help you to decide whether delegation is appropriate.

Improving your own delegating abilities:

Reflect upon factors that could impact on your delegating ability. For example, is your ability hampered by a lack of confidence in either your own abilities or the abilities of others, a fear of losing your authority or control, wanting to avoid risk or merely a lack of ability to provide clear direction to others?

Creating a Supportive Culture

Delegating care appropriately will help you to make the best use of contributions from other team members and can also be an effective way of developing their skills and abilities. As we have already highlighted, contemporary leadership approaches should be less about 'command and control' and more about supporting individuals with their own development, empowering them to identify and address their own learning needs. Offering support and guidance in this way will also help to foster teamwork and collaboration. Coaching and mentoring styles of leadership provide a valuable opportunity to assist colleagues to reflect upon their own practice and performance, identifying potential for improvement, though there are subtle differences between the two.

Table 9.6 below outlines the main similarities and differences between mentoring and coaching.

Table 9.6   Mentoring, training, and coaching

	Mentoring	Coaching
Focus	Career and personal development.	Identifying and achieving specific goals.
Source of expertise	Mentor (usually more experienced and qualified than the 'mentee' and is often a senior person in the organisation who can pass on knowledge, experience and open doors to otherwise out of reach opportunities).	Coachee (a coach does not need same background or experience – could be a superior, subordinate or peer).
Relationship	Ongoing 1:1 relationship that can last for a long period of time.	Tends to be a short-term intervention. A collaborative relationship between both parties – one in which both sides work to reach an agreed destination. Could involve working with individuals or teams.

(Continued)

Table 9.6 Mentoring, training, and coaching (*Continued*)

	Mentoring	Coaching
Goal	Help at point of need Development of individual. Guidance and advice.	To improve an individual's performance and unlock individual potential enabling coachee(s) to transform the quality of their working or/and personal lives.
Agenda	Set by the mentee, with the mentor providing support and guidance to prepare them for future roles.	Typically set by the coachee but in agreement/consultation with the coach.
Stakeholder	Other stakeholders may be involved.	Other stakeholders may be involved.
Setting	Can be informal and can take place as and when the mentee needs some advice, guidance or support.	Generally more structured in nature and meetings are scheduled on a regular basis.
Approach	Based on personal experience.	Ask powerful questions to tap into individuals' vision, wisdom and directed action in service of self-identified agenda.

- What are the similarities and differences between mentoring and coaching?
- What skills might you use and how would these differ depending on your own leadership approach?
- How might you use each of these approaches to help colleagues improve their own practice?

When developing a mentoring or coaching relationship, it is vital for the mentor/coach to consider the importance of organisational culture. The Royal College of Nursing (2012) has developed a useful framework to help create a learning culture for older workers (Figure 9.2) although you could argue that this could equally be applied to all members of the team, irrespective of age.

Developing a Healthy Work Environment

The NMC (2018a) requires you to be able to work cooperatively with other members of staff, sharing your skills and experience and respecting their contribution to the efforts of the team. As a manager or leader, part of your role will involve maintaining a healthy work environment. However, this might not be as easy as it sounds. The population of the UK is changing and along with it, the workforce is becoming more diverse in terms of educational background, roles, professionalisation (e.g., different value systems), ethnicity, gender and age (The Kings Fund, 2018; Office for National Statistics, 2021). All of these factors can influence how people act and communicate with each other – for example, expectations of behaviour or differing styles of

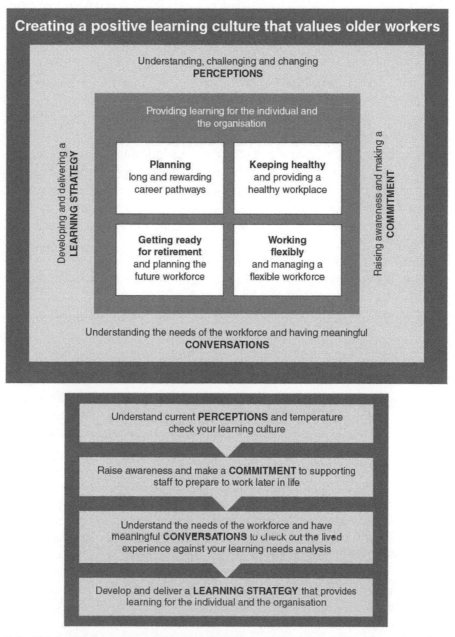

Figure 9.2 Valuing older workers (RCN (Royal College of Nursing), 2012). (Reproduced with the permission of the Royal College of Nursing)

communication. A nurse leader will need to be able to demonstrate cultural intelligence, recognising the importance of creating an environment where everyone feels valued, included and has a sense of belonging, (Richard-Eglin, 2021) alongside an understanding of how diversity can be harnessed to build and maintain a healthy workplace (Stanley, 2010).

However, some argue that the organisational culture in many healthcare settings is toxic, controlling and repressive, where workers are often afraid to speak out due to a worry about reprisal rather than being facilitative and supportive (Francis, 2013; Kirkup, 2018; Ockenden, 2022). A healthy work environment correlates to job satisfaction, which in turn, positively influences recruitment and healthier service-users (Cowden et al., 2011; Wong et al., 2013). Equally, a poor work environment adversely affects health. Employees spiral into burnout leading to frequent absences and recurrent sickness, impacting negatively on professional attitudes and behaviours (De Hert, 2020). Therefore, the workplace culture has a huge influence on how employees carry out their work and this in turn, will affect care delivery. There is a growing call for nurse leaders and managers to embrace the core principles of nursing (e.g., caring and compassion) and translate these into the type of nurse management and leadership needed in today's contemporary healthcare settings (West, 2021). Cummings and Bennett (2012: 11) suggest that 'leaders at every level have a responsibility to shape and lead a caring culture'. Indeed, an effective leader needs to be able to deconstruct a work culture if that becomes necessary (Sherwood, 2003). Hewison and Griffiths (2004) argue that without paying attention to the wider need of transforming a 'sick' organisational culture all the effort placed in developing future leaders could be wasted.

Amina

Amina's first post as a registered nurse was on a 30-bedded rehabilitation ward. She was happy to be joining a well-established team and was looking forward to her new role. The ward appeared well organised and resourced, providing care for older people recovering from surgery or falls at home. The ward manager was a forthright individual who held the belief that healthcare providers sometimes 'had to be cruel to be kind' in a bid to ensure that the rehabilitation process-particularly the remobilisation of individuals receiving care-facilitated their return home as quickly as possible. However, Amina soon began to realise that all was not how it first appeared. Long-serving team members were often seen to apply the 'mantra' of the ward manager inflexibly and sometimes a little too literally when attempting to encourage mobilisation, using behaviour and language that Amina felt lacked compassion and perceived to be bullying. Protests from people were either ignored or resulted in staff labelling some individuals 'uncooperative' or 'lazy.' Amina raised concerns with more experienced members of staff. Some agreed with the approach favoured by the ward manager whilst others appeared more uncomfortable but admitted to having done nothing about it due to a fear of retaliation if they 'stepped out of line.' Amina quickly established that those who challenged the ward manager's approach were labelled as 'soft' or 'unhelpful' or had simply left. Amina subsequently found it difficult to exert authority or establish her role as a 'team leader,' even when the ward manager was not on duty.

- Do you consider the culture of the ward above to be toxic or facilitative? Give your reasons.
- What are the key influencing factors?

According to the International Council of Nurses (2007), positive practice environments are characterised by the following:

- Occupational health, safety and wellness policies that address workplace hazards, discrimination, physical and psychological violence, and issues pertaining to personal security;
- Fair, manageable workloads and job demands;
- An organisational climate reflective of effective management and leadership practices, good peer support, worker participation in decision making and shared values;
- Work schedules and workloads that permit a healthy work–life balance;
- Equal opportunity and treatment;
- Opportunities for professional development and career advancement;
- Professional identity, autonomy, and control over practice;
- Job security, decent pay, and benefits;
- Safe staffing levels;
- Support, supervision and mentorship;
- Open communication and transparency;
- Recognition programmes;
- Access to adequate equipment, supplies and support staff.

Activity 9.5

Considering the International Council of Nurses (2007) list above, is there anything more that you or leaders in your current workplace could do to make sure that the workplace is a healthy one?

Managing Conflict

Managing the delivery of health and social care involves collaborating with a variety of complex organisations and professionals within a diverse workforce. Nowadays, health and social care staff are constantly under pressure to improve services, often when resources are stretched. In certain circumstances this can result in a communication breakdown or poor provision of care which leads to frustration, particularly when this involves service-users and relatives who may be anxious and upset, distressed or angry. Therefore it is inevitable that you will encounter conflict at some stage in your career.

Conflict is defined as:

'a serious disagreement or argument;' 'a state of mind in which a person experiences a clash of opposing feelings or needs;' 'a serious incompatibility between two or more opinions, principles, or interests'. (Oxford English Dictionary, 2018)

Conflict can potentially arise in any situation but particularly where changes have taken place due to restructuring, team working is poor, or there are differing management styles, individual personalities or behaviours. However, although dealing with 'difficult' people or situations can be extremely uncomfortable and stressful, if ignored or handled inadequately conflict can have a negative impact on individuals, organisations and care provision resulting in poor job satisfaction, sickness, and poor staff retention (Brinkert, 2010). Yet conflict is not always unhealthy. A degree of conflict can sometimes increase understanding and problem solving, leading to higher levels of creativity, and can enhance team motivation if handled appropriately (Almost, 2006). To be able to do this effectively you will need to have an appreciation of all the contributing factors and an understanding of ways in which conflict can be resolved successfully.

Sources of conflict can be intrapersonal (e.g., a poor work–life balance or role conflict), interpersonal (e.g., a personality clash or differences in beliefs, values, objectives, and priorities) or organisational (e.g., competing for resources). Perhaps not surprisingly, a common source of interpersonal conflict involves other nurse colleagues (Duddle and Boughton, 2007; Leiter et al., 2010), often resulting in workplace incivility, verbal abuse or bullying (Bambi et al., 2018). Other sources of interpersonal conflict include other healthcare professionals (e.g., nurse–doctor conflict) and individuals or their families, usually because of poor communication or perceived shortcomings in provision of care (Brinkert, 2010).

Activity 9.6

- Identify and list the potential sources of conflict within your current workplace. What are the aggravating or mitigating factors? How would you normally respond to conflict situations?

In stressful circumstances each of us will adopt certain strategies or styles to manage the situation (Almost et al., 2010). Furthermore, there are recognised differences in the way individuals handle conflict. Some commonly use avoidance or accommodating tactics (Duddle and Boughton, 2007) whereas others tend to use power (Almost, 2006).

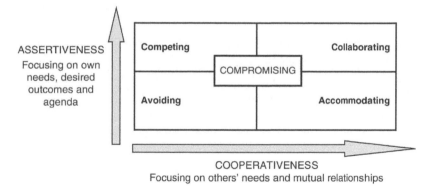

Figure 9.3   Thomas–Kilman conflict modes (1977)

Thomas and Kilman (1977) suggest that there are five common approaches to managing conflict (Figure 9.3):

1   Avoiding (e.g., ignoring or withdrawing from the situation);
2   Competing (e.g., dominating as a way of controlling a situation, using whatever power is at your disposal to achieve your goal);
3   Compromising (e.g., respecting and accepting the needs of others, which involves seeking common ground to find a mutually acceptable solution that partially satisfies both parties);
4   Accommodating (e.g., neglecting your own concerns to satisfy the other person, i.e., yielding to another person's point of view);
5   Collaborating (e.g., working with the other person to find some solution that fully satisfies both parties – this involves a full exploration of underlying concerns from all points of view to understand the needs of others to find a creative solution).

As with other leadership and management styles no one approach is applicable in every situation. However, Friedman et al. (2000) claim that people who use accommodating, compromising, and collaborating styles tend to experience lower levels of conflict and stress. Northouse (2012) also suggests that problem-solving skills (i.e., being able to identify problems and potential solutions and developing effective strategies to deal with conflict) are especially useful. At the very least, taking time to actively identify, explore and discuss differences in a non-threatening environment should help to resolve some tricky situations and reduce workplace stress.

To be able to do this effectively you need to be able to understand your own emotions and those of others and then apply this knowledge and understanding when choosing strategies to deal with conflict as it arises. The five integrated domains of emotional intelligence asserted by Goleman et al. (2013) have already been highlighted earlier in this and previous chapters. However, Huber (2010: 4) interprets these further in relation to the concept of team working as the following:

- **Self-awareness** (e.g., an ability to read your own emotional state and be aware of your own mood and how this might affect relationships);
- **Self-management** (e.g., the ability to take corrective action so as not to transfer your own negative moods on to staff relationships);
- **Social awareness** (e.g., intuitive skill of empathy and expressiveness: being sensitive and aware of the emotions and moods of others);
- **Relationship management** (e.g., using effective communication with others to disarm conflict and an ability to develop the emotional maturity of other team members).

Activity 9.7

Make a list of the qualities, skills, and abilities that you think may be important when dealing effectively with conflict.
- What measures could you take to help minimise the sources of conflict in your workplace?

Being open-minded and listening carefully and empathetically to someone else's point of view, concerns and anxieties will help you to demonstrate fairness, respect, and emotional maturity. Well-developed communication skills should also assist you to negotiate and collaborate with others to attempt to resolve issues and disputes.

Dealing with Unacceptable Behaviour

Unacceptable behaviour is defined by the RCN (2017: 5) as:

> 'behaviour directed towards a person that in any way attempts to belittle, threaten, intimidate, including verbal, written and physical abuse, and harassment.'

Surprisingly, workplace bullying and discrimination does exist in health and social care settings and can be a major contributing factor to unhealthy and toxic environments (Johnson, 2009). Bullying has been identified as a factor that not only affects care outcomes but also increases occupational stress, decreases job satisfaction, and adversely affects staff retention (Carter et al., 2013). According to an employment survey carried out by the Royal College of Nursing (2021), bullying can manifest itself physically (e.g., hitting or pushing), verbally (e.g., name calling or arguing) or psychologically (e.g., being ignored, excluded or undermined) with respondents also reporting incidents of discrimination which occurs when an employer, supervisor or co-worker treats another employee unfairly based on religion, age, ethnicity, gender, sexual orientation, disability, skin colour, nationality or race. Bullying can be very unpleasant and in serious cases may be dealt with legally (e.g., Health and Safety at Work

Act 1974 [www.legislation.gov.uk/ukpga/1974/37] and Protection from Harassment Act 1977 [www.legislation.gov.uk/ukpga/1997/40/contents]). Discrimination is also unlawful (Equality Act 2010 [www.legislation.gov.uk/ukpga/2010/15/contents]). It is worth noting that bullying and discrimination can occur within or outside the normal working environment (e.g., staff social gatherings and away days).

Dealing with discriminatory or negative behaviour – whether you are personally on the receiving end or not – can obviously be particularly challenging. However, Bennett and Sawatzky (2013) argue that individuals with greater emotional intelligence (EI) are not only more able to recognise early signs of negative behaviour but also deal with it more effectively. The aim is to achieve a workplace culture in which everyone treats each other with dignity and respect and where action is taken to help minimise sources of conflict, bullying or discrimination, including:

- Setting out and clearly verbalising behavioural expectations to other members of staff – linking these expectations of local policies (e.g., bullying and maintaining dignity in the workplace);
- Identifying the risks and warning signs (e.g., levels of staff sickness, absence, or staff turn-over);
- Improving reporting mechanisms by facilitating a supportive, non-blame and responsive culture to encourage 'victims' to come forward;
- Treating complaints seriously – enforcing expectations where necessary by reiterating these in line with identified policies and clearly outlining these to all parties.

The challenge for any leader or manager will be to deal with conflict in a way that does not add to the stress of the situation within the workplace. It is worth remembering that there are other sources of help that individuals can turn to if necessary (e.g., a mentor/practice supervisor, line manager, related educational institution if involving learners or trade union representative).

Activity 9.8

Access the following ACAS website at www.acas.org.uk/if-youre-treated-unfairly-at-work and review the discrimination, bullying and harassment guidelines. Afterwards, take a moment to consider the actions you would take if you were to experience or witness unacceptable behaviour in the workplace.

Managing Risk and Safety

Earlier in this chapter, we explored the notion that the work environment is influenced not least by the quality of leadership provided within the placement and organisation. Equally, effective leadership and management play a pivotal role in maintaining safety by creating and maintaining safe working environments and practices (Squires et al., 2010). Critical incidents commonly occur because of poor organisational systems or conditions; for example, a failure to follow good practice, poor communication, poor record keeping or as the result of equipment failure (Berwick, 2013). As a qualified nurse, ensuring that you have sufficient knowledge and critical understanding of the input and resources needed to manage risk effectively will be crucial to help maintain the safety of service users and colleagues. Risk can be predictable or unpredictable, environmental (e.g., linked to levels of cleanliness, light, temperature and/or adequacy of space) or human-related (e.g., working practices or impaired functioning). Unsafe staffing levels or inappropriate skill mix within teams can also put people at risk, impacting the quality-of-care provision (Francis, 2013; National Quality Board, 2016; Royal College of Nursing, 2022).

At this stage, it is important to recognise the difference between 'risk aversion' and 'risk management.' Risk aversion in healthcare relates to an unwillingness to take risks or wanting to avoid risks as much as possible, derived from a belief that risks should be eliminated entirely. Risk averse behaviour can be driven by a fear of litigation or a reluctance to depart from policy. As you can imagine, risk aversion can often stifle innovation and creativity. The term 'risk management,' on the other hand, focuses on understanding and analysing risks, and then taking the appropriate action to avoid or minimise their impact.

Risk assessments comprise a careful examination of what could cause harm to people so that you can decide whether you have taken enough precautions or should do more to prevent harm.

Activity 9.9

Reflecting upon your experience so far:

- Closely examine your current workplace or placement area. Make a list of the common risks and adverse incidents that can occur within this setting.
- Consider the role that you, your colleagues and service users have in creating and maintaining safe working environments.

Common incidents in healthcare settings (Health and Safety Executive or HSE, 2021) are outlined below:

- Slips, trips, and falls;
- Lifting and handling injuries;
- Physical assault/workplace violence;
- Exposure to materials, substances, or infections at work (e.g., soaps, disinfecting agents or latex, viruses);
- Spillages and/or chemical injuries;
- Needle-stick injuries;
- Equipment failure;

- Procedural failure (e.g., resulting in the development of pressure ulcers, incorrect surgery, and drug errors or hospital-acquired infections).

It is important to remember the potential for psychosocial risks for staff that are associated with poor health – for example, work-related stress, lack of influence, discrimination, time and work pressures, working long and irregular hours (HSE, 2021) and the potential impact on care outcomes and healthcare workers as a result of unsafe staffing levels (RCN, 2022).

The term '*risk management*' refers to the process of identifying, assessing/evaluating, and reporting risks to maintain the safety of people as well as improve the quality of care delivery. Risk management is about practicing safely and ensuring that the occurrence of harmful or adverse events is reduced by anticipating and preventing potential problems, learning from incidents, near misses, complaints, and litigation and by introducing systems to help staff to reflect upon and develop their practice. Figure 9.4 demonstrates the process of risk assessment using the five-step process of the HSE (2014).

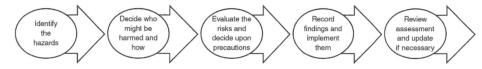

Figure 9.4   The HSE's (2014) five-step process to risk assessment

To practice safely and manage risk effectively, nurses need to ensure that risk assessment and management strategies are both utilised and applied, in and to current work practices.

Critical incident reporting is a system that was introduced with the aim of improving safety. By thorough investigation of an 'incident,' the intention is for practitioners to learn from the event and put additional measures or solutions in place to ensure that the situation is improved. However, fear of reprisals and sometimes a lack of understanding of how these should be reported can sometimes deter individuals from reporting incidents. Nevertheless, all nurses have a statutory duty to report concerns when they believe there is a potential danger. You have a legal responsibility to ensure that no one is harmed because of an act or omission on your part. Indeed, it is important to remember that you can still be pursued for compensation as an individual even if what you are doing is part of your contractual duties and can be prosecuted for criminal damage or negligence. *The Code* demands that you make the care and safety of those in your care your main concern (NMC, 2018b: 6) and that you '*share information to identify and reduce risk*' (NMC, 2018b: 10) and '*act immediately to put right the situation if someone has suffered actual harm for any reason*' (NMC, 2018b: 13). This will involve documenting any concerns carefully as soon as possible, making sure that records are clearly signed, dated, and timed, and asking for additional help where necessary (e.g., from more senior staff and/or risk managers). Therefore, familiarising yourself with local/national risk management policies and the role/functions of numerous safety agencies, as well as required reporting systems, is essential to ensure that appropriate action is taken.

Critical incident analysis

When incidents occur, it is important to ensure that lessons are learned to prevent the same incident occurring again or elsewhere. A root cause analysis framework can be helpful when trying to identify exactly what has happened and more importantly, why. Getting to the root of the problem and understanding why something has happened will help to ensure that the real cause of the incident will be uncovered rather than just the details of the incident itself. You should then be able to focus on identifying and implementing solutions to improve the situation and ensure that the risk of it happening again is minimal. The 'five whys' approach used in the example below is one of the simplest approaches because it is considered one of the easiest to learn and apply.

Root cause analysis using the 'five whys' approach

Step 1: Write down the details of the specific problem. This helps you formalise the problem and describe it accurately. It will also help the team focus on the same problem.
Step 2: Brainstorm to ask why the problem occurs and then write the answer down.
Step 3: If this answer does not identify the source of the problem, ask 'why?' again and write that answer down.
Step 4: Loop back to Step 3 until the team agrees that they have identified the problem's root cause. Again, this may take fewer or more than five 'whys'.

Sabrina

Sabrina, is covering for a colleague who is ill. A busy nurse-led vaccination clinic is taking place and several people waiting have already complained due to the delays in their appointments because of staff shortages. As Sabrina is a little unfamiliar with the clinic processes – and to try to save time – a receptionist has offered to assist with the necessary paperwork (e.g., completing forms and checklists before sending individuals through to the treatment room). Sabrina rapidly calls the first person into the treatment room and quickly checks the paperwork before administering the required injections. However, immediately after doing so Sabrina quickly realises that she has given the person the wrong injection. The paperwork she looked at belonged to a different individual and had been mixed up in the process.

Using the 'five whys' approach outlined above consider the following:
- What is the probable cause of the accident/incident?
- What are the underlying causes – if any?
- What immediate action should be taken?

- How could the incident have been prevented?
- Are there any other issues that need to be considered or addressed?

Several factors most likely contributed to the incident above; for example, staff shortages, escalating waiting times leading to complaints, unfamiliar processes, poor delegation and/or a lack of acknowledgement on Sabrina's part of her limitations. Obviously the most immediate action would be to ensure that the recipient of the injection had not come to any harm because of the mistake. It is also clear that measures could have been taken to prevent this (e.g., informing those waiting of staff shortages, rearranging appointments, ensuring the availability of appropriately experienced staff, or even cancelling the clinic if necessary). Staff education, training and support are also issues that should be considered.

- What opportunities are provided in your placement area to offer staff the chance to critically reflect on such incidents?

Managing Team Performance

Earlier in this chapter we explored some of the leadership approaches that aim to enhance team performance. In your role as a leader you will be responsible for supporting junior staff to fulfil their own professional obligations. Performance management is a continuous process by which managers and employees work together to plan, monitor and review work objectives with the aim of improving their overall contribution to the organisation including:

- Agreeing SMART (specific, measurable, achievable, relevant, and time-bound) objectives, competencies, and development needs;
- Reviewing individual performance against agreed objectives;
- Giving appropriate feedback;
- Agreeing a personal development plan;
- Helping staff to achieve objectives through coaching and providing access to training or other development opportunities.

Occasionally, you will need to address concerns about the underperformance or behaviour of members of your team. However, fear and mistrust could lead to people keeping quiet and not reporting their concerns. Therefore as a nurse leader, one of your key aims should be to build an effective organisational culture in which there is trust and accountability among members of your team, fostering a culture of openness and transparency to build an atmosphere in which everyone is encouraged to identify and report unsafe conditions within a 'non-blame' culture. All organisations should have internal mechanisms for investigating and dealing effectively with complaints or concerns (e.g., robust policies and procedures). Healthcare professionals also have a duty to report any concerns they may have about the quality of care in their organisation or indeed any other organisation with which they have contact (NMC, 2017). Raising and escalating concerns or 'whistleblowing' is *'the act of reporting a concern about a risk, wrongdoing, or illegality at work, in the public interest'* (Brown, 2015) – to someone in authority. It is meant to act as an early warning system which provides an opportunity to put things right before something worse happens. Normally, in the first instance, this would involve informing senior staff or clinical leaders. If unresolved, additional external mechanisms, e.g., reporting concerns to the Care Quality Commission may also be implemented, although if this is necessary it is advisable to follow your organisation's published whistleblowing procedures. In all instances where practice or procedures are brought into question, clear, comprehensive, and unambiguous records will be crucial in determining what has happened. Good record keeping – as well as being a duty of professional practice – will also protect staff.

The NMC's **Code** (NMC, 2018b) sets out what service users, colleagues, families, and carers can expect from nurses:

- What factors could contribute to situations where nurses might fail to meet such expectations?
- Are you confident about the quality of care that you and your colleagues deliver?
- If so, what evidence do you have that this is the case?
- If not, what can you do about it?

Berwick (2013: 10) provides a useful summary of leadership behaviours that are thought to reduce risk and make healthcare provision safer. They include avoiding apportioning blame and instead expecting and insisting on honesty and transparency; seeking out and listening to colleagues and staff; hearing the voice of service users at every level; and using data accurately to support healthcare and continual improvement. He also advocates leading by example through commitment, encouragement, compassion and adopting a learning approach, helping develop the leadership potential in others by providing support and work experiences to enable them to improve their own leadership capability.

Chapter Summary

There is evidence to suggest that effective leadership is positively associated with improved care outcomes. Therefore, the need for strong and effective nurse leadership throughout the whole organisation has never been greater. However, leadership and management activities are complex and multifaceted with many differing theories advocating essential skills, desirable attributes, and approaches. The most effective leaders and managers are those who recognise the importance and impact of emotional intelligence and resilience in developing valuable relationships with others and who can apply well-developed team leadership skills to ensure the delivery of safe and effective practice by every member of the team.

Useful Websites

ACAS: www.acas.org.uk.
NHS Leadership Academy: www.leadershipacademy.nhs.uk/
Royal College of Nursing (Leadership): www.rcn.org.uk/Professional-Development/
    Professional-services/Leadership-Programmes
UK Government Guidance on Whistleblowing: www.gov.uk/whistleblowing

Further Reading

National Institute for Health and Care Excellence (2017) *Healthy Workplaces: Improving Employee Mental Health and Wellbeing*. London: NICE. Available at: www.nice.org.uk/guidance/qs147 (last accessed 29 March 2023).
NHS Scotland (2015) *Clinical and Care Governance Framework*. Available at: www.gov.scot/ publications/clinical-care-governance-framework/ (last accessed 5 July 2022).
Welsh Government (2021) *NHS Quality and Safety Framework: Learning and Improving*. Available at: https://gov.wales/nhs-quality-and-safety-framework (last accessed 5 July 2022).

References

ACAS (2014) *How to Manage Performance*. Available at: https://webarchive.nationalarchives.gov.uk/ ukgwa/20210104113253/https://archive.acas.org.uk/index.aspx?articleid=6608 (last accessed 29 March 2023).
Adair, J. (2009) *Effective Leadership: How to be a Successful Leader*. London: Pan Macmillan.
Almost, J. (2006) 'Conflict within nursing work environments: concept analysis', *Journal of Advanced Nursing*, 53(4): 444–53.
Almost, J., Doran, D.M., McGillis Hall, L.M. and Spence Laschinger, H.K. (2010) 'Antecedents and consequences of intra-group conflict among nurses', *Journal of Nursing Management*, 18: 981–92.
American Psychological Association (2018) *The Road to Resilience*. Available at: www.apa.org/ helpcenter/road-resilience.aspx (last accessed 5 July 2022).
Bambi, S., Foa, C., De Felippis, C., Lucchini, A., Guazzini, A. and Rasero, L. (2018) 'Workplace incivility, lateral violence and bullying among nurses. A review about their prevalence and related factors,' *Acta Biomed for Health Professions*, 89(S6): 51–79.
Barr, J. and Dowding, L. (2012) *Leadership in Healthcare*, 2nd edn. London: Sage.

Bass, B.M. (1990) *Bass and Stodgill's Handbook of Leadership: Theory, Research and Managerial Application*, 3rd edn. New York: Free Press.

Behan, C. (2020) 'The benefits of meditation and mindfulness practices during time of crisis such as COVID-19', *Irish Journal of Psychological Medicine*, 37: 256–8.

Bennett, K. and Sawatzky, J.V. (2013) 'Building emotional intelligence: a strategy for emerging nurse leaders to reduce workplace bullying', *Nursing Administration Quarterly*, 37(2): 144–51.

Berwick, D. (2013) *A Promise to Learn: A Commitment to Act. Improving the Safety of Patients in England*. London: HMSO.

Blanchard, K., Zigarmi, D. and Nelson, R. (1993) 'Situational leadership after 25 years: a retrospective', *Journal of Leadership Studies*, 1(1): 22–36.

Brinkert, R. (2010) 'A literature review of conflict communication causes, costs, benefits and interventions in nursing', *Journal of Nursing Management*, 18: 145–56.

Brown, C. (2015) 'When silence isn't golden', *Primary Care Nursing Review*. Available at: https://pcnr.co.uk/articles/188/when-silence-isnt-golden- (last accessed 5 July 2022).

Carsten, M.K., Uhl-Bien, M., West, B.J., Patera, J.L. and McGregor, R. (2010) 'Exploring social constructions of followership: a qualitative study', *The Leadership Quarterly*, 21: 543–62.

Carter, M., Thompson, N., Crampton, P., Morrow, G., Burford, B., Gray, C. and Illing, J. (2013) 'Workplace bullying in the UK NHS: a questionnaire and interview study on prevalence, impact and barriers to reporting', *BMJ Open*, 3(6): 1–12.

Chaleff, I. (2009) *The Courageous Follower: Standing up to and for Our Leaders*. San Francisco, CA: Berrett-Koehler.

Ciulla, J.B. (2003) *The Ethics of Leadership*. Belmont, CA: Wadsworth/Thompson Learning.

Cocchiara, R.A., Peruzzo, M., Mannocci, A., Ottolenghi, L., Villari, P., Polimeni, A., Guerra, F. and La Torre, G. (2019) 'The use of yoga to manage stress and burnout in healthcare workers: a systematic review', *Journal of Clinical Medicine*, 8(3): E284.

Cowden, T., Cummings, G. and Profetto-McGrath, J. (2011) 'Leadership practices and staff nurses' intent to stay: a systematic review', *Journal of Nursing Management*, 19: 461–77.

Cummings, J. and Bennett, V. (2012) *Compassion in Practice: Nursing, Midwifery and Care Staff: Our Strategy*. Leeds: NHS Commissioning Board.

De Hert, S. (2020) 'Burnout in healthcare workers: prevalence, impact, and preventative strategies', *Local and Regional Anesthesia*, 13: 171–83.

Dimond, B. (2015) *Legal Aspects of Nursing*, 7th edn. Harlow: Pearson Education Ltd.

Duddle, M. and Boughton, M. (2007) 'Intra-professional relations in nursing', *Journal of Advanced Nursing*, 59(1): 29–37.

Fiedler, F.E. (1967) *A Theory of Leadership Effectiveness*. New York: McGraw-Hill.

Francis, R. (2013) *Report of the Mid Staffordshire NHS Foundation Trust Public Inquiry Executive Summary*. Available at: http://webarchive.nationalarchives.gov.uk/20150407084003 or www.midstaffspublicinquiry.com/report (last accessed 5 July 2022).

Francis, R. (2015) *Freedom to Speak Up. An Independent Review into Creating an Open and Honest Reporting Culture in the NHS*. Available at: www.gov.uk/government/publications/sir-robert-francis-freedom-to-speak-up-review (last accessed 5 July 2022).

French, J.P.R., Jr and Raven, B. (1960) 'The bases of social power'. In D. Cartwright and A. Zander (eds), *Group Dynamics*. New York: Harper & Row, pp. 607–23.

Friedman, R.A., Tidd, S.T., Currall, S.C. and Tsai, J.C. (2000) 'What goes around comes around: the impact of personal conflict style on work conflict and stress', *International Journal of Conflict Management*, 11: 32–55.

George, B. (2003) *Authentic Leadership: Rediscovering the Secrets to Creating Lasting Value.* San Francisco, CA: Jossey-Bass.

Goleman, D., Boyatzis, R. and McKee, A. (2013) *Primal Leadership. Unleashing the Power of Emotional Intelligence.* Boston, MA: Harvard Business Review Press.

Goss, S. (2015) *Systems Leadership: A View from the Bridge.* London: Office for Public Management.

Greenleaf, R.K. (1977) *Servant Leadership: A Journey into the Nature of Legitimate Power and Greatness.* New York: Paulist.

Hardacre, J., Cragg, R., Shapiro, J., Spurgeon, P. and Flanagan, H. (2011) *What's Leadership Got to Do with It?* London: The Health Foundation.

Hasson, F., McKenna, H.P., and Keeney, S. (2013) 'Delegating and supervising unregistered professionals: the student nurse experience', *Nurse Education Today*, 33(3): 229–35.

Health and Safety Executive (2014) *Five Steps to Risk Assessment.* Belfast: HSE.

Health and Safety Executive (2021) *Health and Safety Statistics for the Public Services Sector in Great Britain 2021.* Available at: www.hse.gov.uk/sTATIsTICs/index.htm (last accessed 5 July 2022).

Hersey, P. and Blanchard, K.H. (1988) *Management of Organizational Behavior*, 5th edn. Upper Saddle River, NJ: Prentice Hall.

Hewison, A. and Griffiths, M. (2004) 'Leadership development in healthcare: a word of caution', *Journal of Health Organisation and Management*, 18(6): 464–73.

Huber, D.L. (2010) *Leadership and Nursing Care Management*, 4th edn. Missouri, IL: Elsevier.

International Council of Nurses (2007) 'Positive practice environments: Quality workplaces = quality patient care'. *Information and Action Tool Kit.* Available at: www.hrhresourcecenter.org/node/1645.html. (last accessed 4 July 2022).

Johnson, S.L. (2009) 'International perspectives on workplace bullying among nurses: a review', *International Nursing Review*, 56: 34–40.

King's Fund, The (2011) *The Future of Leadership and Management in the NHS: No More Heroes.* London: The King's Fund.

King's Fund, The (2012) *Leadership and Engagement for Improvement in the NHS.* London: The King's Fund.

King's Fund, The (2014) *Culture and Leadership in the NHS*: The King's Fund 2014 Survey, May 2014. Available at: www.kingsfund.org.uk/sites/files/kf/field/field_publication_file/survey-culture-leadership-nhs- may2014.pdf. (last accessed 5 July 2022).

King's Fund, The (2018) *The Health Care Workforce in England. Make or Break?* Available at: www.kingsfund.org.uk/publications/health-care-workforce-england (last accessed 5 July 2022).

Kirkup, B. (2015) *The Report of the Morecambe Bay Investigation.* Available at: www.gov.uk/government/publications (last accessed 5 July 2022).

Kirkup, B. (2018) *Report of the Liverpool Community Health Independent Review.* Available at: https://improvement.nhs.uk/news-alerts/independent-review-liverpool-community-health-nhs-trust-published (last accessed 5 July 2022).

Kouzes, J. and Posner, B. (2017) *The Leadership Challenge*, 6th edn. Hoboken, NJ: Wiley.

Leiter, M.P., Price, S.L. and Spence Lashinger, H.K. (2010) 'Generational differences in distress, attitudes and incivility among nurses', *Journal of Nursing Management*, 18: 970–80.

Marquis, B.L. and Huston, C.J. (2006) *Leadership Roles and Management Functions in Nursing: Theory and Application*, 5th edn. Philadelphia, PA: Lippincott.

Mayo, E. (1949) *Hawthorne and the Western Electrical Company: The Social Problems of an Industrial Civilisation*. London: Routledge & Kegan Paul.

McGregor, D. (1960) *The Human Side of Enterprise*. New York: McGraw-Hill.

Messenger, G. and Pollard, L. (2022) *Leadership for a Collaborative and Inclusive Culture*. London: Department of Health and Social Care. Available at: www.gov.uk/government/publications/health-and-social-care-review-leadership-for-a-collaborative-and-inclusive-future/leadership-for-a-collaborative-and-inclusive-future (last accessed 1 July 2022).

National Quality Board (2016) *Supporting NHS Providers to Deliver the Right Staff, with the Right Skills, in the Right Place, at the Right Time*. Available at: www.england.nhs.uk/publication/national-quality-board-guidance-on-safe-staffing (last accessed 5 July 2022).

NHS Improvement (2022) *Creating a Culture of Compassionate and Inclusive Leadership*. Available at: https://senioronboarding.leadershipacademy.nhs.uk/networks/compassionate-and-inclusive-leadership/ (last accessed 5 July 2022).

NHS Leadership Academy (2022) *Healthcare Leadership Model*. Available at: www.leadershipacademy.nhs.uk/resources/healthcare-leadership-model (last accessed 7 July 2022).

Northouse, P.G. (2012) *Introduction to Leadership Concepts and Practice*, 2nd edn. London: Sage.

Nursing and Midwifery Council (2017) *Raising Concerns: Guidance for Nurses and Midwives*. London: NMC.

Nursing and Midwifery Council (2018a) *Future Nurse: Standards of Proficiency for Registered Nurses*. London: NMC.

Nursing and Midwifery Council (2018b) *The Code: Professional Standards of Practice Behaviour for Nurses and Midwives*. London: NMC.

Nursing and Midwifery Council (2020) *Delegation and Accountability: Supplementary Information to the NMC Code*. London: NMC.

Ockenden, D. (2022) *Final findings, conclusions, and essential actions from the independent review of Maternity Services at the Shrewsbury and Telford NHS Trust*. Available at: www.gov.uk/government/publications/final-report-of-the-ockenden-review. (last accessed 5 July 2022).

Office for National Statistics (2021) *Changing trends and recent shortages in the labour market, UK: 2016 to 2021*. Available at: www.ons.gov.uk/employmentandlabourmarket/peopleinwork/employmentandemployeetypes/articles/changingtrendsandrecentshortagesinthelabourmarketuk/2016to2021 (last accessed 29 March 2023).

Oxford English Dictionary (2018) 'Conflict', Oxford: Oxford University Press. Available at: www.oxfordlearnersdictionaries.com/definition/conflict (last accessed 29 March 2023).

Richard-Eglin, A. (2021) 'The significance of cultural intelligence in nurse leadership', *Nurse Leader*, 19(1): 90–4.

Rose, L. (2015) *Better Leadership for Tomorrow: NHS Leadership Review*. Available at: www.gov.uk/government/uploads/system/uploads/attachment_data/file/445738/Lord_Rose_NHS_Report_acc.pdf (last accessed 5 July 2022).

Rowland, D. (2017) *Still Moving: How to Lead Mindful Change*. Chichester: Wiley & Sons.

Royal College of Nursing (2012) *Valuing Older Workers*. London: RCN.

Royal College of Nursing (2017) *Managing Unacceptable Behaviour. Guidelines for Accredited Representatives and Relevant RCN Staff*. London: RCN.

Royal College of Nursing (2021) *Employment Survey Report 2021: Workforce Diversity and Employment Experiences*. Available at: www.hse.gov.uk/sTATIsTICs/index.htm (last accessed 4 July 2022).

Royal College of Nursing (2022) *Nursing Under Unsustainable Pressure: Staffing for Safe and Effective Care in the UK*. Available at: www.rcn.org.uk/Professional-Development/publications/nursing-under-unsustainable-pressure-uk-pub-010-270 (last accessed 5 July 2022).

Senge, P.M. (1990) *The Fifth Discipline: The Art and Practice of the Learning Organization*. London: Random House/Doubleday.

Sherwood, G. (2003) 'Leadership for a healthy work environment: caring for the human spirit', *Nurse Leader*, Sept/Oct: 36–40.

Sfantou, D.F., Laliotis, A., Patelarou, A.E., Sifaki-Pistolla, D., Matalliotakis, M. and Patelarou, E. (2017) 'Importance of leadership style towards quality-of-care measures in healthcare settings: a systematic review', *Healthcare (Basel)*, Oct 14: 5(4): 73.

Squires, M., Tourangeau, A., Spence Laschinger, H.K. and Doran, D. (2010) 'The link between leadership and safety outcomes in hospital', *Journal of Nursing Management*, 18: 914–25.

Stanley, D. (2010) 'Multigenerational workforce issues and their implications for leadership in nursing', *Journal of Nursing Management*, 18(7): 846–52.

Stein, S.J. (2017) *The EQ Leader*. Hoboken, NJ: Wiley.

Thomas, K.W. and Kilman, R.H. (1977) 'Developing a forced-choice measure of conflict behaviour: the "mode" instrument', *Educational and Psychological Measurement*, 37: 309–25.

Tuffin, R. (2016) 'Implications of complexity theory for clinical practice and healthcare organization', *BJA Education*, 16(10): 349–52.

West, M.A., Eckert, R., Steward, K. and Pasmore, B. (2014) *Developing Collective Leadership for Healthcare*. London: The King's Fund.

West, M., Armit, K., Loewenthal, L., Eckert, R., West, T. and Lee, A. (2015) *Leadership and Leadership Development in Healthcare: The Evidence Base*. London: Faculty of Medical Leadership and Management.

West, M.A. (2021) *Compassionate Leadership: Sustaining Wisdom, Humanity and Presence in Health and Social Care*, UK: The Swirling Leaf Press.

Wong, C.A., Cummings, G.A. and Ducharme, L. (2013) 'The relationship between nursing leadership and patient outcomes: a systematic review update', *Journal of Nursing Management*, 21: 709–24.

10

DEVELOPING PRACTICE AND MANAGING CHANGE

Dianne Burns

Chapter objectives

- Appraise the concept of quality, focusing on quality assurance frameworks and methods of monitoring and improving the quality of care and service provision;
- Outline current legal, ethical and professional drivers for change/service improvement;
- Critically discuss the role of change agents in developing and leading teams to effective change;
- Identify effective strategies for managing change and consider their application to healthcare practice;
- Critically discuss barriers to service improvement and implementation appraising potential solutions to overcome them.

One of the biggest challenges for leaders of healthcare today is how to achieve more for less. Not only do healthcare practitioners have to care for more people – many of whom are highly dependent with complex care needs – but we are also called on to provide high(er) quality care and improve service user satisfaction whilst maintaining and enhancing safe care provision.

For us to be able to deliver safe and effective person-centred healthcare in a timely, cost-effective and efficient manner, we need to continually monitor and improve the way we work. However healthcare provision in the UK is constantly changing and this can be unsettling for everyone.

Yet change is an integral part of service improvement and being able to live with and manage change is an essential skill. Moreover, as a nurse you have a professional responsibility to make a positive contribution towards shaping a healthcare environment that promotes excellent care and service-user satisfaction (NMC, 2018a).

Related Nursing and Midwifery Council (NMC) Proficiencies for Registered Nurses

The overarching requirement of the NMC is that all nurses must be able to contribute effectively to continuous monitoring and quality improvement processes to be able to improve health outcomes for those receiving care (NMC, 2018b).

TO ACHIEVE ENTRY TO THE NMC REGISTER
YOU MUST BE ABLE TO

- Identify the implications of current health policy and future policy changes for nursing and other professions, and understand the impact of policy changes on the delivery and coordination of care;
- Understand how health legislation and current health and social care policies can be used to influence organisational change;
- Demonstrate an understanding of the principles of health economics and their relevance to resource allocation in health and social care organisations and other agencies;
- Demonstrate an understanding of how to monitor and evaluate the quality and effectiveness of care (including service-user experience) and how this can be used to bring about continuous service improvement;
- Demonstrate an understanding of the principles of improvement methodologies, participate in all stages of audit activity and identify appropriate quality improvement strategies;
- Work with people, their families, carers, and colleagues to develop effective improvement strategies for quality and safety, sharing feedback and learning from positive outcomes and experiences, mistakes, and adverse outcomes;
- Demonstrate an understanding of the mechanisms involved in influencing policy development and change including the importance of exercising political awareness and skills to maximise the influence and effect of registered nursing on quality of care, service-user safety and cost effectiveness;
- Demonstrate an understanding of the processes involved in developing a basic business case for additional care funding by applying knowledge of finance, resources, and safe staffing levels.

(Adapted from NMC, 2018b)

Drivers for Change

In Chapter 9, we focused on the leader's role in leading and managing teams. We also explored the importance of improving safety and reducing/managing risk, which are of course important drivers for change. Here, we will begin to explore the nurse's role in managing quality, developing practice and leading change.

It is imperative that healthcare systems across the UK can deliver good quality care, defined by the National Quality Board (2013: 4) as *'care that is effective, safe and provides as positive an experience as possible'*. Considering the failures highlighted by Francis (2013) and others (Andrews and Butler, 2014; Kirkup, 2015; 2018; Ockenden, 2022), monitoring and improving the quality of care we deliver has never been higher on the political or professional agenda. However, it is also a complex and demanding task. Having a working knowledge of the relevant frameworks, policies, tools and techniques alongside an ability to enable and facilitate others is central to leading improvement in the NHS, particularly when dealing with more complex issues (Hardacre et al., 2011). To sustain good quality care nurses (and their co-workers) will need to maintain and enhance safety while also taking action to improve efficiency by managing available resources effectively (NHS England, 2016).

Clinical governance is a term used to define the framework through which NHS organisations are accountable for continuously improving the quality of care and services (Department of Health or DH, 1998). The three components of clinical governance that you will no doubt be involved in are **clinical effectiveness**, **patient safety**, and **patient experience** (Figure 10.1).

This encompasses an entire range of quality improvement activities that fall within the three main strands above. (National Quality Board, 2013). As a qualified nurse you will be accountable for the standard of nursing care, dignity, and wellbeing of those you are providing care for so you will have a vital role to play in putting these into practice (NMC, 2018a). You will also have the responsibility of promoting awareness of essential standards of quality and safety, monitoring the standard of care delivered and taking action to make improvements where necessary. This will involve ensuring that the workplace culture is one in which quality improvement activities flourish and where frontline staff can grasp opportunities to make a positive contribution not only by enhancing their own professional development but also by engaging collaboratively with service users to improve and enhance care delivery.

Good quality care is care that is delivered according to the best evidence of what is clinically effective in improving an individual's health outcomes. Having clear, robust systems and structures in place can help us to identify and report on the quality of care provision. For example, in England the NHS Outcomes Framework (NHS Digital, 2022), the Public Health Outcomes Framework (Office for Health Improvement and Disparities, 2022) and the Adult Social Care Outcomes Framework (NHS Digital, 2021) set out indicators for measuring outcomes within health and social care systems in an effort to ensure continuous improvement in the quality of NHS services across all care providers. Similar strategies have been implemented in Scotland, Northern Ireland, and Wales (NHS Health Scotland, 2019; Department of Health, Social Services and Public Safety or DHSSPS, 2019; NHS Wales, 2022).

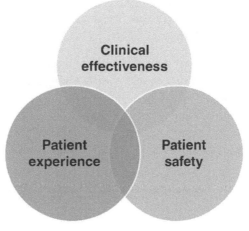

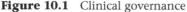

Figure 10.1   Clinical governance

Measuring quality

It is more than 30 years ago since the concept of quality improvement in healthcare settings was introduced by Donabedian (2005) among others, who suggested that by observing *structure* (the setting in which care is delivered, e.g., nurse: patient ratio, staffing levels), *focus* (the process or means by which the end point is achieved, e.g., care pathways) and *outcomes* (the end point, e.g., readmission rates, number of reported falls or hospital-acquired infection rates) we can measure the quality of healthcare. More recently the introduction of agreed standards of care has allowed us to measure the care we deliver against a set standard (e.g., benchmarking). As a bare minimum, current requirements dictate that we should meet essential standards for quality and safety set out by the Care Quality Commission (2018). We should also be aiming to meet standards set by the National Institute for Health and Care Excellence (NICE), and National Service Frameworks which focus on the care of individuals with a particular condition and set out what good quality care looks like for a particular group.

Regular participation in activities that continuously measure and monitor the quality of care delivered in your current workplace is essential. To do this effectively requires the use of robust systems and processes designed to monitor performance. Examples include:

- *Quality indicators* (QIs) – also referred to as *clinical quality indicators* (CQIs) – are reliable and valid measures, which can be used to assess health processes and outcomes (Maintz, 2003);
- *Clinical audit*: a cyclical staged process that seeks to improve standards of care and care outcomes through a systematic review of care measured against explicit criteria (e.g., quality indicators), a course of action taken to improve services and followed by continued monitoring to sustain improvement;
- *Clinical benchmarking*: a systematic process in which current practice and care are compared and amended to attain best practice and care (DH, 2010); it involves sharing evidence of best practice with colleagues and peers;

- *Patient-reported outcome measures* (PROMs) which can be used to evaluate the effectiveness of current service provision, recognise deficits, and assist in the development of new evidence-based services (Weldring and Smith, 2013).

To be successful, healthcare professionals need to fully understand the importance and value of collecting data because the success of such strategies is entirely dependent on the values and behaviours of staff working within the system. For example, some nurses may be a little sceptical about the benefits of time consuming 'number crunching' and do not understand the importance of data collection and how information can be used to improve care. As you continue to read on, you will hopefully begin to see how these data can be used in the drive for service improvement.

Activity 10.1

Access the Healthcare Quality Improvement website at www.hqip.org.uk/

What information is available here?

How might you use this resource to improve your own knowledge and understanding of ways in which you might measure and improve performance?

Clinical effectiveness

Quality care is *'care which is delivered according to the best evidence as to what is clinically effective in improving an individual's health outcomes'*. (National Quality Board, 2013: 13)

The provision of good quality care is of great interest to providers and purchasers of care alike. In recent years the emphasis for care providers has focused on evidence-based practice. Indeed, the NMC's *Code* (NMC, 2018a) demands that you deliver care based on the best available evidence. This requires you to keep your knowledge and skills up to date, ensuring that you have a good understanding of the current evidence base and an ability to apply this to your day-to-day practice. In addition purchasers are keen to ensure that healthcare provision is cost-effective and provides value for money. However concerns about the quality of care within some healthcare settings have continued to attract national publicity and often focus on the failure of organisations to provide services that deliver exacting standards of care. For example, the National Confidential Enquiry into Patient Outcome and Death (NCEPOD) (Healthcare Quality Improvement Partnership, 2022) has identified four areas of inequality – age and disability, social-economic deprivation, organisation of healthcare services and inclusion health groups – potentially impacting on the quality of care provision, care outcomes and death in recent times. Clinical effectiveness is about improving people's care and experience by critically reviewing what you/your team do by considering the following:

- What should be happening? (Identifying evidence of best practice);
- What is happening? (Reviewing current practice);

- How can we do it better? (Comparing your practice with good practice and implementing change);
- Evaluating change (using clinical audit and other measures, i.e., PROMs to demonstrate improvement).

Activity 10.2

Consider how you might begin to improve care and experience in your current practice setting. What would you need to know? What types of data might you need to collect and why? How might you do this?

Service-user experience

According to the World Health Organization (2022), quality care is defined as

"...care that is safe and effective, people-centred, efficient, timely and equitable".

Quality care looks to give an individual as positive an experience of receiving and recovering from illness as possible, including being treated according to what that individual wants or needs with compassion, dignity, and respect. People are encouraged to take more control of their own care (Scottish Government, 2017; NHS England, 2019; DHNI, 2022) and they have an important part to play in determining how services are designed, implemented, and evaluated (King's Fund, 2014). By collaborating closely with individuals and responding appropriately to their feedback, nurses can deliver more appropriate care and ensure that any concerns raised are dealt with quickly and appropriately (Coulter, 2012). This will usually involve collecting and using information provided by service users (e.g., satisfaction surveys or focus groups) to deliver the kind of services they want. Whatever approach is used the key aim is to find out what they really think about the services we offer and provide supporting evidence of this. It is extremely rewarding when you receive compliments from people about their care. However, unfortunately from time-to-time complaints will also feature. When they arise, it is important to ensure that they are not ignored.

Think of some examples currently used in your practice setting to elicit service-user feedback. How effective are these methods? How is the feedback used?

Luxford et al. (2011) suggest that the following factors are critical in assuring the quality of a person's experience of care:

- Strong and committed senior leadership;
- Communication of the strategic vision;

- Engagement of those receiving care and their families;
- A sustained focus on employee satisfaction;
- Regular measurement and feedback reporting;
- Adequate resourcing for care delivery design;
- Building staff capacity to support person-centred care;
- Accountability and an incentives culture that is strongly supportive of change and learning.

Resource management

Although safety and quality care are obvious drivers for change so too is the need to be able to manage resources effectively. As resources are limited we must make choices about how they are used. Resource management is about getting the best value for money and reducing 'unwarranted variations' by addressing overuse, misuse and underuse of treatment (NHS England, 2016). As a nurse, it is important to be able to provide the best quality care in the most efficient and effective way possible. We need to be able to balance available budgets and eliminate waste whilst improving the quality of the services we provide. All areas of expenditure will need to be carefully monitored and scrutinised. This is a huge challenge at a time where current severe funding restraint is accompanied by major reorganisations of health and social care services alongside calls for improvements in care quality too (NHS England and NHS Improvement, 2021). Nevertheless, it is possible. For example, Alderwick et al. (2015) highlight significant savings that have been made using generic medicines and targeted efforts to reduce the length of stays in acute care settings – driven in part by improved cooperation between clinicians and managers redesigning care pathways to maximise good healthcare outcomes, improved data collection/information and 'frontline' support from clinicians in practice.

Lean thinking is a philosophy used widely in manufacturing industries but has been applied more recently in healthcare settings (D'Andreamatteo et al., 2015). It is about simplifying processes, identifying which parts of a process add value to care provision, enabling care to flow more effectively and eliminating waste. The *Lean* framework incorporates six areas of consideration when seeking to manage available resources more effectively: overproduction; inventory; waiting; transportation; staff movement; and unnecessary processing. Some argue that a *Lean* approach is being used effectively to manage safety and improve productivity (Burroni et al., 2021), whereas others suggest that there is conflicting evidence of the outcomes of *Lean* thinking when applied in healthcare settings (Andersen et al., 2014, Mahmoud et al., 2021).

Activity 10.3

Closely observing the care delivered to individuals within a chosen healthcare setting:

1 Record the care processes (from the perspective of a person receiving care) encountered throughout the day (e.g., waiting times, provision of information, contact with other healthcare professionals, investigations and procedures performed).

2 Identify where savings could be made while maintaining or improving service-user safety and service provision.

3 What information or evidence might you need to collect to support your claims?

In response to the previous activity you may have witnessed (or been involved in) practices that include undertaking an activity 'just in case' (*overproduction*) – for example, unnecessary duplication of diagnostic tests; ordering excess material because the supply is unreliable (*inventory*); or using complex equipment to undertake simple tasks – for example, opening a sterile dressing pack to get access to gauze swabs (*overprocessing* or *unnecessary processing*). You may have seen people *waiting* in queues at a GP (General Practitioner) surgery, *waiting* for tests or having treatment delayed due to vital equipment not being available. You may also be familiar with issues related to the *transportation* of individuals receiving care or ways in which staff movement in the workplace seems inefficient (e.g., layout and organisation of the workplace). You could also have witnessed misuse or poor use of services – for example, poor access to end-of-life care in the community resulting in admission to hospital or poor concordance with prescribed medication or preventable health complications (e.g., venous thromboembolism, falls or medication errors).

Many of the current targets and organisational aims require us to make changes to services in order to improve the quality of care or safety (e.g., intervening earlier to avoid the development of possible complications), making more effective use of financial resources by improving stock rotation or ordering processes or perhaps improving management systems to ensure that you can make better use of human resources and available staff (e.g., reducing sickness and absence, providing education and training, motivating and allowing staff to be innovative).

Change Management Theories

Change is not a single action; it is a challenge to experience as well as to plan and manage. It requires a variety of resources – both human and material. Although many argue that change needs to involve a *well-planned, stepwise process* (proactive approach) and include a combination of interventions, linked to specific needs and obstacles to change (Lewin, 1951; Grol and Grimshaw, 2003), others support the view that change can also be *unplanned* (emergent/reactive) or ad hoc – particularly in rapidly changing environments or when triggered by organisational crisis – and that change will always contain complex emergent elements (Olson and Eoyang, 2001), especially in large-scale projects. Approaches can be *top-down* (i.e., from management downwards) or *bottom-up* (i.e., generated by frontline staff upwards). Pearson et al. (2008) suggest that both can be successful in disseminating nursing interventions depending on the requirements and circumstances.

Although there are many change management theories one popular traditional theory is that of Lewin (1951). Within this model (Figure 10.2), the *unfreezing* stage seeks to destabilise the forces that maintain the status quo. Actions of the change agent or leader are focused on gathering data and evidence to support the change, generating an air of discontent among

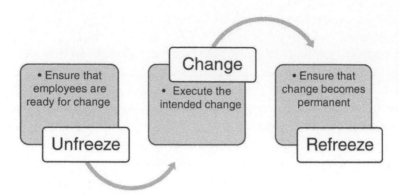

Figure 10.2 Lewin's model of change (1951)

those involved, decreasing the strength of old values, attitudes and behaviours and making others aware of the need for change. Once the need for change is recognised, goals and objectives are agreed, planned, and implemented. The *change* stage requires the leader to identify areas of support and resistance, developing strategies to support those involved or affected by the proposed change, in addition to dealing with resistance effectively. *Refreezing* seeks to stabilise the change, sustaining efforts to ensure that the new ways of working are incorporated into practice on a long-term basis.

However, current health and social care organisations are demanding, complex, challenging, and inter-dependent, and change management processes will often require consideration of a variety of factors (e.g., workplace cultures, availability of technology, workforce and skillsets, service user expectations and experience, the need to manage and reduce risk, competition, government policy and economics). It is worth remembering that seeking to change or improve services will always have an impact on someone. Having a critical understanding of the key issues, influencing factors and potential barriers is crucial if you are going to succeed in managing change and improving services within healthcare settings. The Health Foundation (2015) suggests that the key barriers to improvement in the NHS relate to the *initiative* itself (e.g., insufficient evidence base or usability of interventions), the *skills and attitude of individuals* (e.g., resistance, lack of knowledge and skills, role demarcation), *organisational context* (e.g., lack of leadership and management, culture and stability, lack of funding or time) or are *system wide* (e.g., incentives and funding, NHS culture, lack of stability and partnership working).

Indeed, it would be easy if once a need for change has been identified everyone involved readily accepted this and supported the development. However, it is never that simple even when intended benefits are clear since not everyone will be willing or interested. Changing entrenched clinical styles can be a difficult and lengthy process. Defensive reactions from colleagues, lack of awareness, incentives or training, time pressures or a fear of losing power can all act as barriers (Coulter, 2012). The organisational culture, changes in roles and responsibilities, and policy shifts can also affect the outcome of improvement work.

According to Silber (1993), the degree of resistance from individuals or groups will often depend upon four factors:

1   Their flexibility to change;
2   Their evaluation of the immediate situation;
3   Their anticipated consequences of the change;
4   Their perception of what they may lose and/or gain.

Potential barriers often include organisational politics and conflict that cannot be easily identified or resolved. Therefore to progress with a change idea, all the driving and restraining forces need to be identified (Lewin, 1951). Lewin's force field analysis framework (Figure 10.3) can be a useful tool to assist in the identification of the drivers and restrainers or change within planning and implementation phases.

Several types of forces that you will need to consider include:

- Available resources/funding/costs;
- Current targets and productivity;
- Current and past practices;
- The vested interests of stakeholders and attitudes of those who will be affected by the proposed change;
- Organisational structures/traditions and/or culture;
- Regulations, policies, and procedures (national or local)
- Relationships;
- Personal and/or group needs;
- The values of both the organisation and individuals;
- Opportunities.

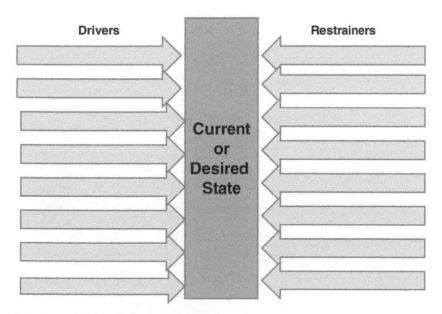

Figure 10.3   Force field analysis (Lewin, 1951)

Activity 10.4

Identify the potential barriers to change in your own workplace and consider how you might overcome these.

By (2005) provides a useful critical review of organisational change management exploring the differences in approaches but concludes that there is still a lack of underpinning evidence to suggest the best approach in any given situation, concluding that more robust research is needed to evaluate organisational change management frameworks. This is particularly vital when considering changes involving healthcare organisations. Traditional approaches as outlined by Lewin (1951) and Kotter (1996) are now considered too simplistic and, although some would argue that they are still relevant today, emergent Agile approaches acknowledging the complexity of working with individuals within multifaceted, inter-dependent organisations are now considered more appropriate (Kotter, 2014; Solid et al., 2019: Franklin, 2021). Unlike traditional and linear change management frameworks, advocates of Agile approaches argue the need to be able to understand, quickly adapt and respond to demands.

Kotter's eight-step change model (Kotter, 2014) comprises eight overlapping accelerators that assist those leading transformational change. He argues that, although strategy, structure, culture, and systems are important, nothing matters more than changing the behaviour of people by dealing with their feelings. This model therefore focuses on how people experience the change process. Updated from previous work (Kotter, 1996; Kotter and Cohen, 2002), it proposes a dual operating system – the hierarchy to take care of business and the network to react quickly to change and opportunities – suggesting that the two operating systems work side by side and are both essential for success.

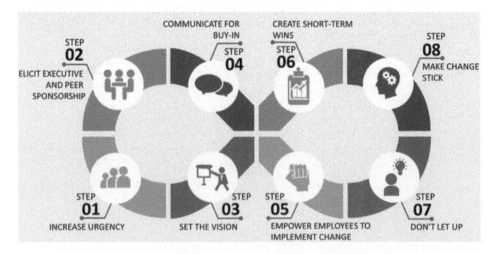

Figure 10.4 Kotter's eight-step model for effective change

Franklin (2021) also recognises the importance of attending to both project management activities and behavioural change. Additionally, they argue that it is much more effective to focus on smaller parts of the identified solution or goal (i.e., a sub-set of priority items), try them out (**apply**), and seek feedback from those affected to see how effective they are (**inspect**) before deciding what element of the overall solution to deliver next (**adapt**). The aim is to achieve these within small 2–4-week iterations **(sprints).** It is also acknowledged that the end goal might be adapted or changed because of this iterative process.

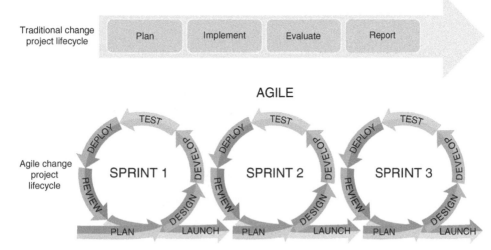

Figure 10.5   Traditional versus Agile change management approaches

Leading and managing change to improve services

Lockitt (2004) provides a useful overview of five broad strategies for affecting change, claiming that each has its advantages, disadvantages, and potential effects (Table 10.1).

Table 10.1   Strategies for affecting change

Strategy	Advantages	Disadvantages	Potential effects
Directive: change is usually imposed by managers with little or no consultation with others (i.e., those affected).	Can be implemented quickly.	Fails to take into consideration the views and feelings of those involved in or affected by the change.	May lead to valuable information or ideas being missed. May cause resentment from staff and those affected.
Expert: management of change is seen as a problem-solving process that needs to be resolved by an 'expert'. Change is normally led by specialist project team or manager.	The 'experts' play a major role in finding the solution and often the solution can be implemented quickly because a small number of 'experts' are involved.	Those affected may have different views from those of the 'experts' and may not appreciate the solution being imposed or the outcomes of the changes made.	

(Continued)

Table 10.1 Strategies for affecting change (*Continued*)

Strategy	Advantages	Disadvantages	Potential effects
Negotiating: recognises the willingness to negotiate and bargain in order to affect change.	Those affected by the change have an opportunity to have a say in what changes are made, how they are implemented. and the expected outcomes; therefore, feeling more involved and more supportive of the changes made.	Negotiating effectively takes time and the outcomes cannot be predicted.	Adjustments and concessions may be required in order to implement change, so the final changes may not meet the. total expectation of the change agent. Relatively slow to implement. More complex to manage. Requires more resources/costs.
Educative: involves changing people's values and beliefs in order for them to fully support the proposed change using a mixture of activities including persuasion, education, training and selection, and led by in-house experts.	Encourages the development of a shared set of organisational values that individuals are willing and able to support.	Takes longer to implement change.	Involves a mixture of activities including persuasion, education, training and selection and is led by in-house experts.
Participative: involves all those affected by anticipated changes. Driven less by managers and more by groups or individuals within an organisation.	All views are taken into account before change is made. Any changes made are more likely to be supported due to the involvement of all those affected. The commitment of individuals and groups within the organisation will increase because those individuals and groups feel ownership over the changes being implemented.	Can be time-consuming and costly due to the number of meetings needed, etc. Outcomes cannot be accurately predicted.	The organisation and individuals also have the opportunity to learn from this experience and will know more about the organisation and how it functions, thus increasing their skills, knowledge and effectiveness to the organisation.

Kouzes and Posner (2017) also maintain that having a leadership or management style that generates a shared purpose across all stakeholders is the most effective strategy to ensure success. They identify the following five leadership behaviours that contribute to a leader's ability to engage and empower others, some of which are considered crucial when attempting to affect change within healthcare settings and can be easily integrated within any of the approaches outlined previously.

Modelling the way involves identifying and clarifying shared values (e.g., the application of evidence-based practice and the provision of excellent standards of care) and then setting an example for others to follow. To be able to do this effectively requires an ability to identify new opportunities and the confidence to be able to speak up, to share fresh ideas and to demonstrate commitment to supporting others in making the change by creating opportunities (e.g., setting interim goals to achieve small wins while working towards larger objectives using pilot studies or small trials).

Inspiring a shared vision involves creating a shared picture of how things might be better with the change imposed. The leader needs to be able to inspire others by making the 'shared vision' appeal to a wider audience. Carefully exploring the interests and aspirations of others, listening to their views and finding a common ground to ensure that the 'vision' is shaped, shared and agreed by team members will help everyone involved to develop a keen sense of ownership. In fact, the ability to build coalitions of support and counter resistance to change is considered crucial to success (King's Fund, 2012) and a good leader will play a key role in enabling others to contribute their views, expertise and ideas.

Challenging the process often involves taking carefully considered risks so it is important for a leader to be able to develop a supportive climate/culture in which trying out innovative approaches is considered normal and safe experimentation is encouraged. Mistakes and failures – while disappointing – are a key component of success because learning from these will help individuals to progress.

Enabling others to act Rogers (2003) suggested that a common process occurs as people adopt a new idea. He identified five categories of adopters of an innovation – **innovators** (eager and adventurous); **early adopters** (respected opinion leaders); **early majority** (may deliberate for some time); **late majority** (sceptical and cautious); and **laggards** (traditionalists who prefer to do things as they have always done) – all of whom will have an impact on success. A variety of approaches may be needed to engage with all those involved as implementing the 'vision' will require collaboration over an extended period. Regularly reviewing and recognising the contribution of other members of your team as you go – encouraging, empowering, and sometimes challenging those involved – can help to develop confidence and competence and in turn generate an overall climate of trust. However, this will often require tolerance and empathy, showing sensitivity to the needs of others to make everyone feel included (Northouse, 2012).

Encouraging the heart Successfully managing change in healthcare organisations often involves a lot of hard work and dedication. People can frequently lose heart, particularly if there are no quick wins. Recognition of the achievements of others as well as yourself (however small) helps to keep optimism and determination alive. Giving praise to others also shows that their support and commitment has been noticed and appreciated. This can involve something as simple as passing an encouraging comment or something a little 'showier,' such as public praise in team meetings, celebration events or 'telling the story.'

In summary, the act of connecting and engaging with others is considered crucial to effect change in healthcare settings.

Service Improvement Models and Frameworks

Improving the quality of care services involves 'the combined and unceasing efforts of everyone to make the changes that will lead to better service-user outcomes (**health**), better system performance (**care**) and better professional development (**learning**)' (Batalden and Davidoff, 2007: 2) (Figure 10.6).

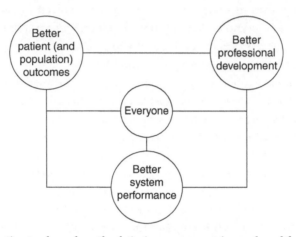

Figure 10.6 Illustrative tools and methods in improvement (reproduced from Batalden and Davidoff, 2007, with the permission of the BMJ Publishing Group)

There is a vast array of service improvement frameworks and tools available to support healthcare practitioners in their quest to improve healthcare services, all of which provide the means to manage and implement sustainable change (Welsh Government/AcademiWales, 2014; NHS England, 2018).

Though the reasons for change in healthcare settings are numerous, the focus should be on improving services for service-users (directly or indirectly). This will often include the effective introduction of new policies and guidelines (in line with an emerging evidence base) the consideration of the safe introduction of innovative technology and equipment, changes to the workforce/team or the need for effective resource management. Safety, care quality and the need to manage resources effectively are all key drivers for change that may be required in response to new government policies or legislation, professional guidance (top-down approach) or because practitioners at ground level recognise the need to influence or change local policies, procedures and practice (bottom-up approach). Whatever the circumstances, being able to 'think differently' about care delivery options is a crucial skill for future healthcare leaders (Bevan, 2013).

The first step towards service improvement is to identify what needs improving. To gain support for a project it is useful to align the proposal to overall organisational aims, clearly illustrating short-term and long-term benefits.

What are the quality/service improvement drivers in your workplace?

Find out about existing targets and/or service and organisational aims.

Service or quality improvement projects can vary from local small-scale schemes to the complete redesign of an organisation (Figure 10.7). As a nurse you will be in an ideal position to identify opportunities to make a positive difference to care delivery or the working environment, getting involved in service improvement initiatives or even taking the lead on change management projects. The task at this stage is to provide a strong rationale for change that is underpinned by supporting evidence and can be used to help create an impetus for movement, creating a vision for why and how things could be different.

LOCAL – SMALL SCALE:	MEDIUM SCALE:	LARGE ORGANISATIONAL SCALE:
e.g. Protected meal or rest times	e.g. The Productive Ward Programme (NHS Institute for Innovation and Improvement)	e.g. Health and Social Care Bill and Reconfiguration of the NHS

Figure 10.7 Levels of change

Stakeholder Engagement

To manage change effectively there is a need to involve others at every stage (e.g., team members, managers, multidisciplinary staff, service users, family/friends/carers, and learners). Early in the life of a project it is critical to identify all the organisations and people who may have an impact on the project. It is useful to remember that a 'stakeholder' is any person or organisation that is actively involved in a project, or whose interests may be affected positively or negatively. Once an area for improvement has been identified, it will need to be clear to others what it is that needs to be improved (e.g., situation, structure, process, treatment pathways, roles, behaviours) and why. We can then effectively share this 'vision' with others by appealing to their values, beliefs, hopes and dreams to come together to form a 'shared vision.' The identification of key stakeholders and their potential influence or resistance are crucial in helping to determine their fears and concerns as well as identifying potential difficulties. To be able to overcome resistance you will not only have to create interest in the proposed project but must also be prepared to face up to and either win over the sceptics or amend the 'vision' in response to their views.

Can you identify all the potential stakeholders who might influence a service improvement project in your current placement area?

How might you engage with *all* of these?

It is important to recognise that not all stakeholders will be found among your immediate colleagues. Stakeholders can be internal or external to the organisation. Depending on the proposed change, this could include service users and carers, team members or other professional groups and employees, suppliers, communities, and representatives from the private or voluntary sector, professional associations, and government regulatory agencies. Once identified it is also worth considering each stakeholder's importance and impact on the project. Stakeholder engagement involves understanding the needs of all the distinct groups or individuals who may be interested or affected by your proposed change and building relationships with them. It also helps to define which stakeholders will be involved while considering a communication strategy that aims to obtain 'buy-in' from all. Table 10.2 provides an overview of the different engagement approaches that could be employed depending on the needs and interests of the individuals, group, or organisation.

Table 10.2 Stakeholder engagement approaches

Engagement approach	Description
Partnership	Shared accountability and responsibility.
Participation	Part of the team engaged in delivering tasks or responsibility for a particular area/activity. Two-way engagement within limits of responsibility.
Consultation	Involved, but not responsible and not necessarily able to influence outside of consultation boundaries. Limited two-way engagement: organisation asks questions, stakeholders answer.
Push communications	One-way engagement: organisation may broadcast information to all stakeholders or target particular stakeholder groups using various channels, e.g., email, letter, webcasts, podcasts, videos, leaflets.
Pull communications	One-way engagement: information is made available, and stakeholders choose whether to engage with it, e.g., web pages or construction hoardings.

Reproduced with the permission of stakeholdermap.com

A clear statement of the need for change and what that will mean is essential for rallying support and commitment from stakeholders. Indeed, you may need to create more than one message if stakeholder priorities are different. Dixon-Woods et al. (2012) suggest that it is important to convince people there is a problem that is relevant to them (i.e., securing emotional engagement) and this can be achieved by using powerful stories and voices.

Service-user Involvement

Service-users and carers can offer valuable first-hand experience of inefficiencies and areas for improvement. There is a growing recognition of the need to involve them in service improvement processes. Service user involvement refers to the process by which people who are using or have used a service become involved in the planning, development and delivery of that service. Levels of involvement can vary, ranging from consultation (e.g., where they are asked their views but have limited influence on decision making), participation (e.g., where their views are sought and have a direct impact on decisions made), partnership working (e.g., contributing as equals – sharing decisions and responsibility) to full control (e.g., controlling the decision-making process).

Consider the role that service users and carers have in service development. What would you consider to be meaningful engagement? Are there any potential barriers? How might these be overcome?

Beresford (2013) suggests that to achieve effective and meaningful involvement with people particularly those whose voices are seldom heard, e.g., those with communication problems, black and ethnic minority groups, travellers, those in residential care or homeless individuals, means exploring, evaluating, and monitoring new and creative ways of engaging with and involving them. He goes on to say that some of the common barriers include:

- Devaluing service users – not valuing or listening to what they say;
- Tokenism – asking for their involvement but not taking it seriously, making it an unproductive experience;
- Stigma – associated with service user identity (e.g., alcohol, drug abuse or ex-offenders), discouraging them from associating themselves with it and getting involved on that basis;
- Low levels of confidence and self-esteem – leaving service users feeling that they do not have much to contribute or are worried about whether they will be able to do it;
- Language and culture – the frequent reliance on jargon and other exclusionary arrangements for involvement, puts off many service users who are not confident in or used to such situations;
- Inadequate information about involvement – this is made worse by the frequent lack of appropriate and accessible information about getting involved, discouraging many from taking the first steps to getting involved.

To overcome these issues Beresford (2013) recommends reaching out directly to service users, communities, and community leaders ensuring that they can gain access to the decision-making structures and collective working opportunities and providing support and practical help to build their skills and confidence so that they can participate effectively.

Activity 10.5

Access and read the following document:

> NHS England (2022) *Accelerated Access Collaborative Patient and Public Involvement Strategy 2021-26*. Available at: www.england.nhs.uk/aac/publication/accelerated-access-collaborative-patient-and-public-involvement-strategy/ (last accessed 19 July 2022).

Consider how this guidance could be used to improve engagement with service users, carers and the public in your own workplace setting.

Target Setting

Capturing all the information generated from engagement activities should help to ensure that the current situation is understood and will provide a focus for the improvement, assisting in the setting of measurable targets (NHS Institute for Innovation and Improvement, 2010). It is important to have measurable quality outcomes (a change is not necessarily an improvement!), so thought must be given right at the start about how the outcomes might be measured, depending on the aims and objectives. It is helpful to remember that there may already be data available that can initially be used as a baseline to set new targets.

At this stage, Dixon-Woods et al. (2012) caution against setting overambitious goals that can alienate people so it is important to try to set and agree realistic targets with the aim to include all stakeholders in order to counteract perceived lack of ownership and subsequent disengagement. Agreeing goals that are aligned with those of the organisation(s) also helps to ensure that individuals do not feel pulled in too many directions. When attempting to make improvements you should try to ensure that your goals are SMART:

- **S**pecific – focused, specific objectives are much easier to manage and execute;
- **M**easurable – you must be able to measure the extent to which your objective has been achieved;
- **A**ttainable – goals within reach but challenging enough to motivate;
- **R**elevant – goals aligned to professional or organisational goals;
- **T**imely – goals have target dates that monitor and maintain progression.

Once the goals have been clarified and agreed, activities need to be planned and implemented. It is important that all of those involved or affected fully understand the demands of the process. This may require provision of detailed explanations and ongoing support to ensure everyone involved has a clear understanding of the future and an agreed action plan (Dixon-Woods et al., 2012). Setting individual and team goals and targets based on the agreed objectives should help to keep the focus. Giving timely constructive feedback should also help to maintain and improve motivation.

Activity 10.6

Identify one area of practice where you think implementing a change (however small) could help improve service user safety, experience, quality of care provision or save valuable resources.

Make a list of the skills and attributes you think could be helpful when attempting to implement change within a healthcare setting and explain how and why they would be useful.

What strategies might you use and why? Think about how you might present ideas in a way that the current situation is understood so that you can obtain support from relevant stakeholders.

The plan–do–study–act (PDSA) cycle (Langley et al., 2009) is advocated for use by NHS England (2018) when attempting to test new change ideas on a small scale by temporarily trialling a change and assessing the impact – for example, trying out a new way to make appointments for clinic or trying out a new information sheet with a selected group of people before introducing the change to all clinics or service-user groups. The cyclical process (Figure 10.8) provides an opportunity to allow assessments to be made of whether the intervention is successful early on in a project, thereby allowing adjustments where necessary as the project moves forward.

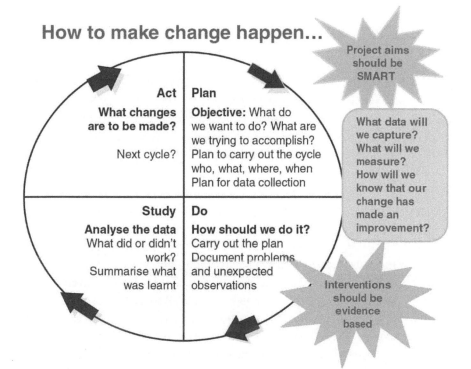

Figure 10.8 Plan–do–study–act cycle

Others argue that *Agile* project management methodology provides clearer design features, additional structure and planning, emphasising innovation and creativity and includes pacing and feedback mechanisms which are thought to offer an advantage over the less structured PDSA model (Williams, 2017). However, there is currently limited data available to illustrate effective application within clinical care settings other than digital health technology development. Similarly, Taylor et al. (2013) report variations in the way PDSA has been implemented in healthcare settings suggesting that the process has not always been used optimally. In addition, Reed and Card (2016) argue that in some cases (particularly where organisational and cultural changes are required) there is a need for an extensive repertoire of skills and knowledge to be able to use it well; thus it's legitimacy as a preferred quality improvement tool remains questionable (Knudsen et al., 2019).

Activity 10.7

Find out a little more about PDSA and AGILE project management tools by accessing and reading the journal articles below:

> Leis, J.A. and Shojania, K.G. (2017) 'A primer on PDSA: executing plan-do-study-act cycles in practice, not just in name', *BMJ Quality & Safety*, 26: 572-7.
> Špundak, M. (2014) "Mixed Agile/traditional project management methodology - reality or illusion?' *Procedia - Social and Behavioral Sciences*, 119: 939-48.

Which approach do you think would be most appropriate/applicable to use in your own setting and why?

When evaluating the impact of a change or service improvement we are seeking to assess how well (or not!) we have managed to achieve all of our aims and objectives. Solberg et al. (1997) suggest there are three characteristics of performance measures; measuring for *improvement*, *accountability*, and *research*. However, unlike research measurements taken where the aim is to extend the available knowledge by means of a systematically defensible process of enquiry, measures for improvement may have a lower threshold than that of research (i.e., 'good enough'). It is often better to have just a few good measures rather than a range of hard to collect details. Accountability measurements often relate to whether services meet a defined standard.

Sustaining improvement whereby innovations are embedded into everyday practice is not always easy. Berwick (2003) suggests that only a third of all innovations are successfully adopted and integrated into practice. Indeed, sustainability is vulnerable when improvement efforts are seen as one-off or time-limited projects or when they rely on certain individuals to ensure compliance or success (Dixon-Woods et al., 2012). Greenhalgh et al. (2005) suggest that the spread of innovation can be passive (e.g., unplanned, and informal diffusion) or active (e.g., by means of a planned and coordinated approach). The NHS Institute for Innovation and Improvement (2010) sustainability model was designed to help address this problem, proposing a strategy to measure the likelihood of sustaining improvement in practice and suggesting actions to take to ensure that this is increased where possible. It's use can also lead to useful discussions about the improvement process.

Activity 10.8

Thinking back to the area of practice you identified in Activity 10.6; how would you evaluate your project effectively?

Access the NHS Institute for Innovation and Improvement (2010) sustainability model at www.england.nhs.uk/improvement-hub/publication/sustainability-model-and-guide/

Once you have read this, consider what you could do to ensure the success of your project.

Factors that are likely to improve the chances of sustainability include:

- Where there are benefits beyond helping people (e.g., making a difference to working lives, reducing waste, duplication, or costs);
- Where benefits to service-users, staff and the organisation are visible, are believed by staff and can be described clearly;
- Where changed processes will continue to meet the need of the organisations and can be maintained when an individual or group of people who initiated it are no longer there;
- When data is easily available to monitor progress or assess improvement and where there are systems to communicate this in the organisation;
- When staff play a part in the implementation of changes to processes and where the training and development of staff are provided to help sustain these changes;
- When staff ideas are taken on board, they are then given the opportunity to test these ideas and their belief that this is a better way of doing things;
- When credible and respected senior and clinical leaders are seen as promoting and investing their own time in changes;
- When the changes being made are seen as an important contribution to the overall organisational aims;
- When staff, facilities, equipment, and policies and procedures are adequate to sustain new processes.

NHS Institute for Innovation and Improvement (2010)

Developing a Business Case

Case Scenario

You are a registered nurse currently leading a nursing team. Over the last 12 months the team have found it difficult to maintain the provision of good quality care provision. More recently, two registered nurse members of your team have left, having managed to secure jobs elsewhere, and despite attempts to recruit replacements their positions remain vacant. Although acknowledging the need to replace your registered nurse colleagues as soon as possible, you think there may also be an opportunity to introduce a wider skill mix into the team by recruiting nursing associates, and you have been asked to produce a business case to support this plan. How would you go about this?

When developing your business case it could be argued that the process would be similar to those outlined earlier. You would need to carry out a fair amount of research into the key issues and to consider and analyse all viable options. A good business case will explain the key issues clearly and identify potential solutions before going on to explain how the proposal would aim to address this. Central to your proposal of course, should be the current and overall potential impact on safety, the quality-of-care provision and service-user experience. You would need to include the benefits, costs, timescale, and the risks associated with both acting and/or doing nothing. For example, you would point out the need to ensure sufficient capacity and capability while also making best use of available resources. Finally, you would need to make recommendations for which option you think is best. You may be able to include convincing measures of impact outcomes and success criteria from similar projects that have been implemented elsewhere, demonstrating the value and benefits your proposal will bring. Relating your proposal back to the organisational strategy or vision is always useful to demonstrate how important it is; convincing the commissioner/funding body that the solution you have proposed is the right one is key.

Political Influencing

As an adult nurse you should be aware of the influence of UK government healthcare policies on our day-to-day practice. Undeniably, political decisions impact every aspect of nursing at every level. Yet it may be of no surprise to learn that many nurses appear disinterested in the political processes despite the need more than ever before to stand together to be able to ensure the best possible care is provided. Speaking up and speaking out on behalf of service users and our profession is a vital role if we wish to influence the future of UK healthcare services. Political activity consists of having the knowledge, skills, ability and will to engage and influence politicians. To do so effectively requires knowledge of current healthcare or nursing issues, laws, and current health policies, in addition to all the leadership and influencing skills highlighted in this and previous chapters.

Boswell et al. (2005) highlight that barriers to political activism are heavy workloads, feelings of powerlessness, time constraints, gender issues and a lack of understanding of the political process.

Activity 10.9

Do you know how the UK government works?

Find out about how you can lobby your elected political representative. Irrespective of whether this person is an MP (UK Parliament), MSP (Scottish Parliament), a member of the National Assembly for

Wales (AM) or a member of the Northern Ireland Assembly, the principles of lobbying and engagement are the same.

Would you know the most effective way to get your key message across? Think about ways in which you can strengthen your case and arguments by using powerful service-user stories to illustrate key issues.

Chapter Summary

The numerous demands placed on us as nurses sometimes challenge our ability to maintain – let alone improve – standards of care. However, nurses will remain the first line of defence in the safeguarding of safe, good quality care underpinning the use of recognised change management and quality improvement tools and techniques to improve care within their own sphere of influence. Dixon-Woods et al. (2012) suggest that being an effective leader or change agent involves a delicate combination of the ability to set out a clear vision while also being sensitive and aware of the needs of others. By acknowledging the complexity of change management we should recognise there is no prescribed linear order to the change process. Instead, frameworks encourage leaders of change to consider and focus on various – interacting factors, ensuring that all the components are aligned for sustained success.

Whichever model or framework you choose to use, understanding the nature of the change or improvement you wish to make and the context in which you are working is important in determining your chosen approach. Having a clear understanding of the people, processes and organisational culture that will be affected by your change is considered crucial to success. Burnes (1996: 13) believes that

> *"successful change is less dependent on detailed plans and projections than on reaching an understanding of the complexity of the issues concerned and identifying the range of available options".*

Whilst this seems a most sensible approach to take, research demonstrates that such factors are often overlooked, ignored, or underestimated by those wishing to implement change (Kotter, 1996; Fernandez and Rainey, 2006). It is vital to also remember that any changes to services should always consider the needs of service-users first. Targets require constant monitoring and revising if necessary to remain valid and meaningful. Therefore, evaluation is an essential part of this process whether or not the change has achieved the desired outcome. Finally, within service improvement or change management initiatives the most effective leadership styles are those that seek to include others, offer clear explanations, and apply gentle persuasion most effectively (Dixon-Woods et al., 2012).

Useful Websites

Care Quality Commission: www.cqc.org.uk
Healthcare Improvement Scotland: www.healthcareimprovementscotland.org
Healthcare Quality Improvement Partnership (HQIP): www.hqip.org.uk/
Information on Quality Improvement in Wales: www.iqi.wales.nhs.uk/home
Improvement Cymru: https://phw.nhs.wales/services-and-teams/improvement-cymru/
NHS England: www.england.nhs.uk/
NHS Improvement Resources: www.england.nhs.uk/improvement-hub/
NHS Northern Ireland: www.health-ni.gov.uk/
NHS Scotland: www.nss.nhs.scot/
NHS Wales: www.wales.nhs.uk/
NICE Guidance on Service Improvement Processes: www.nice.org.uk/about/what-we-do/
    into-practice/audit-and-service-improvement
NICE Quality Standards and indicators: www.nice.org.uk/guidance (Standards and
    Indicators)
Safety and Quality Standards Northern Ireland: www.health-ni.gov.uk/topics/
    safety-and-quality
World Health Organization Quality Toolkit: www.who.int/publications/i/
    item/9789240043879

References

Alderwick, H., Robertson, R., Appleby, J., Dunn, P. and Maguire, D. (2015) *Better Value in the NHS. The Role of Changes in Clinical Practice*. London: The King's Fund.
Andersen, H., Røvik, K.A. and Ingebrigtsen, T. (2014) 'Lean thinking in hospitals: is there a cure for the absence of evidence? A systematic review of reviews,' *BMJ Open*, 4: e003873. doi:10.1136/bmjopen-2013-003873.
Andrews, A. and Butler, M. (2014) *Trusted to Care. An Independent Review of the Princess of Wales Hospital and Neath Port Talbot Hospital at Abertawe Bro Morgannwg University Health Boards* (Executive Summary). Available at: http://gov.wales/topics/health/publications/health/reports/care (last accessed 5 July 2022).
Batalden, P.B. and Davidoff, F. (2007) 'What is "quality improvement" and how can it transform healthcare?' *Quality and Safety in Healthcare*, 16: 2–3.
Beresford, P. (2013) *Beyond the Usual Suspects*. London: Shaping our lives. Available at: https://shapingourlives.org.uk/report-series/beyond-the-usual-suspects/ (last accessed 19 July 2022).
Berwick, D.M. (2003) 'Disseminating innovations in healthcare', *JAMA*, 289(15): 1969–75.
Bevan, H. (2013) *What Can Civil Rights Leaders Teach us about Strategy for Transformation?* Available at: www.hsj.co.uk/opinion/blogs/the-nhs-change-agent/the-nhs-change-agent/5003114.bloglead (last accessed 4 June 2023).

Boswell, C., Cannon, S. and Miller, J. (2005) 'Nurses' political involvement: responsibility versus privilege', *Journal of Professional Nursing*, 21(1): 5–8.

Burnes, B. (1996) 'No such thing as... a "one best way" to manage organizational change,' *Management Decision*, 34(10): 11–18.

Burroni, L., Bianciardi, C., Romagnolo, C., Cottignoli, C., Palucci, A, Fringuelli, F.M., Biscontini, G. and Guercini, J. (2021) 'Lean approach to improving performance and efficiency in a nuclear medicine department', *Clinical and Translational Imaging*, Springer. Available at: https://doi.org/10.1007/s40336-021-00418-z (last accessed 15 July 2022).

By, R.T. (2005) 'Organisational change management: a critical review', *Journal of Change Management*, 5(4): 369–80.

Care Quality Commission (2018) *Essential Standards for Quality and Safety*. London: CQC (Care Quality Commission).Available at: www.cqc.org.uk/what-we-do/how-we-do-our-job/fundamental-standards (last accessed 19 July 2022).

Coulter, A. (2012) *Leadership for Patient Engagement*. Available at: www.kingsfund.org.uk/sites/default/files/leadership-patient-engagement-angela-coulter-leadership-review2012-paper.pdf (last accessed 19 July 2022).

D'Andreamatteo, A., Ianni, L., Lega, F. and Sargiacomo, M. (2015) 'Lean in healthcare: a comprehensive review', *Health Policy*, 119: 1197–209.

Department of Health (1998) *A First Class Service Quality in the New NHS*. London: DH.

Department of Health (2010) *Essence of Care*. London: DH.

Department of Health (Northern Ireland) (2022) *Patient Education/Self-Management Programmes for People with Long term Conditions*. Available at: www.health-ni.gov.uk/topics/doh-statistics-and-research/patient-education-programmes (last accessed 15 July 2022).

Department of Health, Social Services and Public Safety (2019) *Quality 2020: A Ten-Year Strategy to Protect and Improve Quality in Health and Social Care in Northern Ireland*. Available at: www.health-ni.gov.uk/publications/quality-2020-ten-year-strategy-protect-and-improve-quality-health-and-social-care (last accessed 5 July 2022).

Dixon-Woods, M., McNichol, S. and Martin, G. (2012) 'Ten challenges in improving quality in healthcare: lessons from the Healthcare Foundation's programme evaluations and relevant literature', *BMJ Quality & Safety*, 21: 876–84.

Donabedian, A. (2005) 'Evaluating the quality of medical care 1966', *The Milbank Quarterly*, 83(4): 691–729.

Fernandez, R., and Rainey, H.G. (2006) 'Managing successful organisational change in the public sector', *Public Administration Review*, March/April: 168–76.

Francis, R. (2013) *Report of the Mid Staffordshire NHS Foundation Trust Public Inquiry Executive Summary*. Available at: http://webarchive.nationalarchives.gov.uk/20150407084003 or www.midstaffspublicinquiry.com/report (last accessed 5 July 2022).

Franklin, M. (2021) *A practical framework for successful change planning and implementation*, London: Kogan Page.

Greenhalgh, T., Robert, G., Bate, P., Macfarlane, F. and Kyriakidou, O. (2005) *Diffusion of Innovations in Health Service Organisations: A Systematic Literature Review*. Oxford: Blackwell Publishing.

Grol, R. and Grimshaw, J. (2003) 'From best evidence to best practice: effective implementation of change in patients' care', *The Lancet*, 362(9391): 1225–30.

Hardacre, J., Cragg, R., Shapiro, J., Spurgeon, P. and Flanagan, H. (2011) *What's Leadership Got to Do with It?* London: The Health Foundation.

Health Foundation (2015) *What's Getting in the Way? Barriers to Improvement in the NHS*. London: The Health Foundation.

Healthcare Quality Improvement Partnership (2022) *How Data Captured by NCEPOD Supports the Identification of Healthcare Inequalities: A Review – 2022*. Available at: www.hqip.org.uk/wp-content/uploads/2022/04/Ref.-357-NCEPOD-Health-Inequalities-report-FINAL.pdf (last accessed 15 July 2022).

King's Fund, The (2012) *Leadership and Engagement for Improvement in the NHS. Together We Can*. London: The King's Fund.

King's Fund, The (2014) *People in Control of Their Own Health and Care. The State of Involvement*. London: The King's Fund.

Kirkup, B. (2015) *The Report of the Morecambe Bay Investigation*. Available at: https://assets.publishing.service.gov.uk/government/uploads/system/uploads/attachment_data/file/408480/47487_MBI_Accessible_v0.1.pdf (last accessed 19 July 2022).

Kirkup, B. (2018) *Report of the Liverpool Community Health Independent Review*. Available at: www.england.nhs.uk/publication/report-of-the-liverpool-community-health-independent-review/ (last accessed 19 July 2022).

Knudsen, S.V., Laursen, H.V.B., Johnsen, S.P., Bartels, P.D., Ehlers, L.H. and Mainz, J. (2019) 'Can quality improvement improve the quality of care? A systematic review of reported effects and methodological rigor in plan-do-study-act projects,' *BMC Health Services Research*, 19: 683.

Kotter, J.P. (1996) *Leading Change*. Boston, MA: Harvard Business School Press.

Kotter, J.P. (2014) *Accelerate: Building Strategic Agility for a Faster-Moving World*. Boston, MA: Harvard Business Review Press.

Kotter, J.P. and Cohen, D.S. (2002) *The Heart of Change: Real-life Stories of How People Change Their Organisations*. Boston, MA: Harvard Business School Press.

Kouzes, J. and Posner, B. (2017) *The Leadership Challenge*, 6th edn. Hoboken, NJ: Wiley.

Langley, G.L., Nolan, K.M., Nolan, T.W., Norman, C.L. and Provost, L.P. (2009) *The Improvement Guide: A Practical Approach to Enhancing Organizational Performance*, 2nd edn. San Francisco, CA: Jossey-Bass.

Lewin, K. (1951) *Field Theory in Social Science*. New York: Harper & Row.

Lockitt, W. (2004) *Change Management*. Available at: www.scribd.com/doc/50615816/CHANGE-MANAGEMENT (last accessed 19 July 2022).

Luxford, K., Safran, D.B. and Delbanco, T. (2011) 'Promoting patient-centered care: a qualitative study of facilitators and barriers in healthcare organizations with a reputation for improving the patient experience', *International Journal for Quality in Healthcare*, 23(5): 510–15.

Mahmoud, Z., Angele-Halgand, N., Churruca, K., Ellis, L.A. and Braithwaite, J. (2021) 'The impact of lean management on frontline healthcare professionals: a scoping review of the literature', *BMC Health Services Research*' 21(383): 4–11.

Maintz, J. (2003) 'Defining and classifying clinical indicators for quality improvement', *International Journal for Quality in Healthcare*, 15(6): 523–30.

National Quality Board (2013) *Quality in the New Health System: Maintaining and Improving Quality* (Final Report). Available at: www.gov.uk/government/publications/quality-in-the-new-health-system-maintaining-and-improving-quality-from-april-2013 (last accessed 19 July 2022).

NHS Digital (2021) *Adult Social Care Outcomes Framework*. Available at: https://digital.nhs.uk/data-and-information/publications/statistical/adult-social-care-outcomes-framework-ascof (last accessed 19 July 2022).

NHS Digital (2022) *NHS Outcomes Framework*. Available at: https://digital.nhs.uk/data-and-information/publications/statistical/nhs-outcomes-framework (last accessed 5 July 2022).

NHS England (2018) *The Change Model Guide*. Available at: www.england.nhs.uk/wp-content/uploads/2018/04/change-model-guide-v5.pdf (last accessed 19 July 2022).

NHS England (2019) *The NHS Long Term Plan*. N. England: NHS England.

NHS England and NHS Improvement (2021) *Building Strong Integrated Care Systems Everywhere: Guidance on the ICS people function*. Available at: www.england.nhs.uk/publication/integrating-care-next-steps-to-building-strong-and-effective-integrated-care-systems-across-england/ (last accessed 19 July 2022).

NHS Health Scotland (2019) *Development of Health and Social Care Inequality Indicators for Scotland. National overview report*. Available at: www.healthscotland.scot/media/2920/health-and-social-care-overview.pdf (last accessed 5 July 2022).

NHS Institute for Innovation and Improvement (2010) *The Handbook of Quality and Service Improvement Tools*. Coventry: NHS Institute for Innovation and Improvement.

NHS Wales (2022) *NHS Wales Performance Framework 2022-2023*. Available at: https://gov.wales/sites/default/files/publications/2022-06/nhs-wales-performance-framework-2022-2023.pdf (last accessed 5 July 2022).

Northouse, P.G. (2012) *Introduction to Leadership Concepts and Practice*, 2nd edn. London: Sage.

Nursing and Midwifery Council (2018a) *The Code: Professional Standards of Practice Behaviour for Nurses and Midwives*. London: NMC.

Nursing and Midwifery Council (2018b) *Future Nurse: Standards of Proficiency for Registered Nurses*. London: NMC.

Ockenden, D. (2022) *Final findings, conclusions, and essential actions from the Independent review of Maternity Services at the Shrewsbury and Telford NHS Trust*. Available at: www.gov.uk/government/publications/final-report-of-the-ockenden-review (last accessed 5 July 2022).

Office for Health Improvement and Disparities (2022) *Public Health Outcomes Framework*. Available at: www.gov.uk/government/collections/public-health-outcomes-framework (last accessed 5 July 2022).

Olson, E.E. and Eoyang, G.H. (2001) *Facilitating Organizational Change: Lessons from Complexity Science*. San Francisco, CA: Jossey-Bass/Pfeiffer.

Pearson, M.L., Upenieks, V.V., Yee, T. and Needleman, J. (2008) 'Spreading nursing unit innovation in large hospital systems', *Journal of Nursing Administration*, 38(3): 146–52.

Reed, J.E. and Card, A.J. (2016) 'The problem with plan–do–study–act cycles', *BMJ Quality & Safety*, 25: 147–152.

Rogers, E.M. (2003) *Diffusion of Innovations*. New York: Free Press.

Scottish Government (2017) *Health and Social Care Standards. My Support, My Life*. Edinburgh: Scottish Government.

Silber, M.B. (1993) 'The "Cs" in excellence: choice and change', *Nursing Management*, 24(9): 60–2.

Solberg, L., Mosser, G. and McDonald, S. (1997) 'The three faces of performance measurement: improvement, accountability and research', *Joint Commission Journal on Quality Improvement*, 23(3): 135–47.

Taylor, M.J., McNicholas, C., Nicolay, C., Darzi, A., Bell, D. and Reed, J.E. (2013) 'Systematic review of the application of the plan–do–study–act method to improve quality in healthcare', *BMJ Quality & Safety*, 23: 290–8.

Weldring, T. and Smith, S.M.S. (2013) 'Patient-Reported Outcomes (PROs) and Patient-reported Outcome Measures (PROMS)', *Health Service Insights,* 13(6): 61–8.

Welsh Government (2014), *Tools and Techniques for Change. A Leaders Handbook.* Available at: www.wales. nhs.uksitesplus/documents/1096/Change%20Management%20Handbook%20for%20leaders.pdf (last accessed 19 July 2022).

Williams, S.J. (2017) 'Delivering Agile and Person-Centred Care', chapter 4, pp. 45–67. In *Improving Healthcare Operations,* Cham, Switzerland: Springer International Publishing.

World Health Organization (2022) *Quality of Care.* Available at: www.who.int/health-topics/ quality-of-care (last accessed 19 July 2022).

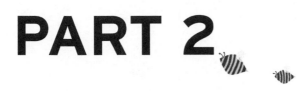

PART 2

CARING FOR ADULTS IN A VARIETY OF SETTINGS

11

SUPPORTING AND PROMOTING HEALTH

Karen Iley, Janice Christie, and Gillian Singleton

Chapter objectives

- Introduce the principles and practice of epidemiology and social determinants of health;
- Outline knowledge that supports registered nurses' action to promote health and wellbeing;
- Consider a range of opportunities available to promote mental, physical, and behavioural health for individuals, families, and populations within contemporary healthcare settings.

Health promotion is an enabling process which supports individuals and groups of people to have more involvement in enhancing their own wellbeing. It can be enacted through supporting individuals to alter their behaviours or perceptions and by initialing changes to social or physical environments (World Health Organization [WHO], 2022a). Public health involves supporting and improving the health and wellbeing of populations instigated through political, social or health care systems (Jarvis et al., 2020).

This chapter will focus on four modifiable lifestyle behaviours (diet, exercise, smoking and alcohol consumption) in relation to cardiovascular disease (CVD), obesity, sexual health, and mental health as these are priority areas for improving the health and wellbeing of the UK population (NHS England, 2019a).

Related Nursing and Midwifery Council (NMC) Proficiencies for Registered Nurses

The overarching requirement of the NMC is that registered nurses must promote health and wellbeing whenever the opportunity arises, irrespective of their practice setting (Nursing and Midwifery Council [NMC], 2018a, 2018b). Health promotion activities should be carried out with individuals, families, communities or population at any life stage to prevent illness and promote or protect health following national or global health agendas (NMC, 2018b).

━━━━━━━━ TO ACHIEVE ENTRY TO THE NMC REGISTER

YOU MUST BE ABLE TO ━━━━━━━━

- Understand the importance of early years' interventions and the impact of adverse life experiences on lifestyle choices and mental and physical wellbeing;
- Understand and explain the contribution of social influences, health literacy, individual circumstances, behaviours and lifestyle choices to mental and physical health outcomes in people, families, and communities;
- Demonstrate knowledge of epidemiology, demography, genomics, and the wider determinants of health, illness, and wellbeing at all stages of life and apply this to an understanding of patterns of health and illness and health outcomes;
- Understand the aims and principles of health promotion and health improvement and be able to apply these when caring for individuals, families, communities, and populations;
- Understand and explain the principles, practice and evidence base for health screening when engaging with individuals, families, and populations to promote and improve mental and physical health outcomes;
- Understand and apply the principles of pathogenesis and immunology, and the evidence base for immunisation, vaccination and herd immunity when engaging with individuals, families, and populations to promote health and avoid ill health;
- Identify and use every appropriate opportunity to discuss with people the impact of lifestyle choices including smoking, substance use, alcohol, sexual behaviours, diet and exercise on mental, physical, cognitive and behavioural health and wellbeing;
- Critically appraise and apply information about health outcomes when supporting people and families to manage their healthcare needs and make health choices;
- Explain and demonstrate the use of up-to-date approaches to behaviour change to enable individuals, families, and populations to use their strengths and expertise, and make informed choices when managing their own health and making lifestyle adjustments.

(Adapted from NMC, 2018b)

While population health can be tackled at community, regional, national, and global levels (WHO, 2022b), a nurse in everyday practice should be able to support public health strategy. For example, a five-minute conversation with a person before their discharge from hospital can help signpost them to resources that they might not know about (e.g., sexual health screening services for the over-55 age group) (DH, 2013). The nurse's approach to health promotion can vary depending on the targeted person, setting and resources available. Health promotion can either be 'planned,' e.g., as part of a wider public health initiative (RCN, 2012), or 'opportunistic', e.g., delivered as the need arises (RCN, 2016). The role of the nurse in *making every contact count'* (PHE, 2016a) is an essential element of the national health promotion strategy (Percival, 2014). Depending on the setting, nurses can form longer-term professional relationships with individuals to support them undertaking a tailored health promotion strategy – for example, using motivational interviewing as part of a smoking cessation package (Karatay et al., 2010). Nurses can also work to improve the health or a group of people such as through the facilitation of a 'support' group for people with diabetes (Gillett et al., 2010) or the delivery of a cardiac rehabilitation programme within the community (Taylor et al., 2010).

Activity 11.1

Access and look at the following document:

NHS Choices (2022) **Better Health - let's do this**. Available at: www.nhs.uk/better-health/

What opportunities can you think of to incorporate health promotion within everyday nursing practice?

The recognition that lifestyle is a major preventable contributor to morbidity and mortality has resulted in the formulation of national public health strategies to achieve healthy lifestyles in the UK (Public Health Wales, 2018; NHS England 2019a; Public Health Scotland, 2022).

It is accepted that a range of factors referred to as *'determinants of health'* impact the health and wellbeing of people (WHO, 2022a). Examples of these determinants include genetics, housing, social connectedness, and wealth which not only affect the health of individuals but are shared among groups of people. Nurses need to have a sound knowledge of the health of the population they care for and what influences their health as well as being able to apply this knowledge to support public health agendas (NMC, 2018b).

Epidemiology is the scientific study of the distribution of health events in different populations and why these occur (Coggon et al., 2020) so that this information can then be applied to the prevention and management of such events (Mulhall, 1996). During the years of sanitary reform (1848 to 1870), the emphasis of public health was on changing or improving the physical environmental conditions in which people lived to improve health – for example, removing the handle of a public-used water pump in London to stop a cholera outbreak

(Gunn and Masellis, 2008). It is still recognised today that the physical environment (e.g., access to clean water and air, and safe housing) is an important determinant of health (WHO, 2022a). In 1974, Lalonde presented the 'Health Field Concept' framework, which identified four key areas impacting health: **human biology**, **the environment**, **lifestyle,** and **healthcare organisation**. This became a key turning point for building more holistic public health policy and practice which considered wider determinants of health (Tulchinsky, 2018).

Determinants of Health and Health Inequalities

In contemporary public health practice, the broad concept of health promotion is underpinned by principles of 'equity,' 'participation' and 'empowerment' (WHO, 2022a).

> *Equity* refers to **fairness and justice** and is distinguished from equality. Where equality means providing the same to all, *equity* means recognising that we do not all start from the same place and must acknowledge and adjust imbalances so that everyone can achieve their potential for good health (WHO, 2021a). For example, people living within socio-economically deprived communities have poorest health and lowest life expectancy (Marmot, 2020) and to tackle this in one area in NW England, there are plans to reduce debt, improve wages, and increase the number of children who can access free school meals (Institute of Health Equity, 2021).

> *Participation* describes a process where the involvement of a population or service users is desired and valued in decisions about services and policy that affect their health (WHO, 2019a). Participation is a significant feature of contemporary UK healthcare policy. An example here would be service users and the public in decisions about what public health services are commissioned for a local area (NHS England, 2017a).

> *Empowerment* is a process that allows people to gain control over things that influence their wellbeing and decision-making about their health (WHO, 1986); for example, the provision of a comprehensive model of personalised care for people with complex needs to enable and support them to make care choices about the management of their health and social wellbeing (NHS England, 2022).

Health inequalities are unjust differences in disease, death and access to health resources between distinct groups of people (The Kings Fund, 2022) arising from variations in determinants of health that impact people throughout their lives.

The Black Report (Townsend et al., 1992), Acheson Report (1998) and Marmot Reviews (Marmot, 2010; 2020) have all shown that differences in determinants of health such as income and living and working conditions contribute to inequalities in health within the UK. For example, the poorest 10% of the UK population will have the lowest life expectancy and healthy life expectancy (Office for National Statistics, 2018a).

Marmot (2010; 2020) argues that adverse socioeconomic circumstances accumulate during a person's life, with health disadvantage beginning at conception and continuing through life for the poorest, resulting in early and avoidable mortality. It is important for nurses to understand the relationship between health and social factors so that they can be sensitive and empathetic when assessing a person's needs, anticipate and plan for targeted health promotion activity and be supportive in signposting them to appropriate resources (Phillips et al., 2020).

Dahlgren and Whitehead (1991) offer a useful visual representation of the various determinants of health (Figure 11.1) which demonstrates that health is not solely dependent on healthcare services but also affected by individuals themselves and their social and material resources, which are in turn influenced by wider national policies (Naidoo and Wills, 2016).

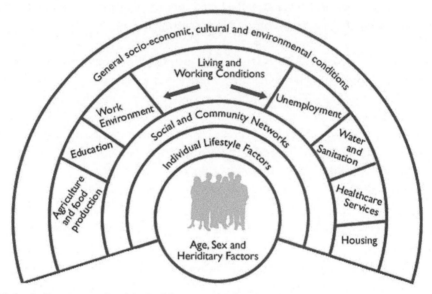

Figure 11.1 Influences on health (Dahlgren and Whitehead, 1991)

As nurses we also need to be aware of the resources that individuals, families and communities have access to when assessing their health needs and planning interventions. For example, if promoting healthy eating we should consider the individual or family budget, the quality of food storage available and facilities for food preparation. The lack of good access to healthy foods within some geographical areas can be problematic so we also need to think about the accessibility, availability, and affordability of culturally appropriate healthy food as this can vary from place to place (Rodney, 2015). It is therefore clear that the nurse's role in health promotion is wide and far-reaching, and in many instances requires committed, joined up working with other agencies (Green and Tones, 2010).

Levels of Prevention

When thinking about the type of health promotion activity we might use we need to consider whether the level of prevention we are aiming for is *'primary,' 'secondary'* or *'tertiary'* (Loveday and Linsley, 2011) to have a realistic expectation of the outcome.

> *Primary*: to prevent disease developing (this might have a population-wide focus);
>
> *Secondary*: to prevent disease from progressing (this could focus on individuals 'at risk' but not currently unwell);
>
> *Tertiary*: to prevent the further consequences of the disease (this could focus on those who are unwell).

Activity 11.2

Consider the different scenarios below. Do you think that the healthcare professionals here are engaging in primary, secondary, or tertiary levels of prevention? Reflect on why you conclude this.

1. The diabetes nurse specialist advises a 22-year-old with type 1 diabetes mellitus on their diet, insulin regimens and glucose monitoring.
2. A 78-year-old is given an annual influenza vaccination by their practice nurse.
3. A 37-year-old is offered annual mammograms after being identified as carrying the *BRCA1* gene.

One key area of primary health prevention that nurses can engage in to promote public health is immunisation (vaccination) programmes. The prevention of communicable disease by mass inoculation can be extremely effective in directly protecting those who have been immunised against an infectious disease (Hamami et al., 2017). When a sufficient proportion of the population has been immunised achieving 'herd immunity' (Fine et al., 2011) (Figure 11.2), it provides some protection to the remaining non-immunised population as the rate of transmission of the disease is slowed or stopped (Vynnycky and White, 2010). The additional benefit of 'herd immunity' is of notable value to those who are immunocompromised (Cesaro et al., 2014). Although 'disease-specific herd immunity thresholds' can vary (Betsch et al., 2017), the World Health Organization (2021b) recommended target for immunisation uptake is 95% for most programmes.

However, to adequately discuss immunisation with people a nurse should be aware that there are several factors that can affect uptake of a vaccine (Vynnycky and White, 2010). For example, health beliefs in relation to the vaccination (and the disease it aims to prevent) can have a significant effect (Funk and Klepac, 2015). In addition, potential recipients may be allergic to some part of the vaccine (Chung, 2013), and those with a compromised immune system due to existing morbidity and/or medical treatment may be unable to receive some vaccinations (UKHSA, 2017).

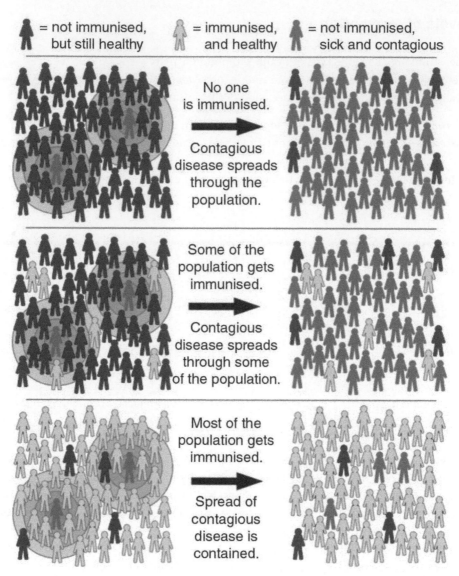

Figure 11.2 Herd immunity (from National Institute of Allergy and Infectious Diseases)

Activity 11.3

Have a look at the current data available on adult immunisation uptake across the
UK: www.gov.uk/government/collections/vaccine-uptake. What is the uptake like
in your area?

What could you do as an adult nurse to positively influence immunisation uptake?

Behaviour Changes for Health

Adult nurses have a role in impacting the health of individuals, families, and communities within a range of settings (NMC, 2018b) and can influence health policy at a local and national level (Naidoo and Wills, 2016). This impact can be enacted through:

1. Supporting an individual or family to change behaviours that impact their health;
2. Involvement in community development and action to support communities to identify and address health issues;
3. Influence change within their healthcare organisation;
4. Public policy change.

Due to the varied nature of the nurse's role in health promotion it can sometimes be difficult to decide how to approach a health promotion opportunity. Fortunately, several health promotion models have been created to make sense of and simplify the complexity of health promotion (Davies and Macdowall, 2006). Models can assist us to select the most relevant type of health promotion activity and decide whether the intervention is individually or collectively focused. For example, the health belief model (Becker, 1974; Rosenstock, 1974) draws on health psychology and focuses on individual belief systems in relation to lifestyle choices meaning an individual may believe jogging contributes to good cardiovascular health. This and some other models are outlined in Table 11.1.

Table 11.1   An overview of models used in health psychology – and their application to health promotion

Nature of model/Approach	Author(s)	Key features
Health belief model	Rosenstock (1974); Becker (1974)	Acknowledge the influence of demographics, social class, gender, age, internal and external cues; Perceived susceptibility and severity of the negative health outcome plays a key role; The perceived benefits and barriers to the behaviour change are also important; Specific 'cues to action'/perception of threat can contribute to a behaviour change; Levels of self-efficacy inform decision to change.
Transtheoretical model	Prochaska and DiClemente (1986)	Suggest that change follows 'sequential' stages; Describe 'processes' which people typically use to facilitate change; Change can be predicted by consideration of the 'decisional balance'; Self-efficacy is described as the person's confidence in their ability to make changes. This model has been applied to a variety of unhealthy behaviours (for example, smoking, alcohol consumption, exercise, diet, drug abuse) with evidence to suggest that health promotion programmes that are designed or tailored around each of the stages above are more effective (Noar et al., 2007).

(Continued)

Table 11.1 An overview of models used in health psychology – and their application to health promotion (*Continued*)

Nature of model/Approach	Author(s)	Key features
Theory of planned behaviour	Ajzen (1991)	An extension of the theory of reasoned action (Ajzen and Fishbein, 1980). Used to study cognitive determinants of health behaviours; Behaviour is determined by the strength of intention and the level of control a person perceives they have; Acknowledges the role of 'subjective norms' in influencing behaviour choices, e.g., perceived social pressure to perform or not perform a behaviour (Ajzen, 1991).
'Model of intervention' and 'Focus of intervention' criteria used to generate four models of health promotion activity	Beattie (1991)	*Focus* of intervention may be *individual* or *collective*. *Mode* of intervention may be *authoritative* (top-down and expert-led) or *negotiated* (bottom-up, individual). Health promotion practice identified as: Health persuasion (authoritative, individual); Legislative action (authoritative, collective); Personal counselling (negotiated, individual); Community development (negotiated, collective).
Three overlapping spheres of activity: health education, prevention and health protection	Tannahill (1990)	*Health education* – communication to enhance wellbeing and prevent ill-health through influencing knowledge and attitudes. *Prevention* – reducing or avoiding the risk of disease and ill health primarily through medical intervention. *Health protection* – safeguarding population health through legislative, fiscal or social measures.
Five approaches to health promotion activity	Ewles and Simnett (2003)	*Medical* approach – treatment, for example drugs. *Behavioural* approach – providing advice and guidance. *Educational* approach – specific information and/or training provided. *Empowerment* approach – life skills approach, for example assertiveness and communication. *Social change* approach – appraisal of services available, lobbying, campaigning.

Table 11.1 summarises the key features of the most well-known models though further reading in relation to each specific model or approach is recommended. These models specifically focus on an area of health promotion and tend to acknowledge both individual and community approaches to public health interventions. The potential scope of health promotion activity goes beyond working with the individual. Therefore, in addition to models that focus on the individual there are also 'collective' models such as community development theory (Fawcett et al., 1995) which acknowledge the importance of harnessing the resources within a community.

Activity 11.4

Although there is only a selection of models highlighted in Table 11.1 you will see that there are several approaches to health promotion practice with a varied emphasis on each component.

Consider which of these models might be useful to use in the following scenarios:

1. A person tells you they have not thought about stopping smoking;
2. A parent tells you that they want their children to eat healthily but there is nowhere locally where they can buy healthy foods.

How could each model be applied to each of these scenarios?
What were the benefits and limitations of them in each scenario?

Health Needs Assessment

Before any nursing activity is commenced we should carry out an effective assessment as highlighted in previous chapters (Kozier, 2008). Engaging in community or population level interventions requires a thorough knowledge of the health issues in any given community (Naidoo and Wills, 2016) and therefore a community health needs assessment should be undertaken. This is a process that systematically reviews the health of a population, informing on priorities and the allocation of resources (Cavanagh and Chadwick, 2005). Although this is particularly relevant to the work of community practitioners (Rowe et al., 2001), knowledge of an individual's local community is important for all nurses since this knowledge also informs effective individual assessment and discharge planning (Timby, 2012).

A good community assessment includes standard measurements such as data about disease, environment, local resources and important services, and the views of service users.

Undertaking a community health needs assessment is not always straightforward, yet it is a key aspect of service planning (Green and Tones, 2010).

There are three main stages:

1 Identifying need;
2 Identifying assets or available resources;
3 Determining which health needs to prioritise actioning.

When determining needs there are different perspectives that can be considered such as:

- The epidemiological perspective regarding diseases and risk factors for disease;
- The population and service providers' perspectives on health and health issues;
- The health economist's perspective – e.g., is the health promotion intervention 'clinically effective' and 'cost effective'?;
- The sociological perspective – e.g., the social determinants of health and health inequalities.

Social epidemiological data helps us identify the main disease-related issues in a particular area (Mulhall, 1996) – for example collecting morbidity rates (the rates of death within a defined population over a defined period) and mortality rates (the rates of death within a defined population over a defined period of time). Social and economic differences between populations use sources such as the Office of National Statistics (ONS) data and deprivation scores (e.g., *Index of Multiple Deprivation* measuring various indicators to obtain a score of relative deprivation). Other sources that also use these measures include the Health Survey for England. Both give useful insight into population demographic data and socioeconomic needs of the population.

What is the difference between 'incidence' and 'prevalence'?

As a nurse you will come across these terms very frequently with implications for your role as an adult nurse. 'Incidence' refers to the number of new cases of a particular disease, condition, or event in a particular population (usually within the previous year). 'Prevalence' refers to the total number of cases in a particular population (at a set point or period), some of which may have been diagnosed for several years.

What can incidence rates tell us about our health promotion practice?
What are the potential health needs of your workplace/placement setting or geographical area? How might these be addressed?

Policy, Legislation, and Health Promotion

In general a healthcare policy is a statement about a goal in healthcare and a plan for achieving that goal (Earle et al., 2007).

Each country within the UK regularly updates their main 'flagship' health policy, which sets out their long-term vision for their health services. In 2021, a government reform to public health and promoting health changed, with two new bodies: the National Institute for Health Protection (subsequently renamed UK Health Security Agency (UKHSA) and the Office for Health Promotion (subsequently renamed the Office for Health Improvement and Disparities (OHID) (Hunter et al., 2022).

Activity 11.5

Select and review at least one of the Government Acts below which is most pertinent to you:

Health and Social Care (Quality and Engagement) (Wales) Act: summary: www.gov.wales/
health-and-social-care-quality-and-engagement-wales-act-summary-html
Health and Care Bill (2021): www.parliament.scot/bills-and-laws/legislative-consent-
memorandums/health-and-care-bill

Health and Care Act (2022): www.legislation.gov.uk/ukpga/2022/31/contents/enacted

Health and Social Care Act (Northern Ireland) 2022: https://statutoryinstruments.parliament.uk/instrument/gV3mVq2h/.

A UK White Paper is an official government report that sets out government policy on a matter that is presented to parliament. Acts on the other hand are laws, for example the Smoking (Northern Ireland) Order (see www.legislation.gov.uk/nisi/2006/2957/contents) or the Tobacco and Primary Medical Services (Scotland) Act (see www.legislation.gov.uk/asp/2010/3/contents). These are usually preceded by a White Paper (Masterson, 2011).

However laws and policies are often insufficient as 'stand-alone' agents to completely change health behaviour although they can play a significant role. For example, despite the Health Act 2006 and subsequent smoking ban people across the UK continue to smoke (ONS, 2020), although the overall prevalence of smoking has reduced (ONS, 2020); fewer people aged 18 to 24 years smoke than older adults (ONS, 2020). Psychological theory suggests that people must want to stop smoking (Prochaska and DiClemente, 1986) and hence there will be a group of people who do not want to stop smoking for a range of reasons such as weight gain and appetite suppression (Ming, 2018). An important consideration in a smoking cessation policy therefore, is how this group of people are accessed and targeted.

E-cigarettes and vaping are an effective intervention to aid quitting smoking and has helped 50,000 people to quit and has some of the highest success rates (PHE, 2021a). Although many young people have tried or use vapes, prevalence has not changed in recent years despite speculation (PHE, 2021a). However, the long-term consequences are unknown, such as variations in the nicotine strengths, and use between socioeconomic groups. PHE (2021a) acknowledges that close monitoring, further research, and greater regulation of sales to young people is needed.

This has implications for targeted health promotion and we must be mindful that smoking can be more prevalent in various parts of the UK and in groups with lower socioeconomic status (ONS, 2020a).

Lifestyle and Public Health

Four lifestyle factors are associated with almost half of the overall 'illness burden' in the UK and the developed world (Everest et al., 2022) – alcohol consumption/drug misuse, smoking, poor diet (including low consumption of fruit and vegetables) and low levels of physical activity. These factors often occur together (PHE, 2020), much like the coexistence of different illnesses in those individuals with long-term conditions (PHE, 2020). Furthermore, the 'clustering' of unhealthy behaviours can have a compound effect on an individual's health outcomes (Meader et al., 2016) and have implications for the approach to health promotion practice and the nurse's role (RCN, 2012). As adult nurses, we come across a range of health issues (both acute and long term) that can be influenced in part by lifestyle choices (NHS England, 2019a) and that play a significant role in health outcomes for adults across the lifespan (Fuller, 2011).

The NHS Long Term Plan (NHS England, 2019a) discusses actions planned to focus on prevention and health inequalities as well as the UKHSA continuing with previous Public Health England's strategies for protecting and improving the nation's health. Current priorities include reducing health inequalities; smoking cessation; tackling Type 2 Diabetes; obesity, healthy weight, and nutrition; mental health; tackling health harms (alcohol and substance misuse); sexual and reproductive health and early years' health and development (NHS England, 2019).

Alcohol intake is a recognised aspect of the British culture and lifestyle and in 2017 across the UK an estimated 29.2 million adults drank alcohol (ONS, 2018a). Current recommendations for low-risk drinking are less than 14 units for women and 20 for men, whereas increasing risk is for women 14–35 units and 20–50 for men and higher risk is over 35 units for women and 50 for men (DHSC (Department of Health and Social Care), 2021). Tackling alcohol misuse is a priority as it is known to cause or contribute to 200 health conditions and led to 1.1 million hospital admissions between 2017–2018 (OHID, 2021). The first national strategy for England was published in 2003 (Prime Minister's Strategy Unit, 2003) but the current *Alcohol, Applying All our Health* strategy (OHID, 2021) focuses on health professionals supporting individuals to reduce their harmful levels of consuming alcohol. Excess alcohol intake has also been linked to a range of public health and social issues (OHID, 2021) with an increased incidence of crime and hospital admissions when binge drinking has occurred (ONS, 2021b). At first glance, we could assume that binge drinking is only a small part of our national lifestyle, yet half of the total alcohol consumption in the UK is attributed to binge drinking (OHID, 2021). Several strategies have been put forward to address this issue.

Scenario

In 2018, the Scottish Government introduced and implemented a 'Minimum Unit Pricing' strategy to reduce alcohol consumption (Scottish Government, 2018).

Relating back to the previous health promotion models outlined, what type of approach is the example above? How could each model be applied to reduce rates of alcohol consumption in this scenario?

We must remember that our role is to promote health and be non-judgemental when working with individuals, groups, and communities (NMC, 2018a). However, despite the need to consider the coexistence of unhealthy behaviours, it does not mean that we should immediately reject any intervention that focuses on just one behaviour (e.g., smoking). Indeed, it may be that coexisting unhealthy behaviours do need to be addressed 'one at a time,' because success in one lifestyle change may empower and motivate an individual to make other changes (Paiva et al., 2012).

Motivational Interviewing

Motivational interviewing (MI) has been increasingly used in healthcare, especially in primary care as a method to help individuals to improve their health. It is a skilful way of having a clinical conversation to enable individuals to assess their own motivation for making changes and to identify their own solutions to improve their health (Rollnick et al., 2007). This approach puts the person at the centre of the process and the role of the nurse is to act as a facilitator rather than educator.

The key element is the 'spirit' of MI, which is to be collaborative, evocative, and honouring individual autonomy (Rollnick et al., 2007). Being collaborative means having a joint active conversation and joint decision making about a behaviour change. The nurse needs to understand the individual's perspective so they can evoke their own good reasons and the motivation to change. Honouring individual autonomy is the most important aspect of the 'spirit' and can sometimes be challenging for nurses as it means allowing a person to make their own choices even if we do not believe it's the correct action to take.

The practice of MI has four guiding principles that healthcare professionals must follow: *Resist*, *Understand*, *Listen* and *Empower*. These all relate to the process of conversations that take place between an individual and the nurse. The overriding concern is that a person will initiate change when they are ready to. We need to try not to influence or push decisions which individuals may resist but to listen and understand their viewpoint and support their choices whatever they may be.

MI has been found to be clinically effective and used successfully to address several health concerns such as alcohol misuse, substance misuse and physical activity (NICE; 2011; 2013; 2017a).

Activity 11.6

Find out more about motivational interviewing by accessing some of the resources below:

1   Wagner, C. and Ingersol, K.S. (2012) *Motivational Interviewing in Groups*. London: Guilford.
2   Miller, W.R. and Rollnick, S. (2012) *Motivational Interviewing: Helping People Change*. London: Guilford.
3   Levounis, P., Arnaout, B. and Marienfel, C. (2017) *Motivational Interviewing for Clinical Practice: A Practical Guide for Clinicians*. Virginia: American Psychiatric Publishing.
4   Motivational Interviewing Network of Trainers (MINT) guidance YouTube videos: https://youtu.be/n263wS6-l24 https://youtu.be/reTb-x6UOmY

We have already acknowledged the value of looking at health issues and lifestyle behaviours, both in clusters and on an individual basis. We will now focus on four specific areas – obesity, cardiovascular disease/coronary heart disease (CVD/CHD), sexual health and mental health – in more detail. These can be impacted by at least one of the four lifestyle behaviours (e.g., smoking, drinking alcohol, diet, and exercise) as outlined by the WHO (2021a) and as such, can be effectively targeted for health promotion intervention (Table 11.2).

Table 11.2 Lifestyle problems in the UK

Health issue	Scale of the problem	Associated lifestyle behaviours – examples
Obesity	Adult morbid obesity has tripled since 1993. Prevalence has increased from 15% in 1993 to 28% in 2019 (HSE, 2020)	Low level of physical activity and poor diet
Cardiovascular disease/coronary heart disease (CVD/CHD)	One of the leading causes of death in England (ONS, 2021a) and across the UK	Poor diet, smoking, low levels of physical activity
Sexual health	Rates of infectious syphilis highest since the 1950s (PHE, 2021b) 45% of pregnancies are unplanned (PHE, 2018)	Excessive alcohol use, substance misuse increases likelihood of risk-taking behaviour
Mental health	Suicide is the most common cause of death in men and women aged 45-49 years in England and Wales (ONS, 2022b). Young people aged 16-24 in England drinking to hazardous levels (ONS, 2018a) 3.1% show signs of drug dependence (Roberts et al., 2016)	Breakdown of relationships, substance misuse, poor mental health

Obesity

Although obesity is an increasing problem, we must also consider safety, comfort, dignity, and respect regarding the nursing care of this group. Obesity can have a range of consequences on both physical and mental health (NHS England, 2019b) and, as such, it is never too late to start or continue any intervention for addressing obesity.

Femi and Agwe

Femi, a 27-year-old with a BMI (body mass index) of 35 (note that BMI is [weight in kg]/ [height in m²]) is married to Agwe, 31, who has a BMI of 21. Both Femi and Agwe are smokers. Femi works as a receptionist but has recently had a prolonged period of absence due to back pain. Agwe is a long-distance lorry driver who works erratic hours. Femi attends an asthma clinic appointment with the practice nurse, and asks for advice about healthy weight loss, disclosing that they would like to start a family.

What are Femi's main health needs?

What are the key influencing factors?

What would be your approach to promoting Femi's health in this scenario?

There are a range of factors that contribute to obesity (e.g., poor diet, physical inactivity and /or alcohol intake – NICE, 2022; NHS England, 2019a). The impact of obesity can have consequences for both an individual and the wider family (Flodgren et al., 2017). This is evident within the previous scenario because there could be an impact on fertility (Reynolds and Gordon, 2018) in addition to an increased risk of heart disease and diabetes (Jenkins et al., 2018). The good news however, is that there are several health promotion strategies to use in cases such as this. For example, as an adult nurse the work you do with Femi and Agwe could be on an individual, family or community basis (Naidoo and Wills, 2016), targeting a range of lifestyle issues. Using the opportunity to discuss health and potential lifestyle changes, however brief, can begin the process by '*Making Every Contact Count*' (PHE, 2016a). Furthermore, motivational interviewing could be implemented as part of an individual weight management programme (NICE, 2022), with the additional benefit of Femi and Agwe supporting each other. In turn, this could facilitate an improvement in the ability to exercise.

However care must be taken when evaluating the success of certain initiatives because any data gathered must be a valid measure of their impact (Flodgren et al., 2017). For example, you may have already come across the difficulty with BMI as a 'universal' measurement, e.g., some individuals with a 'high' BMI may simply have a higher muscle mass (Shah and Braverman, 2012) and/or be from a different ethnic group (NICE, 2022) as opposed to being 'obese'. Individuals should also be encouraged to learn how to record additional measurements such as 'waist: height ratio' (NICE, 2022), as well as a broader, holistic assessment of the individual (Roper et al., 2000).

Cardiovascular Disease/Coronary Heart Disease

CVD is an umbrella term that includes disease involving the heart and/or blood vessels (Mendis et al., 2011). In 2020, 6.6% of all deaths were as a result of CVD (ONS, 2022a). Nevertheless, the overall mortality for CVD has been declining, although death rates are falling more slowly in younger age groups (ONS, 2021a). Mortality from CVD in England is highest in the north-west region (ONS, 2021a).

What are the lifestyle risk factors associated with the development of CVD?

A knowledge of both risk and protective factors can help a nurse to deliver targeted and effective health promotion.

Jay

You are due to assess 60-year-old Jay, who has been referred to you as part of a community rehabilitation programme. Jay is overweight, has type 2 diabetes, a strong family history of CVD and suffered a myocardial infarction two weeks ago. Jay is retired, and lives with retired husband Andy. They have a son, Martin, who lives in Australia. Jay and Andy each smoke 20 cigarettes a day.

What assessment tools would you use to ascertain Jay's health needs?

What health promotion initiatives could be accessed that may be of benefit to Jay?

Jay's case scenario demonstrates the multifactorial nature of CVD (WHO, 2002; Tolstrup et al., 2014) and the implications of this for health promotion practice. The importance of a case-specific assessment is apparent here because the evidence for home and centre-based cardiac rehabilitation services demonstrates a broadly equal level of effectiveness (Taylor et al., 2010). Therefore, further exploration of factors such as personal preference and convenience would enable the nurse to implement an appropriate health promotion initiative (Naidoo and Wills, 2016).

Sexual Health

Sexual health needs vary according to factors such as age, gender, sexuality, and ethnicity. Some individuals are particularly at risk of poor sexual health. However, although individual needs may vary, there are certain core needs that are common to everyone (DH, 2013: 4). Although there is a growing awareness of the importance of sexual health within the UK there are several ongoing issues in England. For example, there has been a steady increase in diagnosis of infection with *Chlamydia* in men who have sex with men (MSM) (MacGregor et al., 2021).

Ricardo and David

Ricardo and partner David have both attended the sexual health clinic as part of the local screening services for MSM. Both Ricardo and David attend the clinic for their results and state that they are happy to obtain their results together. When you access their medical records, you see that David has tested positive for **Chlamydia**, but Ricardo has not.

What are the wider issues involved here?

How could you overcome these challenges to health promotion?

What nursing skills would be required in this scenario?

Now consider the many factors that may affect or inform sexual health. This may include religious beliefs, social norms, drug and alcohol use, and issues of vulnerability, coercion, and abuse.

What strategies could you employ as an adult nurse to address these factors as part of your nursing assessment?

Promoting Mental Health

About one in four people in the UK suffer from mental health problems each year, with many going untreated (MacManus et al., 2016). Mental illness is estimated to account for almost a quarter of the total burden of disease (Parkin and Powell, 2017).

Mental health is more than a lack of mental illness (WHO, 2003). Concepts related to mental health include subjective wellbeing, perceived self-efficacy, autonomy, competence, intergenerational dependence, and recognition of the ability to realise one's intellectual and emotional potential. It has also been defined as a state of wellbeing whereby individuals recognise their abilities, can cope with the normal stresses of life, work productively and fruitfully, and contribute to their communities (WHO, 2003). Keyes (2009) prefers to view mental health at one end of a continuum with mental illness at the other end (Figure 11.3). People may move along this continuum at various times in their lives. Friedli (2009) argues that mental illness should be understood less in terms of individual pathology and more in terms of the response to adversity.

Mental health ———————————————————————————— Mental illness

Figure 11.3   Mental health continuum

In recent years, the government has sought to raise the profile of mental healthcare, treatment and services, achieving parity of esteem between mental and physical health. The government strategy for mental health, *No Health Without Mental Health* (DH, 2011) makes explicit its objective to give equal priority to mental and physical health. The NHS Mental Health Implementation Plan 2019/20–2023/24 (NHS England, 2019b) sets targets to improve mental health throughout the lifespan from pre-conceptual parental mental health through to mental health in old age. This plan aims to ensure wider access to high quality, better choice, and additional dedicated mental health services; all based on the best evidence. It aligns mental health with NHS long-term plans for primary care, justice system care, ageing well/frailty, urgent and emergency care, learning disabilities, long-term conditions, and maternity services (NHS England, 2019b). Another aim is to tackle inequalities in access, experience and outcomes of mental health services for black and minority ethnic people through a Patient and Carer Race Equality Framework (PCREF).

Culture and mental health

The issue of mental health, illness and ethnicity is a complex and controversial one. The term 'minority ethnic group' encompasses many diverse groups with different experiences and beliefs about mental health and illness. For example, there is a long history of higher admission rates to psychiatric hospitals for black men than those for the majority white population (Bignall et al., 2019). Black and black British men are four times more likely to be receiving inpatient care and ten times more likely to have a community treatment order in place than white men (NHS Digital, 2021). In 2011, the Care Quality Commission reported that 23% of people receiving inpatient care in mental health units in England and Wales were from ethnic minority groups with admissions for people from black Caribbean, black African and mixed white/black groups at least twice higher than average. People of Afro-Caribbean origin are also more likely to be subject to compulsory treatment under the Mental Health Act than the majority UK population (DH, 2011), with over four times the rate of detention for black or black British groups over those of the white group (NHS Digital, 2021). The boundary between mental health and mental illness is related to the question of normality, which is culturally relative (Sashidharan and Commander, 1998; Fernando, 2002). Mental health and illness are socially constructed, in terms of both the person suffering from the 'abnormality' and the person making any judgement on 'abnormality' (Helman, 2000), suggesting that cultural misunderstanding may contribute to some misdiagnosis. Helman notes that as well as having a higher rate of mental illness than the majority population in their adopted countries, immigrants also have higher rates of mental illness than the populations of their countries of origin. This suggests that mental health problems among immigrants may be associated with experiences in host countries. The government acknowledges that progress in tackling inequalities for minority ethnic groups has been disappointing (Salway et al., 2016; NHS England, 2020). It is also clear that the role of social disadvantage cannot be ignored as it is known that rates of schizophrenia have been elevated since their migration to the UK in the 1960s. Rates are far higher among second-generation (UK-born) Afro-Caribbean people compared to the white population. There are several associated factors but it has been suggested that this could be because of their greater socioeconomic disadvantage (i.e., poor inner-city housing and higher rates of unemployment) rather than psychiatric misdiagnosis (Sharpley et al., 2018).

Activity 11.7

Find out more about culture and mental health by accessing the following report: Bignall, T., Jeraj, S., Helsby, E. and Butt, J. (2019) *Racial Disparities in Mental Health: Literature and Evidence Review*. Available at: https://raceequalityfoundation.org.uk/wp-content/uploads/2022/10/mental-health-report-v5-2-2.pdf

What does the report show about prevalence of mental health for each ethnic minority group?
What are the barriers faced by ethnic minority service users when trying to access services?
How can nurses help to improve service users' experience and care given?

Labelling and stigma

People with mental health problems often suffer from labelling and social stigma (Bignall et al., 2019). Stigma has connotations of shame and deviations from normal. The process of stigmatising involves making adverse social judgements about a person or a group. People who are stigmatised often experience rejection and exclusion and may be treated as outcasts (Scambler, 2009), so it is not surprising perhaps that current policy aims to raise awareness of mental health and illness and to promote positive views on mental health.

Maladaptive coping strategies

Stressful circumstances can be damaging to health. Ongoing adverse social and psychological circumstances (e.g., low pay and difficulties in supporting a family, paying a mortgage, or rent, difficult working conditions and/or social isolation) can cause long-term stress, which in turn can have a detrimental effect on physical and mental health (Marmot, 2020). In such situations some people might turn to health-damaging behaviours as a way of dealing with their problems. Misuse of drugs and alcohol can then lead to addiction. The Centre for Social Justice (2013) reports the following statistics:

- 1.6 million adults (1 in 20) are dependent on alcohol;
- 380,000 people (1 in 100) are addicted to heroin or crack cocaine;
- 335,000 children (1 in 37) live with a parent who is addicted to drugs;
- 1 in 7 children under the age of one live with a substance-abusing parent.

Drug and alcohol abuse has significant effects on individuals, families, and communities (WHO, 2003; Centre for Social Justice, 2013). Such abuse can lead to child poverty, family breakdown, welfare dependency and severe personal debt as well as crime (Centre for Social Justice, 2013). For example, the WHO (2003) demonstrates how excessive alcohol consumption can result in more money being spent on alcohol, which in turn can lead to financial problems and less money being available to spend on food. Living conditions can deteriorate, the individual and other family members may experience social stigma and the health of the entire family may be affected because of the stigma and poor nutrition. The impact of drug and alcohol abuse is felt particularly in Britain's most deprived communities (Centre for Social Justice, 2013). Drinking alcohol at dangerous levels is increasing and alcohol-related hospital admissions and deaths are rising (Centre for Social Justice, 2013). Furthermore, coping strategies such as smoking are linked to physical health problems (WHO, 2003). Poor mental health can also cause and be the result of being homeless. The rate of mental health problems is higher among the homeless population than the general population and one report found that homeless people were twice as likely to have mental health problems – with the rate of psychosis much higher than in the general population (Rees, 2009). A later report (Sanders and Brianna, 2015) also found that two-thirds of homeless people cited drug or alcohol use as a reason for becoming homeless, and those who used drugs were seven times more likely to be homeless. The Unhealthy State of Homelessness report (Homeless Link, 2022) found that most of the homeless population did not have regular access to health services, resulting in heavy use of acute services, for both physical and mental health. Their data showed that the number of A&E visits per homeless person was three times higher than for the public.

What health promotion activities are targeted towards homeless individuals in your area?

Suicide prevention

The Mental Health Implementation plan (NHS England, 2019) aims to ensure that every local area will have a suicide prevention programme by 2023/24.

Paul

Paul, a 24-year-old, is brought into A&E having self-harmed, by a friend who claims that Paul is suicidal. As a nurse working in the A&E department, what could you do?

Suicide is everyone's business and not just the realm of specialist mental health nurses. Although specialist mental health nurses are expected to use evidence-based models of suicide prevention, intervention, and harm reduction to reduce risk, adult nurses also have their part to play. For example, Scotland has used a combination of local and national strategies to prevent suicide (Public Health Scotland, 2020). This broad approach includes promoting emotional resilience and wellbeing initiatives across schools and the wider public, tackling issues related to discrimination, stigma, and poverty. There have also been measures introduced to improve the knowledge and understanding of suicide among all frontline NHS staff by promoting suicide prevention courses such as: STORM, ASIST, safeTALK of SMHSA. Northern Ireland introduced a Protect-2 life programme based on a similar approach (Department of Health, 2019).

Activity 11.8

Access the Health and Social Care Alliance Scotland *Suicide Prevention Strategy Report* (2018) at: https://media.samaritans.org/documents/suicide-prevention-strategy-report-scotgov.pdf and identify the key issues faced by those at risk of suicide.

You can find out more about the STORM, ASIST and safeTALK programmes by accessing the websites below:

www.healthscotland.scot/health-topics/suicide/suicide-prevention-training-courses-and-resources
https://prevent-suicide.org.uk/training-courses/asist-applied-suicide-interventions-skills-training/

Consider how you could respond sensitively and effectively to those individuals at risk of suicide.

Health Promotion in Prisons

There is a high need for healthcare for individuals in prison arising from social circumstances that contribute to poor health. Long-term conditions, blood-borne viruses, TB, poor mental health, and substance misuse are common (HCHSCC, 2018). It is also estimated that 80% of individuals in prison in England and Wales smoke compared to 15% of the general population (Hutchings and Davies, 2021). A nurse working within a prison setting may come across several challenges. Nevertheless, Hutchings and Davies (2021) contend that the principle of 'equivalence of care' is a policy ideal rather than a reality as the prison population has significantly poorer health and this is a concern as funding has dramatically decreased since 2010. Cardiovascular disease is the leading natural cause of death for individuals in prison (Shaw et al., 2020). This is unsurprising given that the relationship between poor health and social circumstance is well documented. There is, therefore, an opportunity to implement more involved health promotion strategies in such settings.

Travelling Communities

Members of travelling communities are more likely to suffer from poor health and have a lower life expectancy (Parliament UK, 2019). Several health concerns include poor infant and child health, maternal mortality, and high rates of depression, anxiety, and suicide (McFadden et al., 2016). Engaging with travelling communities presents several challenges including cultural beliefs as well as poor access to services (Lhussier et al., 2015). Van Cleemput et al. (2007) highlight the specific cultural beliefs that inform many travellers' health behaviours, including clear rules about what is 'pure' and 'impure' and a notable 'fear of death'. The beliefs about 'pure' and 'impure' extends to the uptake of vaccinations, whereas the 'fear of death' means that a general anaesthetic might be avoided, because it might be considered a 'little death' (Van Cleemput et al., 2007). Accessing services can also be difficult because of a mobile lifestyle or discrimination by staff (McFadden et al., 2016). This can be further compounded by higher levels of illiteracy and mistrust of healthcare professionals (Lhussier et al., 2015). Having no fixed address often means not being registered with a GP (General Practitioner), resulting in limited access to services, which is further complicated by primary healthcare staff who are reluctant to visit Traveller sites or camps (McFadden et al., 2016).

Migrants, Refugees, and Asylum Seekers

In 2019 the World Health Organization (WHO, 2019b) stated that the number of forcibly displaced people had reached its highest-ever level, at an estimated 68.5 million individuals, including 25.4 million refugees. In the UK unprecedented numbers of asylum applications from individuals arriving from countries such as Afghanistan, Iran, Syria, Eritrea, and Sudan have been reported (Home Office, 2023). These individuals often lack basic human rights to freedom of movement, education, and access to healthcare and other social determinants of health (Iqbal et al., 2021).

Activity 11.9

Take some time out to enhance your own understanding of the health needs of migrants, refugees, and asylum seekers.

Why do people migrate or become displaced from a country? Read WHO (2023) at www.who.int/tools/
   refugee-and-migrant-health-toolkit/essential-knowledge-health-and-migration#About

Who is granted asylum in the UK? Read the Migration Observatory at https://migrationobservatory.ox.ac.
   uk/resources/briefings/migration-to-the-uk-asylum/

What are the potential health and social inequalities associated with migration? Read WHO
   (2023) at https://www.who.int/tools/refugee-and-migrant-health-toolkit

After reading the above, you will no doubt be aware of the associated significant risks to health faced by such individuals and families. As a nurse there is an expectation that you will have the required knowledge and understanding to promote the health of all individuals, whatever their personal circumstances or settings.

Scenario

An individual presents at your local Accident and Emergency Department. They cannot speak English and they point to a large wound in their leg and say something that you recognise to be spoken in Arabic. You ask for a translator. The translator tells you that the person has just arrived in the UK from Syria where there is an ongoing conflict, and they are seeking asylum and refugee status in the UK. The individual is asking for advice about the health resources available to them in the UK.

Using the information below, identify the health support available for migrants in the UK and consider how you will respond.

Office for Health Improvement and Disparities (2022) www.gov.uk/government/collections/migrant-health-guide

Promoting the Health of Mothers and Babies

The health of a mother during pregnancy is vital to the health of the unborn baby. The foundations of adult health are laid before birth and during early childhood (Marmot, 2010; 2020). Unfavourable circumstances during pregnancy, for example poor nutrition, stress, smoking, the misuse of drugs and alcohol, can affect the developing baby and set the scene for poor health in later life (Marmot, 2010; 2020) so ensuring a good start means supporting mothers and young children especially as health outcomes have become worse since 2010 (Marmot, 2020). Most families are receptive to help and advice during this period because most parents will want their children to have the best possible start in life. Therefore, healthcare professionals are in a prime position to make use of this opportunity to provide support to families and give advice about a healthy lifestyle during pregnancy (PHE, 2016b).

Nutrition in pregnancy

A healthy diet is important during pregnancy to meet the needs of both the mother and developing fetus since it has been found that maternal under-nutrition during fetal life or immediately after birth can have lasting consequences on the child and may extend into adulthood (Wyness et al., 2013). The general advice for nutrition during pregnancy is to find a balance of eating a wide variety of foods, appropriate weight gain and physical exercise (Wyness et al., 2013). As an adult nurse you should familiarise yourself with the advice that is offered to expectant mothers concerning their diets.

Activity 11.10

Locate *The Pregnancy Book* (DH, 2022) at www.publichealth.hscni.net/publications by placing the term 'The Pregnancy Book' in the website's search engine.

Read the section 'Your health in pregnancy' (pages 31-38). You should ensure that you are able to pass on this advice to expectant mothers if required.

Smoking cessation in pregnancy

In pregnancy the adverse effects of smoking include the risk of miscarriage, a premature birth, a low birth weight, stillbirth, and sudden infant death (Wisborg et al., 2000; Anderson et al., 2005; Duaso and Duncan, 2012; Percival, 2013). Furthermore, mothers who are exposed to environmental smoke – including second-hand smoke – are more likely to give birth to babies with low birth weights (Duaso and Duncan, 2012). Children who are exposed to passive smoking are at an increased risk of developing pneumonia, bronchitis, and asthma. Guidelines on quitting smoking in pregnancy and after childbirth (NICE, 2021a) state that anyone planning a pregnancy, who is already pregnant or has an infant under 12 months, should receive smoking cessation support. Therefore, healthcare professionals should assess expectant mothers' exposure to cigarette smoke, inform them of the dangers of smoking, ask smokers if they would like to stop smoking and refer them to NHS Stop Smoking Services appropriately.

Vulnerable families

Women who experience stress during pregnancy may give birth to babies of low birth weight and as they grow up these children may have emotional and behavioural problems (Wilkinson, 2005). Thus, alongside the mainstream services for pregnant women and young children are some initiatives that focus on more vulnerable families. Women living in complex social situations (e.g., those at risk from substance abuse, recent migrants with language barriers, and victims or potential victims of domestic abuse) often avoid antenatal care so there is a need to reach out to such women. Many healthcare organisations have specialist midwives with a responsibility to target and support vulnerable women. The Healthy Start programme is a UK-wide government scheme to improve the health of low-income pregnant women and families on benefits and tax credits. The programme provides vouchers for healthy food, for example milk, fresh or frozen fruit and vegetables. Another initiative that aims to help vulnerable, young, first-time mothers across the UK is the Family Nurse Partnership Programme (FNP, 2021). This programme aims to improve pregnancy outcomes, improve child health and development, and improve parents' economic self-sufficiency. All first-time mothers aged 19 and under at conception are eligible and participation in the programme is voluntary. Healthcare professionals use theory and expertise to engage in behaviour change methods to foster the adoption of healthier lifestyles by the families.

Vaccinations for pregnant women

The pertussis (whooping cough) vaccine is recommended for all pregnant women from 16 weeks' gestation (ideally around 20 weeks after the anomaly scan). This was commenced in 2012 in response to the increase in morbidity and mortality rates of newborn infants contracting pertussis before the normal vaccination age of around 8 weeks (PHE, 2016b). The influenza vaccine is now offered to all pregnant women and can be given at any stage of pregnancy. This was introduced in 2012 after the Confidential Enquiry into Maternal Deaths 2009–2012 which reported that 36 women died during pregnancy from flu-related problems (Hinton, 2014). Both vaccines are safe for pregnant women and the unborn child, providing immunity to the fetus and protecting the newborn for the first two months of life.

Postnatal care and transition to the community

Before being discharged from hospital mothers will receive a postnatal examination by a midwife. This examination includes an assessment of the mother's emotional state and her physical wellbeing (Kinge and Gregory, 2011). All newborn babies are examined within 72 hours of birth by a competent practitioner. New mothers are offered advice on contraception and are advised to make an appointment for a postnatal check-up with their GP in six weeks' time for themselves and their babies. A health visitor will also visit the mother and baby at home between 10 and 14 days after the birth and will advise where and how often to take the baby for regular assessments.

The period of six to eight weeks after childbirth is referred to as the puerperium and it is a time of enormous adjustment (Kinge and Gregory, 2011). NICE (2021b) has developed a quality standard (QS37) for postnatal care, outlining the care and support that every woman should receive during the postnatal period. This care should be individualised to meet the needs of the mother and baby (including partners and family as appropriate). The midwife will normally visit the family at home following discharge from hospital until 10–14 days postnatal. However, this care and support can be extended beyond the 6 to 8 week period if necessary. The health visitor will visit from day 7 postnatal. NICE (2021b) recommends the provision of postnatal education programmes delivered by a multidisciplinary team which provides advice, information and support for new mothers and their families (Kinge and Gregory, 2011).

Physical health

Women who have just given birth should be provided with information about how to look for signs that they are becoming ill. For example, if they have flu-like symptoms they should report this immediately to their midwife or GP (NICE, 2021b). Other symptoms such as persistent headache and aches and pains should not be ignored. Maternal sepsis has been a leading cause of maternal death (Knight et al., 2018). It can affect women during pregnancy and in the first few weeks after birth. Women and their families need to remain aware of early warning signs:

- Elevated temperature (>38.3°C);
- Low temperature (<36°C);
- Chills and shivering;
- Fast heartbeat;
- Fast breathing, breathlessness;
- Headache;
- Severe abdominal pain;
- Extreme sleepiness (Hinton, 2014: 3).

If any of these symptoms appear, urgent medical advice should be sought.

Perinatal mental health

Perinatal mental health problems are those that occur during pregnancy or in the first year after the birth of a child, affect up to 20% of women and cover a wide range of conditions. If left untreated, they can have significant and long-lasting effects not only on the woman but also on her children's emotional, social, and cognitive development. The NICE clinical guidelines

(NICE, 2021b) require that at a pregnant woman's first contact with services, healthcare professionals should ask questions about past and present severe mental illness, previous treatment by mental health professionals and family history of perinatal mental illness. The aim here is early detection and treatment. It is important to be aware of the mental health problems that can arise in the postnatal period and to be able to differentiate 'baby blues' (e.g., irritability, anxiety and tearfulness three to four days after childbirth, stopping by the time the baby is about ten days old), postnatal depression (e.g., a depressive disorder that can affect women in the months after childbirth (Robertson, 2010) and postpartum (or puerperal) psychosis (e.g., a severe episode of mental illness representing a psychiatric emergency, with a sudden onset during the days or weeks after childbirth (Royal College of Psychiatrists, 2018).

Activity 11.11

Access the NHS website's 'Postpartum Psychosis' (NHS, 2020). Available at: www.nhs.uk/mental-health/conditions/post-partum-psychosis/

Consider how useful this information might be when educating new mothers about postnatal mental health.

Breastfeeding

Breast milk supplies all the nutrients a baby needs for around the first six months of life (NHS, 2015). Policies on breastfeeding across the UK promote feeding babies solely on breast milk for the first six months of life, after which time it is suggested that breastfeeding can continue as long as the mother and baby wish while gradually introducing a more varied diet (NICE, 2014b). Breastfeeding contributes to the health of both mother and baby. It has been found that babies who are not breastfed are more likely to acquire infections such as gastroenteritis and respiratory problems during their first year of life (NICE, 2014b). Women who are disadvantaged are less likely to breastfeed than their better-off counterparts.

Activity 11.12

Read the following document: NHS (2015) *Off to the Best Start.* Available at: https://www.unicef.org.uk/babyfriendly/baby-friendly-resources/breastfeeding-resources/off-to-the-best-start/

Promoting the Health of Children and Young People (CYP)

As a registered nurse you may encounter children or young people while working in an Accident and Emergency department, primary care, secondary care setting or in your personal day-to-day life. The United Nations' convention on the Rights of the Child (UN, 1989; ratified by the UK in 1991) defines a child as anyone under the age of 18. The General Medical Council (GMC) defines young people as 'older or experienced children who could make important decisions for themselves' (GMC, 2018). Currently, 18.9% of the UK population is aged under 15 years though this may decrease to about 17.7% by 2046 as the current population ages (ONS, 2017a). Nonetheless, children and young people are any country's future and each of the four UK countries (England, Scotland, Wales, and Northern Ireland) has a Commissioner for Children and Young People. These Commissioners work independently to uphold children's rights under the UN convention and represent the views of children and young people to policy makers and other stakeholders with a view to improving the lives of all children, particularly the most vulnerable.

The UN's Convention stresses that the family (as the natural place for nurturing children) should be afforded the necessary protection and assistance to fulfil its responsibilities (UN, 1989). The ONS defines a family as 'married, civil partnered or cohabiting couple with or without children, or a lone parent, with at least one child, who live at the same address' (ONS, 2018b: 2). Families come in all 'shapes and sizes' including co-habiting, lone parent, same sex and reconstituted (where parents with existing children unite to create a new family) forms. All types of families are important for meeting children's and young people's psychological and physical needs, providing behavioural support and finances for shelter, food, health, development, protection, and socialisation; thus, enabling children to learn about identity, roles, values, and culture (Berger and Font, 2015). Ideals about family life and child rearing may vary according to the family structure, cultural beliefs, and values. It is important to develop cultural competency (e.g., understanding, appreciating, and effectively communicating with people from diverse cultures) so that care for families is neither too intrusive nor so lax that it results in children's needs being overlooked (Akilapa and Simkiss, 2012). Despite the importance of families to children's wellbeing, families living in difficult circumstances such as domestic violence/intimate partner violence, drug or alcohol dependency, and other adverse childhood experiences, can negatively impact on children's lives and subsequent health and wellbeing in adulthood.

Activity 11.13

If you have access to Open Athens, you may wish to undertake cultural competence training: www.E-lfh. org.uk/programmes/cultural-competence. If not, you can read more about it here:
   www.ncbi.nlm.nih.gov/pmc/articles/PMC7011228/

Universal services

Current UK policies aim to ensure that all children and young people have the best start in life (HSC Public Health Agency, 2011; Welsh Government, 2013; Scottish Government, 2017; NHS England, 2019).

Universal services are those that are provided to everyone. Every child and young person in the UK are offered a range of universal health, education and welfare support. A child or young person can have needs for additional education, health, or social care support (i.e., resulting from learning difficulties, disabilities, or abuse) and require a comprehensive assessment to ensure that additional targeted services are provided to meet their needs. The whole family may also need additional support when their child is ill or has additional needs. Thomas and Price (2012) explored the experiences of some mothers caring for children with complex needs. They identified that parents felt physically burdened and isolated, and experienced emotional turmoil, yet they valued additional support services.

The Healthy Child Programme offers universal services from pregnancy to 19 years and is part of 'giving every child the best start in life' initiative (PHE, 2016b). The programme offers children, young people, and their families' health promotion, such as immunisations, or advice and support about physical or emotional wellbeing, health and developmental reviews, and screening (e.g., the UK newborn screening programme for various disorders).

Universal health and development reviews are a key feature of the Healthy Child Programme (PHE, 2016b). These reviews are carried out by healthcare professionals who have skills in assessing child development, and an understanding of the factors that influence family health and wellbeing. One of the aims of the review is to support keeping children and the family healthy (e.g., good oral health, nutrition, or safety) and detecting any potential health issues early so that appropriate support can be offered to the child and the family (early intervention). The Healthy Child Programme 0–5 years offers the following health and development reviews:

- Prenatal: at 28 weeks of pregnancy;
- Within 14 days of birth;
- The baby's 6- to 8-week examination;
- At 9–12 months old;
- Between 2 and 2½ years old.

Keeping children healthy

UK policy documents emphasise the importance of good child health, for example through encouraging families to have their children immunised and by encouraging healthy lifestyles.

Activity 11.14

What vaccinations are children given in the UK and what diseases do they prevent?

Follow this link to find out: www.nhs.uk/conditions/vaccinations/nhs-vaccinations-and-when-to-have-them/

Childhood obesity is a national concern because around a third of children are overweight or obese and this can negatively impact on their health and wellbeing as children and adults (Office for Health Improvement and Disparities, 2022). However the government has a child obesity action plan (Department of Health, 2017a). As part of 'making every contact count' we should encourage everyone to make healthy lifestyle choices (Health Education England, 2018), encouraging healthy diets and daily moderate-to-vigorous physical activity for children (Office for Health Improvement and Disparities, 2022). We can also help children and their parents to understand what child-size portions are (Marteau et al., 2015).

Activity 11.15

Get familiar with NHS choices. What advice does the website offer for parents with overweight children? Check out: https://www.nhs.uk/live-well/healthy-weight/childrens-weight/advice-for-parents-overweight-children/

The importance of play and early education

Protective factors in early childhood such as secure attachment, consistent parenting, appropriate play and learning opportunities, contribute to children's emotional wellbeing and chances of reaching their potential (Fearn and Howard, 2012). Play is internationally recognised as a child right, under article 31 of the Rights of a Child (UN, 1989: 10) to 'rest and leisure, to engage in play and recreational activities appropriate to the age of the child and to participate freely in cultural life and the arts'. Fearn and Howard (2012) found that play can provide a healing experience for children affected by war and conflict and encourages the growth of resilience.

During play children create imaginary worlds and through play can develop a range of adaptive capacities and strategies to help them cope or adapt with abuse, conflict, displacement and/or poverty (Lester and Russell, 2010). Preschool education can also enhance a child's intellectual, social, and behavioural development and subsequent educational attainment – particularly for those children from challenging social environments (Cebolla-Boadoet et al., 2016). A key component in 'giving every child a good start in life' is preparing children to be ready to learn and to be ready for school (Public Health England, 2016b).

Safeguarding children

Safeguarding is any action taken to promote the wellbeing of children or young people and to protect them from harm (National Society for the Prevention of Cruelty to Children (NSPCC), 2022). All nurses have a responsibility to raise concerns with an appropriate person for anyone who is vulnerable, at risk and needing protection (NMC, 2018a). There are clear guidelines in the UK about how to raise a safeguarding concern about a child. The first Government Act to prevent cruelty to children was passed in 1889, but UK policies were strengthened after the death of Victoria Climbié. The Laming Report (DH, 2003) identified poor communication, inter-professional working and team work as being among the factors that contributed to the failure of professional services to protect Victoria. This report influenced the establishment of local children's Trusts, consisting of multidisciplinary teams of health, education, and social service professionals. Other policy developments included The Children Act 2004 (www.legislation.gov.uk/ukpga/2004/31/contents), which defined the duties of agencies working with children to promote health and wellbeing, as well as protecting children from harm (Powell, 2013).

Despite these policy changes, there have still been subsequent high-profile and shocking cases of child abuse and neglect. Below, we encourage you to consider the case of Daniel Pelka, an incredibly sad case which resulted in his death at the hands of his mother and her male partner. Daniel's case was extensively covered in the media and in a Serious Case Review (Coventry Safeguarding Children Board, 2013).

A Serious Case Review (SCR) is commissioned to determine what can be learned from a case about the way in which local professionals and organisations worked individually and together to safeguard children.

Daniel Pelka

Daniel was aged 4 years and 8 months at the time of his death. He had one older and one younger sibling. His family had migrated to the UK from Poland in 2005. Daniel was born in the UK in 2007. His family life was chaotic – his mother had relationships with three different partners whilst in the UK. All these relationships involved high alcohol consumption and abuse. The family was known to the police who were called to the home on many occasions, including 27 reported incidents of domestic abuse. In 2011 Daniel was taken to A&E with a spiral fracture to his arm. As the fracture had occurred on the previous day (the mother and stepfather had delayed taking Daniel to hospital) – and with the knowledge that this type of fracture is associated with non-accidental injury – the hospital referred the case to the police. Although a social worker carried out an assessment, professionals accepted the mother's account of what led to the fracture and no continuing need for intervention was identified.

In September 2011, Daniel started school and over the ensuing months his attendance was poor. He grew thinner, was constantly hungry, stopped growing and went to school with bruises. His teachers reported seeing facial injuries, black eyes and bruises on his neck and head. Daniel was found scavenging in bins at school for food but when the school staff spoke to his mother about his hunger, she told them he had an eating disorder that caused him to feel constantly hungry. She also told them that they should not give him any food.

It is reported that Daniel spoke little English, had few friends, often played in isolation and sometimes displayed ritualistic behaviours. He did however, have a strong bond with his older sibling. When teachers asked him how he got his injuries, he looked down at the ground and did not answer.

Daniel's mother and stepfather were both sentenced to life imprisonment when he died of a subdural haematoma after a severe blow to the head in March 2012. The trial and SCR revealed that, for at least six months before his death, Daniel had been starved, assaulted, neglected, and abused. Daniel was frequently locked in a 'box room' without a window, heating, or toys. The only 'furniture' in this room was a soiled mattress. Daniel was plunged into cold baths, he was beaten and denied meals. He was force fed salt until he vomited. A postmortem examination found him to be emaciated, grossly malnourished and dehydrated with bruising over his body – a total of 40 injuries. There was evidence of long-standing neglect.

The SCR reported that his mother and stepfather set out to deliberately harm Daniel and deceive professionals. The professionals who had contact with Daniel and his family included teachers, classroom assistants, school nurses, an education welfare officer, a general practitioner, a community paediatrician, social workers, and the police. Teachers variously described Daniel as 'losing weight,' 'pale,' 'ashen' and 'a bag of bones'. There was poor communication between the professionals who met Daniel and professional concerns were not well recorded. As in previous cases, there were many missed opportunities to protect Daniel. The SCR claims that no professional tried hard enough to engage with Daniel about his eating habits or home life and concluded that all professionals need to 'think the unthinkable' and believe and act on what they see and not accept parents' versions of events without challenging.

Having read the case study about Daniel, can you identify any areas where professionals might have identified concerns or 'professional curiosity'?

Apart from Daniel's visible injuries there are several issues that you might have identified. For example, Daniel was not growing well. Growth is an important indicator of a child's health and wellbeing and slow growth during childhood can have psychosocial causes (Wilkinson, 2005). Daniel's apparent isolation or bin scavenging might have also caused you concern. You might have considered his lack of response when asked about his injuries in terms of 'professional curiosity,' you might have asked the question 'What eating disorder?' in response to his mother's explanation of Daniel losing weight and being constantly hungry.

Many of the professionals who were in contact with Daniel were concerned about him but they did not act adequately on those concerns and the various professional groups did not communicate with each other. The revised document *Working Together to Safeguard Children: A Guide to Inter-agency Working to Safeguard and Promote the Welfare of Children* (HM Government, 2022) emphasises that safeguarding children is everyone's responsibility; everyone who encounters children and their families has a role to play. The document stresses that a child's needs remain paramount (primarily). Professionals' failures to protect children are often the result of losing sight of the needs of children or placing the interests of adults ahead of those of children (HM Government, 2022). Acknowledging that no single professional can have a full picture of a child's needs and circumstances, the document stresses the need to share information. Lack of sharing information has often resulted in a failure to protect children.

Activity 11.16

Please look at the NSPCC Protecting Children from Neglect resources:
  https://learning.nspcc.org.uk/child-abuse-and-neglect/neglect

Can you identify common factors associated with neglect?
What is your role as a nurse to support families and what should you do if you suspect a child is at risk of being neglected?

The nurse's role in relation to safeguarding children

HM Government (2022) identifies that safeguarding is everyone's responsibility, everyone should have a child-centred approach and good understanding of the needs and views of children and all professionals should share information in a timely way and discuss their concerns. This means that no one should assume that someone else will pass on information about a child and everyone should share information about concerns as soon as possible to ensure early intervention and prevention of any further difficulties for the child. Early and effective communication is key to protecting children and young people. Children are best protected when professionals are clear about what is required of them individually, and how they need to work together (HM Government, 2022: 7).

As a nurse you will need to be aware of the factors that might place a child at risk of maltreatment (HM Government, 2022: 13); these are children who:

- Are disabled and have specific additional needs;
- Have special educational needs;
- Are a young carer;
- Are showing signs of engaging in antisocial or criminal behaviour;
- Are in family circumstances presenting challenges for the child, such as substance abuse, adult mental health, domestic violence;
- Are showing early signs of abuse and/or neglect (see the next section).

Are you aware of the distinct types of maltreatment? Are you familiar with the procedures for safeguarding the welfare of children in your area?

Child and young person maltreatment: what is it and what do you need to do?

Child maltreatment can involve physical, emotional, or emotional abuse, neglect or exploitation of children or young people (WHO, 2020). Maltreatment causes significant harm to a child's or young person's current and future health, development, and wellbeing; the health and social effects of such abuse can last a lifetime (NICE, 2017a; 2017b).

Activity 11.17

Read the WHO's (2020) document about child maltreatment at: www.who.int/news-room/fact-sheets/detail/child-maltreatment:

What are some of the different forms of maltreatment?
What are the characteristics of a child who may suffer maltreatment?
What are the characteristics of a parent or care giver that may increase the risk of maltreatment?
Think about how **you** might prevent child maltreatment.

It is important that a child's needs are paramount (considered first) and are child-centred (e.g., focused on their needs, concerns and wishes). To protect, safeguard and promote the wellbeing of children and young people effectively, everyone in education, health or social care organisations needs to do their part in identifying concerns and promptly sharing information with appropriate, child-safeguarding professionals. This is because no one professional will know everything about a child and the family (HM Government, 2022).

There are some regional and national variations in child safeguarding policies in the UK; it is, therefore, important to be aware of your local policies and to keep yourself up to date with policy through regular training. There are two important things to know no matter where you work. The first is to be aware of the types of child maltreatment, so that you can be vigilant and identify signs that may indicate that a child is being maltreated. The second is to know to whom, and how to communicate any concerns.

Recognising child maltreatment

Although maltreatment is often classified as neglect, physical, sexual, or emotional, it is important to remember that children or young people can experience more than one type of maltreatment.

Types of maltreatment

Neglect happens when there has been a failure to meet a child's basic needs over a period (e.g., neglect of a child's health, education, emotional development, food, or safety needs);

Physical abuse is the intentional use of physical force (e.g., hitting, beating, kicking, shaking, biting, scalding, pinching, poisoning, or suffocating a child);

Emotional or psychological abuse occurs when there is a persistent failure to provide an appropriate environment for mental wellbeing (e.g., by telling a child that they are not loved, or not good enough, by belittling, blaming, threatening, frightening, discriminating, ridiculing, rejecting, or showing hostility to a child);

Sexual abuse happens when a child is involved in inappropriate sexual activity (this includes physical contact or non-contact activities such as forcing children to watch sexual images), which the child does not understand and is not developmentally prepared for.

(Adapted from WHO and ISPCAN, 2006; HM Government, 2020)

How can you recognise maltreatment?

NICE have produced two guidelines of what you might see or hear that can suggest maltreatment (NICE calls these 'alerting features'). NICE (2017b; 2017c; 2019) describes these alerting features as either 'suspect' or 'consider'. 'Suspect' is an alerting feature that should trigger a 'serious level of concern' that maltreatment might be occurring, and 'consider' is where maltreatment may be an explanation for a child's injury or presentation.

Activity 11.18

Read the alerting features section of the following NICE guidelines: physical maltreatment (NICE, 2019) and NICE (2017b; 2017c) for alerting features to other forms of maltreatment.

Make a note of what should alert you to consider or suspect maltreatment.

Children and young people may be maltreated by parents or other family members, caregivers, people in authority, strangers, friends, or other children (HM Government 2022). If a child tells you that they are being maltreated, you should listen to them, pay attention and respect what they are saying. Then you should reassure the child that you will 'act to keep them safe' by enacting your local safeguarding guideline (HM Government, 2022). It is also important to be alert for 'unsuitable explanations' where a child/young person's, carer's or parent's account about an injury or presentation is not adequate or plausible, or if explanations are contradictory or inconsistent (NICE, 2019).

Communicating and recording

You need to become familiar with procedures for safeguarding the welfare of children in your area and know whom to contact to express any concerns you might have. Every NHS trust has a named member of staff who takes the lead on concerns relating to child maltreatment and safeguarding. If you suspect that a child is being maltreated, you should report your concerns; if you are a student you may report to your practice supervisor or an experienced colleague. He or she may well refer the matter to the named nurse for safeguarding children who could then make a referral to social services. You must record your concerns clearly – exactly what you observed and heard from whom and when. In addition, record why this is of concern and what you did about your concerns.

The focus of this section has been on maintaining health during childhood so that everyone can have 'the best start in life.' We have considered the importance of assessing every child's needs and how being vigilant and effective communication with appropriate professionals can support vulnerable children and young people.

Promoting the Health of Adults with Learning Disabilities

A learning disability can be mild, moderate, severe, or profound (RCN, 2013) and some people may have more than one disability and complex healthcare needs (Brown et al., 2010). NICE (2021c) estimates that there are around 950,000 adults and 300,000 children with learning disabilities currently living in England. Traditionally, services for people with learning disabilities were based around long-stay institutions (Leaning and Adderley, 2016). There has been a move away from institutional care for people with learning disabilities towards practices that promote more ordinary lives (Health Foundation, 2018). People with learning disabilities may live in a wide range of settings but the majority live in their own home or the family home (Burt, 2015), some may live in supported housing provided by social services, the private sector, or the voluntary sector.

An increasing number of people with a learning disability live into old age; however, because of additional health problems they can become frequent users of health services (Brown et al., 2010; Phillips, 2012). Individuals with significant or complex disabilities can need full-time care and support with most aspects of daily life.

All UK Governments promote the provision of mainstream healthcare services for people with learning disabilities, supported by specialist services as appropriate (Gibson, 2009). However, evidence suggests that the needs of people with learning disabilities are often not met sufficiently in general healthcare services (LeDer, 2021), resulting in inequalities in healthcare provision. Having a learning disability is associated with a significantly reduced expectancy, extended hospital stays and overmedication (NICE, 2021b). It is important to promote the health and wellbeing of people with learning disabilities as they are more likely to prematurely die from preventable heart disease and respiratory problems, have higher risk of epilepsy and constipation than the general population (LeDer, 2021) and many suffer with unrecognised mental health problems (MENCAP, 2020).

Activity 11.19

Review NICE (2021c) www.nice.org.uk/about/what-we-do/into-practice/measuring-the-use-of-nice-guidance/impact-of-our-guidance/nice-impact-people-with-a-learning-disability. Then consider the actions you might need to take to ensure that you are able to promote the health of patients with learning disabilities within healthcare settings.

Chapter Summary

In this chapter, we have considered the registered nurse's role in promoting the health of individuals, groups and communities and have also identified health needs arising from social disadvantage. There are many different issues that need to be considered when promoting health but the most important principle to remember is to consider the whole person – physical, developmental, social, and mental health – whenever the opportunity arises.

All registered nurses are expected to be able to engage in health promotion activities regardless of the practice setting (RCN, 2012; NMC, 2018b). You should always refer to the most up-to-date and best available evidence to inform your health promotion activities and be able to appraise the effectiveness of your interventions – with individuals, families, and communities (NMC, 2018b).

Useful Websites

Public Health Agency, Northern Ireland: www.publichealth.hscni.net/
Department of Health (NI), Health Promotion Website: www.health-ni.gov.uk/topic
    s/public-health-policy-and-advice/health-promotion
Public Health Scotland: www.healthscotland.scot/
Public Health Wales: https://phw.nhs.wales/
World Health Organization: www.who.int/

Further Reading

NHS England (2019) *NHS Long Term Plan*. London: NHS England.

Robinson, S. (2022) *Priorities for Health Promotion and Public Health. Explaining the Evidence for Disease Prevention and Health Promotion*. London: Routledge.

References

Acheson, D. (1998) *Independent Inquiry into Inequalities in Health Report*. London: The Stationery Office.

Akilapa, R. and Simkiss, D. (2012) 'Cultural influences and safeguarding children', *Paediatrics and Child Health*, 22(11): 490–5.

Anderson, M.E., Johnson, D.C. and Batal, H.A. (2005) 'Sudden infant death syndrome and prenatal maternal smoking: rising attributed risk in the back to sleep era', *BMC Medicine*. Jan 11; 3:4. doi: 10.1186/1741-7015-3-4. PMID: 15644131; PMCID: PMC545061.

Becker, M.H. (ed.) (1974) 'The Health Belief Model and personal health behaviour', *Health Education Monographs*, 2: 324–508.

Berger, L.M. and Font, S.A. (2015) 'The role of the family and family-centered programs and policies', *Future Child*. Spring, 25(1): 155–76.

Betsch, C., Bohm, R., Korn, L. and Holtmann, C. (2017) 'On the benefits of explaining herd immunity in vaccine advocacy', *Nature Human Behaviour*, 1, 0056.

Bignall, T., Jeraj, S., Helsby, E. and Butt, J. (2019) *Racial Disparities in Mental Health: Literature and evidence review*. London. Available at: https://raceequalityfoundation.org.uk/wp-content/uploads/2020/03/mental-health-report-v5-2.pdf (last accessed 24 June 2022).

Brown, M., MacArthur, J., McKechanie, A., Hayes, M. and Fletcher, J. (2010) 'Equality and access to general healthcare for people with learning disabilities: reality or rhetoric?' *Journal of Research in Nursing*, 15(4): 351–61.

Burt, A. (2015) *Understanding the Needs of People with Learning Disabilities*. Available at: www.gov.uk/government/speeches/understanding-the-needs-of-people-with-learning-disabilities (last accessed 27 February 2023).

Cavanagh, S. and Chadwick, K. (2005) *Summary: Health Needs Assessment at a Glance*. London: Health Development Agency/NICE.

Cebolla-Boado, H., Radl, J. and Salazar, L. (2016) 'Preschool education as the great equalizer? A cross-country study into the sources of inequality in reading competence', *Acta Sociologica*, [online]. 60(1): 41–60.

Centre for Social Justice (2013) *No Quick Fix: Exposing the Depth of Britain's Drug and Alcohol Problem*. London: CSJ. Available at: www.centreforsocialjustice.org.uk/library/no-quick-fix-exposing-depth-britains-drug-alcohol-problem (last accessed 20 February 2023).

Cesaro, S., Giacchino, M., Fioreda, F., Barone, A., Battisti, L., Bezzio, S., Frenos, S., De Santis, R., Livadiotti, S., Marinello, S., Zanazzo, A.G. and Caselli, D. (2014) 'Guidelines on vaccinations in paediatric haematology and oncology patients', *Biomedical Research International*, doi:10.1155/2014/707691. PMC 40205020. PMID 24868544.

Chung, E.H. (2013) 'Vaccine allergies', *Clinical and Experimental Vaccine Research*, 4(3): 50–7.

Coggon, D., Rose, G. and Barker, D.J.P. (2020) 'Epidemiology for the uninitiated' 4th edition, *The BMJ* (2020, October 26). Available at: www-bmj-com.manchester.idm.oclc.org/about-bmj/resources-readers/publications/epidemiology-uninitiated (last accessed 19 December 2022).

Coventry Safeguarding Children Board (2013) *Serious Case Review: Daniel Pelka*. Available at: https://pdscp.co.uk/wp-content/uploads/2020/02/SCR-Daniel-Pelka-2013.pdf (last accessed 28 February 2023).

Dahlgren, G. and Whitehead, M. (1991) *Policies and Strategies to Promote Social Equity in Health*. Stockholm: Institute for Future Studies.

Davies, M. and Macdowall, W. (2006) *Health Promotion Theory*. Maidenhead: Open University Press.

Department of Health (2003) *The Victoria Climbié Inquiry: Report of an Inquiry by Lord Laming*. Cm5730. London: DH.

Department of Health (2011) *No Health Without Mental Health*. London: HMSO.

Department of Health (2013) *A Framework for Sexual Health Improvement in England*. London: HMSO.

Department of Health (2014) *Better Care for People With 2 or More Long Term Conditions*. London: HMSO.

Department of Health (2017) *Childhood Obesity: A plan for action*. [online] GOV.UK. Available at: www.gov.uk/government/publications/childhood-obesity-a-plan-for-action/childhood-obesity-a-plan-for-action (last accessed 1 March 2023).

Department of Health (2019) *Protect Life 2. Suicide Prevention Strategy*. Available at: www.health-ni.gov.uk/protectlife2 (last accessed 18 February 2023).

Department of Health (2022) *The Pregnancy Book*. London: DH. Available at: www.publichealth.hscni.net/sites/default/files/2022-04/The%20pregnancy%20book%202022%20chapter%205%20pages%2031%20to%2053.pdf [online]. (last accessed 1 March 2023).

Department of Health and Social Care Social Care (2021) *Guidance Chapter 12: Alcohol*. Available at: www.gov.uk/government/publications/delivering-better-oral-health-an-evidence-based-toolkit-for-prevention/chapter-12-alcohol (last accessed 20 February 2023).

Department of Health, Social Services and Public Safety (DHSSPS) (2012) *A Fitter Future for All: Framework for Preventing and Addressing Overweight and Obesity in Northern Ireland 2012–2022*. Belfast: DHSSPS.

Department of Health Social Services and Public Safety (DHSSPS) (2014) *Making Life Better – A Whole System Framework for Public Health 2013-2023*. Available at: www.health-ni.gov.uk/sites/default/files/publications/dhssps/making-life-better-strategic-framework-2013-2023_0.pdf (last accessed 1 March 2023).

Duaso, M.J. and Duncan, D. (2012) 'Health impact of smoking and smoking cessation strategies: current evidence', *British Journal of Community Nursing*, 17(8): 356–63.

Earle, S., Lloyd, C.E., Sidell, M. and Spur, S. (2007) *Theory and Research in Promoting Public Health*. London: Sage.

Everest, G., Marshall, L., Fraser, C. and Briggs, A. (2022) Addressing the leading risk factors for ill health. A review of government policies tackling smoking, poor diet, physical inactivity, and harmful alcohol use in England. London: The Health Foundation.

Family Nursing Partnership (2021) *Enabling Parents to Give Their Children the Best Start in Life*. Available at: www.fnp.nhs.uk/ (last accessed 20 February 2023).

Fawcett, S.B., Paine-Andrews, A., Francisco, V.T., Schultz, J.A., Richter, K.P., Lewis, R.K., Williams, E.L., Harris, K.J., Berkley, J.Y., Fisher, J.L. and Lopez, C.M. (1995) 'Using empowerment theory in collaborative partnerships for community health and development', *American Journal of Community Psychology*, 23(5): 677–97.

Fearn, M. and Howard, J. (2012) 'Play as a resource for children facing adversity: an exploration of indicative case studies', *Children and Society*, 26: 456–68.

Fernando, S. (2002) *Mental Health, Race and Culture*, 2nd edn. Basingstoke: Palgrave.

Fine, P., Eames, K. and Heymann, D.L. (2011) '"Herd immunity": a rough guide', *Clinical Infectious Diseases*, 52(7): 911–16.

Flodgren, G., Gonçalves-Bradley, D.C. and Summerbel, C.D. (2017) 'Interventions to change the behaviour of health professionals and the organization of care to promote weight reduction in children and adults with overweight or obesity "'(Review)"', *Cochrane Database of Systematic Reviews*. Available at: https://pubmed.ncbi.nlm.nih.gov/29190418/ (last accessed 14 February 2023).

Friedli, L. (2009) *Mental Health, Resilience, and Inequalities*. Copenhagen: WHO. Available at: www.euro.who.int/__data/assets/pdf_file/0012/100821/E92227.pdf (last accessed 1 March 2023).

Fuller, E. (2011) *Smoking, Drinking and Drug use among Young People in England in 2010*. London: Information Centre for Health and Social Care.

Funk, S. and Klepac, P. (2015) 'Nine challenges in incorporating the dynamics of behavior in infectious disease models', *Epidemics*, 10(15): 21–5.

General Medical Council (2018) *Who are Children and Young People?* [Online]. London: General Medical Council. Available at: www.gmc-uk.org/ethical-guidance/ethical-guidance-for-doctors/protecting-children-and-young-people/definitions-of-children-young-people-and-parents (last accessed 1 March 2023).

Gibson, T. (2009) 'Learning disabilities education in the common foundation programme', *Nursing Standard*, 23(46): 35–9.

Gillett, M., Dallosso, H.M., Dixon, S., Brennan, A., Carey, M.E., Campbell, M.J., Heller, S., Khunti, K., Skinner, T.C. and Davies, M.J. (2010) 'Delivering the diabetes education and self-management for ongoing and newly diagnosed (DESMOND) programme for people with newly diagnosed type 2 diabetes', *British Medical Journal*, Aug 20, 341: c4093.

Green, J. and Tones, K. (2010) *Health Promotion: Planning and Strategies*, 2nd edn. London: Sage.

Gunn, S.W. and Masellis, M. (2008) *Concepts and Practice of Humanitarian Medicine*. New York: Springer.

Hamami, D., Cameron, R., Pollock, K.G. and Shankland, C. (2017) 'Waning immunity is associated with periodic large outbreaks of mumps: a mathematical modeling study of Scottish data', *Frontiers in Physiology*, 8(233).

Health and Care Act (2022). Available at: www.legislation.gov.uk/ukpga/2022/31/contents/enacted (last accessed 29 February 2023).

Health and Social Care (Quality and Engagement) (Wales) Act: summary. Available at: www.gov.wales/health-and-social-care-quality-and-engagement-wales-act-summary-html (last accessed 19 February 2023).

Health and Social Care Public Health Agency (2011) *Give Every Child the Best Start in Life* [Online]. Available at: www.publichealth.hscni.net/directorate-public-health/health-and-social-wellbeing-improvement/give-every-child-best-start-life (last accessed 26 February 2023).

Health Education England (2018) Making Every Contact Count (MECC) [Online]. Available at: www.hee.nhs.uk/our-work/population-health/our-resources-hub/making-every-contact-count-mecc (last accessed 16 June 2023).

Health Foundation (2018) *The Better Services for the Mentally Handicapped.* Available at: https://navigator.health.org.uk/theme/better-services-mentally-handicapped-white-paper (last accessed 26 February 2023).

Health Survey for England (2020) *Health Survey for England 2019.* Available at: https://digital.nhs.uk/data-and-information/publications/statistical/health-survey-for-england/2019 (last accessed 18 February 2023).

Helman, C.G. (2000) *Culture, Health and Illness,* 4th edn. Oxford: Butterworth-Heinemann.

HM Government (2022) *Working Together to Safeguard Children, A Guide to Inter-agency Working to Safeguard and Promote the Welfare of Children.* London: HM Government.

Hinton, L. on behalf of the MBRRACE-UK Lay Summary Writing Group (2014) *Saving Lives, Improving Mothers' Care* – Lay Summary 2014. Report of MBRRACE (Mothers and Babies Reducing Risk through Audits and Confidential Enquiries across the UK). Available at: www.npeu.ox.ac.uk/assets/downloads/mbrrace-uk/reports/Saving%20Lives%20Improving%20Mothers%20Care%20report%202014%20Lay%20Summary.pdf (last accessed 6 July 2022).

Homeless Link (2022) *The Unhealthy State of Homelessness.* London: Homeless. Available at: https://homelesslink-1b54.kxcdn.com/media/documents/Unhealthy_State_of_Homelessness_2022.pdf (last accessed 1 March 2023).

Home Office (2023) *Immigration System Statistics Year Ending Dec 22.* Available at: www.gov.uk/government/statistics/immigration-system-statistics-year-ending-december-2022/summary-of-latest-statistics#why-do-people-come-to-the-uk (last accessed 1 March 2023).

House of Commons Health and Social Care Committee (2018) *Prison Health Twelfth Report of Session 2017–19.* Available at: https://publications.parliament.uk/pa/cm201719/cmselect/cmhealth/963/963.pdf (last accessed 18 February 2023).

Hunter, D.J., Littlejohns, P. and Weale, A. (2022) 'Reforming the public health system in England', *The Lancet Public Health,* 7(9), e797–e800. Available at: https://doi.org/10.1016/s2468-2667(22)00199-2 (last accessed 1 March 2023).

Hutchings, R. and Davies, M. (2021) *How Prison Health Care in England Works.* Available at: www.nuffieldtrust.org.uk/resource/prison-health-care-in-england (last accessed 18 February 2023).

Institute of Health Equity (2021) *Build Back Fairer in Greater Manchester: Health Equity and Dignified Lives, Report 06/21.* Available at: www.instituteofhealthequity.org/resources-reports/build-back-fairer-in-greater-manchester-health-equity-and-dignified-lives (last accessed 14 February 2023).

Iqbal, M.P., Walpola, R., Harris-Roxas, B., Li, J., Mears, S., Hall, J. and Harrison, R. (2021) 'Improving primary health care quality for refugees and asylum seekers: asystematic review of interventional approaches', *Health Expectations,* 25:2065–94 [open access]. Available at: https://doi.org/10.1111/hex.13365 (last accessed 29 March 2023).

Jarvis, T., Scott, F., El-Jardali, F. and Alvarez, E. (2020) 'Defining and classifying public health systems: a critical interpretive synthesis', *Health Research Policy and Systems,* 18(1) [Open Access]. Available at: https://health-policy-systems.biomedcentral.com/articles/10.1186/s12961-020-00583-z (last accessed 1 March 2023).

Jenkins, D., Bowden, J., Robinson, H., Sattar, N., Loos, R.J.F., Rutter, M. and Sperrin, M. (2018) 'Adiposity-mortality relationships in type 2 diabetes, coronary heart disease and cancer populations in the UK Biobank, and their modification by smoking', *Diabetes Care*, 41(9): 1878–86.

Karatay, G., Kublay, G. and Emiroglu, O.N. (2010) 'Effect of motivational interviewing on smoking cessation in pregnant women', *Journal of Advanced Nursing*, 66(6): 1328–37.

Keyes, C.L.M. (2009) *Atlanta: Brief Description of the Mental Health Continuum Short Form (MHC-SF)*. Available at: https://peplab.web.unc.edu/wp-content/uploads/sites/18901/2018/11/MHC-SFoverview.pdf (last accessed 1 March 2023).

Kinge, S. and Gregory, I. (2011) 'Maternity focus: postnatal classes and effective care', *British Journal of Healthcare Assistants*, 5(8): 399–400.

Knight, M., Nair, M., Tuffnell, D., Shakespeare, J., Kenyon, S. and Kurinczuk, J.J. (eds) (2018) *Saving Lives, Improving Mothers' Care*. MBRRACE-UK. Available at: www.npeu.ox.ac.uk/assets/downloads/mbrrace-uk/reports/MBRRACE-UK%20Maternal%20Report%202018%20-%20Web%20Version.pdf (last accessed 1 March 2023).

Kozier, B. (2008) *Fundamentals of Nursing: Concepts, Process and Practice*. London: Pearson.

Lalonde, M. (1974) *A New Perspective on the Health of Canadians. A working document*. Ottawa: Government of Canada.

Leaning, B. and Adderley, H. (2016) 'From long-stay hospitals to community care: reconstructing the narratives of people with learning disabilities', *British Journal of Learning Disabilities*, 44(2): 167–71.

(LeDeR) (2021) *Learning Disability Mortality Review. Action from learning report 2020/21*. Available at: www.england.nhs.uk/wp-content/uploads/2021/06/LeDeR-Action-from-learning-report-202021.pdf (last accessed 1 March 2023).

Lester, S. and Russell, W. (2010) *Children's right to play: an examination of the importance of play in the lives of children worldwide* (Working paper no. 57). The Hague, The Netherlands: Bernard van Leer Foundation.

Lhussier, M., Carr, S.M. and Forster, N. (2015) 'A realist synthesis of the evidence on outreach programmes for health improvement of Traveller Communities', *Journal of Public Health*, 38(2): e125–e132.

Loveday, I. and Linsley, P. (2011) 'Implementing interventions: delivering care to individuals and communities'. In P. Linsley, R. Kane and S. Owen (eds), *Nursing for Public Health: Promotion, Principles and Practice* pp. 134–43. Oxford: Oxford University Press.

MacGregor, L., Speare, N., Nicholls, J., Harryman, L., Horwood, J., Kesten, J.M., Lorenc, A., Horner, P., Edelman, N.L., Muir, P., North, P., Gompels, M. and Turner, K.M.E. (2021) 'Evidence of changing sexual behaviours and clinical attendance patterns, alongside increasing diagnoses of STIs in MSM and TPSM', *British Medical Journal*, 97(7): 507–13.

Marmot, M. (2010) *Fair Society, Health Lives. The Marmot Review*. Available at: www.instituteofhealthequity.org/resources-reports/fair-society-healthy-lives-the-marmot-review (last accessed 29 June 2022).

Marmot, M. (2020) *Health Equity in England. The Marmot Review 10 years on*. Available at: www.instituteofhealthequity.org/resources-reports/marmot-review-10-years-on (last accessed on 29 June 2022).

Marteau, T.M., Hollands, G.J., Shemilt, I. and Jebb, S.A. (2015) 'Downsizing: policy options to reduce portion sizes to help tackle obesity', *British Medical Journal*, 351: h5863.

Masterson, A. (2011) 'The importance of nursing to public health: the political and policy context'. In P. Linsley, R. Kane and S. Owen (eds), *Nursing for Public Health: Promotion, Principles and Practice* pp. 89–97. Oxford: Oxford University Press.

McFadden, A., Atkin, K., Bell, K., Innes, N., Jackson, C., Jones, H., MacGillivary, S. and Siebelt, L. (2016) 'Community engagement to enhance trust between Gypsy/Travellers, and maternity, early years' and child dental health services: protocol for a multi method exploratory study', *International Journal for Equity in Health*, 15: 183.

McManus, S., Bebbington, P., Jenkins, R. and Brugha, T. (2016) *Mental Health and Wellbeing in England: Adult Psychiatric Morbidity Survey 2014*. Available from: http://content.digital.nhs.uk/catalogue/PUB21748/apms-2014- full-rpt.pdf (last accessed 20 February 2023).

Meader, N., King, K., Moe-Byrne, T., Wright, K., Graham, H., Petticrew, M., Power, C., White, M. and Sowden, A.J. (2016) 'A systematic review on the clustering and co-occurrence of multiple risk behaviours', *BMC Public Health*, 16: 657.

Mencap (2020) *Mental Health*. Available at: www.mencap.org.uk/learning-disability-explained/research-and-statistics/health/mental-health

Mendis, S., Puska, P. and Norrving, B. (2011) *Global Atlas on Cardiovascular Disease Prevention and Control*. Geneva: WHO, 3–18.

Ming, D.L. (2018) 'Tobacco Smoking, Food Intake, and Weight Control'. In *Tobacco Smoking Addiction: Epidemiology, Genetics, Mechanisms, and Treatment*. Singapore: Singapore.

Mulhall, A. (1996) *Epidemiology, Nursing and Healthcare: A New Perspective*. Basingstoke: Macmillan.

Naidoo, J. and Wills, J. (2016) *Foundations for Health Promotion*, 4th edn. London: Elsevier.

National Institute for Health and Care Excellence (2011) *Alcohol-use disorders: diagnosis, assessment, and management of harmful drinking (high-risk drinking) and alcohol dependence. Clinical guideline [CG115]*. Available at: www.nice.org.uk/guidance/cg115 (last accessed 1 March 2023).

National Institute for Health and Care Excellence (2013) *Physical Activity: Brief advice for adults in primary care. Public health guideline [PH44]*. Available at: www.nice.org.uk/guidance/ph44 (last accessed 1March 2023).

National Institute for Health and Care Excellence (2014) *Maternal and Child Nutrition, NICE Public Health Guidance 11*. Available at: www.nice.org.uk/guidance/ph11 (last accessed 6 July 2022).

National Institute for Health and Care Excellence (2017a) *Drug Misuse Prevention: Targeted interventions. NICE guideline [NG64]*. Available at: www.nice.org.uk/guidance/ng64 (last accessed 27 February 2023).

National Institute for Health and Care Excellence (2017b) *Child Maltreatment: When to Suspect Maltreatment in under 18s (Clinical guideline CG89; last updated 2017)*. London: NICE.

National Institute for Health and Care Excellence (2017c) *Child Abuse and Neglect. NICE Guideline NG76*. Available at: www.nice.org.uk/guidance/ng76 (last accessed 20 February 2023).

National Institute for Health and Care Excellence (2019) *Child Abuse and Neglect. NICE Guideline QS179*. Available at: www.nice.org.uk/guidance/qs179 (last accessed 20 February 2023).

National Institute for Health and Care Excellence (2021a) *Quality Standard 37. Postnatal Care*. Available at: www.nice.org.uk/guidance/ng194: (last accessed 6 July 2022).

National Institute for Health and Care Excellence (2021b) *NICE Impact People with a Learning Disability*. Available at: www.nice.org.uk/about/what-we-do/into-practice/measuring-the-use-of-nice-guidance/impact-of-our-guidance/nice-impact-people-with-a-learning-disability (last accessed 17 November 2023).

National Institute for Health and Care Excellence (2022) *Obesity: Identification, assessment, and management Clinical guideline (CG189)*. Available at: https://cks.nice.org.uk/topics/obesity/background-information/causes-risk-factors/ (last accessed 14 February 2023).

National Society for the Prevention of Cruelty to Children (2021) *Protecting Children from Neglect*. Available at https://learning.nspcc.org.uk/child-abuse-and-neglect/neglect (last accessed 20 February 2023).

National Society for the Prevention of Cruelty to Children (NSPCC) (2022) *NSPCC Learning*. Available at: https://learning.nspcc.org.uk/safeguarding-child-protection (last accessed 3 July 2022).

National Health Service (NHS) (2015) *Off to the Best Start: Important Information about Feeding Your Baby*. Available at: www.unicef.org.uk/babyfriendly/wp-content/uploads/sites/2/2010/11/otbs_leaflet.pdf (last accessed 6 July 2022).

National Health Service (NHS) (2020) *Postpartum Psychosis*. Available at: www.nhs.uk/mental-health/conditions/post-partum-psychosis/ (last accessed 6 July 2022).

NHS Digital (2021) *Mental Health Act Statistics, Annual Figures: 2020–21, Experimental Statistics*. Available at: https://digital.nhs.uk/data-and-information/publications/statistical/mental-health-act-statistics-annual-figures/mental-health-act-statistics-annual-figures-2016-17-experimental-statistics (last accessed 1 March 2023).

NHS England (2017a) *Framework for Patient and Public Participation in Public Health Commissioning*. Available at: www.england.nhs.uk/wp-content/uploads/2017/01/ph-participation-frmwrk.pdf [website] (last accessed 26 January 2023).

NHS England (2019a) *NHS Long Term Plan*. London: NHS England. Available at: www.longtermplan.nhs.uk/ (last accessed 14 February 2023).

NHS England (2019b) *NHS Mental Health Implementation Plan 2019/20–2023/24*, Available at: www.longtermplan.nhs.uk/wp-content/uploads/2019/07/nhs-mental-health-implementation-plan-2019-20-2023-24.pdf (last accessed 1 March 2023).

NHS England (2020) *Advancing Mental Health Equalities Strategy*. London: NHS England.

NHS England (2022) *NHS England Comprehensive Model of Personalised Care*. Available at: www.england.nhs.uk/personalisedcare/comprehensive-model-of-personalised-care (last accessed 19 December 2022).

Nursing and Midwifery Council (2018a) *The Code: Professional Standards of Practice and Behaviour for Nurses and Midwives*. London: NMC.

Nursing and Midwifery Council (2018b) *Future Nurse: Standards of Proficiency for Registered Nurses*. London: NMC.

Office for Health Improvement and Disparities (2021) *Alcohol: Applying All Our Health*. Available at: www.gov.uk/government/publications/alcohol-applying-all-our-health/alcohol-applying-all-our-health (last accessed 23 June 2022).

Office for Health Improvement and Disparities (2022) *Childhood Obesity: Applying All Our Health*. [online] GOV.UK. Available at: www.gov.uk/government/publications/childhood-obesity-applying-all-our-health/childhood-obesity-applying-all-our-health#:~:text=Overweight%20and%20obesity%20prevalence%20(including,2018%20to%202019%20NCMP%20data (last accessed 5 August 2022).

Office for National Statistics (2017) *Overview of the UK Population: July 2017*. London: ONS. Available at: www.ons.gov.uk/peoplepopulationandcommunity/populationandmigration/populationestimates/articles/overviewoftheukpopulation/july2017 (last accessed 1 March 2023).

Office for National Statistics (2018a) *Adult Drinking Habits in Great Britain: 2017*. London: ONS. Available at: www.ons.gov.uk/releases/adultdrinkinghabitsingreatbritain2017 (last accessed 1 March 2023).

Office for National Statistics (2018b) *Families and Households: 2017*. London: ONS. Available at: www.ons.gov.uk/peoplepopulationandcommunity/birthsdeathsandmarriages/families/bulletins/familiesandhouseholds/2017 (last accessed 1 March 2023).

Office of National Statistics (2020) *Adult Smoking Habits in the UK: 2019*. Available at: www.ons.gov.uk/peoplepopulationandcommunity/healthandsocialcare/health andlifeexpectancies/bulletins/adultsmokinghabitsingreatbritain/2019 (last accessed 23 June 2022).

Office of National Statistics (2021a) *Deaths Registered in England and Wales: 2020* Available at: www.ons.gov.uk/peoplepopulationandcommunity/birthsdeathsandmarriages/deaths/bulletins/deathsregistrationsummarytables/2020 (last accessed 23 June 2022).

Office for National Statistics (2021b) *Alcohol-specific Deaths in the UK: Registered in 2020*. Available at: www.ons.gov.uk/peoplepopulationandcommunity/healthandsocialcare/causesofdeath/bulletins/alcoholrelateddeathsintheunitedkingdom/registeredin2020 (last accessed 19 February 2023).

Office for National Statistics (2022a) *Estimating the Number of People with Cardiovascular or Respiratory Conditions Living in Poverty, England: 2021*. Available at: www.ons.gov.uk/vestimatingthenumberofpeoplewithcardiovascularorrespiratoryconditionslivinginpoverty england/2021#:~:text=Out (last accessed 19 February 2023).

Paiva, A.L., Prochaska, J.O., Yin, H.G., Rossi, J.S., Redding, C.A., Blissmer, B., Robbins, M.L., Velicer, W.F., Lipschitz, J., Amoyal, N., Babbin, S.F., Blaney, C.L., Sillice, M.A., Fernandez, A., McGee, H. and Horiuchi, S. (2012) 'Treated individuals who progress to action or maintenance for one behaviour are more likely to make similar progress on another behaviour: coaction results of a pooled data analysis of three trials', *Preventive Medicine*, 54(5): 331–4.

Parkin, E. and Powell, T. (2017) *Mental Health Policy in England*. London: House of Commons.

Parliament UK (2019) *Tackling Inequalities faced by Gypsy, Roma, and Traveller Communities*. London: HM Government. Available at: https://publications.parliament.uk/pa/cm201719/cmselect/cmwomeq/360/report-files/36005.htm (last accessed 24 June 2022).

Percival, J. (2013) 'Smoking cessation: reducing harm and improving the health of children', *Journal of Health Visiting*, 1(12): 689–95.

Percival, J. (2014) 'Promoting health: making every contact count', *Nursing Standard*, 28(29): 37–41.

Phillips, J., Richard, A., Mayer, K.M., Shilkaitis, M., Fogg, L.F. and Vondracek, H. (2020) 'Integrating the social determinants of health into nursing practice: nurses' perspectives', *Journal of Nursing Scholarship*, 52(5), 497–505.

Phillips, L. (2012) 'Improving care for people with learning disabilities in hospital', *Nursing Standard*, 26(23): 42–58.

Powell, J. (2013) 'Use of the common assessment framework in an acute setting', *Nursing Children and Young People*, 25(5): 24–8.

Prime Minister's Strategy Unit (2003) *Alcohol Misuse: How much does it cost?* UK Parliament.

Prochaska, J.O. and DiClemente, C.C. (1986) 'Towards a comprehensive model of change'. In W.R. Miller and N. Heather (eds), *Treating Addictive Behaviors: Processes of Change*. New York: Plenum, 3–27.

Public Health England (2016a) *Making Every Contact Count (MECC) Consensus Statement.* Available at: www.england.nhs.uk/wp-content/uploads/2016/04/making-every-contact-count.pdf (last accessed 17 February 2023).

Public Health England (2016b) *Health Matters: Giving every child the best start in life.* [online] GOV. UK. Available at: www.gov.uk/government/publications/health-matters-giving-every-child-the-best-start-in-life/health-matters-giving-every-child-the-best-start-in-life (last accessed 5 August 2022).

Public Health England (2018) *Health Matters: Reproductive health and pregnancy planning.* Available at: www.gov.uk/government/publications/health-matters-reproductive-health-and-pregnancy-planning/health-matters-reproductive-health (last accessed 23 June 2022).

Public Health England (2019) *Executive Summary 2020-2025.* Available at: https://assets.publishing. service.gov.uk/government/uploads/system/uploads/attachment_data/file/830105/PHE_Strategy__2020-25__Executive_Summary.pdf (last accessed 28 February 2023).

Public Health England (2020) *The Burden of Disease in England Compared with 22 Peer Countries. A report for NHS England.* Available at: https://assets.publishing.service.gov.uk/government/uploads/system/uploads/attachment_data/file/856938/GBD_NHS_England_report.pdf (last accessed 19 February 2023).

Public Health England (2021a) *Vaping in England: 2017 evidence update summary.* Available at: www. gov.uk/government/publications/vaping-in-england-evidence-update-february-2021/vaping-in-england-2021-evidence-update-summary (last accessed 19 February 2023).

Public Health England (2021b) *Tracking the Syphilis Epidemic in England: 2010 to 2019.* Available at: www.gov.uk/government/publications/tracking-the-syphilis-epidemic-in-england (last accessed 23 June 2022).

Public Health Scotland (2020) *Suicide Prevention Overview.* [online] Available at: www.healthscotland. scot/health-topics/suicide/suicide-prevention-overview (last accessed 5 August 2022).

Public Health Scotland (2022) *A Scotland Where Everybody Thrives: Public Health Scotland's three-year plan: 2022–25.* Available at: www.publichealthscotland.scot/media/16485/public-health-scotland-strategic-plan-2022-2025.pdf (last accessed 1 March 2023).

Public Health Wales (2018) *Working to Achieve a Healthier Future for Wales.* Available at: https:// phw.nhs.wales/about-us/our-priorities/long-term-strategy-documents/public-health-wales-long-term-strategy-working-to-achieve-a-healthier-future-for-wales/ (last accessed 1 March 2023).

Rees, S. (2009) *Mental Ill Health in the Adult Single Population. A Review of the Literature.* London: Crisis.

Reynolds, R.M. and Gordon, A. (2018) 'Obesity, fertility and pregnancy: can we intervene to improve outcomes?', *Journal of Endocrinology*, 239(3): R47–R55.

Robertson, K. (2010) 'Understanding the needs of women with postnatal depression', *Nursing Standard*, 24(46): 47–55.

Rodney, A. (2015) 'Food Deserts'. In *The Wiley Blackwell Encyclopedia of Consumption and Consumer Studies*, 1–2.

Rollnick, S., Miller, W.R., Butler, C.C. and Rollnick, S.P. (2007) *Motivational Interviewing in Health Care: Helping Patients Change Behavior.* New York: Guilford Publications.

Roper, N., Logan, W.W. and Tierney, A.J. (2000) *The Elements of Nursing.* Edinburgh: Churchill Livingstone.

Rosenstock, I.M. (1974) 'Historical origins of the health belief model', *Health Education Monographs*, 2: 328–35.

Rowe, A., McClelland, A. and Billingham, K. (2001) *Community Health Needs Assessment: An Introductory Guide for the Family Health Nurse in Europe*. Geneva: World Health Organization.

Royal College of Nursing (2012) *Going Upstream: Nursing's Contribution to Public Health: RCN Guidance for Nurses*. London: RCN.

Royal College of Nursing (2013) *Meeting the Health Needs of People with Learning Disabilities: RCN Guidance for Nursing Staff*. London: RCN. Available at: www.complexneeds.org.uk/modules/Module-4.1-Working-with-other-professionals/All/downloads/m13p040b/meeting_health_needs_people_with_ld.pdf (last accessed 1 March 2023).

Royal College of Nursing (2016) *Nurse 4 Public Health: Promote, Prevent and Protect: The Value and Contribution of Nursing to Public Health in the UK: Final Report*. London: RCN.

Royal College of Psychiatrists (2018) *Postpartum Psychosis*. Available at: www.rcpsych.ac.uk/mental-health/problems-disorders/postpartum-psychosis (last accessed 6 2022).

Salway, S., Mir, G., Turner, D., Ellison, G.T.H., Carter, L. and Gerrish, K. (2016) 'Obstacles to "race equality" in the English National Health Service: insights from the healthcare commissioning arena', *Social Science and Medicine*, 152: 102–10.

Sanders, B. and Brianna, B. (2015) *I Was on My Own: Experiences of Loneliness and Isolation amongst Homeless People*. London: Crisis.

Sashidharan, S.P. and Commander, M.J. (1998) 'Mental health'. In S. Rawaf and V. Bahl (eds), *Assessing Health Needs of People from Minority Ethnic Groups*. London: Royal College of Physicians.

Scambler, G. (2009) 'Health-related stigma', *Sociology of Health and Illness*, 31(3): 441–55.

Scottish Government (2017) *Our Children have the Best Start in Life and are Ready to Succeed* [online]. Available at: www.gov.scot/publications/scotland-performs-update-2017/pages/21/ (last accessed 1 March 2023).

Scottish Government (2018) *Minimum Unit Pricing*. Scotland: The Scottish Government. Available at: www.mygov.scot/minimum-unit-pricing (last accessed 1 March 2023).

The Scottish Parliament (2021) *Health and Care Bill*. Available at: www.parliament.scot/bills-and-laws/legislative-consent-memorandums/health-and-care-bill (last accessed 19 February 2023).

Shah, N.R. and Braverman, E.R. (2012) 'Measuring adiposity in patients: the utility of body mass index (BMI), percent body fat, and leptin', *PLoS ONE*, 7(4): e33308.

Shaw, J., Talbot, J., Norman, A., Lyon, J., Heathcote, L., Bernard, A. and Worthington, N. (2020) *Avoidable Natural Deaths in Prison Custody: Putting things right. Independent Advisory Panel on Deaths in Custody and Royal College of Nursing*.pdf. Available at: www.rcn.org.uk/-/media/royal-college-of-nursing/documents/clinical-topics/nursing-in-justice-and-forensic-healthcare/prevention-of-natural-deaths-in-custody-final-nov-2020.pdf?la=en&hash=0992599A705070ED06C9821DDE97B505 (last accessed 18 February 2023).

Sharpley, M., Hutchinson, G., Murray, R.M. and McKenzie, K. (2018) 'Understanding the excess of psychosis among the African-Caribbean population in England. Review of current hypotheses', *The British Journal of Psychiatry*, 178, suppl. 40: s60–s68.

Taylor, R.S., Dalal, H., Moxham, T. and Zawada, A. (2010) 'Home-based versus centre-based cardiac rehabilitation', *Cochrane Database of Systematic Reviews*, (1): CD007130. doi: 10.1002/14651858.CD007130.pub2

The King's Fund (2022) *What are Health Inequalities?* Available at: www.kingsfund.org.uk/publications/what-are-health-inequalities (last accessed 26 January 2023).

Thomas, S. and Price, M. (2012) 'Respite care in seven families with children with complex care needs', *Nursing Children and Young People*, 24(8): 24–7.

Timby, B.K. (2012) *Fundamental Nursing Skills and Concept*, 10th edn. Philadelphia, PA: Lippincott, Williams & Wilkins.

Tolstrup, J.S., Hvidtfeldt, U.A., Flachs, E.M., Spiegelman, D., Heitmann, B.L., Balter, K., Goldbourt, U., Hallmans, G., Knekt, P., Liu, S., Pereira, M., Stevens, J., Virtamo, J. and Feskanich, D.(2014) 'Smoking and risk of coronary heart disease in younger, middle-aged, and older adults', *American Journal of Public Health*, 104(1): 96–102.

Townsend, P., Davidson, N. and Whitehead, M. (eds) (1992) *Inequalities in Health: The Black Report: The Health Divide*. London: Penguin Books.

Tulchinsky, T.H. (2018) 'Marc Lalonde, the Health Field Concept and Health Promotion', *Case Studies in Public Health*, 523–41. doi: 10.1016/B978-0-12-804571-8.00028-7. Epub 2018 Mar 30.

UK Health Security Agency (2017) *Contraindications and Special Considerations: the green book, chapter 6. Information for public health professionals on immunisation*. Available at: www.gov.uk/government/publications/contraindications-and-special-considerations-the-green-book-chapter-6 (last accessed 14 February 2023).

United Nations (UN) (1989) *Convention on the Rights of the Child*. Available at: www.ohchr.org/EN/ProfessionalInterest/Pages/CRC.aspx (last accessed 14 February 2023).

Van Cleemput, P., Parry, G., Thomas, K., Peters, J. and Cooper, C. (2007) 'Health-related beliefs and experiences of Gypsies and Travellers: a qualitative study', *Journal of Epidemiology and Community Health*, 61(3): 205–10.

Vynnycky, E. and White, R.G. (2010) *An Introduction to Infectious Disease Modelling*. Oxford: Oxford University Press.

Welsh Government (2013) *Building a Brighter Future: Early Years and Childcare Plan* [online]. Available at: www.gov.wales/written-statement-publication-early-years-and-childcare-plan (last accessed 1 March 2023).

Wilkinson, R.G. (2005) *The Impact of Inequality: How to Make Sick Societies Healthier*. London: Routledge.

Wisborg, K., Kesmodel, U., Henriksen, T.B., Olsen, S.F. and Secher, N.J. (2000) 'A prospective study of smoking during pregnancy and SIDS', *Archives of Disease in Childhood*, 83: 203–6.

World Health Organization (1986) *First International Conference on Health Promotion, Ottawa, 21 November: Track 1 Community empowerment*. Available at: www.who.int/teams/health-promotion/enhanced-wellbeing/first-global-conference (last accessed 26 January 2023).

World Health Organization (2002) *The World Health Report 2002: Reducing Risks, Promoting Healthy Life*. Geneva: WHO.

World Health Organization (2003) *Investing in Mental Health*. Geneva: WHO. Available at: https://apps.who.int/iris/handle/10665/42823 (last accessed 1 March 2023).

World Health Organization (2019a) *Participation as a Driver of Health Equity*. Available at: https://apps.who.int/iris/handle/10665/324909 [website] (last accessed 26th January 2023).

World Health Organization (2019b) *World Health Assembly Update, 27 May 2019* [press release]. 2019 May 27. Available at: www.who.int/news-room/detail/27-05-2019-world-health-assembly-update-27-may-2019 (last accessed 1st March 2023).

World Health Organization (2020) *Child Maltreatment*. Available at: www.who.int/news-room/fact-sheets/detail/child-maltreatment (last accessed 14 February 2023).

World Health Organization (2021a) *Health Equity*. Available at: www.who.int/health-topics/health-equity#tab=tab (last accessed 19 December 2022).

World Health Organization (2021b) *Non-Communicable Diseases*. Geneva: WHO. Available at: www.who.int/news-room/fact-sheets/detail/noncommunicable-diseases (last accessed 24th June 2023).

World Health Organization (2022a) *Health Promotion*. Available at: www.who.int/health-topics/health-promotion#tab=tab_1 (last accessed 14 February 2023).

World Health Organization (2022b) *Determinants of Health*. Available at: www.who.int/news-room/questions-and-answers/item/determinants-of-health (last accessed 19 December 2022).

Wyness, L., Stanner, S. and Buttriss, J. (2013) *Nutrition and Development: Short and long term consequences for health*. British Nutrition Foundation. London: John Wiley & Sons.

12

SPECIALIST CARE OF THE OLDER PERSON: A PERSON-CENTRED, BIOGRAPHICAL APPROACH

Emma Stanmore and Christine Brown Wilson

Chapter objectives

- Outline the specialist needs and challenges around planning and delivering high-quality care to pre-frail and frail older people, and supporting their carers in a variety of settings;
- Consider the principles of anti-discriminatory practice through examining myths and stereotypes that may detrimentally influence the care of older people, including those with dementia;
- Explain the importance of preventative care and health promotion for older people, including those with dementia with reference to physical activity and falls prevention;
- Explore the principles of independence, empowerment, and choice for the delivery of care, and the role of technology in supporting these principles;
- Identify how dignity and compassion might be promoted for older people in everyday practice;
- Evaluate the role of the nurse in establishing the needs and preferences of older people and their carers using person-centred and biographical care planning.

This chapter considers the knowledge, skills and attitudes required by nurses for the optimum care of older adults and how we as nurses might promote person-centred care in everyday practice. We explore how the principles of health promotion (with reference to physical activity and falls prevention) can be applied to promote independence and improve the quality of life for older people. We address important topics such as dignity in care, empowerment and choice in relation to the care of older people, including people with dementia or 'frailty.' We also consider the role of carers of older adults and how we might support their needs, including those caring for people living with dementia. A key aim is for readers to question current perceptions of ageing, using examples of myths and stereotypes that can often influence how ageing is viewed and valued in our society. The chapter promotes an understanding of the principles of anti-discriminatory practice with reference to age and considers how this is applied in practice. Most importantly, we also demonstrate the importance of using biography throughout the assessment process, appreciating the experience, skills, and wisdom of older people to both enrich our nursing practice and enhance person-centred care.

Related Nursing and Midwifery Council (NMC) Proficiencies for Registered Nurses

The overarching NMC requirements are that all registered nurses should be able to

> manage the complex nursing and integrated care needs of people at any stage of their lives; supporting and enabling them to make informed choices about how to manage health challenges to maximise their quality of life and improve health outcomes.

> Working in partnership with people, be able to use information obtained during assessments (i.e., considering their circumstances, characteristics, wishes and preferences) to identify the priorities and requirements for person-centred and evidence-based nursing interventions. Assess risks to safety or experience and take appropriate action to manage those, putting the best interests, needs and preferences of people first across a range of organisations and settings.
>
> (Nursing and Midwifery Council [NMC], 2018)

▬▬▬▬▬ TO ACHIEVE ENTRY TO THE NMC REGISTER
YOU MUST BE ABLE TO ▬▬▬▬▬

- Understand the principles and processes involved in supporting people and families with a range of care needs to maintain optimal independence and avoid unnecessary interventions and disruptions to their lives;

- Consider knowledge of body systems and homoeostasis, human anatomy and physiology, biology, pharmacology, social, physical, behavioural, and cognitive health conditions, medication usage and treatments when undertaking full and accurate person-centred nursing assessments;
- Demonstrate the ability to accurately process all information gathered during the assessment process (including an understanding of co-morbidities and the need to meet people's complex nursing and social care needs) to individualise nursing care, developing and applying person-centred evidence-based plans for nursing interventions with agreed goals;
- Demonstrate the ability to work in partnership with people, families, and carers (encouraging shared decision making) to continuously monitor, evaluate and reassess the effectiveness of all agreed nursing care plans and care, readjusting agreed goals, documenting progress and decisions made to support individuals, their families, and carers to manage their own care when appropriate;
- Effectively assess a person's capacity to make decisions about their own care, to give or withhold consent, and understand and apply the principles and processes for making reasonable adjustments and best interest decisions where people do not have capacity;
- Recognise and assess people at risk of harm and the situations that may put them at risk, using a range of contemporary assessment and improvement tools, and ensuring that prompt action is taken to safeguard those who are vulnerable;
- Demonstrate knowledge of when and how to refer people safely to other professionals or services for clinical intervention or support.

(Adapted from NMC, 2018)

It is a cause for celebration that people in the UK are living longer, reflecting our advancement in areas such as healthcare technologies, pharmacology, education, and reduced childhood mortality. For the first time in history we have more people over the age of 60 than those under the age of 18 (ONS (Office for National Statistics, 2020) with the 'oldest old' (over the age of 85) being the fastest growing demographic. In addition, the number of years spent in good health without disability, is declining; this is now 62.4 years for men and 60.9 years for women (ONS, 2020). It is for this very reason that all adult nurses need to be educated in the specialism of care of older people to ensure that their individual needs are met.

It would be logical to think that as older people are the core users of the NHS, this would lead to more expertise and improved care within this field. However, recent reports repeatedly highlight a picture of poor or variable care for older people (Humphries et al., 2016; Care Quality Commission, 2022). A notable example was the Mid Staffordshire inquiry that highlighted the need for the delivery of compassionate care for older people. This public inquiry and other similar reports (Andrews and Butler, 2014) revealed a negative culture of disengagement, low morale, tolerance of poor care and long-term understaffing which led to high mortality rates, undignified care, and excessive levels of unaddressed complaints. Since then, issues of quality of care for older people have consistently been in the public eye (Age UK, 2019).

The positive side of these perturbing reports is that they have led to an unparalleled opportunity to transform services for older people, in which nurses have a key role. As older people account for most adults in receipt of nursing care, all adult nurses should be educated in this specialism, including the awareness and skills in working with individuals who are frail or cognitively impaired (such as those with dementia). There have been several government actions to help put the care of older people at the centre of healthcare, which include an improved publicly available ratings system for the inspection of healthcare organisations with a greater emphasis on compassionate care. There has been a governmental drive to promote more innovation and research and improve standards for the care of older people with dementia (NHS England, 2019). Similarly, following the recognition that mild frailty or pre-frailty is potentially reversible, the e-frailty index tool has been implemented to highlight those at risk with a view to preventing frailty progression (National Institute for Health and Care Excellence [NICE], 2016). Tailored education and support should be offered for nursing staff to promote the values of compassion, dignity and respect, and there should be a reduction in unnecessary bureaucracy through streamlining inspections, data sharing and the improved use of technology among frontline staff, to give more time to and emphasis on caring (NHS England, 2019).

There has also been a governmental push to recruit people into the care workforce who demonstrate a desire and ability to care for others (Government Office for Science, 2016). Therefore because of these policies, we may see some important leadership changes in the care of older people, with a greater recognition of the skills required for competent and compassionate care, and nurses need to seize these opportunities to make a difference.

Identify the key nursing skills required to care effectively for older people to overcome the shortcomings of the public inquiries mentioned above.

- When providing care to an older adult, how could you ensure that you are able to develop your clinical skills outlined in annexes A and B of the NMC (2018) proficiency framework?
- How might you demonstrate these skills in everyday practice?
- Provide one or two examples where you might implement these skills.

Myths and Stereotypes of Older People

Before discussing the challenges of caring for older people further, it is important to recognise the value of older people as individuals with beneficial societal roles and influences. Ageing should not signify decline and disease. Many older adults continue to perform at exceptionally high levels and learn new skills, as well as coping with major life changes such as retirement and bereavement. With age comes a wealth of experience, wisdom and skills that are a rich resource for all generations. At present, these skills do not seem to be fully realised by society at large, although since 2011 older people can if they wish, continue working past the age of 65. A 2015 Eurobarometer report found that people in the UK are the second most likely in Europe to see ageism as a problem, with those in the 50–64 and 65–74 age groups most likely to be worried that employers will show preference to those in their 20s (European Commission,

2015; Government Office for Science, 2016; Age UK, 2017). Older people can be as productive as younger generations and we need to discard any stereotypes about what we think it means to be 'old' (Bowers et al., 2013). Older people should not be seen as a homogeneous group with burdensome needs but as diverse individuals with the ability to contribute to society and the same right to dignified, personalised care as any other generation.

Myths can be described as stories propagated within a society and were often a means of educating people about the values and morals of society. In the global society in which we currently live, myths now emerge from advertising through a range of media. In terms of ageing, myths portray old age either as a sign of decline and increasing decrepitude or as a heroic point in life, where older adults overcome adverse effects of ageing to do things that would be expected of younger members of society such as running marathons. Neither of these views are particularly helpful for older people because they do not recognise the individual nature of ageing or the context in which people live their later years (Minkler, 1996). These views have been perpetuated by early sociological research, resulting in the disengagement and activity theories and more latterly, the theory of successful ageing (for a discussion on these theories, please see Bond et al., 2007).

We stereotype people by placing them in a group with others whom we believe all have similar traits and so will behave in similar ways, and this is often used as a mechanism to mentally organise workload. In addition, by stereotyping people in this way, we risk seeing them as 'different' and so can justify treating them differently. For older people, this may mean treating them with less dignity than other groups of people in our care. The language we use often refers to the stereotypes to which we subscribe (Oliver, 2013; Gendron et al., 2018). For example, referring to older people as 'the elderly' suggests we believe that all older people have limited capacity for development because they are in a period of decline. This may be used to justify nursing older people in bed for longer periods because they already have limited mobility and limited capacity to recover. However, when we consider the personal nature of ageing, we cannot assume that all older people age in the same way (Bond et al., 2007). We might conclude that myths and stereotypes of ageing in our society may have an adverse impact on older people in healthcare environments. For example, nurses in busy environments may unknowingly use stereotypes to make quick decisions when faced by an increasing workload. Learners have recounted how some qualified nurses can make assumptions based on these stereotypes, such as the expectation that an older person will be incontinent or have dementia (Brown Wilson, 2013). These decisions may have an adverse impact on care because nurses are often the gatekeepers for referrals to other healthcare professionals/services.

Consider two older people you know or have cared for who are similar ages.

- What influences their approach to their ageing?
- Are there similarities and differences?
- What do you attribute these to?
- What do you think this means for your care of the older person?

No one will be immune from societal stereotypes but an awareness of when myths or stereotypes are being used to make judgements about care is the first step in minimising the potential harm they may cause (Gendron et al., 2018). In addition, adopting an approach to care that focuses on the person and enables a practitioner to see the condition in context to the person will also lessen the impact negative stereotypes may have. As nurses, we must challenge stereotypes of ageing as a period of decline and support older people to maintain and enhance their quality of life by improving their health in ways that are meaningful to them.

The Opportunities and Challenges of Caring for Older People

Older people are the main users of health services in both hospitals and the community, and this trend is likely to continue. With increasing age, the risk of living with one or more long-term condition increases. And hospitals are struggling to cope with fewer beds and increasing numbers of emergency admissions due to the increase in older people (CQC, 2022). The Office for Budget Responsibility (2015) projects total public spending to increase by almost 5% of GDP between 2019–20 and 2064–65 – equivalent to £79 billion in today's terms – due to the ageing population. The growing number of older people will bring new challenges to nurses as well as new opportunities to ensure high-quality care is experienced and maintained.

Traditionally, care of the older person has been seen as a less attractive career pathway compared with other nursing specialisms, but it is a rewarding, challenging field of nursing that is ripe for further development and innovation. There are opportunities for nurses to pioneer and transform services designed to support older people to live longer in their own homes using assistive technologies and to deliver better preventative care or specialist care that incorporates their needs and preferences. For example, there are growing numbers of 'virtual wards and 'smart homes' with embedded health devices such as movement and fall sensors, programmes to manage complex medication regimens, and microprocessors in appliances, furniture and clothing that collect health-monitoring data. Social media, ubiquitous computing, and digital health technologies such as mobile health apps are proving to be of immense value to healthcare. People are increasingly using social media such as Twitter and Facebook to post medical problems and seek help finding diagnoses, and apps are commonly used to provide information about conditions and support self-management of care.

Furthermore, the Covid-19 pandemic accelerated the adoption of telehealth (also known as telecare or remote monitoring) to enable more older people to receive care under the remote supervision of a healthcare team, reducing infection risks, costly home visits and extending access to care as well as potentially preventing accidents and crises.

Despite these technological advances which aim to enable people to remain active at home for longer, benefits achieved to date still require further research (Greenhalgh and Papoutsi, 2019). The NHS Long Term Plan (NHS, 2019) outlined a commitment to every individual having the right to be offered digital-first primary care by 2023/24. It should be noted however, that a digital-first approach may increase workload and with workforce shortages could worsen issues of access. Therefore, new digital initiatives should be implemented in a staged way alongside careful evaluation (Salisbury et al., 2020). The process of developing and implementing tele-health technologies requires coordination and commitment between numerous professions and organisations. However, nurses are in a key position to support, implement and evaluate inno-vative technologies to ensure that they are introduced using the best evidence, with joined-up service provision and, most importantly, what older people want.

- Consider an older person that you know - what technology do they use in everyday life? How might this or similar technology be used to enhance their health or maintain their independence as they age?

The care of older people can be emotionally demanding and requires qualities such as compas-sion, empathy, and patience, alongside specialist gerontological education to ensure that nurses are equipped to meet the complex care needs using a person-centred approach. Caring for older people requires an understanding of the physiological changes that take place as we age, with in-depth knowledge of long-term conditions such as diabetes, depression, arthritis, cardiovascular disease, respiratory conditions and dementia, to name but a few (see Arking (2006) for more information about the biology of ageing and Goodwin et al. (2010), to learn more about the long-term condi-tions affecting older people).

We know that older people, given the right help and support, would prefer to live in their familiar homes and communities for as long as possible. However, Smith et al. (2011) argue that undergraduate nurse education programmes are often more focused on acute hospital care for those individuals with single organ or infectious diseases, whereas many older people have com-plex care needs and multiple co-morbidities and use primary care services as well as hospitals. Indeed, the current model of acute care is geared to treatment and cure and is not well suited to older people living with complex needs. There is also the consideration of the complexities of polypharmacy, (i.e., the interaction between multiple medications and their side effects), and the need to give preventative care to enable older people to stay independent and disease free. As a registered nurse you will need to develop your knowledge and understanding of these issues to be able to support those with complex, often interrelated co-morbidities, the frail 'oldest old' and the growing number of people with dementia in an already over-stretched health service. This may require you to undertake additional gerontological courses in the future to gain the skills required for the care of older people.

Developing the specialised skills and knowledge to care for older people and a positive atti-tude to ageing at the individual as well as the organisational level should drive a sustainable improvement in service provision and improve dignity in care.

Maintaining Dignity for the Older Person

Dignity in care refers to the care and support in any setting that promotes and maintains a person's self-respect whatever their circumstances, health, age or any other such difference. The Social Care Institute for Excellence (2020) defines dignity as a state, quality or manner worthy of esteem or respect and (by extension) self-respect. Although dignity may be difficult to define, it is clear to an older person when they have not received dignified care and this can result in feelings of embarrassment and humiliation. From the perspective of the older person in hospital, it can be the small actions such as finding out their usual routines, needs and preferences rather than conforming to standardised hospital routines, that can make an older person feel like a valued individual (Tauber-Gilmore et al., 2018). Being thoughtful, polite, and caring not only enriches the care that is delivered but can also reduce the person's anxiety and increase their confidence. For example, simply reading an excerpt from a book that is of interest to a person who is blind shows that you are trying to do what really matters to them.

Nordenfelt and Edgar (2005) describe four ways of understanding dignity (Figure 12.1): dignity we earn by our actions (Dignity of Merit) and for whom we are in society (Dignity of Identity), dignity we feel within ourselves (Dignity of Moral Status) and dignity we deserve because we are human (Menschenwürde). These are interrelated concepts with Dignity of Merit and Dignity of

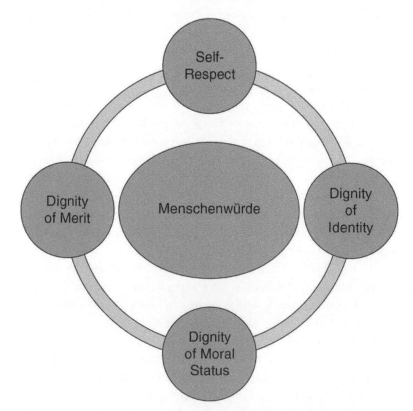

Figure 12.1 Four ways of understanding dignity (Nordenfelt and Edgar, 2005)

Identity conferred on us by others. If people treat us with dignity because they feel our position in society warrants this, then this will support our own sense of worth, leading to self-respect. Each of these notions is underpinned by the respect we should show to all people because they are human beings. However, if this respect is not shown, then our sense of dignity becomes eroded which then impacts adversely on our self-respect (Nordenfelt and Edgar, 2005).

In their meta synthesis of the concept of dignity, Clancy et al. (2021) describe dignity as either 'absolute' or 'relative' with relative dignity being able to be promoted or violated through the confirmation of others. Examples of how dignity might be compromised include when older adults' views are not respected by healthcare professionals or they do not feel valued as a person (Tauber-Gilmore et al., 2018). Such actions implied a lack of respect. Autonomy is a key issue and involves supporting older people to maintain independence wherever possible, ascertaining a person's wishes to be involved in their care and then involving them in the decision-making process (Tauber-Gilmore et al., 2018). Overall, maintaining dignity is about treating people as people, not as objects. This demonstrates respect for the person and builds trust between the professional and the person receiving care.

Box 12.1 (Levenson, 2007)

- Dignity in care is inseparable from the wider context of dignity as a whole;
- Dignity is about treating people as individual persons;
- Dignity is not just about physical care;
- Dignity thrives in the context of equal power relationships;
- Dignity must be actively promoted;
- Dignity is more than the sum of its parts.

When older people are admitted to hospital, the dignity of the person can be undermined while they are unwell because their key focus is recovering (Jacelon, 2003; Goodrich, 2011). However, as they transition from the acute phase of their illness, they become more aware of such assaults on their dignity. Jacelon (2003), in her observational study, found that many older people attempted to address this by interacting with staff and developing reciprocal relationships. One interpretation of this study might be that healthcare professionals become so focused on one approach to care that they do not always realise the impact their actions have on a person's dignity. If we return to the four notions of Dignity (see Figure 12.1), we might understand such actions as an effort by the older person to enhance their dignity of moral status (because they were trying to help staff) because the dignity conferred by others has not been forthcoming.

Furthermore, people with dementia are more likely to suffer assaults on their dignity because they may not be able to communicate in a way that is understandable to busy healthcare professionals. This is often compounded by them being in an unfamiliar environment and having their usual routines disrupted. Moreover, many people with dementia may be admitted to a healthcare environment with an underlying medical problem such as an infection that is not recognised due to the overlying symptoms of dementia, which then results in poor consequences for the person (van der Geugten and Goossensen, 2020).

Ada

Consider the needs of Ada, a 70-year-old with impaired hearing and poor eyesight, admitted to hospital for treatment for viral pneumonia.

Think of the practical ways in which nursing and hospital staff could work to maintain Ada's dignity.

Consider simple methods such as keeping Ada informed and being polite, for example. How would you communicate effectively, considering Ada's needs and preferences. What would you need to consider to assist Ada to maintain her personal hygiene needs? What difficulties could you face in a busy acute hospital? Write down your thoughts and reflections. There are some websites listed at the end of this chapter that contain useful information when considering dignity and the care of older people.

Compassion, choice, and empowerment in healthcare

Previous chapters have highlighted the value of compassion, personal choice and empowerment in healthcare provision. However, we feel this is important enough to reiterate it again here in relation to caring for the older person.

Compassion in nursing care is defined as 'how care is given through relationships based on empathy, respect and dignity – it can also be described as intelligent kindness and is central to how people perceive their care' (DH, 2013). Compassionate and effective care for the older person requires nurses to be able to respond in an ever-changing environment and place the care of the older person and their individual needs at the forefront. We also need to focus on the things that matter to older people and their families and not just their medical care.

The Care Quality Commission (CQC) regularly inspects hospitals, care homes and primary care centres in Scotland, England, and Wales to ensure that services are effective, safe, and compassionate. In Northern Ireland, the Regulation and Quality Improvement Authority (RQIA) has a similar remit for their province. All regulatory authorities across the UK publish their findings from these inspections and encourage services to make improvements where shortfalls in care are identified. In terms of the care of the older person, the CQC in England and Wales has made recommendations to several NHS services including the recruitment of specialist care nurses for the older person, more consultant geriatricians, increasing staffing levels and the introduction of the compassionate care training programme for all staff working with older people.

However, it is often difficult from these reports to identify what is meant by terms such as 'caring' and 'compassion.' If we examine these in more detail, we see examples of nurses telling older people to use an incontinence aid rather than being taken to the toilet (Tauber-Gilmore et al., 2018). Similarly, research reports comparable issues such as nurses or carers assuming that an older person is not hungry rather than finding out the underlying reason they are not eating (Tadd et al., 2011). These reports describe everyday occurrences observed in busy ward environments that imply a lack of dignity. Such practices may occur when we fail to consider the impact of our approach to care when we care for older people.

Consider how you might improve your practice in each of the following areas - Care, Compassion, Courage, Communication, Commitment and Competence - and how any improvements that you introduce could be measured to demonstrate change.

The measurement of compassion may be difficult because compassion is not always visible. Think about novel ideas such as collecting case studies where compassion was demonstrated or introducing short feedback forms in your work setting, which could be used to recognise good examples of care or areas that need further improvements.

The responsibility for improving the quality of older people's care needs to be taken at the individual level as well as by nurses in leadership positions. As nurses lead by best example, the culture and environment of undervaluing older people can be changed to one of empowerment and putting their perspective first. Many older people are reliant on support from family carers, and it is these carers who often raise concerns and complaints about the quality of care.

Nurses need to be proactive in involving older people in their care decisions from the onset; giving explanations, managing expectations, and involving families in decision making and discharge planning. In a study on the views of older people in the choice of care for intermediate care services, there appeared to be mixed views from the people on whether they received choices about their care and about how much they wanted to be involved in the decisions about this (Stanmore, 2011). An early study by Pickard and Glendinning (2002) recommends that older carers should receive real choice about the extent of their involvement in care giving, that healthcare professionals should anticipate the needs of older carers and provide a more proactive service when offering help. The implementation of this advice would ensure that older carers would feel more supported and valued.

In a systematic review of the literature, carers' needs are described in two key areas: meeting the needs of the person receiving care and meeting their own needs (McCabe et al., 2016). Although professionals may recognise and support carers in how to provide care and meet the needs of the person receiving care, it is rare that they also consider the needs of the carers themselves. For example, the health of carers demonstrated that they are more likely to experience worse physical and mental health than those without caregiving duties living in the community (Pinquart and Sorensen, 2003). Depression is associated with the amount of caregiving per week, alongside the care recipients' physical impairment in the absence of dementia, with stronger associations found for spouses than for adult children (Pinquart and Sorensen, 2003). However, those caring for a person with dementia are more likely to experience poorer physical and mental health than other carers (Pinquart and Sorensen, 2004). Differences also exist between groups of carers, with spouses experiencing worse physical and mental health than adult children who provide care (Pinquart and Sorensen, 2011).

The subjective wellbeing of carers may be encouraged by enabling carers with time to continue activities that contribute to their subjective wellbeing or ensuring that they are still experiencing the 'uplifts' of caregiving rather than reducing their burden. For example, positive pre-caregiving relationships have been associated with better outcomes, suggesting that interventions that consider the context of family relationships may support improved outcomes for the caregiving and the person receiving the care (Quinn et al., 2012).

In the UK, the Care Act 2014 (www.legislation.gov.uk/ukpga/2014/23/contents/enacted) provides family carers with the same recognition in their need for support as the person they are caring for (Department of Health and Social Care, 2016). The carer assessment might be undertaken by a social worker or another trained professional such as a registered nurse (district/community or psychiatric) and may occur together with the assessment of the person receiving care. The assessment covers caring responsibilities, housing, work, study, leisure opportunities, relationships, and social activities, as well as the goals of the caregiver (Carers UK, 2016). This may result in services such as support with meals, help around the home, replacement care or gym membership, depending on the outcome of the assessment (Department of Health and Social Care, 2016). However, looking at the literature, we can see the importance of understanding that different carers have unique needs. For example, spousal carers may benefit from respite care to reduce burden whereas adult children may benefit from interventions that strengthen their relationship with the person receiving care (Pinquart and Sorensen, 2011; Gaugler et al., 2018). Adult children might also have caring responsibilities for young children alongside their responsibilities for an ageing parent, suggesting they will have dissimilar needs to adult children with no additional caregiving responsibilities (Gaugler et al., 2016). In addition, the more recent phenomenon of adult children staying at home for longer delays the transition to adulthood, further compounding stressors for those caring for ageing parents as well (Mitchell et al., 2015).

As nurses supporting carers, we also need to understand the impact of the conditions experienced by care recipients on the needs of carers. Dementia is one such condition that creates additional issues for carers due to the nature of the condition. It is estimated that the number of people living with dementia would increase from 57.4 million people globally in 2019 to 152.8 million people in 2050 with more women than men being affected (Nichols et al., 2022). There are currently around 900,000 people living with dementia in the UK with this projected to rise to 1.6 million in the UK by 2040 (Wittenberg et al., 2019). This means that 34% of the UK population are affected by dementia in their family, with 700,000 people involved in caregiving (Alzheimer's Research UK, 2015a). Of these, 60–70% are women with 20% having to drop from full-time to part-time work due to caregiving responsibilities (Alzheimer's Research UK, 2015b). Over a third of carers provide over 100 hours per week in caregiving and 30% of caregivers had been providing care for a person with dementia for over five years (SACE, 2017). Of dementia caregivers, 15% say that they are not in paid work due to caregiving commitments (SACE, 2017). The nature of dementia being a progressive loss of the person's identity alongside their cognitive and physical abilities creates additional stressors for these carers, and subsequently impacts on the life decisions of other members of the family. In this way, the caregiving trajectory in dementia has been likened to a 'career' due to the transition points of diagnosis, behavioural changes, institutionalisation and bereavement (Gaugler et al., 2005). Understanding this caregiving 'career' is vital for nurses and other healthcare professionals in supporting dementia carers. For example, the nature of dementia alters the dynamics of family relationships and so may impact on the caregiver's social support as well as their wellbeing. There is limited literature that considers the wider family dynamics, although these altered relationships may impact on the level of support received and, subsequently, the caregiving trajectory (Gaugler et al., 2018).

However, we must beware of engaging in substitute decision making because we believe the older person or the person with dementia is unable to engage in the decision-making process. We must endeavour to provide opportunities for involvement and where necessary facilitate supported decision making, ensuring that information is provided at times when the person is alert and not medicated, the environment is conducive, and the information is provided in accessible language. If people wish to opt out of the decision-making process, then they will be able to make this known, but it is also important to support people in identifying an advocate until they wish to be involved in the decision-making process. Person-centred care does not stop at assessment and should be incorporated throughout the person's care. People are entitled to be involved in their healthcare decisions and their involvement should be embedded in the structures of all aspects of health and social care.

Biographical Approach to Care

So, how can we ensure that older people receive the person-centred care that they deserve? It is by valuing the older person for whom they are, understanding what is important and ensuring that significant routines are maintained in their care that we deliver person-centred care. We start this by developing an understanding of the biography of the older person which supports us in valuing them as a person first and then considers their needs as a recipient of care in this context (Box 12.2).

Box 12.2 Biographical Approach to Care Planning

- Encourage individuals to talk about how they approach their life;
- Develop rapport by talking about everyday events and people during care routines;
- Use personal belongings and photos as triggers for discussion;
- Recognise unique assets and characteristics of each person and build on these when care planning;
- Build on lifelong interests to offer individuals opportunities to experience new things and interests in context to their care.

We may think we do this, but as busy healthcare professionals we often focus on the condition the person presents with first, with the needs of the older person a secondary consideration. It is when focusing on the condition rather than the person becomes established practice that we begin to see examples of poor care as described by The Health Foundation (2021), and inquiries such as Francis (2013). These reports highlight established practice which results in care that lacks compassion and dignity, and often provide examples of older people and/or people with dementia. As nurses are often in the frontline of care provision, it is their care that comes under scrutiny, with reports about nurses not having time to care or losing their compassion.

Promoting Person-Centred Care with Older People and those with Dementia

Person-centred care has been identified as a way of improving the care of older people (McCormack and McCance, 2021) and those with dementia (Brooker, 2004).

Dementia is not one condition but a syndrome characterised by decline of mental and physical abilities, including recent memory, problem solving, language, visuospatial skills, and orientation (Alzheimer's Society, 2021). There are many types of dementia, the most common being Alzheimer's disease accounting for two-thirds of people living with dementia. Vascular dementia is the second most common cause, with dementia with Lewy bodies being the third most common (Alzheimer's Society, 2022). Although most people affected by dementia are aged over 65, there is a hidden population of over 70,000 people under this age affected by early onset dementia in the UK (Carter, 2022). A high proportion of people living with dementia will have co-morbid conditions (Dowrick and Southern, 2014), with those aged over 65 likely to have four co-morbid conditions when compared with people aged over 65 without dementia (Poblador-Plou et al., 2014). (For further details of the aetiology of dementia, see SCIE resources at the end of this chapter.)

Older lesbian, gay, bisexual, transgender, queer and intersex (LGBTQI+) individuals have greater challenges in accessing healthcare where heterosexuality is considered the norm (Crameri et al., 2015). Treating LGBTQI+ older people as the 'same' as other older people does not acknowledge the history of the lives they have lived, usually experiencing discrimination, stigma, and potential imprisonment or forced 'cures' (Crameri et al., 2015). This collective experience contributes to a culture of shared values, beliefs, and behaviours, which is distinct from the shared experience of the heterosexual population. This perspective supports us in recognising that older LGBTQI+ people have additional needs and requires us to provide a culturally safe environment in the delivery of services. LGBTQI+ older people's fear about discrimination may result in delay in accessing services with greater dependency and strain on intimate partners, particularly when one partner has dementia (Barrett et al., 2015). In speaking with LGBTQI+ couples (some of whom had dementia) and service providers, it is evident that older people do not change their sexuality or gender recognition following dementia (Barrett et al., 2015). LGBTQI+ individuals will require additional support to maintain their support structures with their intimate partners and 'family of choice,' to prevent social isolation and depression when entering services. Indeed, it can be the attitudes of service providers and families of origin that can be more damaging to a person's identity than dementia itself (Barrett et al., 2015). Many older people who identify as LGBTQI+ wish to remain in their own homes yet fear or experience discrimination from home care services, suggesting mandatory LGBTQI+ sensitivity training for workers (Smith and Wright, 2021). Developing culturally safe services requires engagement with LGBTQI+ people in planning of services, organisational leadership, staff education and inclusive service literature where LGBTQI+ people are visible (Crameri et al., 2015).

Not all older people will have dementia, but the risk of some dementias such as Alzheimer's disease, increases with age. This suggests that increased longevity may also increase the number of people diagnosed with dementia. Person-centred care, as developed by Tom Kitwood (1997), aims to focus the attention of professionals on the person rather than the condition. Kitwood believed that considering the emotional needs of the person alongside their physical needs would enhance the care of people with dementia. Brooker developed these principles into the VIPS model (valuing the person with dementia, providing individualised care, recognising the perspective of the person with dementia, and examining the social environment in which the person is located) (Røsvik et al., 2011). Recognising that the individual is a person first is now considered a guiding principle across all models of healthcare. For example, the Institute of Medicine's (2001) definition of person-centred care includes respecting needs, values, and preferences, as well as providing emotional and physical support. However, many of these models lack specific guidance as to how these models might be put into practice (Dewing, 2004), with Goodrich and Cornwell (2008) finding that few healthcare professionals in the UK could describe what was meant by person-centred care.

Activity 12.1

Draw a timeline of your life and consider how some of the events that have been significant in your life have shaped how you approach your life today.

- Consider an older person you know in your personal life. How have events in their life shaped how they make decisions about their health?
- For this older person, what are the significant routines in their life that might be interfered with if they required health and social care support?
- How might you as a concerned relative try to influence their care?

Person-centred care is an approach that nurses should use with all older people and is characterised by understanding the biography of the person and seeing beyond the immediate context of illness (McCormack and McCance, 2021). A systematic review of personal experience in acute hospitals suggests that older people and their families want health and social care staff to recognise who they are and what is important to them, to involve them in decision making and to support them in maintaining links with their community while in hospital (Bridges et al., 2010). This is of particular importance for older LGBTQI+ people who may not have traditional social support networks as reflected in the heterosexual population. Intimate partners and wider friendships in the LGBTQI+ community are often the only environments where LGBTQI+ people feel safe to be themselves, with such networks becoming 'families of choice' (Barrett et al., 2015). However, it is also important not to treat all LGBTQI+ people as the same, particularly people of Trans or non-binary experience who may require additional support for personal care and grooming (Ansara, 2015).

Brown Wilson (2013) develops the use of biography to consider what is significant in a person's life, including day-to-day routines that give the older person's life meaning, or for the person with dementia, provides an understandable structure to their day. Nurses often develop insights into this biographical information through the daily contact they have with individuals in providing care, such as giving out medication, bathing, dressing, and supporting people at mealtimes. This information may not be shared as routine because it might not be considered relevant to the nursing care of this person (Brown Wilson, 2013). The challenge for nurses at this point is how to document information such as this so it becomes part of accepted practice for the older person and not dependent on one nurse being on duty for that older person.

Sexuality and intimacy are another important aspect of ageing and one often neglected both in the literature and in practice, which suggests that older people are not seen as sexual beings (Simpson et al., 2017a). As nurses, we might feel extremely uncomfortable in speaking about these issues, but older people speak about their needs to engage in ongoing intimate and sexual relationships (Simpson et al., 2017b). Indeed, the highest incidence of sexually transmitted infections are now in the over-60 age group (Lee, 2016), suggesting a vital role for nurses in speaking to older people about their sexual health. This work suggests that we need to move away from the perspective that sexuality is only about providing choice in what an older person wishes to wear or how they express their gender. However, this element of care is of particular importance for transgender and intersex people who do not necessarily conform to the binary gender of male or female (Ansara, 2015). Also maintaining connection with LGBTQI + networks and safe spaces for the continuation of intimate relationships are aspects of care important to LGBTQI+ individuals as they age and enter services (Barrett et al., 2015). However, the need to maintain intimate and sexual relationships is ignored in the design of care systems (Simpson et al., 2017a) with staff identifying the structural barriers in addressing such needs (Simpson et al., 2017b). A first step in addressing the sexuality and intimacy needs of older people might be finding out what important relationships they have and developing trusting relationships, enabling older people to feel comfortable in speaking about these issues.

Implementing person-centred care

So far, we have suggested several ways in which the principles of person-centred care can be implemented as a mechanism by which to promote dignity when working with and/or caring for older people. However, it is recognised that the environment in which care is delivered and organised also has an impact on the implementation of approaches such as person-centred care (Brown Wilson, 2013; McCormack and McCance, 2021).

McCormack and McCance (2021) identify the care environment as a key feature of their model of person-centred nursing, suggesting that a range of factors such as organisational systems, physical environment, skill mix and staff relationships, needs to be taken into consideration. Each of these factors will contribute or act as a barrier to the implementation of person-centred care. Often person-centred care may be considered something additional because some of these factors may require additional work and sometimes be beyond the control of ward-based staff. Brown Wilson (2009) suggests several considerations to be considered when seeking to support health and social care staff in implementing a person-centred approach by integrating the following into current practice:

- Leadership;
- Staff motivation;
- Teamwork;
- A consistent approach to care;
- Continuity of care.

To develop person-centred services, nurses need to consider how to use their leadership irrespective of their position in the organisation. Indeed, nurses may be working at every level in some organisations and as such, have the power to influence person-centred care, whether it be at the bedside or at the executive level (Brown Wilson, 2017). As we have already established in Chapter 9, leadership that is approachable, able to generate trust, supportive of staff in resolving conflict and promotes an exchange of information to support staff in their decision making is more likely to develop positive relationships in the workplace (Anderson et al., 2003). Brown Wilson (2009) suggests that this style of leadership can also come from those delivering day-to-day care in ways such as role modelling good practice.

To get to know a person and then to implement significant changes to their care plan requires the continuity of staff who will adopt a person-centred approach. Initially, sharing biographical knowledge may be dependent on developing relationships with specific members of staff but, once this information has been disseminated, continuity can be promoted even when the same nursing staff are on duty through a consistent approach to care. This is possible even when staffing levels and skill mix may be suboptimal.

The personal philosophy of staff, their beliefs and values are integral to a person-centred approach (Brown Wilson and Davies, 2009; McCormack and McCance, 2021). This has been represented in Figure 12.2, as staff motivation with a 'do unto others' philosophy is more likely to create a focus on the person. This means that the staff consider what the older person considers important in their care and seeks to implement care in this way. In her work, Brown Wilson (2009) found that a critical mass of staff working with the same philosophy was more likely to result in a focus on the person. Therefore, this implies that developing a culture in the work environment where the older person is listened to, and their needs are acted on is more likely to deliver a person-centred approach to care.

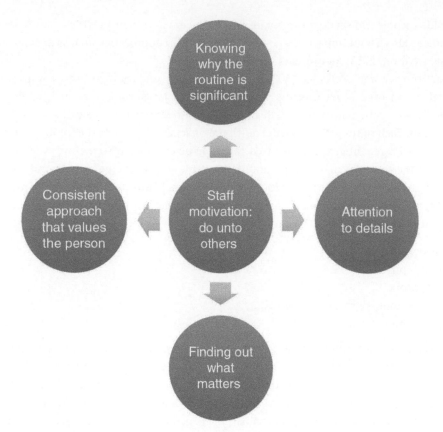

Figure 12.2 Brown Wilson's (2013) person-centred approach

Older people and families often seek to make a direct contribution to or influence their care through the development of relationships with staff (Jacelon, 2003; Brown Wilson, 2009). Adopting a biographical approach to care planning is one way of recognising and valuing this contribution. This may highlight reasons behind different behaviours, supporting staff in making sense of these given their workload.

Joseph

Joseph's pain had been attributed to age and whilst currently being treated for depression Joseph appeared withdrawn. Following an exploratory conversation, the nurse found out that Joseph had always been an active and outgoing person and enjoyed volunteering at the local hospital but was unable to continue this due to the knee pain which restricted mobility. Finding out what was significant to Joseph, he was then transferred into action by referring to other members of the multidisciplinary team to investigate the cause of the pain. In the meantime, the nurse arranged for transport for him to attend a day centre, which was enjoyed immensely.

Understanding Frailty in the Older Person

One of the key challenges for supporting people as they age is the increasing level of frailty. Frailty is a complex, age-related health state in which people progressively lose their in-built reserves and ability to recover from minor events or illness (Kojima et al., 2019). Frailty as a term is often used but remains poorly defined with little consensus on definitions (Rockwood and Koller, 2013). Some have defined frailty as a collection of deficits – the more people have wrong with them, the frailer they are (Mitnitski et al., 2005) – with some researchers suggesting it is a specific syndrome represented by weight loss, exhaustion, low physical activity, and slowness (Fried et al., 2004). Despite these different definitions there is increasing recognition that frailty is a physiological syndrome that causes an older person to be more vulnerable to adverse health outcomes (Kojima et al., 2019). This is due to a decline in physiological function across multiple systems often caused by co-morbid conditions. This results in the older person's body system having limited ability to respond to internal stressors such as viruses or environmental stressors such as changes in temperature. This approach suggests that frailty is not simply a result of the ageing process and so should not be defined by chronological age, but by how the older person's body responds to different stressors.

Rockwood et al. (2006) undertook a large-scale study testing the hypothesis that at a given age, frailty can be defined in relation to how many deficits an older person has, such as problems with mobility, nutrition and the ability to undertake activities of daily living. The accumulation of deficits is important because it may tip the balance between an older person being able to live independently in the community or requiring institutional care (Rockwood et al., 1994). A Frailty Index has been developed to summarise a person's health status by counting the number of deficits which is then used to infer relative frailty of an individual (Mitnitski et al., 2005). This has more recently been further developed and implemented as an electronic frailty index (eFI) in many GP (General Practitioner) practices throughout the UK (Clegg et al., 2016). The work undertaken by Rockwood et al. (2006) and Clegg et al. (2016) suggests that it is the accumulation of these deficits that is important for health outcomes, rather than the individual nature of each deficit. This is important for nurses in healthcare because we often focus on the nature of the deficit.

It is very tempting to think about frailty as a fixed condition, e.g., once you become frail there is no going back. However, frailty can be reversed even in old age as the trajectory of frailty varies according to the individual (Kojima et al., 2019). Rockwood et al. (1994) consider frailty as a balance (Figure 12.3). For older people, the scales are tipped towards the side of the assets (medical and social). Increasing frailty then brings the scales into alignment until one additional problem may tip the scales in favour of the deficits. However, the nature of those deficits may be amenable to treatment to enable the balance between asset and deficit to change. Although no standard treatment exists for frailty, the use of multicomponent exercise interventions with a resistance component has been consistently successful (Kojima, et al., 2019).

There is substantial evidence that older people benefit from a comprehensive geriatric assessment (CGA) in acute settings (Ellis et al., 2017) although the evidence is less clear for older people experiencing frailty in community environments (Briggs et al., 2022). The CGA benefits older people with frailty as it is an assessment and intervention that is whole person

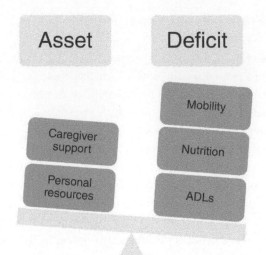

Figure 12.3 Interpretation of the 'Frailty Balance' based on Rockwood et al. (1994)

centred, multidisciplinary, iterative, and case managed (Conroy et al., 2019). Physiological function, the reactions of the body to pharmaceutical treatments, and responses to health challenges and injury all change with age. The syndromes frequently presenting in older people – cognitive impairment, stroke, fragility fractures, falls, syncope and incontinence – are different from those in younger populations.

When using the CGA to assess frailty (Box 12.3) (Jones et al., 2004), the more deficits the older person has, then the greater their risk of poor outcomes. However, when health and social care professionals consider these domains, they tend to consider each issue as an isolated problem. Considering issues of nutrition, mobility, and continence, for example, as indicators of frailty may promote a more holistic assessment of the person. In any assessment, it is vital that we understand the significance of presenting issues to the older person themselves. So, we need to consider the clinical significance of these issues from the person's perspective, i.e., what is most important to that person and what intervention is required to support that person in achieving his or her personal goal. By doing this, we place the older person at the centre of the assessment process and provide an opportunity to learn more about individuals, their current situation, and their desires for the future.

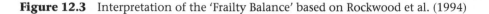

Box 12.3 Assessing Frailty Using CGA Domains Based On Jones et al. (2004)

Cognitive status (no cognitive impairment = no problem; cognitive impairment/no dementia = mild problem; delirium or dementia = severe problem).
Mood and motivation.
Communication (vision, hearing, speech).

Mobility, balance (scored at the highest level of independence with aids where used).

Bowel function.

Bladder function.

IADLs (instrumental activities of daily living) and ADLs (activities of daily living) (rated as no impairment = no problem; IADL impairment = mild problem; ADL impairment = major problem).

Nutrition.

Social resources (scored as a problem if there was need for additional help).

Instructions:

For a Frailty Index, score problems in each domain were scored as 0 (no problem); 1 (a minor problem); or 2 (a major problem). For evaluating the contribution of each domain, the mode of the three ratings determined the value for each subject.

Sami

Sami has been admitted to your ward as a well 88 year-old unable to get out of bed this morning. The community nurses could not find a specific problem but were unable to move Sami from the bed and so arranged admission to hospital. On further assessment, Sami suggests regular meals are taken but admits to weight loss over the past three months. The light meals eaten are those that can be prepared in a microwave because Sami has lost interest in cooking. Sami walks the dog once a day but is only able to shuffle along slowly for a short distance. Additionally, Sami admits to struggling with housework and needs help with the garden but wishes to remain at home.

Using the domains of the Comprehensive Geriatric Assessment, identify how frail you think Sami is and why. What are the risks for Sami if these deficits are not addressed? What nursing actions do you think Sami would benefit from and how would these enable independence to be retained?

Health Promotion for Older People

Caring for older people is not just about treating them during illness. It is also about keeping them well and educating them about how to stay healthy and active for as long as possible. Although it is widely understood that health promotion for older people may encompass activities such as blood pressure control, flu immunisation or smoking cessation, it should be recognised that every contact with an older person may present an opportunity to promote healthy behaviour and lifestyles.

Opportunities for nurses to promote health may be related to screening for the early detection of conditions, identifying whether the older person would benefit from preventative advice or assessment for asymptomatic disease such as hypertension or osteoporosis. Early identification of dementia is also important to ensure that treatment, support, and follow-up can be put into place so that sufferers and their families can receive ongoing care and review. Likewise, recognising through assessment the need for screening for cancers such as breast, prostate, and colon (which are increasingly remediable through surgery or chemotherapy) can lead to much improved outcomes when these diseases are identified early on in their natural history. Similarly, being on the lookout for signs of depression – another common condition in older people – can lead to early diagnosis and treatment that can improve the quality of life in older people.

Simple health-promoting measures such as checking when an older person last had his or her vision or hearing ability checked and referring to appropriate services can improve their general health and wellbeing and assist in maintaining their ability to remain independent. Similarly, establishing whether an older person is experiencing difficulties with urinary incontinence can lead to effective prevention and treatment that also impacts positively on the person's self-esteem. Although urinary incontinence is treatable, fewer than half of individuals with urinary incontinence report their symptoms to a physician and suffer in silence (Orrell et al., 2013). This is usually because they are too embarrassed; they consider their problem a normal part of ageing, absorbent devices are readily available, or they have low expectations of treatment or fear surgery. Developing positive, therapeutic relationships by listening, developing rapport, and displaying empathy with older people may enhance engagement and communication, thus leading to improved care outcomes (Kornhaber et al., 2016).

Educating older people to manage long-term conditions optimally, such as arthritis or diabetes, should also be a key part of nurses' health-promoting role. For instance, reinforcing healthy dietary advice or encouraging physical activity will not only improve the condition but also reduce the likelihood of developing other co-morbid diseases. Diet and lifestyle influences can have a considerable influence on health during the life course (WHO (World Health Organization), 2010). In a study of dietary patterns and lifestyle among individuals aged 70–90 years, adherence to a Mediterranean diet and healthy lifestyle was associated with a more than 50% lower rate of all cause and cause-specific mortality (Knoops et al., 2004). Similarly, there is now good evidence for twelve modifiable risk factors that can prevent the onset of dementia that include low education, obesity, smoking, hypertension, diabetes, hearing loss, excessive alcohol intake, traumatic brain injury, air pollution, depression, physical inactivity, and low social contact (Livingston et al., 2020). The prevailing health promotion messages are to modify these risk factors, even in later life, with the recommendation to keep physically, socially, and cognitively active. Although these may not guarantee that a person will not develop dementia the brain will be in better health with greater cognitive reserves to deal with the condition if it develops.

Health-promoting activities may also encompass the reassessment or review of an individual's medication, considering ongoing needs or their understanding of safe administration and potential side effects. For older people taking four or more medicines (known as polypharmacy), referral to the GP or pharmacist for a medication review has been shown to be beneficial in reducing medication-related complications. These increase with the number of medications consumed, both prescribed and over the counter. Medication management studies in older people have shown that they are more likely to experience adverse consequences and have lower tolerance of drug side effects, and be at greater risk of inappropriate prescribing, more likely to be uncertain about physician instructions, more likely to have greater difficulties ordering and collecting their medicines, and prone to have difficulties administering their medicines because of cognitive, sensory or physical impairment (Rogers et al., 2014). Therefore, taking the time to assess a person's needs in managing their medication, teaching about the safe administration and side effects could save much distress, reduce hospital admissions and potentially be lifesaving.

Marta

Marta, a 78-year-old with coronary heart disease, congestive heart failure and hypertension lives at home with another family member. Marta has decided to stop taking diuretics due to continence problems and is admitted to hospital with worsening heart failure. The nursing assessment has revealed that several general practitioners had visited Marta and adjusted prescribed medication to improve control of heart failure. One of the community nurses had also visited to assess and manage continence problems but neither the doctors nor the nurse was aware of each other's visits.

- In your area of practice, do you think that medication management is considered within the nursing assessment and organisation of care?
- What additional training would you find useful in enabling you to support older people to manage their medicines effectively?
- What nursing and health promoting actions do you think would benefit Marta? How would these actions enable Marta to return home safely and manage prescribed medication effectively?
- What could be done to improve multidisciplinary communication to prevent incidents like this case from occurring again?

Promoting Physical Activity in Older People

For many older people an inactive life can lead to poor mental health and feeling dissatisfied, depressed and socially isolated. Participation in meaningful activity is important for maintaining relationships and feelings of purpose, as well as improving physical and mental health (NICE, 2008). Research over the last 25 years has shown that physically active older people experience a better quality of life and less social isolation, and maintain their function and independence compared with those who remain sedentary (Wilmoth and Ferraro, 2013).

Current evidence suggests that nurses should be encouraging older people to remain active and independent rather than disempowering them or overly increasing their reliance on health and social care professionals.

There are several important reasons for encouraging physical activity or exercise in older people. It can be health promoting, for instance resistance exercises (those that incorporate strength training) can maintain or improve bone health to prevent osteoporosis. Exercise can also be disease preventing, for example it can lower blood pressure and cholesterol, prevent heart disease and diabetes, and has also been associated with preventing certain types of cancer (Centers for Disease Control and Prevention [CDC], 1996; WHO, 2007; British Heart Foundation, 2010).

There are further myths and stereotypes about older people being unable to remain physically fit and active. Those working in exercise science could inform us that older people are capable of functioning at exceptionally high levels and that decline occurs on an individual basis, dependent on factors such as lifestyle and genetics. We know from research studies that older people, even in their 90s, can reverse the effects of ageing through regular muscle-strengthening and balance exercises (Fiatarone et al., 1990). Therefore, it is important for nurses to encourage activity and exercise with older people whatever their ability, and to assist them to find local facilities or give advice on home-based exercises that will maintain and improve their physical function.

Some of the benefits that can be used to encourage older people to become more active and remain active are listed in Table 12.1. The most important points listed here are the benefits in maintaining independence and a social network, losing these abilities are some of the biggest fears of older people. When talking to individuals about staying active and not sitting for longer than an hour they may not be highly motivated to do so, but if it is explained that this could be the difference in staying independent at home for longer they may be much more motivated to increase their physical activity.

Table 12.1 Advantages of physical activity and risks associated with sedentary behaviour

Physically active behaviour	Sedentary behaviour
Increases ability to maintain social network. Reduces fatigue. Improves ability to maintain a stable weight. Better quality of life. Possible improved survival. Improves bone density and lower risk of osteoporosis. Improves muscle strength and balance. Quicker reaction time. Improves proprioception. Improves mental health and cognitive function.	Reduces postural stability. Decreases function and independence. Decreases quality of life. Increases risk of pressure ulcers. Significantly decreases bone density and increases risk of osteoporosis. Can negatively affect mental health. Increases risk of obesity and associated morbidities (e.g., cardiovascular disease, type 2 diabetes, cancer).

Based on Chief Medical Officer (2011) and Sherrington et al. (2019).

As a nation we are becoming increasingly sedentary and this is the first generation to need to make a conscious decision to build physical activity into daily lives (Public Health England [PHE], 2016). Societal changes (such as fewer manual jobs, increased car use and automation) have designed physical activity out of our lives, and there have been many recent governmental campaigns aimed at getting people to be more active to target obesity, social isolation and encourage longer working lives (DH, 2009; PHE, 2016). Sedentary behaviour accelerates the loss of performance and sarcopenia (loss of muscle mass), and older people already lose 1–2%

of functional ability each year. Just one week of bed rest reduces a person's strength by approximately 20% and spine bone density by 1% (LeBlanc et al., 1987). If you consider how much time older people in care homes spend either sitting down or in bed you can understand their increased risk of fractures and falls. All older adults should minimise the amount of time spent being sedentary (sitting) for extended periods, and nurses can educate and encourage older people to be as active as possible.

The question is how active should older people be? This very much depends on the individual, taking into consideration their current health and how active they already are. In 2011, the first ever UK-wide, published guidelines (Chief Medical Officer, 2011) outlined the amount of physical activity older adults (65 years and over) should be doing to benefit their health:

- Older adults who participate in any amount of physical activity gain some health benefits, including maintenance of good physical and cognitive function;
- Some physical activity is better than none, and more physical activity provides greater health benefits;
- Older adults should also undertake physical activity to improve muscle strength on at least two days a week;
- Older adults at risk of falls should incorporate physical activity to improve balance and coordination on at least two days a week.

Research also suggests that there are many barriers (actual and perceived) for older people to overcome to be able to effectively participate in physical activity; some individuals are just too unwell, and others may think that exercise is not good due to their condition. In fact, their health would benefit if they did increase their physical activity (e.g., people needing cardiac rehab or those with rheumatoid arthritis; Stanmore et al., 2013). Some individuals try exercise but do not see any immediate observed positive effects – this is because some of the benefits are not immediately obvious and the person may need to become a little fitter before they experience any improvements in health. Other people may not like the social contact in classes or find they get too fatigued or feel pain, whereas others struggle with motivation or feel they have other more important priorities in their life. For some there may be practical difficulties such as getting to an available class. These barriers can be overcome with help and an individualised approach, so when encouraging an older person to exercise involve them in developing a programme and help them to find a class or sport that they can take part in. Remember there is something for everyone. Skelton et al. (2005) demonstrated in their strength and balance training study of older people that in three months 65 to 90-year-olds were able to rejuvenate 20 years of lost strength.

Exercise should incorporate some kind of aerobic or endurance tasks, some flexibility and resistance exercises, e.g., weight bearing, in particular the lower limb, and some functional task training that is individualised according to the needs and preferences of the person. There is even published research about the benefits of Wii fit, Xbox Kinect and other virtual reality gaming systems for exercise which are being found to be beneficial for older people in the home or care home environment (van Diest et al., 2013).

Consider the types of exercise facilities, classes or services suitable for older people in your local community.

• What do you think might be the barriers to the attendance of older people at each of these activities? How might these barriers be overcome, using an individualised approach, and considering the person's significant routines?

Activity 12.2

Visit your library or search the internet for facilities local to you that are suitable for older people – remember the importance of finding out what the older person's interests are and the need to tailor this to their preferences. There are also some websites listed at the end of this chapter that contain useful information when considering physical activity and older people.

Falls Prevention for Older People

A common myth or stereotype of older people is that falling is often accepted as a natural part of the ageing process. When we look at the research, we find that many falls can be predicted and prevented (Montero-Odasso et al., 2022) but this message needs to reach older people (and some health professionals) who continue to think that falls are inevitable. The National Council on Aging (2013) produced a list of the ten most common misconceptions about falls in older adults such as 'It won't happen to me', 'It's just a normal part of growing older', 'If I limit my activity, I won't fall', 'As long as I stay at home, I can avoid falling', 'Muscle strength and flexibility can't be regained' and 'Taking medication doesn't increase my risk of falling'. So, we can conclude that older people also need re-educating about these misconceptions and we, as nurses, should be reiterating the positive message that with support, falls can be prevented.

It is true however, that falls are common in older people, yet many older people are unaware of their risk of falling. Around one in three people aged over 65, and half of those aged over 80, fall at least once a year and this rate increases with age and in those living in care homes (American Geriatrics Society, British Geriatrics Society, and American Academy of Orthopaedic Surgeons Panel on Falls Prevention [AGS/BGS], 2010). Approximately 10% of falls will result in fractures, and most concerning is that falls resulting in hip fractures commonly lead to death or institutional care within a year. Fear of falling is also an important concern that can restrict social activity and lead to older adults becoming more sedentary and isolated. The risk of falls is exacerbated due to the resulting muscle weakness and balance difficulties. Therefore, it is imperative that nurses raise awareness of the importance of falls risk screening and assessment of older people with other health and social care professionals, older people, and their carers/relatives.

We can easily identify those who are most at risk of a fall by asking questions related to the most important risk factors. Fall risk factors for older people can be categorised as biological, behavioural and psychosocial (Figure 12.4). A history of a previous fall is the best predictor of a future fall and any older person who responds positively to this question should receive support in preventing further falls. For some older people, reduced physical activity causes their balance and muscle strength to deteriorate, and their reaction time and gait speed slow so the ability to remain steady and upright becomes much more challenging. We know that older people are more sedentary and this can increase the likelihood of a fall.

Having poor strength and balance, gait problems and fear of falling also increase the risk of falls. Some diseases such as Parkinson's disease, stroke, rheumatoid arthritis, and dementia also increase the likelihood of falls, as does having poor vision, foot pain and incontinence (WHO, 2007; Stanmore, 2013). We know that taking more than four types of medicine and certain types of medicine (antidepressants, diuretics, analgesics, and antipsychotic medicines) is also a contributing factor. A person's environment can also increase the likelihood of falls, for instance if there were lots of tripping hazards or uneven surfaces in the home (NICE, 2013).

Over the last three decades, researchers have conducted fall prevention trials with older people and have shown that exercise reduces the number of falls by around a quarter (23%) to up to 42%. A Cochrane Systematic Review (Sherrington et al., 2019) assessed the effects of exercise interventions to reduce the incidence of falls in older people living in the community and included 108 clinical trials. They concluded that exercise programmes carried out in a group

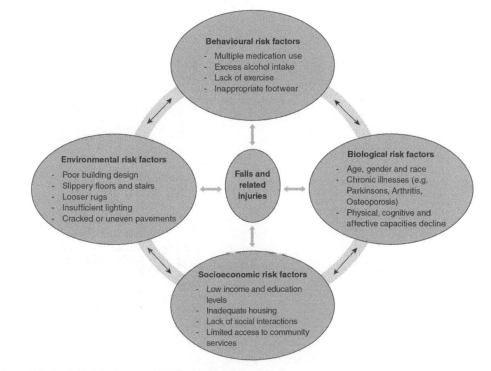

Figure 12.4   Fall risk factors (WHO, 2007; NICE, 2013)

class or at home prescribed by a health professional (such as a physiotherapist) or a trained exercise leader were effective and those with resistance exercise such as using weights to make the exercises harder worked best. The reviewers also concluded that fall prevention strategies can be cost saving (Sherrington et al., 2019). This evidence could be used by nurses to reduce the risk of falling and improve the quality of life for older people.

A first-line approach for nurses (in any setting) to identify older individuals at considerable risk of falls would be to ask if the individual has fallen in the last year and, if so, the frequency, injuries, and circumstances of the fall(s). What older people and health professionals classify as a fall can differ. A stumble or trip where the person can respond, and recover is not a fall. The following wording is recommended when asking older people about falls, 'In the past month, have you had any fall including a slip or trip in which you lost your balance and landed on the floor or ground or lower level?' (Lamb et al., 2005). A positive history of falls should trigger an in-depth assessment to identify modifiable risk factors that can be dealt with by the health professional (Figure 12.5).

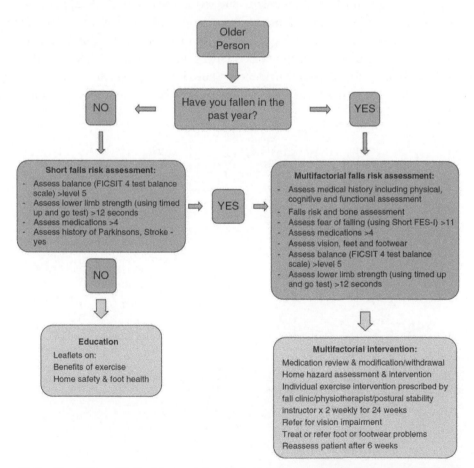

Figure 12.5   Algorithm of falls risk-screening tool. (Adapted from Nandy et al., 2004; AGS/ BGS, 2010; Stanmore, 2013)

To target those who are at an elevated risk of falls but who have not yet fallen, a short assessment of the individual's functional and physical ability may be carried out. In-depth guidance on how to assess, prevent and manage falls has recently been published by a Global Taskforce on falls prevention (see Montero-Odasso et al., 2022).

Strength and balance exercises are particularly good at reducing the risk of falls, increasing bone health (therefore reducing the risk of fractures) and can have other beneficial properties such as improving mood and social contact. To find out more about trained postural stability instructors or therapists who deliver strength and balance exercises for older people, nurses should contact their local community physiotherapy departments or visit the website of Later Life Training, for a directory of trained staff within local regions (www.laterlifetraining. co.uk/falls-directory). Recent reviews suggest that the higher the dose of exercise and the more challenging it is to balance, the greater the reduction in rate of falls (Sherrington et al., 2019). Referrals to physiotherapists, specialist falls services, occupational therapists, postural stability instructors and GPs (General Practitioners) (for medication review) could be carried out by nurses to ensure that evidence-based practice is carried out for older people. A home assessment by an occupational therapist or community nurse would also be invaluable to highlight any fall hazards that may be present in the person's home environment.

Ensuring that older people receive regular eyesight checks and treatment for visual problems (e.g., cataract surgery) can be helpful in preventing falls, as can wearing well-fitting, anti-slip shoes. As many older people can be taking several types of medicines, it is important that they receive a regular review of their medication (especially psychotropic medicines) so that they can be modified if necessary.

Fear of falling can negatively affect individuals and their ability to maintain social networks and maintain independence. A simple measure of fear of falling, such as the validated Short Falls Efficacy Scale – International (Kempen et al., 2008) can be undertaken to identify those with low levels of confidence. People who fall recurrently would benefit from a more detailed multi-factorial assessment, and an individual falls prevention programme from a trained clinician or at a fall prevention clinic.

Florence

Florence is a 79-year-old independent person and lives at home with frail husband Paulo who has Parkinson's disease. Florence has been having difficulties sleeping and has recently had a couple of falls during the night, resulting in some minor bruising and a small laceration to the right shin. As a registered nurse, you are requested to visit and assess.

- How would you conduct a bio-psychosocial assessment with Florence, thinking about individual needs and care?
- What is normal for Florence? What has changed?

Physical assessment: past medical history, current health status, co-morbidities; nocturia: detailed falls assessment (see Figure 12.5); medications: prescribed and use of over the counter, type, and frequency; sleep duration, quality, difficulties falling asleep/staying asleep/un-refreshing sleep/daytime sleepiness, sleep apnoea; wound assessment.

Psychological assessment: assess mood, anxiety, cognition.

Social assessment: lifestyle; formal and informal support; environment; exercise levels; husband's needs; what is important to Florence and her husband, their interests, past occupations, hobbies, family, etc.

How could you ensure a biographical approach is incorporated into the assessment?

Dementia and Delirium

The most important issue for nurses is to understand that the behaviour exhibited by people living with dementia will be dictated by the type of dementia they have and the area of the brain most affected. The deterioration of abilities will also vary from person to person, which further instils the need for individualised, person-centred care as an example, Alzheimer's dementia is characterised by a progressive deterioration of brain function, whereas people with a diagnosis of vascular dementia may experience a stepped decline in function, alongside cognitive symptoms such as apathy, anxiety or depression, and mood swings (Alzheimer's Society, 2022). As with the general population, people with dementia will require hospital treatment for conditions as they age. However, the rate of short-stay emergency admissions of people living with dementia is increasing, representing 32.4% of all emergency admissions (Government Office, 2020). During an emergency admission, the person with dementia will be exposed to the confusing effects of waiting for long periods, moving between departments and/or wards and seeing a number of different people, when they may be used to seeing only one or two people per day. Equally, they may be experiencing pain or feeling ill and being bombarded with information from multiple sources, which may cause stress with the person's behaviour being adversely impacted. This may present challenges for staff in acute and busy environments because people with dementia are not able to communicate in the same way as older people without dementia. Quite often it may be the situation impacting on a person with dementia's behaviour and, if we can create a more appropriate environment, the behaviour may create fewer challenges for staff (Table 12.2).

Table 12.2 Common responses to hospital environment for people with dementia

Psychological	Physical
Stress	Disturbance in relation to activities of living,
Fear	e.g.,
Agitation and/or aggression	Sleep patterns
Vocalisations	Nutrition
Wandering or excessive walking	Hydration
Searching	Elimination
Wanting to go home	Mobility

Clarke et al. (2003) undertook a pilot investigation into how staff understanding the life history of a person with dementia might improve person-centred care in an acute context. The philosophy of this project emphasised that attitudes, desires, and interests of older people are a culmination of life experience and sought to support staff in viewing later decades as a time of ongoing development and self-determination. By encouraging older people to talk about their life experiences staff can gain a fuller appreciation of people's needs, concerns and aspirations (Clarke et al., 2003). Life story work is being used more widely across dementia care and usually involves the construction of a life storybook (McKeown et al., 2006). However, a practice development project undertaken with staff in a dementia environment suggests that the focused use of biographical information can also promote person-centred practice (Brown Wilson et al., 2013).

It is important that nurses do not make assumptions about the behaviour of people living with dementia, attributing it solely to their dementia. Changes in behaviour may also be a result of underlying physical issues such as pain or the onset of infection. For example, a urinary tract infection (UTI) continues to be a reason for older people being admitted to hospital. Using questionnaires to document the cues an older person might exhibit to suggest a change in their condition has been found to be acceptable to both nurses and care recipients in acute services (Hill, 2012). Infection in older people may result in delirium, which often presents as cognitive confusion and may be misdiagnosed as dementia. The key difference between the two conditions is that the cognitive confusion that presents with delirium is acute in onset and improves with appropriate treatment.

Delirium is often unrecognised, undiagnosed, and poorly managed by healthcare professionals. Despite this, delirium is often avoidable and reversible (Lieow et al., 2019). When experienced by older people, delirium can potentially lead to long-lasting physical and cognitive symptoms and premature death (Ospina et al., 2018). This situation may be further compounded if nurses subscribe to the myth that all older people are likely to be confused because of their age rather than a result of underlying and treatable conditions. Delirium is different from dementia because it is acute in onset, often with families telling healthcare staff that their family members are not normally confused. There are several risk factors associated with delirium, for example: age, fever, co-morbidities, malnutrition, dehydration, and low serum albumin (Siddiqi et al., 2016). A comprehensive assessment and a multi-factorial approach are required to treat the underlying causes of delirium but there is now compelling evidence that multicomponent interventions prevent delirium in hospitalised individuals (Siddiqi et al., 2016). Therefore, healthcare professionals need to be better prepared to have the necessary confidence and skills to prevent, identify and manage delirium (Lieow et al., 2019; Mitchell et al., 2021).

In undertaking a practice development project, Hill (2012) found that nurses can identify and treat the early onset of delirium when patients and relatives identify early behavioural or cognitive changes that might go unrecognised by staff.

Jeffrey

Jeffrey has been sent by the GP to the emergency department due to second-degree burns on the right leg from his electric fire. On initial assessment Jeffrey appears unkempt, is wearing soiled clothes, is in a confused state, and is disorientated to time and place. The doctor requests an urgent care home placement and prescribes painkillers and non-adhesive, antimicrobial wound care dressings. You are asked to assist the social worker to set up the care home package and to contact the family. On contacting the family, you discover that Jeffrey is usually self-caring, but since the loss of his partner 6 weeks ago he has not been coping at home, has not been eating and drinking and has stopped going out bowling with friends.

What further assessments need to be carried out to gain a comprehensive and systematic nursing assessment of Jeffrey's needs? What acute problems or illnesses could have led to his delirium? What nursing actions do you think would benefit Jeffrey to enable him to return home with the aim of maintaining his independence?

Chapter Summary

Nurses must be aware of the myths and stereotypes of ageing and ensure that these are not influencing key decisions in how they support older people. Subscribing to the myths of ageing or stereotyping older people may precipitate decisions leading to lack of dignity in care giving. Seeing the person not the condition is essential to ensure that the dignity of older people, including those living with dementia, is maintained.

Person-centred care challenges the nurse to see the person rather than the condition and is a further mechanism whereby dignity can be enhanced in care giving. Adopting a biographical approach to care planning is a first step in identifying what is important to the older person and how this might be integrated into their care. For people living with dementia, knowing their usual routines and working to ensure that these are maintained in unfamiliar environments will enable staff to understand their responses.

Healthy lifestyles are as influential as genetic factors in helping older people avoid the decline traditionally associated with ageing. Many chronic diseases can also be prevented by maintaining a healthy and active lifestyle throughout the course of life. Nurses are well placed to advise on health promotion factors such as physical activity, healthy diets, smoking cessation, immunisation uptake, and optimum management of chronic diseases to prevent deterioration in health. Regular physical activity has been shown to contribute to both improvements in physical and psychological function, including a reduction in depressive symptoms. It contributes to a healthier independent lifestyle by significantly improving the functional capacity and quality of life for older people. Older people also need to be aware of the considerable risk of falls and should be encouraged to undertake strength and balance exercises to try to reduce falls and fall-related fractures and injuries as well as improve their functioning. Those people with a history of falls should be referred to a fall prevention clinic or a trained therapist for a comprehensive assessment of risk factors and a tailored programme to prevent further falls.

Not all older people are frail, but the risk of frailty increases with age and sometimes a small loss of function may precipitate a crisis with a risk of poor outcomes. Frailty is a physiological syndrome characterised by multiple deficits in system functioning. Some of the manifestations such as reduced walking speed or gait problems are reversible even at advanced age.

Registered nurses may be the first contact when a person struggles with memory problems or the one with whom families discuss their concerns when a relative is not coping. They need to be aware of the support available, encourage those with early signs of dementia to seek a diagnosis and recognise the impact on the person and family when a diagnosis of dementia is made. Nurses also need to understand the differences between acute delirium and dementia and act as advocates for older people to ensure that they receive a comprehensive assessment and person-centred care. The behaviour exhibited by people living with dementia will vary from person to person, so personalised care needs to be given to ensure that individual needs are met.

In summary, there is still much to explore about caring effectively for older people but we hope that this chapter will encourage adult nurses to use approaches that value the older person and achieve positive changes that will affect us all as we grow old.

Useful Websites

Age UK website for information on health and wellbeing for older people:
    www.ageuk.org.uk
British Geriatric Society resources on diagnosis and treatment of delirium: www.bgs.org.uk
Dignified Revolution: www.dignifiedrevolution.org.uk
Healthcare Quality Strategies website for more information about the issues of medication
    and falls: www.hqsi.org/index/providers/Adverse-Drug-Events/Medication-and-Falls.html
The King's Fund project on dementia: www.kingsfund.org.uk/projects/
    enhancing-healing-environment/ehe-design-dementia
Later Life Training website for online support and audio files on specific exercises and
    training programmes for falls prevention: www.laterlifetraining.co.uk
Prevention of Falls Network for dissemination website for resources, updates and an online
    forum for advice and discussion: http://profound.eu.com
Royal College of Nursing's dignity campaign: www.rcn.org.uk/professional-development/
    publications/pub-003292
Royal College of Nursing Dementia Resources: www.rcn.org.uk/development/practice/
    dementia
Social Care Institute for Excellence Dementia Resources: www.scie.org.uk/publications/
    dementia/index.asp

Further Reading

Almack, K. and King, A. (2019) 'Lesbian, Gay, Bisexual, and Trans Aging in a U.K. Context: Critical Observations of Recent Research Literature', *The International Journal of Aging and Human Development*, 89(1): 93–107. doi:10.1177/0091415019836921.

Arking, R. (2006) *The Biology of Aging: Observations and Principles*, 3rd edn. Oxford: Oxford University Press.

Baillie, L., Gallagher, A. and Wainwright, P. (2008) *Defending Dignity: Challenges and Opportunities*. London: Royal College of Nursing.

Brown Wilson, C. (2013) *Caring for Older People: A Shared Approach*. London: Sage.

Elvish, R., Burrow, S., Cawley, R., Harney, K., Pilling, M., Gregory, J. and Keady, J. (2016) '"Getting to know me": the second phase roll-out of a staff training programme for supporting people with dementia in general hospitals', *Dementia: The International Journal of Social Research and Practice*, doi:10.1177/1471301216634926.

McCormack, B. and McCance, T. (2021) The Person-Centred Nursing Framework. In: Dewing, J., McCormack, B. and McCance, T. (eds), *Person-centred Nursing Research: Methodology, Methods, and Outcomes*. Cham: Springer.

Montero-Odasso, M. Velde, van der N. and Martin C.F. (2022) and the Task Force on Global Guidelines for Falls in Older Adults, World guidelines for falls prevention and management for older adults: a global initiative. *Age and Ageing* (51)9: afac205. doi: 10.1093/ageing/afac205. PMID: 36178003; PMCID: PMC9523684.

National Institute for Health Research (2017) *Comprehensive Care: Older People Living with Frailty in Hospitals*. London: NIHR. Available at: https://evidence.nihr.ac.uk/themedreview/comprehensive-care-older-people-with-frailty-in-hospital/ (last accessed 1st March 2023).

Reed, J., Clarke, C. and McFarlane, A. (2011) *Nursing Older People: A Textbook for Nurses*. Milton Keynes: Open University Press.

Tolson, D., Booth, J. and Schofield, I. (eds) (2011) *Evidence Informed Nursing with Older People*. Oxford: Blackwell.

References

Age UK (2017) *Ageism* Available at: www.ageuk.org.uk/information-advice/work-learning/discrimination-rights/ageism/ (last accessed 11 November 2022).

Age UK (2019) *Briefing: Health and Care of Older People in England 2019 July 2019*. Available at: www.ageuk.org.uk/our-impact/policy-research/publications/reports-and-briefings/ (last accessed 11 November 2022).

Alzheimer's Research UK (2015a) *Dementia in the Family: The Impact on Carers*. Available at: www.alzheimersresearchuk.org/about-us/our-influence/policy-work/reports/carers-report/ (last accessed 28 February 2023).

Alzheimer's Research UK (2015b) *Women and Dementia: A Marginalized Majority*. Available at: www.alzheimersresearchuk.org/about-us/our-influence/policy-work/reports/women-dementia/ (last accessed 28 February 2023).

Alzheimer's Society (2021) *What is Dementia?* Factsheet 400LP. Available at: www.alzheimers.org.
uk/download/downloads/id/3416/what_is_dementia.pdf (last accessed 28 January 2023).

Alzheimer's Society (2022) *Vascular Dementia*. Factsheet 402LP. Available at: www.alzheimers.org.
uk/download/downloads/id/2427/factsheet_what_is_vascular_dementia.pdf (last accessed 28
January 2023).

American Geriatrics Society, British Geriatrics Society, and American Academy of Orthopaedic
Surgeons Panel on Falls Prevention (AGS/BGS) (2010) 'Clinical practice guideline: prevention
of falls in older persons', *Journal of the American Geriatric Society*. Available at: www.archcare.org/
sites/default/files/pdf/2010-prevention-of-falls-in-older-persons-ags-and-bgs-clinical-practice-
guideline.pdf (last accessed 28 February 2023).

Anderson, R.A., Issel, L.M. and McDaniel, Jr, R.R. (2003) 'Nursing homes as complex adaptive
systems: relationship between management practice and resident outcomes', *Nursing Research*,
52(1): 12–21.

Andrews, A. and Butler, M. (2014) *Trusted to Care. An Independent Review of the Princess of Wales
Hospital and Neath Port Talbot Hospital at Abertawe Bro Morgannwg University Health Boards*
(Executive Summary). Available at: http://gov.wales/topics/health/publications/health/reports/
care (last accessed 28 February 2023).

Ansara, Y.G. (2015) 'Challenging cisgenderism in the ageing and aged care sector: meeting the
needs of older people of trans and/or non-binary experience', *Australasian Journal on Ageing*,
34(Suppl 2): 14–18.

Arking, R. (2006) *The Biology of Aging: Observations and Principles*. New York: Oxford University
Press.

Barrett, C., Crameri, P., Lambourne, S., Latham, J.R. and Whyte, C. (2015) 'Understanding the
experiences and needs of lesbian, gay, bisexual, and trans Australians living with dementia, and
their partners', *Australasian Journal on Ageing*, 34(Suppl 2): 34–8.

Bond, J., Peace, S.M., Dittmann-Kohli, F. and Westerhof, G. (2007) *Ageing in Society: European
Perspectives on Gerontology*. London: Sage.

Bowers, H., Lockwood, S., Eley, A., Catley, A., Runnicles, D., Mordey, M., Barker, S., Thomas, N.,
Jones, C. and Dalziel, S. (2013) *Widening Choices for Older People with High Support Needs*. York:
Joseph Rowntree Foundation.

Bridges, J., Flatley, M. and Meyer, J. (2010) 'Older people's and relatives' experiences in acute care
settings: systematic review and synthesis of qualitative studies', *International Journal of Nursing
Studies*, 47: 89–107.

Briggs, R., McDonough, A., Ellis, G., Bennett, K., O'Neill, D. and Robinson, D. (2022) 'Comprehensive
geriatric assessment for community-dwelling, high-risk, frail, older people', *Cochrane Database
of Systematic Reviews 2022*, Issue 5. Art. No.: CD012705. doi:10.1002/14651858.CD012705.pub2
(last accessed 29 January 2023).

British Heart Foundation (2010) *A Toolkit for the Design, Implementation and Evaluation of Exercise
Referral Schemes*. Loughborough: BHF National Centre, Loughborough University.

Brooker, D. (2004) 'What is person centred care in dementia?', *Reviews in Clinical Gerontology*, 13:
215–22.

Brown Wilson, C. (2009) 'Developing community in care homes through a relationship-centred
approach', *Health and Social Care in the Community*, 17(2): 177–86.

Brown Wilson, C. (2013) *Caring for Older People: A Shared Approach*. London: Sage.

Brown Wilson, C. (2017) *Caring for People with Dementia: A Shared Approach*. London: Sage.

Brown Wilson, C. and Davies, S. (2009) 'Using relationships in care homes to develop relationship centred care: the contribution of staff', *Journal of Clinical Nursing*, 18: 1746–55.

Carers UK (2016) *Factsheet e-1029 Assessments: Getting the Help you Need*. Available at: www.carersuk.org/help-and-advice/practical-support/getting-care-and-support/carers-assessment (last accessed 28 February 2023).

Care Quality Commission (2022) *The State of Health Care and Adult Social Care in England 2021/22*. Available at: www.cqc.org.uk/publications/major-report/state-care (last accessed 11 November 2022).

Carter, J. (2022) 'Prevalence of all cause young onset dementia and time lived with dementia: analysis of primary care health records', *The Journal of Dementia Care*, 30(3): 1–5.

Centers for Disease Control and Prevention (1996) *Physical Activity and Health: A Report of the Surgeon General Executive*. Summary. Atlanta, GA: US Department of Health and Human Services.

Chief Medical Officer (2011) *Public Health Guidelines on Physical Activity for Older Adults*. London: DH.

Clancy, A., Simonsen, N., Lind, J., Liveng, A. and Johannessen, A. (2021) 'The meaning of dignity for older adults: a meta-synthesis', *Nursing Ethics*, 28(6): 878–94.

Clarke, A., Hanson, E.J. and Ross, H. (2003) 'Seeing the person behind the patient: enhancing the care of older people using a biographical approach', *Journal of Clinical Nursing*, 12: 697.

Clegg, A., Bates, C., Young, J., Ryan, R., Nichols, L., Teale, E.A., Mohammed, M.A., Parry, J. and Marshall, T. (2016) 'Development and validation of an electronic frailty index using routine primary care electronic health record data', *Age and Ageing*, 45(3): 353–60.

Conroy, S.P., Bardsley, M., Smith, P., Neuburger, J., Keeble, E., Arora, S. et al. (2019) 'Comprehensive geriatric assessment for frail older people in acute hospitals: the HoW-CGA mixed-methods study'. University of Leicester. Available at: https://hdl.handle.net/2381/11662947.v2 (last accessed 1 March 2023).

Crameri, P., Barrett, C., Latham, J.R. and Whyte, C. (2015) 'It is more than sex and clothes: culturally safe services for older lesbian, gay, bisexual, transgender and intersex people', *Australasian Journal on Ageing*, 34(Suppl 2): 21–5.

Department of Health (2009) *Be Active, Be Healthy. A Plan for Getting the Nation Moving*. London: DH.

Department of Health (2013) *Patients First and Foremost: The Initial Government Response to the Report of The Mid Staffordshire NHS Foundation Trust Public Inquiry*. London: DH.

Department of Health and Social Care (2016) *Making a Difference in Dementia: Nursing Vision and Strategy*. London: DH.

Dewing, J. (2004) 'Concerns relating to the application of frameworks to promote person-centredness in nursing older people', *International Journal of Older People Nursing*, 13(3a): 39–44.

Dowrick, A. and Southern, A. (2014) *Dementia 2014: Opportunity for Change*. London: Alzheimer's Society. Available at: www.alzheimers.org.uk/sites/default/files/migrate/downloads/dementia_2014_opportunity_for_change.pdf (last accessed 28 Feburary 2023).

Ellis, G., Gardner, M., Tsiachristas, A., Langhorne, P., Burke, O., Harwood, R.H., Conroy, S.P., Kircher, T., Somme, D., Saltvedt, I., Wald, H., O'Neill, D., Robinson, D. and Shepperd, S. (2017) 'Comprehensive geriatric assessment for older adults admitted to hospital', *Cochrane Database of Systematic Reviews*. Sep 12; 9(9):CD006211. doi: 10.1002/14651858.CD006211.pub3. PMID: 28898390; PMCID: PMC6484374.

European Commission (2015) *Eurobarometer on Discrimination 2015: General Perceptions, Opinions on Policy Measures and Awareness of Rights*. Available at: http://ec.europa.eu/justice/fundamental-rights/files/factsheet_eurobarometer_fundamental_rights_2015.pdf (last accessed 28 February 2023).

Fiatarone, M.A., Marks, E.C., Ryan, D.T., Meredith, C.N., Lewis, A., Lipsitz, M.D. and Evans, W.J. (1990) 'High-intensity strength training in nonagenarians', *Journal of the American Medical Association*, 263(22): 3029–34.

Francis, R. (2013) *Report of the Mid Staffordshire NHS Foundation Trust Public Enquiry*. London: HMSO.

Fried, L.P., Ferrucci, L., Darer, J., Williamson, J.D. and Anderson, G.F. (2004) 'Untangling the concepts of disability, frailty, and comorbidity: implications for improved targeting and care', *Journals of Gerontology: Series A Biology, Science and Medical Science*, 59A: M255–63.

Gaugler, J.E., Kane, R.L., Kane, R.A. and Newcomer, R. (2005) 'The longitudinal effects of early behavior problems in the dementia caregiving career', *Psychology and Aging*, 20(1): 100–16.

Gaugler, J.E., Reese, M. and Mittelman, M. (2016) 'Effects of the Minnesota adaptation of the NYU caregiver intervention on primary subjective stress of adult child caregivers of persons with dementia', *The Gerontologist*, 56(3): 461–74.

Gaugler, J.E., Reese, M. and Mittelman, M.S. (2018) 'The effects of a comprehensive psychosocial intervention on secondary stressors and social support for adult child caregivers of persons with dementia', *Innovation in Aging*, 2(2): 1–10 igy015.

Gendron, T.L., Inker, J. and Welleford, E. (2018) 'A theory of relational ageism: a discourse analysis of the 2015 White House Conference on Aging,' *The Gerontologist*, (58)2: 242–50.

Goodrich, J. and Cornwell, J. (2008) *Seeing the Person in the Patient: The Point of Care Review Paper*. London: The King's Fund.

Goodrich, J. (2011) *The Point of Care Programme: Consultation on Improving Dignity in Care Submission from The King's Fund to the Partnership on Dignity in Care* (AGE UK, NHS Confederation and Local Government Group). London: The King's Fund.

Goodwin, N., Curry, N., Naylor, C., Ross, S. and Duldig, W. (2010) *Managing People with Long-term Conditions: An Inquiry into the Quality of General Practice in England*. London: The King's Fund. Available at: www.kingsfund.org.uk/sites/default/files/field/field_document/managing-people-long-term-conditions-gp-inquiry-research-paper-mar11.pdf (last accessed 29 March 2023).

Government Office (2020) *Statistical Commentary: Dementia profile, April 2020 data update*. Available at: www.gov.uk/government/statistics/dementia-profile-updates/statistical-commentary-dementia-profile-april-2020-data-update (last accessed 29 January 2023).

Government Office for Science (2016) *Future of an Ageing Population*. London: Government Office for Science.

Greenhalgh, T. and Papoutsi, C. (2019) 'Spreading and scaling up innovation and improvement', *British Medical Journal*, 365: l2068.

Hill, K. (2012) *Critical to Care: Improving the Care to the Acutely Ill and Deteriorating Patient*. Foundation of Nursing Studies Project Report. Available at: http://fons.org/library/report-details.aspx?nstid=18132 (last accessed 29 March 2023).

Humphries, R., Thorlby, R., Holder, H., Hall, P. and Charles, A. (2016) *Social Care for Older People: Home Truths*. London: The King's Fund and the Nuffield Trust. Available at: www.kingsfund.org.uk/sites/default/files/field/field_publication_file/Social_care_older_people_Kings_Fund_Sep_2016.pdf (last accessed 28th February 2023).

Institute of Medicine (IOM) (2001) *Crossing the Quality Chasm: A New Health System for the 21st Century*. Washington, DC: National Academy Press.

Jacelon, C. (2003) 'The dignity of elders in acute care hospital', *Qualitative Health Research*, 13(4): 543–56.

Jones, D., Song, X. and Rockwood, K. (2004) 'Operationalizing a frailty index from a standardized comprehensive geriatric assessment', *Journal of the American Geriatric Society*, 52: 1929–33.

Kempen, G.I., Yardley, L., van Haastregt, J.C., Zijlstra, G.A., Beyer, N., Hauer, K. and Todd, C. (2008) 'The Short FES-I: A shortened version of the falls efficacy scale-international to assess fear of falling', *Age and Ageing*, 37(1): 44–50.

Kitwood, T. (1997) *Dementia Reconsidered: The Person Comes First*. Milton Keynes: Open University Press.

Knoops, K.T., de Groot, L.C., Kromhout, D., Perrin, A.E., Moreiras-Varela, O., Menotti, A., and van Staveren, W.A. (2004) 'Mediterranean diet, lifestyle factors, and 10-year mortality in elderly European men and women: the HALE project', *Journal of the American Medical Association*, 292(12): 1433–9.

Kojima, G., Liljas, A. and Iliffe, S. (2019) 'Frailty syndrome: implications and challenges for health care policy', *Risk Management and Healthcare Policy*, 12: 23–30.

Kornhaber, R., Walsh, K., Duff, J. and Walker, K. (2016) 'Enhancing adult therapeutic interpersonal relationships in the acute health care setting: an integrative review', *Journal of Multidisciplinary Healthcare*, Oct 14, 9: 537–46.

Lamb, S.E., Jorstad-Stein, E.C., Hauer, K. and Becker, C. (2005) 'Development of a common outcome data set for fall injury prevention trials: the prevention of falls network Europe consensus', *Journal of the American Geriatric Society*, 53: 1618–22.

LeBlanc, A., Schneider, V., Krebs, J., Evans, H., Jhingran, S. and Johnson, P. (1987) 'Spinal bone mineral after 5 weeks of bed rest', *Calcified Tissue International*, 41: 259–61.

Lee, D. (2016) 'Sexual health'. In M. Moore (ed.), *Annual Report of the Chief Medical Officer, 2015. On the State of the Public's Health Baby Boomers: Fit for the Future*, pp. 137–56. Available at: https://assets.publishing.service.gov.uk/government/uploads/system/uploads/attachment_data/file/654806/CMO_baby_boomers_annual_report_2015.pdf (last accessed 28 February 2023).

Levenson, R. (2007) *The Challenge of Dignity in Care. Upholding the Rights of the Individual*. London: Help the Aged.

Lieow, J.L.M., Chen, F.S.M., Song, G., Tang P.S., Kowitlawakul, Y. and Mukhopadhyay, A. (2019) 'Effectiveness of an advanced practice nurse-led delirium education and training programme.', *International Nursing Review*, 66(4): 506.

Livingston, G., Huntley, J., Sommerlad, A. et al. (2020) 'Dementia prevention, intervention, and care: 2020 report of the Lancet Commission', *Lancet*, 396: 413–46.

McCabe, M., You, E. and Tatangelo, G. (2016) 'Hearing their voice: a systematic review of dementia family caregivers' needs', *Gerontologist*, 56(5): e70–e88. doi:10.1093/geront/gnw078

McCormack, B. and McCance, T. (2021) 'The Person-Centred Nursing Framework'. In J. Dewing, B. McCormack and T. McCance (eds), *Person-centred Nursing Research: Methodology, Methods, and Outcomes*. Cham: Springer.

McKeown, J., Clarke, A. and Repper, J. (2006) 'Life story work in health and social care: systematic literature review', *Journal of Advanced Nursing*, 55(2): 237–47.

Minkler, M. (1996) 'Critical perspectives on ageing: new challenges for gerontology', *Ageing and Society*, 16: 467–87.

Mitchell, G., Scott, J., Carter, G. et al. (2021) 'Evaluation of a delirium awareness podcast for undergraduate nursing students in Northern Ireland: a pre–/post-test study', *BMC Nurs*, 20 (2021). https://doi.org/10.1186/s12912-021-00543-

Mitchell, W., Brooks, J. and Glendinning, C. (2015) 'Carers' roles in personal budgets: tensions and dilemmas in front line practice', *British Journal of Social Work*, 45(5): 1433–50.

Mitnitski, A., Song, X., Skoog, I., Broe, G.A., Cox, J., Grunfeld, E. and Rockwood, K. (2005) 'Relative fitness and frailty of elderly men and women in developed countries and their relationship with mortality', *Journal of the American Geriatric Society*, 53: 2184–9.

Montero-Odasso, M., van der Velde, N., Martin, C.F. et al. (2022) 'Task force on global guidelines for falls in older adults, world guidelines for falls in older adults, a global initiative', *Age and Ageing* (51)9. afac205. doi: 10.1093/ageing/afac205. PMID: 36178003; PMCID: PMC9523684.

Nandy, S., Parsons, S., Cryer, C., Underwood, M., Rashbrook, E., Carter, Y., Eldridge, S., Close, J., Skelton, D., Taylor, S. and Feder, G. on behalf of the falls prevention pilot steering group (2004) 'Development and preliminary examination of the predictive validity of the falls risk assessment tool (FRAT) for use in primary care', *Journal of Public Health*, 26(2): 138–43.

National Council on Aging (2013) *Debunking the Myths of Older Adult Falls*. Available at: www.ncoa. org (last accessed on 28 February 2023).

National Institute for Health and Care Excellence (2008) *Mental Wellbeing and Older People*, NICE Public Health Guidance 16. Available at: www.nice.org.uk/guidance/ph16 (last accessed 28 February 2023).

National Institute for Health and Care Excellence (2013) *Falls: Assessment and Prevention of Falls in Older People*: NICE Public Health Guidance CG161. Available at: www.nice.org.uk/guidance/ CG161 (last accessed 28 February 2023).

National Institute for Health and Care Excellence (2016) *Multimorbidity: Clinical Assessment* and *Multimorbidity: Clinical Assessment and Management*. NICE guidelines. Available at: www.nice. org.uk/guidance/ng56 (last accessed 11 November 2022).

NHS England (2019) *The NHS Long Term Plan. 2019*. Available at: www.longtermplan.nhs.uk/ (last accessed 11 November 2022).

Nichols, E., Steinmetz, J.D., Vollset, S.E., Fukataki, K., et al. (2022) 'Estimation of the global prevalence of dementia in 2019 and forecasted prevalence in 2050: an analysis for the Global Burden of Disease Study 2019', *The Lancet Public Health*, 7(2), e105–e125. PIIS2468-2667(21)00249.

Nordenfelt, L. and Edgar, A. (2005) 'The four notions of dignity', *Quality in Ageing* 6(1): 17–21.

Nursing and Midwifery Council (2018) *Future Nurse: Standards of Proficiency for Registered Nurses*. London: NMC.

Office for Budget Responsibility (2015) *Fiscal Sustainability Report June 2015*. Available at: http:// budgetresponsibility.org.uk/fsr/fiscalsustainability-report-june-2015 (last accessed 28 February 2023).

Office for National Statistics (2020) *National Population Projections: 2020-based interim*. Available at: www.ons.gov.uk/peoplepopulationandcommunity/populationandmigration/ populationprojections/bulletins/nationalpopulationprojections/2020basedinterim#changing-age-structure (last accessed 11 November 2022).

Oliver, D. (2013) *We Must End Ageism and Age Discrimination in Health and Social Care*. London: The King's Fund. Available at: www.kingsfund.org.uk/blog/2013/05/we-must-end-ageism-and-age-discrimination-health-and-social-care (last accessed 28 February 2023).

Orrell, A., McKee, K., Dahlberg, L., Gilhooly, M. and Parker, S. (2013) 'Improving continence services for older people from the service-providers' perspective: a qualitative interview study', *BMJ Open*, 3: 7.

Ospina, J., King, F., Madva, E. and Celano, C. (2018) 'Epidemiology, mechanisms, diagnosis and treatment of delirium: a narrative review', *Clinical Medicine and Therapy*, 1: 3.

Pickard, S. and Glendinning, C. (2002) 'Caring for a relative with dementia: the perceptions of carers and CPNs', *Quality in Ageing*, 2: 3–11.

Pinquart, M. and Sorensen, S. (2003) 'Predictors of caregiver burden and depressive mood: a meta-analysis', *Journal of Gerontology, Psychological Sciences*, 58: 112–28.

Pinquart, M. and Sorensen, S. (2004) 'Associations of caregivers' stressors and uplifts with subjective well-being and depressive mood: a meta-analytic comparison', *Aging & Mental Health*, 8(5): 438–49.

Pinquart, M. and Sorensen, S. (2011) 'Spouses, adult children, and children-in-law as carers of older adults: a meta-analytic comparison', *Psychology of Aging*, 26(1): 1–14.

Poblador-Plou, B., Calderón-Larrañaga, A., Marta-Moreno, J., Hancco-Saavedra, J., Sicras-Mainar, A., Soljak, M. and Prados-Torres, A. (2014) 'Comorbidity of dementia: a cross-sectional study of primary care older patients', *BMC Psychiatry*, 14: 84.

Public Health England (2016) *Guidance Health Matters: Getting Every Adult Active Every Day*. Available at: www.gov.uk/government/publications/health-matters-getting-every-adult-active-every-day/health-matters-getting-every-adult-active-every-day#:~:text=Adults%20in%20England%20should%20aim,the%20UK%20Chief%20Medical%20Officers (last accessed 28 February 2023).

Quinn, C., Clare, L., McGuinness, T. and Woods, R. (2012) 'The impact of relationships, motivations, and meanings on dementia caregiving outcomes', *International Psychogeriatrics*, 24(11): 1816–26.

Rockwood, K., Fox, R., Stolee, P., Robertson, B. and Beattie, L. (1994) 'Frailty in elderly people: an evolving concept', *Canadian Medical Association Journal*, 150(4): 489–95.

Rockwood, K. and Koller, K. (2013) 'Frailty in older adults: implications for end-of-life care', *Cleveland Clinic Journal of Medicine*, 80(3): 168–74.

Rockwood, K., Mitnitski, A., Song, X., Steen, B. and Skoog, I. (2006) 'Long-term risks of death and institutionalization of elderly people in relation to deficit accumulation at age 70', *Journal of the American Geriatric Society*, 54(6): 975–9.

Rogers, S., Martin, G. and Rai, G. (2014) 'Medicines management support to older people: understanding the context of systems failure', *BMJ Open*, 4: 7.

Røsvik, J.J., Kirkevold, M., Engedal, K., Brooker, D., and Kirkevold, Ø. (2011) 'A model for using the VIPS framework for person-centred care for persons with dementia in nursing homes: a qualitative evaluative study', *International Journal of Older People Nursing*, 6: 227–36.

SACE (2017) *Personal Social Services Survey of Adult Carers in England, 2016–17*. London: NHS Digital. Available at: https://digital.nhs.uk/catalogue/PUB30045 (last accessed 28 February 2023).

Salisbury, C., Murphy, M. and Duncan, P. (2020) 'The impact of digital-first consultations on workload in general practice: modeling study', *Journal of Medical Internet Research*, 16, 22(6): e18203.

Sherrington, C., Fairhall, N.J., Wallbank, G.K., Tiedemann, A., Michaleff, Z.A., Howard, K., Clemson, L., Hopewell, S. and Lamb, S.E. (2019) 'Exercise for preventing falls in older people living in the community', *Cochrane Database of Systematic Reviews*, Issue 1. Art. No.: CD012424.

Siddiqi, N., Harrison, J.K., Clegg, A., Teale, E.A., Young, J., Taylor, J. and Simpkins, S.A. (2016) 'Interventions for preventing delirium in hospitalised non-ICU patients', *Cochrane Database of Systematic Reviews*, Issue 3. Art. No.: CD005563. DOI: 10.1002/14651858.CD005563.pub3 (last accessed 29 January 2023).

Simpson, P., Horne, M., Brown, L.J.E., Brown Wilson, C., Dickinson, T. and Torkington, K. (2017a) 'Old(er) care home residents and sexual/intimate citizenship', *Ageing and Society*, 37: 243–65.

Simpson, P., Brown Wilson, C., Horne, M., Brown, L.E.J. and Dickinson, T. (2017b) '"We've had our sex life way back": older care home residents, sexuality, and intimacy', *Ageing and Society*, 37(2): 243–65.

Skelton, D.A., Dinan, S.M., Campbell, M.G. and Rutherford, O.M. (2005) 'Tailored group exercise (Falls Management Exercise – FaME) reduces falls in community-dwelling older frequent fallers (an RCT)', *Age and Ageing*, 34: 636–9.

Smith, M.E., Dunphy, L.M. and Mainous, R.O. (2011) 'Innovative nursing educational curriculum for the 21st century'. In National Research Council (ed.), *The Future of Nursing: Leading Change, Advancing Health*. Washington, DC: The National Academies Press.

Smith, R. and Wright, T. (2021) 'Older lesbian, gay, bisexual, transgender, queer and intersex people's experiences and perceptions of receiving home care services in the community: A systematic review', *International Journal of Nursing Studies*, 118, 103907 https://doi.org/10.1016/j.ijnurstu.2021.103907.

Social Care Institute for Excellence (2020) *Dignity*. Available at: www.scie.org.uk/dignity/care/defining (last accessed 11 November 2022).

Stanmore, E.K. (2011) 'Choice, appropriateness, and adequacy of care for older people: utilising patients and professionals views to identify future service improvements', *International Journal of Person-Centered Medicine*, 1(3): 522–6.

Stanmore, E.K. (2013) 'The importance of falls assessment in patients with rheumatoid arthritis', *Journal of Health Visiting*, 1(2): 5.

Tadd, W., Hillman, A., Calnan, S., Calnan, M., Bayer, T. and Read, S. (2011) *Dignity in Practice: An Exploration of the Care of Older Adults in Acute NHS Trusts*. Service Delivery and Organisation Programme. Available at: www.sdo.nihr.ac.uk/files/project/SDO_FR_08-1819-218_V01.pdf (last accessed 11 November 2022).

Tauber-Gilmore, M., Addis, G., Zahran, Z., Black, S., Baillie, L., Procter, S. and Norton, C. (2018) 'The views of older people and health professionals about dignity in acute hospital care', *Journal of Clinical Nursing*, Jan; 27(1–2): 223–34. doi: 10.1111/jocn.13877.

The Health Foundation (2021) *Caring for Older Adults with Complex Needs*. Available at: www.health.org.uk/publications/long-reads/caring-for-older-patients-with-complex-needs (last accessed on 11 November 2022).

van der Geugten, W. and Goossensen, A. (2020) 'Dignifying and undignifying aspects of care for people with dementia: a narrative review', *Scandinavian Journal of Caring Sciences*, 34(4): 818–38. doi: 10.1111/scs.12791. Epub 2019 Nov 21. PMID: 31750569; PMCID: PMC7754132.

van Diest, M., Lamoth, C.J., Stegenga, J., Verkerke, G.J. and Postema, K. (2013) 'Exergaming for balance training of elderly: state of the art and future developments', *Journal of Neuroengineering and Rehabilitation*, 10: 101.

Wilmoth, J.M. and Ferraro, K.F. (eds) (2013) *Gerontology Perspectives and Issues.* New York: Springer Publishing Co.

Witenberg, R., Hu, B., Barraza-Araiza, L., and Rehill, A. (2019) *Projections of Older People Living with Dementia and Costs of Dementia Care in the United Kingdom, 2019–2040.* London School of Econoics and political science. Available: https://www.lse.ac.uk/cpec/assets/documents/cpec-working-paper-5.pdf (last accessed 30 August 2023).

World Health Organization (2007) *WHO Global Report on Falls Prevention in Older Age.* Geneva: WHO.

World Health Organization (2010) *A Healthy Lifestyle: WHO Recommendations.* Available at: www.who.int/europe/news-room/fact-sheets/item/a-healthy-lifestyle—who-recommendations (last accessed 11 November 2022).

13

CARING FOR ADULTS WITH LONG-TERM CONDITIONS

Judith Ormrod and Dianne Burns

Chapter objectives

- Identify the common problems encountered by individuals living with a long-term condition;
- Recognise the adult nurse's role in supporting individuals (and their carers) living with long-term conditions in the UK;
- Identify treatment and care pathways that provide the evidence base used to underpin your practice;
- Identify relevant government policies that aim to support self-management, personalised care planning, and working in partnership with individuals and their carers;
- Demonstrate how the concepts of *empowerment* and *shared decision making* can be used to inform the adult nurse's role in partnership working.

Introduction

This chapter aims to offer an introduction to the role of the registered adult nurse in supporting individuals who are living with a chronic illness or a long-term condition (LTC). Chronic illness is defined by the Department of Health (DH, 2012) as a long-term health condition that cannot at present be cured but can be controlled by medication and other therapies.

Reading and completing the activities in Chapter 11 you will be aware of the nurse's public health role, the importance of identifying and reducing risk factors, and educating individuals and their families to help them stay healthy, thereby preventing or minimising (as far as possible) the impact on health of many LTCs. This chapter will help you to build on this knowledge, requiring you to draw on it when considering the role of the nurse in supporting people suffering from a variety of LTCs.

Although it is beyond the remit of this chapter to include every LTC you might encounter during your pre-registration programme we intend to focus on some common conditions, since it could be argued that many of the associated issues/problems encountered are shared across a wide spectrum of conditions.

Related Nursing and Midwifery Council (NMC) proficiencies for Registered Nurses

The overarching requirements of the Nursing and Midwifery Council (NMC) are that all registered nurses must be able to provide nursing care that is person-centred, safe, and compassionate. They should support and enable people at all stages of life and in all care settings to make informed choices about how to manage health challenges to maximise their quality of life and improve health outcomes. They need to prioritise the needs of people when assessing and reviewing their mental, physical, cognitive, behavioural, social, and spiritual need, and use the information obtained during assessments to identify the priorities and requirements for person-centred and evidence-based nursing interventions and support. They should work in partnership with those in their care to develop person-centred care plans that consider their circumstances, characteristics, and preferences, supporting people of all ages in a range of care settings. They also need to work in partnership with families and carers to evaluate whether care is effective and the goals of care have been met in line with the individual's wishes, preferences and desired outcomes; coordinating and managing the complex nursing and integrated care needs of individuals at any stage of their lives, across a range of organisations and settings (NMC, 2018a).

━━━━━━━━━━ **TO ACHIEVE ENTRY TO THE NMC REGISTER**

YOU MUST BE ABLE TO ━━━━━━━━━━

- Understand and recognise the complexities of providing mental, cognitive, behavioural, and physical care services across a wide range of integrated care settings and the need to respond to the challenges of providing safe, effective, and person-centred care for people who have co-morbidities and complex care needs;

- Demonstrate the ability to process accurately all information gathered during the assessment process (including an understanding of co-morbidities and the need to meet a person's complex nursing and social care needs) to individualise nursing care, developing and applying person-centred, evidence-based plans for nursing interventions with agreed goals;
- Demonstrate the ability to work in partnership with individuals, families, and carers (encouraging shared decision making) to monitor, evaluate and reassess continuously the effectiveness of all agreed nursing care plans and care, readjusting agreed goals, documenting progress and decisions made to support individuals, their families, and carers to maintain optimal independence and manage their own care when appropriate;
- Facilitate equitable access to healthcare for people who are vulnerable or have a disability and demonstrate the ability to advocate on their behalf when required; make necessary reasonable adjustments to the assessment, planning and delivery of care;
- Use up-to-date approaches to influence behaviour change to encourage and enable people to make informed choices when managing their own health, and making lifestyle adjustments to have satisfying and fulfilling lives within the limitations caused by reduced capability, ill health, and disability;
- Understand and apply the principles of partnership, collaboration, and interagency working across all relevant sectors;
- Understand the principles and processes involved in planning and facilitating the safe discharge and transition of individuals across caseloads, settings, and services, and demonstrate the ability to coordinate and undertake the processes and procedures involved in routine planning and management of safe discharge home or transfer of people between care settings.

(Adapted from NMC, 2018a)

Long-term Conditions

Long-term conditions (LTCs) are health problems which are managed with medications or other forms of therapy. There is no cure and they present a large burden on individuals, their family, friends and health and social care services. Approximately 26 million people in England are living with one LTC; 10 million have two or more LTCs (Sanderson and White, 2018; ONS, 2020). In Scotland, around 2 million adults are living with a long-term physical or mental health condition (Scottish Public Health Observatory, 2022), whilst in Wales, the Covid-19 pandemic may account for a further 900,000 people of working age developing a LTC (Janke et al., 2020). In Northern Ireland, the NICVA (2016) suggest 20,000 people are living with dementia, 37,000 are living with COPD, 84,000 are living with Diabetes Mellitus and 400,000 experience long-term chronic pain together with an estimated 1 in 5 people who have a mental health condition. Furthermore, there are groups of people within the UK who have been given scant attention. These include those from ethnic minority groups and members of the lesbian, gay, bisexual, transsexual, questioning/queer, intersex, allies, asexual and pansexual (LGBTQ+) community (LGBT Foundation, 2020). In 2011, 15% of individuals living in England and Wales identified themselves as belonging to an ethnic minority group (Office for National Statistics, 2022a). Ethnicity is regarded as a social construct frequently used to describe a distinct population – but it is subjective and based upon a person's self-definition. The concept itself is multi-dimensional and includes language, cultural traditions, origins, and shared history (Raleigh and Holmes, 2021). There are significant differences between the health patterns of different minority groups and between different minority groups and the white population (Stafford et al, 2022). Experiencing racism and racial discrimination has a damaging impact on health together with increased inequalities in housing, employment, and the criminal justice system (Becares, 2013; Toleikyte and Salway, 2018; Moriaty, 2021). Other influences affecting health include biological factors such as gender, genetics and age.

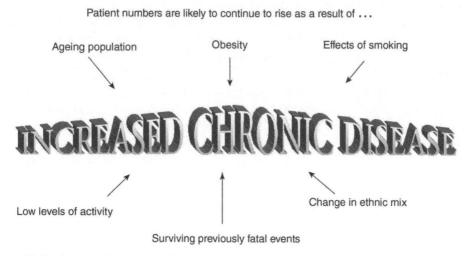

Figure 13.1 Causes of increased chronic disease

Activity 13.1

Access and read at least one of the following articles:

1 Moriarty, J. (2021) *Long term conditions – briefing paper*. Available at:
   https://raceequalityfoundation.org.uk/health-and-care/long-term-health-conditions-collaborative/
2 Raleigh, V. and Holmes, J. (2021) The *health of people from ethnic minority groups in England*. The King's Fund. Available at: www.kingsfund.org.uk/publications/
   health-people-ethnic-minority-groups-england.

What do you think are the key reasons for the omission of information on ethnicity and long-term conditions?

Why do you think it is important that we are able to identify the needs of under-represented groups?

There is a need for better information and data on ethnicity and LTCs (Moriaty, 2021; Raleigh and Holmes, 2021) since good quality data is crucial for practitioners and policy makers to identify the specific needs of different ethnic groups, to provide strategies to reduce inequalities and to evaluate the impact of the strategies over time.

Sexually minority individuals (LGBTQ+) also experience significant difference in LTC management when compared with their heterosexual peers. In 2018, the Government Equalities Office (GEO) received over 108,000 responses, highlighting significant discrimination and poorer experiences when individuals sought healthcare (GEO, 2018)

Activity 13.2

Read the following articles and consider the effects of stigma on health:

1   Kneale, D., Henley, J., Thomas, J., and French, R. (2021) 'Inequalities in older LGBT peoples' health and care needs in the United Kingdom: a systematic scoping review', *Aging and Society*, 41 (3): 493–515.
2   LGBT Foundation (2020) *Hidden figures: LGBT Health Inequalities in the UK*. Manchester: LGBT Foundation.
      • What are the common sources of stigma?
      • What are the social effects of stigma?

Make a list of the common experiences faced by people from the LGBTQ+ community when seeking healthcare.

Chronic neurological conditions

Brain Research UK (nd) estimate that there are around 11 million people in the UK living with a neurological condition. Neurological conditions cause around 140,000 deaths annually and are a leading cause of disability. Examples of long-term neurological conditions include Alzheimer's disease and dementia, epilepsy, multiple sclerosis (MS), motor neurone disease (MND), Parkinson's disease, cerebrovascular accident/stroke (CVA), traumatic brain injury, and chronic fatigue syndrome/myalgic encephalomyelitis (CFS/ME).

Dementia is a leading cause of death and is responsible for almost 1 in 10 of all deaths (80,000) every year in the UK (ONS, 2021a). Furthermore, Moriarty et al. (2011) found 25,000 people from ethnic minority groups were living with dementia in England and Wales, with Wittenberg et al. (2019) suggesting that the number of people living with dementia in the UK will increase to over 1.6 million by 2040. Also, people from ethnic minority backgrounds are less likely to receive support or an early diagnosis (Alzheimer's UK, 2019). Individuals living with a learning disability also appear to have a higher risk of dementia (Hamadelseed et al., 2022).

Activity 13.3

Find out more about how common neurological conditions currently affect people in the UK.

- Alzheimer's Society: www.alzheimers.org.uk
- Epilepsy Society: www.epilepsysociety.org.uk;
- Multiple Sclerosis Society: www.mssociety.org.uk;
- Stroke Association: www.stroke.org.uk/;
- Parkinson's UK: www.parkinsons.org.uk;
- Traumatic Brain Injury: www.headway.org.uk;
- ME Association: www.meassociation.org.uk;
- Motor Neurone Disease: www.mndassociation.org/.

Make a list of the potential problems encountered by individuals suffering from a neurological LTC (remember to include physical/motor, sensory, cognitive, communication, psychosocial and emotional effects).

Heart and circulatory disease

Cardiovascular disease (CVD) is an umbrella term that describes all diseases of the heart and circulation. Although CVD is preventable and the incidence is falling across the UK, it remains a leading cause of illness and death (Table 13.1) (British Heart Foundation, 2022), particularly in Scotland where there is a high prevalence of associated risk factors such as smoking, poor diet and physical inactivity (SIGN, 2017). Furthermore, it is estimated that 7.6 million UK residents are living with the condition (4 million males and 3.6 million females). In addition, it is estimated that as many as 920,000 people across the UK are living with heart failure (British Heart Foundation, 2022).

Table 13.1 Deaths from cardiovascular disease (CVD) and numbers living with CVD

	No. of CVD deaths, 2016	No. of CVD deaths at age <75, 2016	Estimated no. of people living with CVD, 2016
England (2016–17)	124,615	33,812	5.9 million
Scotland (2015–16)	15,131	4644	685,000
Wales (2016–17)	8655	2495	375,000
Northern Ireland (2016–17)	3629	1070	225,000
UK	152,465	42,311	7 million+

Hypertension (high blood pressure) is one of the most preventable causes of premature illness and death across the UK. It is estimated that 28% of adults across the UK have high blood pressure, with at least half of these not receiving treatment (British Heart Foundation, 2022). It is a major risk factor for stroke, heart disease, heart failure, chronic kidney disease and cognitive decline. Lowering blood pressure reduces the risk of long-term ill health (Ettehad et al., 2016).

Activity 13.4

Access and read the resources identified below:

> NHS Wales (no date) *Cardiovascular Disease.* Available at: https://phw.nhs.wales/
>   services-and-teams/observatory/data-and-analysis/cardiovascular-disease/
> NICE (2019) *Hypertension in Adults: Diagnosis and Management.* Available at:
>   www.nice.org.uk/guidance/ng136
> Scottish Intercollegiate Guidelines Network (SIGN) (2016) *Management of Chronic Heart Failure.*
>   Available at: www.sign.ac.uk/o
>   ur-guidelines/management-of-chronic-heart-failure/
> Walthall, H., Floegel, T., Boulton, M. and Jenkinson, C. (2019) 'Patients' experience of fatigue in
>   advanced heart failure', *Contemp Nurse*, Feb; 55(1):71–82.

Using the resources above and relating to CHD/CVD, hypertension, and heart failure (HF):

- Outline the development of each condition and list the contributing lifestyle factors and common symptoms;
- List the treatment options/aims for each condition;
- List the short- and long-term complications of each of the above.
- Identify the key issues faced by individuals with CHD/CVD conditions.

Cancer

Cancer can develop at any age, but it is most commonly diagnosed in older people aged 75 years and above. Cancer Research UK (2023) suggests that between 2016 and 2018 there were 375,000 new cancer cases across the UK each year. The most prevalent cancers (breast, prostate, lung, and bowel cancer) accounted for over 53% of all new cases. Delon et al. (2022) suggest that the incidence rates of cancer are reduced in people of mixed or multiple ethnicities and in Asian and Black ethnic groups.

Activity 13.5

1   Access the Cancer Research UK website (www.cancerresearchuk.org) and identify the potential contributing factors to the incidence of cancer in the UK and the presenting symptoms for all common UK cancers.
2   Look at the National Institute for Health and Care Excellence (NICE) website (www.nice.org.uk) and review guidelines and NICE pathways for breast, prostrate, lung, liver, and bowel cancers.
3   Access the National Cancer Patient Experience Survey website (www.ncpes.co.uk/reports) and review the latest report of firsthand experiences of cancer services and care provision.

Identify the key issues faced by individuals who have survived cancer.

Respiratory disease

Chronic respiratory diseases such as Chronic Obstructive Pulmonary Disease (COPD), asthma, pulmonary hypertension, and occupational lung disease are incurable and affect the everyday lives of people living with these conditions. Risk factors include air pollution, inhaling tobacco smoke, occupational chemicals, and dust (WHO (World Health Organization), 2022). About 10,000 people in the UK are newly diagnosed with a lung disease each week (British Lung Foundation, 2022). According to NHS England (2022), respiratory disease affects approximately 1 in 5 people and is the third highest cause of death in England. The largest incidence is found in people from disadvantaged groups and areas of social deprivation since those living in the most deprived communities have elevated levels of smoking, poor housing conditions (such as damp), exposure to occupational hazards and air pollution. Furthermore, the Office of National Statistics (2022b) estimate that 2.8% of the population in the UK are experiencing long-covid symptoms (defined as lasting over 4 weeks from the initial infections) with symptoms including fatigue, shortness of breath (dyspnoea), loss of smell (anosmia) and muscle ache. Those most affected are people living in socially deprived areas, women aged between 25–69 years of age with previous occupations such as healthcare, social care, and education.

Activity 13.6

Look at the following guidelines:

1   COPD guidelines at www.nice.org.uk
2   British Thoracic Society and Scottish Intercollegiate Guidelines Network (SIGN) (2019)
    British Guidelines on the Management of Asthma. Available at: www.sign.ac.uk/our-guidelines/british-guideline-on-the-management-of-asthma/

3 NICE (2022) *Covid-19 rapid guidelines: managing the long-term effects of Covid-19.*
   Available at: www.nice.org.uk/guidance/ng188/resources/covid19-rapid-guideline-
   managing-the-longterm-effects-of-covid19-pdf-51035515742

Access the following and view some of the patient video stories (www.blf.org.uk/support-for-you/copd/
stories-and-videos; https://youtu.be/r88ILzNHY6Q) before making a list of the issues faced by people
living with COPD.

Diabetes

Approximately 3.9 million people across the UK are living with diabetes (an estimated 9% of the population) and around one million people are living with type 2 diabetes but are yet to be diagnosed (Diabetes UK, 2019). Those from black ethnic groups are more likely to have undiagnosed diabetes than people from white British backgrounds. The risks of developing type 2 diabetes mellitus include being overweight, although family history, ethnicity and age also increase the risk. Black African-Caribbean populations have also been reported to exhibit pronounced insulin resistance and higher rates of hypertension compared to other ethnic groups (Diabetes UK, 2019).

Activity 13.7

Go to the NICE website (www.nice.org.uk) and review the latest guidelines for the diagnosis and management of type 1 and type 2 diabetes.

- Identify the factors that contribute to the onset of type 1 and type 2 diabetes;
- Outline the main symptoms of undiagnosed or poorly controlled diabetes;
- Summarise the main treatment aims and make a list of the short- and long-term complications of type 1 and type 2 diabetes mellitus.

Review the nutritional guidance below and consider how you could use this to provide information, education, and support for adults with diabetes: *Evidence Based Nutrition Guidelines for the Prevention and Management of Diabetes* (Diabetes UK, 2018). Available at: www.diabetes.org.uk/professionals/position-statements-reports/food-nutrition-lifestyle/evidence-based-nutrition-guidelines-for-the-prevention-and-management-of-diabetes

Chronic liver disease

The ONS (2021b) report for the UK indicated liver disease has become the second leading cause of death in people between the working ages of 16–64 in both men and women. Liver disease is almost entirely preventable, with the major risk factors – alcohol, obesity, and hepatitis B and C – accounting for up to 90% of cases (Office for Health Improvement and Disparities, 2022).

Activity 13.8

Access the following information sources to find out more about caring for individuals with liver disease:

British Liver Trust: britishlivertrust.org.uk/information-and-support/living-with-a-liver-condition/liver-conditions/

Royal College of Nursing (2019) *Caring for People with Liver Disease: A Competency Framework for Nursing*, revised edn. Available at: www.rcn.org.uk/Professional-Development/publications/pub-007733

NICE Guidelines: www.nice.org.uk/guidance/conditions-and-diseases/liver-conditions/chronic-liver-disease.

Chronic kidney disease

Chronic kidney disease (CKD) is a term used to describe abnormal kidney function and/or structure. It is common, frequently unrecognised and often exists together with other conditions (e.g., CVD and diabetes). According to Kidney Research UK (2023), it is estimated that there are 60,000 premature deaths each year from CKD, and in the UK 64,000 people are being treated for kidney failure. Furthermore, according to Caskey and Dreyer (2018), there are also an estimated 1 million people with CKD who remain undiagnosed and people from lower socioeconomic groups are not only more likely to develop kidney disease but they also progress faster towards kidney failure and die earlier. Those individuals from black, Asian and minority ethnic populations are less likely to receive a transplant.

Activity 13.9

Access and review the following journal articles:

1   Kovesdy, C.P. (2022). Epidemiology of Chronic Kidney Disease: an update', *Kidney International Supplement*, 12 (1): 7-11. Available at: https://pubmed.ncbi.nlm.nih.gov/35529086/

2   Du, Y., Dennis, B., Ramirez, V. et al (2022), Experiences and disease self-management in individuals living with chronic kidney disease: qualitative analysis of the National Kidney Foundation's online community', *BMC. Nephrology,* 23, 88.

Make a list of the risk factors associated with the development of CKD. Outline the associated health burdens and complications of CKD.

Go to the NICE website (https://www.nice.org.uk/guidance/ng203) and review the latest guidelines for the diagnosis and management of CKD.

Chronic musculoskeletal conditions

The term 'musculoskeletal' describes conditions that affect the joints, muscles and bones. Although the prevalence of musculoskeletal (MSK) conditions tends to increase with age, they can affect any age group and account for 40% of all disabilities across the UK. Conditions include those caused by an abnormal inflammatory process (e.g., rheumatoid arthritis and ankylosing spondylitis), rare autoimmune conditions such as lupus, general 'wear and tear' (e.g., osteoarthritis), and bone disease (osteoporosis). Fibromyalgia is a common condition characterised by widespread muscle and joint pain and stiffness. According to Versus Arthritis (2021), there are estimated to be around 10.2 million people between the ages of 35–64 and 7.4 million people over the age of 65 living with arthritis.

Activity 13.10

Review the following article Versus Arthritis (2021) *The State of Musculoskeletal Health*. Available at: https://www.versusarthritis.org/about-arthritis/data-and-statistics/the-state-of-musculoskeletal-health/

Make some notes on the report's key findings and then reflect upon what adult nurses could do to help.

Mental health issues

Around one in four people in the UK suffer from mental health problems each year, with many going untreated. Mental illness is estimated to account for almost a quarter of the total burden of disease yet NHS spending on mental health services only accounts for 13.8% of the total budget which includes spending for learning disabilities and dementia (NHS England, 2021a). Moreover, people living with long-term depression are also at risk of developing co-morbidities (Bobo et al., 2022).

Activity 13.11

Access the following website and explore some of the '*your stories*' blogs to gain a better understanding of how long-term mental health conditions impact on the lives of people and the care they receive at www.mind.org.uk

Multimorbidity

The number of people living in the UK and globally who are living with multiple conditions (often referred to as *multimorbidity*) is increasing. This brings about increasing challenges for the individual regarding the navigation of health and social care services when there has been a tendency for services to focus on conditions and symptoms rather than consider what may matter most to the individual, failing to notice any emotional wellbeing and mental health concerns (NIHR, 2021). The Academy of Medical Sciences (2018) define 'multiple long-term conditions' as the existence of two or more long-term conditions in one individual and clearly encompasses the psychological and physical needs of the whole person. It is also important to note the interconnectedness of physical and mental health needs – one can impact the other leading to significant consequences for health and wellbeing. Those living with multiple conditions frequently have a reduced quality of life and a higher risk of mortality in comparison with the general population (Williams and Egede, 2016).

As a nurse, it is important that you continue to update your knowledge and understanding, making sure that the care you deliver is based on the best available evidence (NMC, 2018b). Having undertaken all the activities in this chapter thus far you should have a satisfactory level of knowledge and understanding of the common LTCs that affect individuals living in the UK, and the lifestyle factors that often contribute to the onset of some of these conditions. This knowledge and understanding will prove crucial when we focus upon the role of the nurse in supporting people with LTCs later in this chapter.

Activity 13.12

At this point it would also be worth accessing annexes A and B of the NMC *Proficiency Framework* (NMC, 2018a) and identifying all the clinical skills required of registered nurses.

Within a supportive care environment, how could you ensure that you are able to develop your clinical skills to meet the required competencies outlined above?

Living with a Long-term Condition

Most people must learn to live with rather than die from a chronic illness. Therefore, we need to consider the psychosocial impact that living with an LTC can have on individuals and their families.

Activity 13.13

Using the notes you made when undertaking the previous activities, consider the potential impact that a LTC has on job prospects, lifestyle, and relationships with family or significant others, as well as the physical, psychological, and behavioural aspects of life. This is a good opportunity to explore some of these issues with those you care for too (although you will need to do this sensitively).

Make a list of as many impact factors you can think of (including those that you identified earlier). Points you might want to consider include the following:

- If admitted to hospital, what factors led to the admission (e.g., a link to hospital or community care provision)?
- Are there any contributing factors that may have led to other admissions?
- If looked after in a community setting, what care interventions were required and how often?

Think about how the person's ability to work or their choice of job, lifestyle, hobbies, holidays taken, family and social interactions are affected.

Over the years researchers have sought to describe the lived experiences of those living with chronic illness (Stenberg et al., 2016; Aberg et al., 2020; Porter et al., 2020; Hayanga et al., 2021) and although many of these studies focus on a specific disease or condition, there are a number of frequently occurring issues and symptoms that appear to be present no matter what the diagnosis or condition may be. Most commonly, these include:

- Symptoms (e.g., tiredness/fatigue, increasing disability, anxiety, or depression);
- Perceived loss (e.g., in terms of independence and social activity linked to increasing disability affecting daily activities, occupation, confidence, self-worth/value, intimacy, role within family, control and individuality);
- Feelings (e.g., fear, frustration, blame, denial, and sometimes anger).

Associated mental health issues

Those living with an LTC are two to three times more likely to experience mental ill health such as anxiety and depression than those in the general population. Carswell et al. (2022)

found that those living with severe mental illness and LTCs struggled in managing their day-to-day life. Furthermore, the relationship between mental and physical health is a complex one. Several studies highlight how depression can exacerbate the distress, pain, sleeplessness, and fatigue experienced by many people living with a LTC. Awan et al. (2022) found that many South Asian people who were living with LTCs experienced elevated levels of anxiety, emotional distress, and depression. Those living with two or more LTCs are much more likely to have depression than a healthy person.

Many would argue that this aspect of care is often overlooked and that individuals suffering from chronic medical conditions and co-occurring depression or anxiety are often never diagnosed or treated for their psychiatric conditions (Melek and Norris, 2008). The impact of this can be a reduced quality of life, poorer self-care, and adverse health behaviours, as well as poorer health outcomes and overall prognosis (Naylor et al., 2012) (Figure 13.2). Mental health problems can also negatively impact a person's ability to self-manage their condition (HM Government/DH, 2011). Stenberg and Furness (2017) suggest that positively adapting to chronic illness requires both mental adjustments and the ability to gain control by developing coping strategies, and that individuals may need additional support from adult nurses and other external sources to positively adapt to their changed health status.

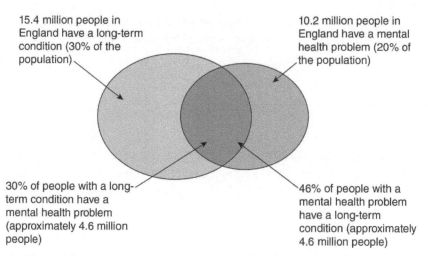

15.4 million people in England have a long-term condition (30% of the population)

10.2 million people in England have a mental health problem (20% of the population)

30% of people with a long-term condition have a mental health problem (approximately 4.6 million people)

46% of people with a mental health problem have a long-term condition (approximately 4.6 million people)

Figure 13.2 The overlap between long-term conditions and mental health problems (Naylor et al., 2012)

Fatigue

Fatigue is commonly experienced by people suffering from a variety of chronic illnesses. The concept of fatigue was initially used in the sixteenth century to describe a tedious duty, although nowadays fatigue is regarded as feeling tired for 'no reason.' Barsevick et al. (2010) have described it as being subjective, a feeling unrelated to being tired after exercise and being relieved after rest.

It may be regarded as exhaustive, unpredictable in its course and affecting cognitive ability. Fatigue is often described as multidimensional and disabling, affecting the quality of life of those living with it. Negative emotions such as anxiety, numbness and vulnerability may also be experienced, and are likely to have an impact on social relationships and family life, often leading to withdrawal and social isolation. A qualitative meta-analysis undertaken by Whitehead et al. (2016) suggests that many individuals feel that others (including healthcare professionals) do not always understand the overwhelming nature of their symptoms. Indeed, Wilson et al. (2006) suggest that gaining an understanding of how a person conceptualises their own unique experience would be a good starting point for nurses, allowing them to tailor interventions that would best suit those they care for rather than merely suggesting strategies for successful living.

Chronic insomnia

Chronic insomnia is defined as difficulty initiating and/or maintaining sleep, early waking and sleep that is non-restorative, together with daytime fatigue and poor concentration lasting over six months (Matin and Benca, 2012). Chronic insomnia is often found in individuals suffering from chronic illness (Roach et al., 2021). However, according to Kay-Stacey (2016) it may be difficult to determine the cause because predisposing conditions, precipitating circumstances and perpetuating factors may be included. Examples include:

- A person who has an anxious personality trait may predispose to sleep problems, resulting in hyperarousal;
- A precipitating event (e.g., a decline in health);
- A stressful event;
- Insomnia that is maintained by perpetuating factors, such as having a nap during the day or having an extended lie-in;
- Use of prescribed medications, alcohol, or other stimulants (e.g., caffeine);
- Pain.

Social isolation and loneliness

Loneliness is a complex concept and a variety of definitions exist, although those with poor health report experiencing loneliness more often (ONS, 2018). Loneliness is associated with an increased mortality risk of 26% (Holt-Lunstad et al., 2015; Hakulinen et al., 2018; Jaspal and Breakwell, 2022). Predisposing factors include partnership status, ethnicity, gender, disability, physical and mental health issues, access to technology, the internet, and social media, being a carer and having a limited income that restricts opportunities (ONS, 2018). It appears crucial for nurses to be able to identify those who are lonely, although this may be problematic due to the degree of stigma attached to the concept. There is obviously a need for nurses to facilitate discussion once a rapport has been established with an individual living with a chronic condition. Individuals who have experienced major losses (e.g., loss of a loved one or having a chronic health condition) are at increased risk of loneliness. An early indicator is the difference in everyday activities, although the need to assess for low mood is also important because changes in everyday activities are one indicator of depression.

Activity 13.14

Access and listen to the podcast below:

> National Institute for Health and Care Research (NIHR) (2021) *How can we reduce the toll of loneliness in older adults? [podcast]* Available at https://evidence.nihr.ac.uk/collection/how-can-we-reduce-the-toll-of-loneliness-in-older-adults/

Take some time out to think about some of these issues might be addressed within your own workplace setting.

Management of Long-term Conditions

Many individuals with an LTC will require support from a range of professionals. As a nurse you will need to be able to work in partnership with other organisations and services (including those in the statutory, voluntary, community and independent sectors) to ensure streamlined and integrated care delivery. This will include working across organisational boundaries and demands effective communication and collaborative multi-agency working skills. Guthrie et al. (2012) argue that clinical guidelines focusing on single conditions do little to assist healthcare practitioners in supporting people with multiple LTCs as they need to take account of multi-morbidity, emphasising the need to ensure that an individual personalised approach is taken.

Although there is no single definitive model of integrated care, the WHO (2016) provides a useful overview of various models and suggests that irrespective of the model used, the concept is likely to be shaped by the views and expectations of several stakeholders. The expanded chronic care model (Barr et al., 2003) highlights the essential components of care, suggesting that the best outcomes for those we care for are achieved when these components are integrated, joint professional working is accomplished and a person–centred approach is adopted – thus moving away from the more traditional 'single disease silo' approach that can sometimes result in duplication or people 'falling through the gaps' as they attempt to navigate their way through the complex array of services via a series of uncoordinated interactions or care pathways.

The NHS Long Term Plan (NHS, 2019) includes a commitment to ensure health and social care is personalised. Personalised healthcare aims to ensure that an individual's strengths and needs are considered when their care is being planned and delivered. This approach includes the potential, capacity and strengths of the person concerned, their family members and wider community to ensure integration of physical and mental health across the lifespan. The aim is to develop a shift in power and decision making from health and social care providers to individuals; ensuring they have a voice which is heard, and they remain connected to their communities and each other.

The Comprehensive Model for Personalised Care (NHS England, 2018) has six components which all need to be delivered together to ensure maximum impact;

1　Shared decision making;
2　Personalised care and support planning;
3　Choice (including the legal right to disagree);
4　Social prescribing and community-based support;
5　Personal health budgets;
6　Supported self-management which includes some key concepts such as patient activation, health coaching, peer support, self-management education and measuring and evaluating supported self-management.

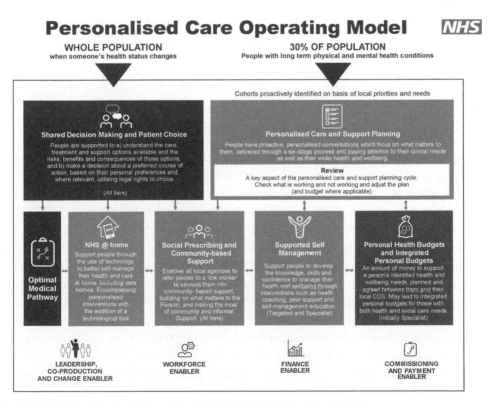

Figure 13.3　Personalised Care Operating Model (NHS England, 2018)

1. Shared Decision Making

People with a LTC are encouraged to work in partnership with health and social care profession-als, taking an active role in managing their condition. Partnership working is a fundamental aspect of the registered nurse's role, requiring an ability to develop an inclusive and mutually beneficial relationship with people and their carers to improve the quality and experience of care. In the past, a paternalistic/maternalistic relationship (reflecting a medical model of care) often meant that the nurse would **tell** individuals what they needed. Nowadays, however, the power relationship between healthcare professionals and those receiving care is more equal. The concept of 'empowerment' has many facets that can differ depending upon on whether this is applied to a community, organisational or individual context. However, in this case we refer to it as being suggestive of the nurse handing over or 'giving power' to the person they are car-ing for. It is a process that aims to change the nature and distribution of power in therapeutic relationships with the intention of increasing a person's control over their own health. People are considered as active partners in the management of their own condition (e.g., planning care and deciding on and evaluating treatment options). By acknowledging that an individual is an expert in terms of their own experience and condition, a more equal and facilitative relationship is established.

Reflecting on the care that you have provided for someone you have cared for recently, think about what you did and how you did it.

- Was it possible to take every opportunity to empower this person? If so, how? If not, why not?
- How did this impact on the care provided?

Working in partnership involves acknowledging and respecting another person's viewpoint, cir-cumstances, and preferences for care. Barriers to partnership working can include lack of confi-dence or experience, lack of cultural awareness/competence, lack of time, or personal attitudes of those involved (Millard et al., 2006; Zoffmann and Kirkevold, 2005, 2007; Upton et al., 2011). To be able to empower the individuals we care for, nurses must be able to communicate effectively, take the time to listen and develop a good understanding of their personal values and goals. A nurse also needs to help individuals access the information they need for them to be able to make appropriate decisions about their care. Most importantly, there is a need to regard the person as an individual who is living with a condition but not defined by it. Conversely, the person cared for needs to be motivated to change and be able to engage in the process. Zoffmann and Kirkevold (2012) suggest that the use of a guided self-determination (GSD) model can assist healthcare prac-titioners to establish meaningful therapeutic relationships and help those they care for identify, express, and share the unique and unexpected difficulties they face while living with an LTC. Using a life-skills approach, the five-stage process involves:

1   The establishment of an I–you sorted relationship;
2   Self-exploration;
3   Self-understanding;
4   Action;
5   Feedback from action.

2. Personalised Care Planning

The *'House of Care'* model provides a framework to deliver holistic, person-centred, preventative, and proactive care starting with a shared decision-making process involving the active participation of people in the development of their care plans with clinicians (Coulter et al., 2016). Planning, implementation, and evaluation of care is an ongoing process with the healthcare provider recognising the personal strengths and the lived experiences of the individual being cared for. This involves helping them to identify their desired outcomes and then setting agreed goals, action planning, problem solving; providing information and access to additional support and treatments where necessary to help them achieve their goals. This process can help people understand the aims of the care and support they are receiving, as well as any actions they may need to take if their condition worsens (e.g., emergency or crisis planning). It involves discussion, negotiation, shared decision making and review. Benefits of a care plan include greater concordance with agreed treatment plans and an increased sense of control for those receiving care. Care plans (written or otherwise) should include information on the individuals' concerns, their wellbeing needs, actions, goals, information relating to support organisations and any other specific needs they may have. Developing a personal care plan in partnership with individuals and carers will call on all the knowledge, skills, attributes, values, and behaviours outlined in previous chapters that are considered crucial when attempting to build a therapeutic relationship.

Another key aspect of the model is to ensure that the care planning for individuals and commissioning for local populations are intricately linked. The aim is for local services, community resources, social care, and healthcare – together with more traditional health services – to work together (Coulter et al., 2016), creating a more interdependent and coordinated health and social care system which aims to help individuals stay active as long as possible (Cook and Grant, 2020).

3. Choice

Individuals across the UK have the right to make informed choices about any healthcare offered (Scottish Government, 2019; Department of Health and Social Care, 2021; Northern Ireland DHSC/HSCNI Strategic Planning & Performance Group, 2022) and access to advocacy services as needed to help them to make the right choices for them.

4. Social prescribing and community-based support

The term *'social prescribing'* relates to the concept of non-medical-based approaches to enhance a person's overall well-being which Polley and Sabey (2022) argue have a positive impact on physical and mental health and an associated reduction in health service use and costs. Activities such as gardening, exposure to green space and nature are thought to have numerous health benefits, although causal mechanisms are not yet fully understood (Mughal et al., 2022).

The voluntary and community sector has key roles in terms of providing advice and information about equipment and tools to help people self-care and maintain their independence. Housing and care services, such as home improvement agencies, will install aids and adapt and repair people's homes to help them live independently (Department of Health and Social Care, 2021).

Activity 13.15

Find out what programmes, courses or voluntary groups are available to people in your area.

- What referral criteria are used?

Consider how you might use this information to help you to support people with LTCs in your workplace.

---

5. Personal health budgets

Personal health budgets are funds allocated to certain individuals to facilitate personalised care and support plans with the overall aim of providing the recipient greater choice and flexibility (Scottish Government, 2019; NHS England, 2021; Northern Ireland DHSC/HSCNI Strategic Planning & Performance Group, 2022). However, the British Medical Association (BMA, 2021) suggest that whilst having the potential to improve quality of life evidence of improved clinical outcomes is limited.

Muriel

Muriel lives with 76 year-old Clive in a ground-floor maisonette in an inner-city area. Clive has been living with COPD and type 2 diabetes for over 28 years and had to retire early from a job as a joiner due to increased breathlessness and poorly controlled diabetes. Since then Clive has, until recently, enjoyed socialising with friends, trying to keep an allotment going and remain the head of an extended family. Muriel has tried to support Clive both physically and emotionally while still taking on some cleaning jobs in the city. Clive admits to being stubborn regarding dietary control, alcohol intake and occasional cigarette smoking. However, the development of a leg ulcer has led to a prolonged period of physical inactivity, disturbed sleep and increasing social isolation. Clive confides in you, reporting feeling tired, lonely, isolated, and depressed, which has resulted in 'comfort eating.' Clive is becoming increasingly breathless and informs you of the occasional secret cigarette, smoked in the back garden. Clive's grandchildren visit after school and try to provide some company but both Muriel and Clive wonder (for varied reasons) if Clive will be able to resume previous levels of activity. In your role as an adult nurse, you have been asked to provide support for Muriel and Clive.

- How would you assess the bio-psychosocial needs of this family?
- What do you consider to be the principal areas of concern?
- What information might Clive and Muriel (and you) need to ensure an evidence-based approach to care?
- How could you encourage personalised care planning, working in partnership and self-management?
- Are there any issues connected with Muriel being a carer for Clive as well as working part-time? How may this dual role affect Muriel physically, emotionally, and socially?
- Compare your answers by discussing this case scenario with your peers and/or colleagues. Is there anything they would do differently?

You will no doubt have identified several key issues that need addressing to improve Clive's health. However, primarily the most important thing to do would be to begin to try to build a therapeutic relationship with Clive and Muriel. To do this, you will need to be available and communicate effectively with them to establish their key concerns. Clive exhibits several physical illnesses, exacerbating symptoms and unhealthy lifestyle choices and reports a deterioration in mental health and social activity. As nurses we are often driven by the need to 'make things better' and so there is a temptation to jump right in and begin to plan the care we think is needed to address all the health issues we have identified. Yet, by listening carefully to Clive and Muriel, you will be able to ascertain their priorities for care. You will then need to consider what valid and reliable assessment tools you might use to assist in this process. For example, how might you assess Clive's sleeping difficulties, fatigue, loneliness, and emotional distress?

By assessing and discussing Clive's needs in more depth and providing information about how identified issues could be addressed, you can empower Clive to take an active role in any agreed interventions which are more likely to be successful. For example:

- Use an integrated approach to assessment to ensure that social and psychological factors are also considered;
- Refer to local/national guidelines and evidence-based care pathways;
- Explore how access to a wider multi-agency team, private or voluntary agencies could help;
- Negotiate and agree on a culturally sensitive, person-centred action plan.

Muriel's needs should also be considered. Carers can often feel overlooked and as a nurse you will be responsible for ensuring that Muriel also receives individualised information, advice, and support, thereby adopting a family rather than an individual focused approach.

6. Supported Self-Management

There are a wide range of initiatives aimed at supporting self-care (Figure 13.4), varying from the provision of information and education to developing technical skills and proactive strategies aimed at changing behaviour and increasing self-efficacy. All these approaches are important but there is evidence to suggest that adopting proactive strategies is the most effective (De Silva, 2011).

Patient activation aims to encompass the skills, knowledge, and confidence a person living with a LTC has in managing their own health and care. It is believed that with support an increase in activation can lead to better health outcomes, fewer unplanned admissions to hospital and a reduction in GP (General Practitioner) appointments together with an improved care experience.

Health coaching is defined as '*helping people gain and use the knowledge, skills, and confidence to become active participants in their care so that they can reach their self-identified health and wellbeing goals*' (NHS England & NHS Improvement, 2020: 6) and involves the use of health coaching skills targeted towards specific groups of people with LTCs. Published studies on health coaching and those living with LTCs have considered the impact of quality of life, self-care behaviours and hospital admission (Bower et al., 2018; Long et al., 2019).

Peer support involves people sharing individual experiences with each other to help increase mental or physical health and reduce isolation. Peer support may be formal or informal, delivered by trained volunteers or peer support staff and can be on a formal or more informal ad hoc basis. For some individuals, a referral to a self-help group or a lay-led educational programme may be beneficial. Entwistle and Cribb (2013) suggest that proactive, behaviourally focused, self-management support can have a positive impact on clinical symptoms, attitudes and behaviours, quality of life and the use of healthcare resources. If successful it can have individual and cost benefits (Price et al., 2022).

Self-management education encompasses all actions taken by people to recognise, treat and manage our own health. This can be achieved independently or in partnership with the healthcare system. Self-management education is any form of training or formal education that people living with a LTC undertake to increase confidence in managing their own care. The NHS Constitution (Department of Health and Social Care, 2021) sets out a commitment to offer easily accessible, reliable, and relevant information to enable people to participate fully in healthcare decisions and support them in making choices. In Chapter 11, we explored the role of the adult nurse in helping people to make healthy lifestyle choices, particularly in terms of taking adequate exercise, good nutrition, and the avoidance of unhealthy behaviours, such as excessive alcohol consumption and smoking. There is also a clear need to ensure that people can access the information and support needed to gain the knowledge and confidence to communicate effectively with healthcare workers. This could include the provision of written or electronic information, videos/DVDs, online courses, person-held records or care plans, and the use of web-based technologies such as the internet or e-health initiatives. Evidence suggests that self-management behaviours can be facilitated through the exchange of health information and disease experience (Willis, 2013).

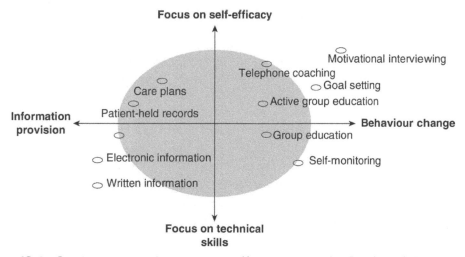

Figure 13.4 Continuum strategies to support self-management. (De Iongh et al. (2015), reproduced with permission of the Health Foundation)

Tools and self-monitoring devices can help individuals play an integral role in monitoring their LTCs. This can involve the monitoring of physiological measurements (e.g., blood pressure or blood glucose/cholesterol levels) via electronic devices or written self-management plans that help patients to self-medicate and self-refer when appropriate. In chapter 5, you may recall how we discussed the use and impact of tele-healthcare that has evidence of benefits to individuals as well as healthcare professionals (Zanaboni et al., 2017; Mounessa et al., 2018; Janjua et al., 2021). Examples include closed circuit TV/video conferencing, the use of email and remote monitoring. Other approaches such as M-health involve the use of mobile apps or personalised systems downloaded to phones or personal computers which are used for the personal monitoring of chronic conditions. These systems can communicate with remote call centres, thereby providing data for a professional review.

Activity 13.16

Make a list of the equipment and tools you have come across that assist those you have cared for to self-care and maintain their independence.

- Do you (and those you provide care for) know how to use these properly?
- Are there any other devices or tools that you or they might be able to access?
- How would you/they gain access to these?

(Remember that in addition to devices related to health and social care, you should consider the contribution of other aids and adaptations that can be accessed via the voluntary and private sectors.)

Measurement and evaluation in supporting self-management can assess the support and self-management needs, evaluate interventions, and assess the confidence and knowledge of people living with LTCs and their carers since it is important to measure what any form of self-management intervention is, or what it claims to achieve; such as effects, properties, values, or qualities. Self-management programmes have been shown to reduce costs and improve health (Price et al., 2022). Reported positive health outcomes include reductions in depression, anxiety, pain and fatigue, fewer GP visits and increased use of cognitive symptom management techniques (e.g., goal setting, exercise, and relaxation). However, the Mental Health Foundation (2012) has called for improvements in the access, quality and professional support provided to peer support schemes aimed at addressing the mental health needs of individuals with LTCs, an aspect of care that is often overlooked.

Activity 13.17

Review two of the following papers and make some brief notes about how nurses can help people living with LTCs cope with potential challenges to facilitate a return to the workplace:

1 Almutairi, N., Hosseinzadeh, H. and Gopaldasani, V. (2020) 'The effectiveness of patient activation intervention on type 2 diabetes mellitus glycaemic control and self-management behaviors: a systematic review of RCTs', *Prim Care Diabetes*, Feb;14(1):12-20.

2 Carswell, C., Brown, J.V.E., Lister, J., Ajjan, R.A., Alderson, S.L., Balogun-Katung, A., Bellass, S., Double, K., Gilbody, S., Hewitt, C.E., Holt, R.I.G., Jacobs, R., Kellar, I., Peckham, E., Shiers, D., Taylor, J., Siddiqi, N. and Coventry, P. (2022), The lived experience of severe mental illness and long-term conditions: a qualitative exploration of service user, carer, and healthcare professional perspectives on self-managing co-existing mental and physical conditions', *BMC Psychiatry*, Jul 19; 22(1):479.

3   Hemming, S. and Munir, F. (2022) 'Using the patient activation measure to examine the self-management support needs of a population of UK workers with long-term health conditions', *Chronic Illn.*, Sep; 18(3): 702–7.
4   Lawless, M.T., Drioli-Phillips, P., Archibald, M.M., Ambagtsheer, R.C. and Kitson, A.L. (2021),Communicating with older adults with long-term conditions about self-management goals: a systematic review and thematic synthesis', *Patient Educ Couns,* Oct; 104(10): 2439–52.

The following papers focus on health practitioners' experiences of patient activation. Highlight the key points and reflect upon how you can incorporate these into your own clinical practice.

1   Heggdal, K., Stepanian, N., Oftedal, B.F., Mendelsohn, J.B., and Larsen, M.H. (2021), Health care professionals' experiences of facilitating patient activation and empowerment in chronic illness using a person-centered and strengths-based self-management program', *Chronic Illn.*, Dec 14.
2   Lawless, M.T., Drioli-Phillips, P., Archibald, M.M., Ambagtsheer, R.C. and Kitson, A.L. (2021) 'Communicating with older adults with long-term conditions about self-management goals: a systematic review and thematic synthesis', *Patient Educ Couns,* Oct; 104(10): 2439–52.

The Role of Carers

A carer is an individual who:

> "looks after a family member, partner or friend who needs help because of their illness, frailty, disability, a mental health problem or an addiction and cannot cope without their support. The care they give is unpaid".

> www.england.nhs.uk/commissioning/comm-carers/carers/

Immediate family members are often seen as a primary resource for managing the impact of long-term ill health across all cultures and groups (Knowles et al., 2016), although we should remember that cultural concepts of caring are not universal. It is estimated that there are around 10.6 million carers in the UK (Carers UK, 2022) and an estimated 800,000 people in Scotland (Carers Trust, 2023). Many carers report a significant negative impact on their own health as a result (Carers UK, 2022).

Registered nurses play a vital role in ensuring that the health needs of carers are addressed so that they can maintain their own health and wellbeing.

Activity 13.18

Access a copy of The Department of Health and Social Care (2018) *Carers action plan 2018 to 2020* at: www.gov.uk/government/publications/carers-action-plan-2018-to-2020.

- What are the responsibilities of local authorities in terms of promoting wellbeing and assessing the needs of individuals and their carers?
- What support services are available to carers in your area (e.g., financial entitlement, respite care/carer breaks and all other forms of support available in the locality)?
- How can you use this knowledge to provide information and support to carers?

Patrick

Patrick is 79 years old and lives at home with Michael. They have known each other since childhood and have lived together for almost 40 years. Patrick is admitted to hospital after suffering a cerebrovascular accident (CVA) associated with left-sided weakness. Patrick has a catheter, can mobilise for short distances with the aid of a frame and can understand what is being said but has difficulty with verbal expression because of dysphasia caused by the CVA. More recently, Patrick has been diagnosed with type 2 diabetes and Michael has been diagnosed with Parkinson's disease. Patrick is Michael's main carer. They have no other close relatives. They live in a house with stairs where the only bathroom and toilet are upstairs. They both want to stay together in their own home.

- What are the overall health and social needs that you would need to consider to plan for Patrick's discharge?
- Which other healthcare professionals and organisations would need to be involved?
- How would you reach an agreed plan of care for Patrick and Michael?

Effective Discharge Planning

The term 'revolving door syndrome' is often used for the readmission of people to hospital within a few days of their discharge. Although some of these readmissions may be difficult to prevent, often they are a result of poor communication, a fragmented care system or inadequate discharge planning. British Red Cross (2019) report on a variability in consistency in effective discharge processes between nations and local areas and suggest that whilst some individuals might appear well enough for discharge, wider non-clinical needs are often unmet. Furthermore, they argue that poor transitions from hospital to home can have a long-lasting negative impact on an individual's experience.

Activity 13.19

Look at the following YouTube video 'Home from Hospital' in which people describe their experiences of hospital discharge:

https://youtu.be/8KC3q9KUXcQ

How do you think the experiences of hospital discharge described here could have been improved?

Most people with LTCs will be cared for in a community setting. However, there will be occasions when admission or transfer to and from acute, intermediate or respite care will be required. Individualised discharge planning has been identified as having the potential to reduce the length of stay in hospital and readmission rates (Kim and Covey, 2022). To ensure continuity of care, the Department of Health, and Social Care (2022) has outlined several key steps involved in the transfer of care process:

1   Supporting people to go home is considered the priority, with consideration for an alternative pathway if this is not possible;
2   Involving the person and their carer in the decision-making process, and respecting their knowledge and opinions when considering the best option so that they can make informed decisions and choices that will deliver a personalised care pathway and maximise their independence;
3   Undertake a rapid and effective assessment of need to mobilise required services;
4   Providing easy access to information, advice, and services to promote self-care/management where possible;
5   Secure consent for sharing of information across partners to enable relevant information to 'move' seamlessly with the person;
6   Plan discharges and transfers to take place over seven days to deliver continuity of care.

Planning a person's discharge or transfer from any care setting is an important part of a person-centred care plan and will ensure that individuals and their families continue to be supported. As a registered nurse, you must be able to liaise effectively with individuals, their families and all other agencies involved to achieve a smooth transition of care. Safe and effective discharges/transfers rely on robust decision-making processes and reaching a consensus with people and their families/carers, as well as other members of the multidisciplinary team. People with LTCs often have complex needs and, as such, this process is reliant on therapeutic engagement and a shared philosophy of care where ethical principles are identified as vital to the nursing endeavour, in terms of doing good, avoiding harm, promoting autonomy, and affording justice.

- What skills do you have that will assist you in supporting individuals and their families through this process?
- What additional knowledge and skills might you need to access to develop and/or review a person-centred care plan?

Chapter Summary

This chapter has encouraged you to find out more about common LTCs that affect adults across the UK and the evidence-based interventions that aim to help people to manage their conditions. We have explored the impact that many LTCs have on individuals and their families. We have also examined some of the contemporary approaches aimed at providing help and support to individuals and families in our role as registered nurses. The concept of person-centred, supported self-care, and the importance of integrated care provision to deliver good quality effective nursing care have also been highlighted.

Useful Websites

Department of Health: www.england.nhs.uk/ourwork/clinical-policy/ltc/
National Voices: www.nationalvoices.org.uk/ (a registered charity that stands up for the rights of individuals, service users and carers).

Further Reading

Egan, G. and Reece, R.J. (2019) *The Skilled Helper. A Problem-Management and Opportunity-Development Approach to Helping*, 11th edn. UK: Cengage.
RCN (Royal College of Nursing) (2016) *Caring for Lesbian, Gay, Bisexual or Trans Clients or Patients – Guide for nurses and health care support workers on next of kin issues*. Available at: www.rcn.org.uk/Professional-Development/publications/pub-005592. (last accessed 25 January 2023).

Skills for Health (2017) *Person-Centred Approaches: Empowering people in their lives and communities to enable an upgrade in prevention, wellbeing, health, care, and support.* Available at: www. skillsforhealth.org.uk/wp-content/uploads/2021/01/Person-Centred-Approaches-Framework. pdf (last accessed 25th January 2023).

References

Åberg, C., Gillsjö, C., Hallgren, J. and Berglund, M. (2020) '"It is like living in a diminishing world": older persons' experiences of living with long-term health problems – prior to the STRENGTH intervention', *Int J Qual Stud Health Well-being*, Dec;15(1):1747251.

Alzheimer's UK (2019) *Black, Asian and Minority Ethnic Communities and Dementia Research.* Available at: www.alzheimers.org.uk/for-researchers/black-asian-and-minority-ethnic-communities-and-dementia-research (last accessed 6 February 2023).

Awan, H., Mughal, F., Kingstone, T., Chew-Graham, C.A. and Corp, N. (2022) 'Emotional distress, anxiety, and depression in South Asians with long-term conditions: a qualitative systematic review', *British Journal of General Practice*, March, e179-189. Available at: https://bjgp.org/content/bjgp/72/716/e179.full.pdf (last accessed 6 February 2023).

Barr, V. J., Robinson, S., Marin-Link, B., Underhill, L., Dotts, A., Ravensdale, D. and Salivasra, S. (2003) 'The expanded Chronic Care Model: an integration of concepts and strategies from population health promotion and the Chronic Care Model', *Hosp Q.*, 7(1): 73–82.

Barsevick, A., Beck, S.L., Dudley, W.N., Wong, B., Berger, A.M., Whitmer, K., Newhall, T., Brown, S. and Stewart, K. (2010) 'Efficacy of an intervention for fatigue and sleep disturbance during cancer chemotherapy', *J Pain Symptom Manage*, Aug; 40(2): 200–16.

Bécares L. (2013) *Which Ethnic Groups Have the Poorest Health? Ethnic health inequalities 1991 to 2011.* Manchester: ESRC Centre on Dynamics of Ethnicity (CoDE)

Bobo, W.V., Grossardt, B.R., Virani, S., St Sauver, J.L., Boyd, C.M. and Rocca W.A. (2022) 'association of depression and anxiety with the accumulation of chronic conditions', *JAMA Netw Open*, May 2; 5(5): e229817.

Bower, P., Reeves, D., Sutton, M., Lovell, K., Blakemore, A., Hann, M., Howells, K., Meacock, R., Munford, L., Panagioti, M., Parkinson, L.R., Sidaway, M., Lau, Y., Warwick-Giles, L., Ainsworth, J., Blakeman, T., Boaden, R., Buchan, I., Campbell, S., Coventry, P., Reilly, S., Sanders, C., Skevington, S., Waheed, W. and Checkland, K. (2018) *Improving care for older people with long-term conditions and social care needs in Salford: the CLASSIC mixed-methods study, including RCT.* Available at: https://livrepository.liverpool.ac.uk/3149509/1/Bookshelf_NBK519984.pdf (last accessed 6 February 2023).

Brain Research UK (nd) *Neurological Conditions.* Available at: www.brainresearchuk.org.uk/info/neurological-conditions (last accessed 6 February 2023).

British Heart Foundation (2022) *UK CVD Factsheet.* Available at: www.bhf.org.uk/-/media/files/research/heart-statistics/bhf-cvd-statistics—uk-factsheet.pdf. (last accessed 25 January 2023).

British Lung Foundation (2022) *Lung Disease in the UK.* Available at: https://statistics.blf.org.uk/ (last accessed 6 February 2023).

British Medical Association (2021) *Personal Health Budgets.* Available at: www.bma.org.uk/advice-and-support/nhs-delivery-and-workforce/commissioning/personal-health-budgets (last accessed 3 February 2023).

British Red Cross (2019) *Home to the Unknown: Getting hospital discharge right*. Available at: www.redcross.org.uk/about-us/what-we-do/we-speak-up-for-change/more-support-when-leaving-hospital/getting-hospital-discharge-right (last accessed 2 January 2023).

Cancer Research UK (2023) *Cancer Statistics for the UK*. Available at: www.cancerresearchuk.org/health-professional/cancer-statistics-for-the-uk.(last accessed 6 February 2023).

Carers Trust (2023) *Our Work in Scotland*. Available at: https://carers.org/our-work-in-scotland/our-work-in-scotland (last accessed 6 February 2023).

Carers UK (2022) *State of Caring*. Available at: www.carersuk.org/policy-and-research/state-of-caring-survey/ (last accessed 6 February 2023).

Carswell, C., Brown, J.V.E., Lister, J., Ajjan, R.A., Alderson, S.L., Balogun-Katung, A., Bellass, S., Double, K., Gilbody, S., Hewitt, C.E., Holt, R.I.G., Jacobs, R., Kellar, I., Peckham, E., Shiers, D., Taylor, J., Siddiqi, N.and Coventry, P. (2022) 'The lived experience of severe mental illness and long-term conditions: a qualitative exploration of service user, carer, and healthcare professional perspectives on self-managing co-existing mental and physical conditions', *BMC Psychiatry*, Jul 19; 22(1): 479.

Caskey, F. and Dreyer, G. (2018) *Kidney Health Inequalities in the United Kingdom: Reflecting on the past, reducing in the future*. Kidney Research UK: Peterborough.

Cook, A. and Grant, A. (2020, *From Fixer to Facilitator. Evaluation of the House of Care Programme in Scotland*. Matter of Focus: Edinburgh.

Coulter, A., Kramer, G., Warren, T. and Salisbury, C. (2016) 'Building the House of Care for people with long-term conditions: the foundation of the House of Care framework', *Br J Gen Pract*, Apr; 66(645): e288-90.

Delon, C., Brown, K.F., Payne, N.W.S. et al. (2022) 'Differences in cancer incidence by broad ethnic group in England, 2013–2017', *Br J Cancer*, 126: 1765–73.

de Iongh, A., Fagan, P., Fenner, J. and Kidd, L. (2015) *A Practical Guide to Self-management Support*. London: Health Foundation. Available at: www.health.org.uk/publications/a-practical-guide-to-self-management-support. (last accessed 6 February 2023).

De Silva, D. (2011) *Helping People Help Themselves*. London: The Health Foundation.

Department of Health (2012) *Long Term Conditions Compendium of Information* (3rd edn). Available at: www.gov.uk/government/publications/long-term-conditions-compendium-of-information-third-edition (last accessed 6 February 2023).

Department of Health (2022) *Quick Guide: Discharge to Assess*. Available at: www.nhs.uk/NHSEngland/keogh-review/Documents/quick-guides/Quick-Guide-discharge-to-access.pdf (last accessed 6 February 2023).

Department of Health & Social Care (2021) *The NHS Constitution for England*. Available at: www.gov.uk/government/publications/the-nhs-constitution-for-england/the-nhs-constitution-for-england (last accessed 3 February 2023).

Department of Health and Social Care/HSCNI Planning & Performance Group (2022) *Self-Directed Support*. Available at: https://online.hscni.net/sds/. (last accessed 3 February 2023).

Diabetes UK (2019) *Diabetes Statistics*. Available at: www.diabetes.org.uk/professionals/position-statements-reports/statistics. (last accessed 23 January 2023).

Entwistle, V.A. and Cribb, A. (2013) *Enabling People to Live Well: Fresh Thinking about Collaborative Approaches to Care for People with Long-term Conditions*. London: The Health Foundation.

Ettehad, D., Emdin, C.A., Kiran, A., Anderson, S.G., Callender, T., Emberson, J., Chalmers, J., Rodgers, A. and Rahimi, K. (2016) 'Blood pressure lowering for prevention of cardiovascular disease and death: a systematic review and meta-analysis', *The Lancet*, 387: 957–67.

Government Equalities Office (2018) *National LGBT Survey*. Available at: www.gov.uk/government/publications/national-lgbt-survey-summary-report. (last accessed 25 February 2023).

Guthrie, B., Payne, K., Alderson, P., McMurdo, M.E.T. and Mercer, S.W. (2012) 'Adapting clinical guidelines to take account of multimorbidity', *British Medical Journal*, 345: e6341. doi:10.1136/bmj. e6341.

Hakulinen, C., Pulkki-Råback, L., Virtanen, M., Jokela, M., Kivimäki, M. and Elovainio, M. (2018) 'Social isolation and loneliness as risk factors for myocardial infarction, stroke and mortality: UK Biobank cohort study of 479 054 men and women', *Heart*, 104 (18): 1536–542.

Hamadelseed, O., Elkhidir, I.H. and Skutella, T. (2022) 'Psychosocial risk factors for Alzheimer's disease in patients with down syndrome and their association with brain changes: a narrative review', *Neurol Ther*, Sep;11(3): 931–53.

Hayanga, B., Stafford, M. and Bécares, L. (2021) 'Ethnic inequalities in healthcare use and care quality among people with multiple long-term health conditions living in the United Kingdom: a systematic review and narrative synthesis', *Int. J. Environ. Res. Public Health*, 18: 12599.

Health and Social Care Northern Ireland (2022) *Shaping the Integrated Care System Northern Ireland*. Available at: https://hscboard.hscni.net/download/PUBLICATIONS/unnamed-file.ics/Integrated-Care-System-Factsheet-01.pdf. (last accessed 27 January 2023).

HM Government/Department of Health (2011) *No Health Without Mental Health: A Cross Government Mental Health Outcomes Strategy for People of All Ages*. London: DH.

Holt-Lunstad, J., Smith, T.B., Baker, M., Harris, T. and Stephenson, D. (2015) 'Loneliness and social isolation as risk factors for mortality: a meta-analytic review', *Perspectives on Psychological Science*, 10(2): 227–37.

Janjua, S., Carter, D, Threapleton, C. J., Prigmore, S. and Disler, R.T (2021) 'Telehealth interventions: remote monitoring and consultations for people with chronic obstructive pulmonary disease (COPD)', *Cochrane Database Syst Rev*, Jul 20;7(7): CD013196.

Janke, K., Lee, K., Propper, C., Shields, K. and Shields, M. (2020) *Macroeconomic Conditions and Health in Britain: Aggregation, dynamics, and local area heterogeneity*. Institute of Labor Economics. Available at: www.iza.org/publications/dp/13091/macroeconomic-conditions-and-health-in-britain-aggregation-dynamics-and-local-area-heterogeneity (last accessed 6 February 2023).

Jaspal, R. and Breakwell, G.M. (2022) 'Socio-economic inequalities in social network, loneliness and mental health during the COVID-19 pandemic', *International Journal of Social Psychiatry*, 68(1): 155–65.

Kay-Stacey, M. (2016) 'Advances in the management of chronic insomnia', *British Medical Journal*, 354: i2123.

Kidney Research UK (2023) *Chronic Kidney Disease*. Available at: www.kidneyresearchuk.org/conditions-symptoms/chronic-kidney-disease/ (last accessed 6 February 2023).

Kim, A. and Covey, C. (2022) 'Benefits of individualized discharge plans for hospitalized patients', *Am Fam Physician*. Nov; 106(5): 500–1.

Knowles, S., Combs, R., Kirk, S., Griffiths, M., Patel, N. and Sanders, C. (2016) 'Hidden caring, hidden carers? Exploring the experience of carers for people with long-term conditions', *Health Soc Care Community*, Mar;24(2): 203–13.

LGBT Foundation (2020) *Hidden Figures: LGBT Health Inequalities in the UK*. Manchester: LGBT Foundation.

Long, H., Howells, K., Peters, S. and Blakemore, A. (2019) 'Does health coaching improve health-related quality of life and reduce hospital admissions in people with chronic obstructive pulmonary disease? A systematic review and meta-analysis', *Br J Health Psychol*, Sep, 24(3): 515–46.

Matin, C. and Benca, R. (2012) 'Chronic insomnia', *The Lancet*, 379: 1129–41.

Melek, S. and Norris, D. (2008) *Chronic Conditions and Co-morbid Psychological Disorders*. Seattle, WA: Milliman.

Mental Health Foundation (2012) *Developing Peer Support for Long Term Conditions (Final Report)*. Edinburgh: Mental Health Foundation.

Millard, L., Hallett, C.E. and Luker, K.A. (2006) 'Nurse–patient interaction and decision-making in care: patient involvement in community nursing', *Journal of Advanced Nursing*, 55(2): 142–50.

Mounessa, J.S., Chapman, J., Braunberger, T., Qin, R., Lipoff, J.B., Dellavalle, R.P. and Dunnick, C.A. (2018) 'A systematic review of satisfaction with teledermatology', *Journal of Telemedicine and Telecare*, 24(4): 263–70.

Moriarty, J. (2021) *Long term conditions – briefing paper*. Available at: https://raceequalityfoundation. org.uk/health-and-care/long-term-health-conditions-collaborative/ (last accessed 6 February 2023).

Moriarty, J, Sharif, N. and Robinson, J. (2011) *Black and minority ethnic people with dementia and their access to support and services. Research Briefing*. Available at: https://kclpure.kcl.ac.uk/portal/files/13501330/SCIE_briefing.pdf (last accessed 6 February 2023).

Mughal, R., Seers, H., Polley, M., Sabey, A. and Chatterjee, H.J. (2022) *How the natural environment can support health and wellbeing through social prescribing*. NASP.

National Health Service (2019) *NHS Long Term Plan*. Available at: www.longtermplan.nhs.uk/publication/nhs-long-term-plan/ (last accessed 6 February 2023).

NHS England (2018) *Comprehensive Model of Personalised Care*. Available at: www.england.nhs.uk/publication/comprehensive-model-of-personalised-care/ (last accessed 6 February 2023).

NHS England (2021) *Personal Health Budgets in NHS Continuing Healthcare (CHC)*. Available at: www.england.nhs.uk/personalisedcare/personal-health-budgets/personal-health-budgets-in-nhs-continuing-healthcare/ (last accessed 6 February 2023).

NHS England (2021a) *NHS Mental Health Dashboard*. Available at: www.england.nhs.uk/mental-health/taskforce/imp/mh-dashboard/ (last accessed 6 February 2023).

NHS England (2021b) *Measuring Supported Self-management: Five steps to help teams choose approaches*. Available at: www.england.nhs.uk/publication/measuring-supported-self-management-five-steps-to-help-teams-choose-approaches/ (last accessed 6 February 2023).

NHS England (2022) *Respiratory disease*. Available at: www.england.nhs.uk/ourwork/clinical-policy/respiratory-disease/ (last accessed 6ᵗ February 2023).

NHS England (nd) *House of Care – a framework for long term condition care*. Available at: www.england.nhs.uk/ourwork/clinical-policy/ltc/house-of-care/ (last accessed 27 January 2023).

NHS England & NHS Improvement (2020) *Health Coaching Implementation and Quality Summary Guide*. Available at: www.england.nhs.uk/wp-content/uploads/2020/03/health-coaching-implementation-and-quality-summary-guide.pdf (last accessed 6 February 2023).

Naylor, C., Parsonage, M., McDaid, D., Knapp, M., Fossey, M. and Galea, A. (2012) *Long-term Conditions and Mental Health: The Cost of Co-morbidities*. London: The King's Fund. Available at: www.kingsfund.org.uk/publications/long-term-conditions-and-mental-health (last accessed 6 February 2023).

(NICVA (2016) *Long Term Conditions Alliance Northern Ireland*. Available at: www.nicva.org/sites/default/files/d7content/attachments-articles/printers_ltcani_printer.pdf (last accessed 6 February 2023).

NIHR Collection (2021) *Multiple Long-term Conditions (multimorbidity): Making sense of the evidence*. Available at: https://evidence.nihr.ac.uk/collection/making-sense-of-the-evidence-multiple-long-term-conditions-multimorbidity/ (last accessed 6 February 2023).

Nursing and Midwifery Council (2018a) *Future Nurse: Standards of Proficiency for Registered Nurses*. London: NMC.

Nursing and Midwifery Council (2018b) *The Code*. London: NMC.

Office for Health Improvement and Disparities (2022) *Liver Disease Profiles, January 2022 update*. Available at: www.gov.uk/government/statistics/liver-disease-profiles-january-2022-update/liver-disease-profiles-january-2022-update (last accessed 6 February 2023).

Office for National Statistics (2011) *People, Population and Community Health and Social Care: Health and wellbeing*. Available at www.ons.gov.uk/peoplepopulation andcommunity/healthandsocialcare/healthandwellbeing/articles/generalhealth inenglandandwales/2013-01-30 (last accessed 6 February 2023).

Office for National Statistics (2018) *Loneliness: What Characteristics and Circumstances are Associated with Feeling Lonely?* Available at: www.gov.uk/government/statistics/loneliness-what-characteristics-and-circumstances-are-associated-with-feeling-lonely (last accessed 6 February 2023).

Office for National Statistics (2020) *People with Long term Health Conditions, UK: January to December 2019*. Available at: www.ons.gov.uk/peoplepopulationandcommunity/healthandsocialcare/conditionsanddiseases/adhocs/11478peoplewithlongtermhealthconditionsukjanuarytodecember2019 (last accessed 6 February 2023).

Office for National Statistics (2021a) *Monthly Mortality Analysis, England, and Wales: Dec 2022*. Available at: www.ons.gov.uk/peoplepopulationandcommunity/birthsdeathsandmarriages/deaths/bulletins/monthlymortalityanalysisenglandandwales/december2022 (last accessed 6 February 2023).

Office for National Statistics (2021b) *Alcohol-specific deaths in the UK: Liver diseases and the impact of deprivation*. Available at: www.ons.gov.uk/peoplepopulationandcommunity/healthandsocialcare/causesofdeath/datasets/alcoholspecificdeathsintheunitedkingdomsupplementarydatatables (last accessed 6 February 2023).

Office for National Statistics (2022a) *Population of England and Wales - Ethnicity facts and figures*. Available at: www.ethnicity-facts-figures.service.gov.uk/uk-population-by-ethnicity, (last accessed 25 January 2023).

Office for National Statistics (2022b) *Prevalence of Ongoing Symptoms Following Coronavirus (COVID-19) Infections in the UK*. Available at: www.ons.gov.uk/peoplepopulationand community/healthandsocialcare/conditionsanddiseases/bulletins/prevalence of ongoingsymptomsfollowing coronaviruscovid19infectionintheuk/4august2022. (last accessed 6 February 2023).

Polley, M. and Sabey, A. (2022) *An Evidence Review of Social Prescribing and Physical Activity*. Available at: https://socialprescribingacademy.org.uk/media/udfpf5o3/review-of-social-prescribing-and-physical-activity_.pdf (last accessed February 2023).

Porter, T., Ong. B.N. and Sanders, T. (2020) 'Living with multimorbidity? The lived experience of multiple chronic conditions in later life', *Health (London)*, Nov; 24(6): 701–18.

Price, A., de Bell, S., Shaw, N., Bethel, A., Anderson, R. and Thompson Coon, J. (2022) 'What is the volume, diversity, and nature of recent, robust evidence for the use of peer support in health and social care? An evidence and gap map,' *Campbell Systematic Reviews*, John Wiley & Sons Ltd.

Raleigh. V. and Holmes, J. (2021) *The Health of People from Ethnic Minority Groups in England*. London: The King's Fund.

Roach, M., Juday, T., Tuly, R., Chou, J.W., Jena, A.B. and Doghramji, P.P. (2021) 'Challenges and opportunities in insomnia disorder', *International Journal of Neuroscience*, 131(11): 1058–65.

Sanderson, J. and White, J. (2018) *Making the Case for a Personalised Approach*. Available at: www.england.nhs.uk/blog/making-the-case-for-the-personalised-approach/ (last accessed 6 February 2023).

Scottish Government (2019) *Self-directed Support Strategy 2010-2020: implementation plan 2019-2021*. Available at: www.gov.scot/publications/self-directed-support-strategy-2010-2020-implementation-plan-2019-21/ (last accessed 3 February 2023).

Scottish Public Health Observatory (2022) *Scottish Health Survey* (2019), Available at: www.scotpho.org.uk (last accessed 6 February 2023).

Stenberg, U., Haaland-Øverby, M., Fredriksen, K., Westermann, K.F. and Kvisvik, T. (2016) 'A scoping review of the literature on benefits and challenges of participating in patient education programs aimed at promoting self-management for people living with chronic illness', *Patient Education and Counseling*, 99(11), November: 1759–71.

Stenberg, N. and Furness, P.J. (2017) 'Living well with a long-term condition: service users' perspectives of a self-management intervention', *Qual Health Res.*, Mar; 27(4): 547–58.

Stafford, M., Knight, H., Hughes, J., Alarilla, A., Mondor, L., Pefoyo Kone, A., Wodchis, W.P., Deeny, S.R. (2022), Associations between multiple long-term conditions and mortality in diverse ethnic groups. *PLoS One*. Apr 1;17(4): e0266418.

The Academy of Medical Sciences (2018) *Multimorbidity: a priority for global health research*. The Academy of Medical Sciences. Available at: https://acmedsci.ac.uk/file-download/82222577. (last accessed 6 February 2023).

Toleikyte, L. and Salway, S. (2018) *Local Action on Health Inequalities: Understanding and reducing ethnic inequalities in health*. London: Public Health England.

Upton, J., Fletcher, M., Madoc-Sutton, H., Sheikh, A., Caress, A.-L. and Walker, S. (2011) 'Shared decision making or paternalism in nursing consultations? A qualitative study of primary care asthma nurses' views on sharing decisions with patients regarding inhaler device selection,' *Health Expectations*, 14(4): 374–82.

Versus Arthritis (2021) *The State of Musculoskeletal health* Available at: https://versusarthritis.org/about-arthritis/data-and-statistics/the-state-of-musculoskeletal-health/ (last accessed 6 February 2023).

Whitehead, L.C., Unahi, K., Burrell, B., and Crowe, M.T. (2016) 'The experience of fatigue across long-term conditions: a qualitative meta-synthesis', *Journal of Pain & Symptom Management*, 52: 131e143.

Williams, J.S. and Egede, L.E. (2016) 'The association between multimorbidity and quality of life, health status and functional disability', *American Journal of Medical Science*, 32: 45–52.

Willis, E. (2013) 'The making of expert patients: the role of online health communities in arthritis self-management', *Journal of Health Psychology*, 0: 1–13.

Wilson, P.M., Kendall, S. and Brooks, F. (2006) 'Nurses' responses to expert patients: the rhetoric and reality of self-management in long-term conditions: a grounded theory study', *International Journal of Nursing Studies*, 43(7): 803–18.

Wittenberg, R., Hu, B., Barraza-Araiza, I. and Rehill, A. (2019) *Projections of older people with dementia and costs of dementia care in the United Kingdom 201 -2040.* Care Policy and Evaluation Centre, LSE, and Political Science. CPEC Working Paper 5.

World Health Organization (2016) *Integrated Care Models: An Overview.* Copenhagen: WHO.

World Health Organization (2022) *Chronic Respiratory Disease.* Available at: www.who.int/health-topics/chronic-respiratory-diseases (last accessed 6 February 2023).

Zanaboni, Z., Hanne Hoaas, H., Aarøen Lien, L.A., 3rd, Hjalmarsen, A. and Wootton, R. (2017) 'Long-term exercise maintenance in COPD via telerehabilitation: a two-year pilot study', *Journal of Telemedicine and Telecare*, 23(1): 74–82.

Zoffmann, V. and Kirkevold, M. (2005) 'Life versus disease in difficult diabetes care: conflicting perspectives disempower patients and professionals in problem solving', *Qualitative Health Research*, 15: 750–65.

Zoffmann, V. and Kirkevold, M. (2007) 'Relationships and their potential for change developed in difficult type 1 diabetes', *Qualitative Health Research*, 17: 625–38.

Zoffmann, V. and Kirkevold, M. (2012) 'Realizing empowerment in difficult diabetes care: a guided self-determination intervention', *Qualitative Health Research*, 22(1): 103–18.

14

CARING FOR THE ACUTELY ILL ADULT

Claire Burns, Trudy Hadcroft and Janet Roberts

Chapter objectives

- Define the aims of acute care and identify a variety of settings in which it takes place;
- Identify the knowledge and skills required to work effectively in acute care settings;
- Summarise the components of a comprehensive assessment of an acutely ill adult;
- Explain how to recognise and respond to acutely ill adults using appropriate evidence-based strategies;
- Define the characteristics of an effective communication strategy when caring for acutely ill adults;
- Highlight the importance of using medical devices safely;
- Explore the use of effective pain assessment and management strategies when caring for adults in pain;
- Consider ways in which a nurse could enhance the experience of adults receiving care within acute settings.

All adults, regardless of the setting, have the potential to become acutely unwell. With the general trend of those in hospital being older, sicker, and having more complex health issues, the need for skills in recognising and responding to the deteriorating adult are becoming increasingly important. Nurses in all clinical areas, and not just those working in acute care environments, should have the knowledge and skills to recognise and respond competently and confidently to the needs of an acutely ill adult.

Caring for acutely ill adults can be challenging, not least because it often involves the use of high-tech equipment and monitoring technology which can be worrying to those unfamiliar with such devices. By exploring the evidence base for the management of acute illness we will provide you with the underpinning knowledge necessary to be able to provide safe and effective care for unwell adults. The use of clinical scenarios and reflective guidance will also help you consider and acknowledge your own limitations, thereby recognising the need to develop your skills further.

Related Nursing and Midwifery Council (NMC) Proficiencies for Registered Nurses

The overarching requirements of the NMC (2018) are that all registered nurses should be able to lead in providing evidence-based, compassionate, and safe nursing interventions. They are required to prioritise the needs of people when assessing and reviewing their mental, physical, cognitive, behavioural, social, and spiritual needs.

They should use information obtained during assessments to identify the priorities and requirements for person-centred and evidence-based nursing interventions, and are responsible for managing nursing care, being accountable for the appropriate delegation and supervision of care provided by others in the team (including lay carers). Nurses are required to play an active and equal role in the multi-disciplinary team, collaborating and communicating effectively with a range of colleagues (NMC, 2018).

━━━━━━ TO ACHIEVE ENTRY TO THE NMC REGISTER
YOU MUST BE ABLE TO ━━━━━━

- Demonstrate and apply knowledge of all commonly encountered mental, physical, behavioural and cognitive health conditions, medication usage and treatments when undertaking full and accurate assessments of nursing care needs, and when developing, prioritising, and reviewing person-centred care plans;
- Demonstrate the ability to manage commonly encountered devices and confidently carry out related nursing procedures to meet people's needs for evidence-based, person-centred care;
- Demonstrate the knowledge and skills required to identify and initiate appropriate interventions to support people with commonly encountered symptoms including anxiety, confusion, discomfort, and pain;
- Demonstrate the ability to undertake accurate risk assessments in a range of care settings using a range of contemporary assessment and improvement tools;
- Interpret results from routine investigations, taking prompt action when required by implementing appropriate interventions, requesting additional investigations, or escalating to others;

- Demonstrate the knowledge and ability to respond proactively and promptly to signs of deterioration or distress in mental, physical, cognitive, and behavioural health, and use this knowledge to make sound clinical decisions;
- Demonstrate knowledge of when and how to refer people safely to other professionals or services for clinical intervention or support;
- Demonstrate the ability to co-ordinate and undertake the processes and procedures involved in routine planning and management of safe discharge home or transfer of people between care settings.

(Adapted from NMC, 2018)

Acute illness is usually defined as an illness of short duration and is often classified as either minor or major acute (Jones et al., 2010). Examples of major acute illnesses include exacerbations of long-term conditions (e.g., epilepsy or chronic obstructive pulmonary disease), the new onset of a previously undiagnosed problem (e.g., a stroke or appendicitis) or recovering from a serious accident/trauma or surgery. Minor acute illnesses comprise illnesses such as minor infections, skin rashes and minor injuries, though these can develop to become major acute illnesses.

Acute care environments include the following (Organisation for Economic Co-operation and Development, 2021):

- Intensive care beds
- Acute care units
- All gynaecological and obstetric services
- Surgical units
- Acute psychiatric beds

Activity 14.1

Access the NHS (National Health Service) digital website (https://digital.nhs.uk/) for hospital accident and emergency activity statistics and identify the profile of those who attend A&E (gender and age), and when they attend (e.g., most common time of arrival at A&E).

England has seen a reduction of 44% in the number of overnight general and acute NHS hospital beds in the past 30 years. In contrast, the number of day beds has increased by 530% in this time, reflecting the rise in day-case surgery (The King's Fund, 2020). The reduction in available hospital beds and an increase in inpatient day care activity has resulted in greater demands for many acute care services. This has led to the introduction of a variety of emergency and urgent care services across the UK, including Emergency departments (EDs) - also called Accident and Emergency (A&E) - which are classified as type 1, 2, 3 and 4 (NHS Digital, 2021a) as shown in Table 14.1, out-of-hours services and NHS 111. During the Covid-19 pandemic there was a decrease in people presenting to A&E (NHS Digital, 2021a). However, this is not representative of the increase seen in previous years or the current picture of a rise in A&E attendances and emergency admissions as the UK emerges from the pandemic (NHS Digital, 2021b). The need to manage acute hospital admissions safely has led to the introduction of medical assessment units (MAUs) and surgical assessment units (SAUs) in some areas which aim to provide fast-track routes to assessment, diagnosis, and subsequent referral to the appropriate specialty.

Adults are admitted to hospital for many reasons. Admissions can be planned (e.g., for elective surgery or medical investigations/treatment) or maybe because of an emergency (e.g., accident or injury, acute sudden illness, or an exacerbation of a long-term condition).

Whatever the clinical setting, registered nurses must be able to provide timely, safe, and effective care which includes an ability to recognise the needs of acutely ill adults, the potential for deterioration in their condition and the ability to respond appropriately. It is acknowledged here that you will need to access other specialist literature to develop specific knowledge and understanding relating to the care of adults undergoing specific medical treatments and surgical interventions (see 'Further reading' at the end of this chapter). The focus for this chapter is the systematic assessment and management of an acutely ill adult.

Acute assessment units are often busy environments, and their aim is to make sure unwell adults are appropriately assessed to ensure that the right care is provided at the right time by the most appropriate caregiver (e.g., facilitating timely referral to inpatient care within the relevant specialty or on to relevant support teams working in primary care settings). As a nurse working in an acute environment, you will need to have a good understanding of the altered physiology of illness and the capacity to rapidly observe, assess, and monitor individuals in your care, interpreting and evaluating observations and assessments to make sound decisions based on your clinical judgement. Team working and the ability to communicate effectively with people and their families, as well as other members of the multi-disciplinary team will be crucial to help to relieve stress and anxiety experienced by the acutely ill adult and ensure continuity of care.

Table 14.1 Accident and emergency department types (NHS Digital, 2021b)

Type	Department
1.	Emergency departments are a consultant-led 24-hour service with full resuscitation facilities.
2.	Consultant-led single specialty A&E service (e.g., ophthalmology, dental).
3.	Other type of A&E/minor injury, which may be doctor-led or nurse-led treating at least minor injuries and illnesses, and can be routinely accessed without appointment.
4.	Other types of A&E/Minor Injury Units (MIUs)/Walk-In Centres (WiC)/Urgent Treatment Centres (UTC) primarily designed for receiving accident and emergency patients.

Acute Medicine

Acute medical emergencies are the most common reason for admission to hospital (Royal College of Physicians, 2007; NHS Digital, 2020). Most UK hospitals have established acute medical units (AMUs) - also known as Medical Assessment Units (MAUs), acute assessment units (AAUs) and early assessment units (EAUs). Scott et al. (2009) suggest that AMUs may reduce inpatient mortality and length of stay and improve service-user and staff satisfaction. AMUs are defined by the Royal College of Physicians (2018) as a dedicated facility within a hospital that acts as the focus for acute medical care for those who have presented as medical emergencies to hospitals or who have developed an acute medical illness while in hospital.

The West Midlands Quality Review Service and the Society for Acute Medicine (2012) recommend that all registered nurses working in such environments should be clinically competent in the following:

Immediate life support (ILS);
Performing an Early Warning Score (EWS) assessment, its interpretation and escalation as appropriate;
Recording an ECG;
Venepuncture;
Intravenous (IV) drug administration;
Urinary catheterisation (male and female);
Aseptic non-touch technique;
Point-of-care testing (e.g., use of small bench analysers for blood glucose, blood gases, coagulation tests);
End of life care;
Handover, transfer, and discharge.

Additionally, Casey et al. (2016) recommend all registered nurses working in the AMU (Acute Medical Unit) should possess core skills including caring for adults with:

*   Ischaemic heart disease;
*   Diabetes;
*   Respiratory illness;
*   Frailty;
*   Cerebrovascular disease;
*   Acute infections.

---

*   As outlined in Chapter 2, the NMC (2018) requires adult nurses to be able to demonstrate numerous additional clinical competencies effectively to achieve entry to the register. Within an acute placement area, what additional skills might you need to the ones outlined above?
*   How could you ensure that you are able to develop your clinical skills within an acute area to meet the required NMC (2018) proficiencies?

Surgery

There have been significant changes in how surgery is performed in the modern healthcare setting. Just like the medical context, adults are getting older, sicker and have more co-morbidities. There have been considerable modifications to the management of surgical wound techniques and advances in the use of technology (e.g., robotic surgery and artificial intelligence), microsurgery and minimally invasive surgical techniques (e.g., 'keyhole' or laparoscopic surgery). As alluded to earlier, there has also been a significant increase in surgery performed as day cases after recommendations from the NHS Modernisation Agency (2004) suggesting that day surgery should be considered the norm for elective surgery rather than inpatient surgery. The increased use of day surgery has several potential economic and service user benefits, including:

- Shorter hospital stays;
- Release of facilities for more complex and emergency cases;
- Fixed scheduling, reducing cancellations and therefore more efficient theatre use;
- Staff reductions (as overnight staffing is usually not necessary);
- A decrease in both the time taken to perform surgical procedures and their cost, taking advantage of advances in surgical and anaesthetic care;
- Better use of high-cost operating room apparatus and supplies (World Health Organization [WHO], 2007a)

Common surgical procedures include abdominal surgery (e.g., cholecystectomy and bowel resection), vascular surgery (e.g., varicose vein surgery, aortic repair, insertion of stents), surgical oncology (e.g., resection of tumours), orthopaedic surgery (e.g., joint replacements or fracture repair) and plastic surgery (e.g., skin grafts, surgical repair, or reconstruction).

Nursing in a surgical setting involves caring for people before, during and after surgery, and requires the knowledge and skills outlined above in addition to those in the following list:

- Preoperative and postoperative care;
- Anaesthesia;
- Pain management;
- Infection prevention and control (relevant to every setting but particularly important here);
- Wound care and dressings, wound healing and the management of wound drains.

Enhanced recovery pathways (ERPs) are an approach used to support individuals to recover more quickly after elective surgery. The approach involves pre-operative assessment of the individual before admission and measures to reduce the physical stress of the surgery, sometimes called 'pre-habilitation.' Pre-habilitation involves interventions such as nutritional support and the management of iron deficiency anaemia to help ensure an individual is in the best condition possible prior to their surgery. Post-operatively, a structured approach to care and appropriate pain management is followed to further enhance recovery (National Institute for Health and Care Excellence [NICE], 2020). ERPs have been shown to reduce hospital length of stay, post-operative pain scores and reduce post-operative complications (UK National Guideline Centre, 2020). Elements of the Enhanced Recovery Pathway can be seen in Figure 14.1 (Enhanced Recovery Partnership Programme, 2010).

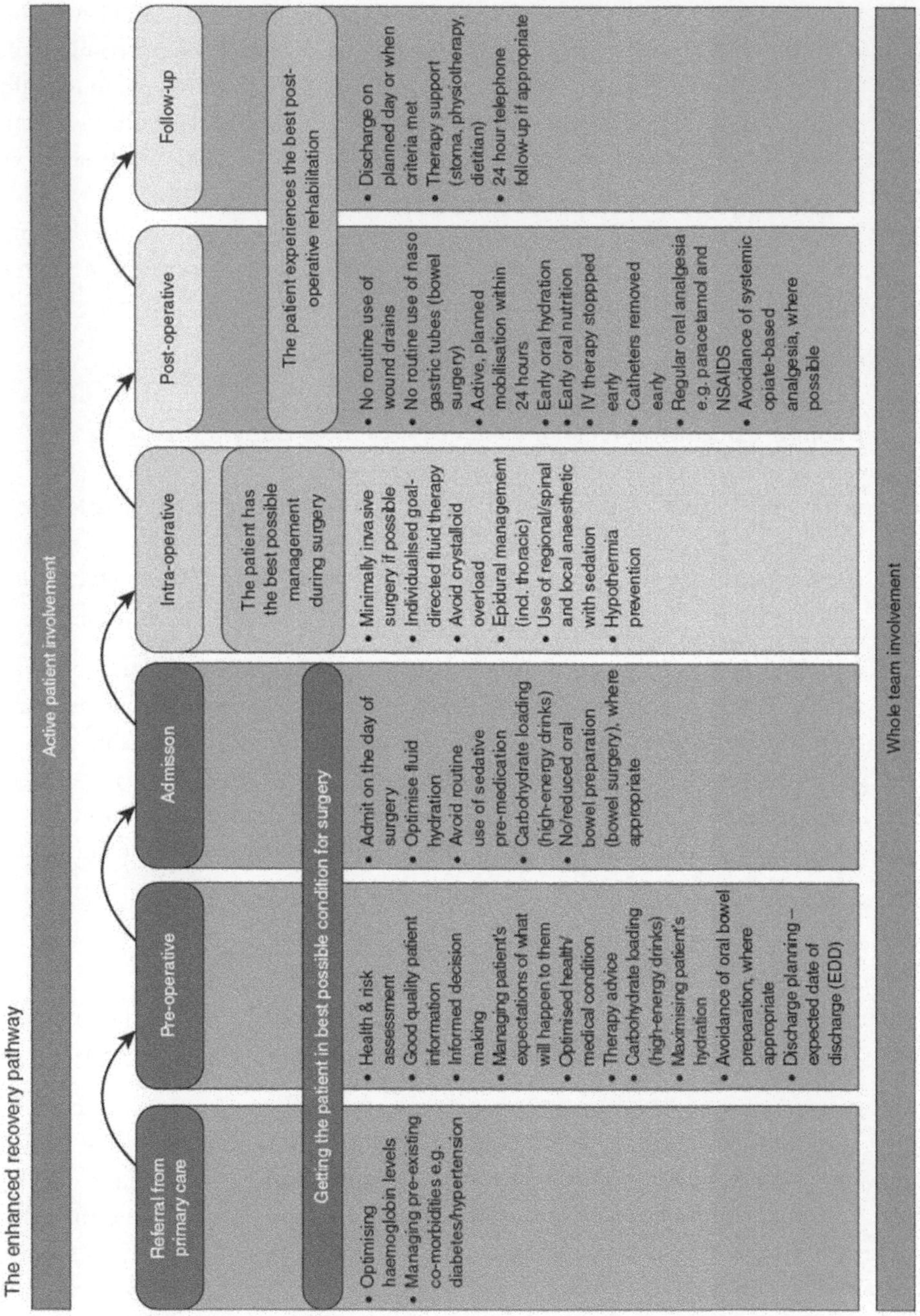

The enhanced recovery pathway

Figure 14.1 The Enhanced Recovery Pathway (© Crown copyright)

There is a growing body of evidence to support the use of enhanced recovery programmes (Aning et al., 2010; Ibrahim et al., 2013; Zhuang et al., 2013; Dwyer et al., 2014; UK National Guideline Centre, 2020). The Enhanced Recovery Partnership now consider that enhanced recovery should be standard practice for most people having major surgery, and it has already been implemented in other areas such as emergency surgery and acute medicine (NHS Improving Quality, 2013). Although not all surgery can be planned, whether a person is undergoing scheduled or emergency surgery nurses have a key role in ensuring people are fully informed about their planned procedure, know what to expect and are fit enough for surgery.

Providing Acute Hospital Care for an Older Person

Conroy and Cooper (2010) recognise that the acute clinical problems and needs of older people are often substantially different from those of younger people. The King's Fund (2014: 27) report, *Making Our Health and Care Systems Fit for an Ageing Population*, emphasises that 'acute hospital care must meet the needs of older patients with complex co-morbidities, frailty and dementia'. The older adult may be considered at higher risk of issues concerning safety while in the acute setting. For example, inpatient falls are the most reported hospital safety incident (Royal College of Physicians, 2016) and adults over the age of 60 suffer the greatest number of fatal falls (WHO, 2022).

Older adults can present with non-specific symptoms, making diagnosis difficult. History taking in the older person can also be problematic due to sensory impairment, dementia, or delirium. Additionally, older people are at a higher risk of adverse outcomes compared to younger individuals and the presence of co-morbidities increases the complexity of caring for the older person (Blomaard et al., 2021; Conroy and Thomas, 2021). One approach to improving the assessment and subsequent care of the older adult requiring acute hospital care is the Comprehensive Geriatric Assessment (GCA) (Parker et al., 2017). The GCA is a multi-disciplinary diagnostic and treatment process that takes a more holistic approach to the assessment and management of the older person than the traditional medical model. According to Ellis et al. (2017) GCAs typically have several key features:

- Specialty expertise;
- Assessment of medical, socioeconomic/environmental, function and psychological issues;
- Co-ordinated multi-disciplinary meetings;
- The development of a care plan around person-centred goals;
- Delivery of the care plan, including rehabilitation;
- Review of progress and care planning.

Adapted from Ellis et al. (2017)

A Cochrane systematic review of CGA for older adults admitted to hospital found that GCA improved the likelihood of older people being alive and discharged to their own homes at follow-up (Ellis et al., 2017).

In 2019, the Healthcare Quality and Improvement Partnership (Corrado et al., 2019) published a national audit report of dementia care in general hospitals, highlighting that at any one time people living with dementia occupy 1 in 4 hospital beds. Several areas of carer dissatisfaction were identified in the report including a lack of person-centred care, a lack of communication from staff and poor discharge planning and transfer of care. Additionally, people living with dementia are likely to experience inpatient falls, delayed discharges, and readmissions to the acute care setting. The report also provides several recommendations to support people living with dementia in hospital; the list below summarises several of these recommendations:

- Delirium assessment of the person living with dementia and that pain is considered as a contributory factor;
- Initial routine assessment including information about factors that cause the person living with dementia distress or agitation and measures that can be taken to prevent these;
- Clear ongoing communication with the families and carers of people living with dementia;
- Mandatory dementia training for all staff providing care for people living with dementia;
- Nutrition and hydration needs of people living with dementia are included in nurse shift handovers;
- Availability of snacks and finger foods for people living with dementia;
- Hospital discharge teams liaise with people living with dementia and their carers about discharge.

Activity 14.2

Conduct a review of care provision in your own clinical setting. Does the provision of care to those living with dementia meet the recommendations outlined above?

Assessing Individuals in an Acute Care Setting

Irrespective of the care setting, it is imperative that as a registered nurse you can assess the needs of people in your care. This demands an ability to accurately assess and monitor a person's condition accurately (on admission and continuously thereafter), develop individualised care plans, and safely administer oxygen therapy, IV fluids, medications and pain relief as needed.

So far in this book, we have introduced you to some of the systematic frameworks that can assist you in carefully assessing the needs of adults in your care. Here, we will focus in more depth on the history taking and observation element of assessment.

Taking a clinical history

History taking is a key component of assessment and is essential in enabling the delivery of high quality care. In the context of the acutely ill adult, this may need to be brief and focused. The scope and depth of the process will need adjusting according to the clinical urgency of the situation. Previously, in Chapter 3 we established that history taking is not just simply a fact finding mission or a way of seeking answers to a list of questions, but is important in the process of establishing a therapeutic relationship and as such, a person-centred approach must be followed, recognising the need for people to feel listened to whilst also acknowledging the need for focus. Information may also need to be gathered about the acutely ill adult from friends or family members, particularly in situations where a person is in pain or cognitively impaired. When taking a clinical history you should always introduce yourself to the person, inform them of why you need the information requested and, where possible, gain consent. Information such as the person's presenting complaint, the history of their presenting complaint and their past medical history should be obtained.

There are several mnemonics such as 'OLD CARTS,' 'PQRST' or 'SOCRATES' that can be used to elicit more specific information from a person in relation to a complaint such as pain or any other symptom (e.g., dyspnoea, palpitations, nausea).

OLD CARTS (**o**nset, **l**ocation, **d**uration, **c**haracter, **a**ggravating/relieving factors, **r**adiation, **t**iming, **s**everity);

PQRST (**p**rovoking or relieving factors, **q**uality, **r**adiation, **s**everity, **t**iming);

SOCRATES (**s**ite, **o**nset, **c**haracter, **r**adiation, **a**ssociations, **t**iming, **e**xacerbating/relieving factors, **s**everity).

Table 14.2 gives an example of some of the questions you may need to consider in taking a history of a person with chest pain using the 'OLD CARTS' mnemonic.

Nurses have long been relied on to monitor the condition of individuals in their care, thus ensuring the prompt detection of deterioration or delays in recovery. This demands an ability to be able to recognise and interpret subtle and/or significant changes in the normal physiological parameters of a person by undertaking specific clinical observations (e.g., blood pressure, pulse and respiratory rate, oxygen saturation, temperature, and level of consciousness).

Table 14.2 Example of 'OLD CARTS' mnemonic

Onset

What brought this on?
Did it start suddenly or gradually?

Location

Where exactly is the pain?
Can you point to where it is?

Duration

How long has it been there?
Is it constant or intermittent?

Character

What is the pain like? Can you describe it to me?
Consider offering some examples - sharp, dull, aching, stabbing, burning, heavy. It is important however to avoid 'leading' the person.

Aggravating/relieving factors

Have you noticed anything that makes it better (e.g., painkillers, other medication such as antacids, positioning)?
Have you noticed anything that makes it worse (e.g., inspiration, movement, lying down)?

Radiation

Does the pain radiate to any other location? (To the abdomen, arm, jaw etc.?)

Timing

When did it start?
Is it getting better, worse or staying the same?

Severity

How severe is it?
Consider using a pain scale as discussed later in this chapter

Other useful questions may ask about associated symptoms, e.g., Do you have any other symptoms with the pain (e.g., dizziness, dyspnoea, nausea)?

---

1   Do you know how to undertake the following clinical observations correctly?

- Blood pressure;
- Pulse rate;
- Respiratory rate;
- Oxygen saturation level;
- Blood glucose level;
- Temperature;
- Level of consciousness.

2   Are you aware of the normal parameters for all the above?

Activity 14.3

Many of the clinical observations above can be measured using medical monitoring equipment.

Make a list of all the medical monitoring equipment available in your clinical area.

Are you familiar with the use of this equipment?

Can you think of any risks/disadvantages that can be associated with relying on the use of such equipment?

What would you need to do to ensure that this risk was minimised?

Access and read your local trust policy relating to the safe use of medical equipment.

Although we will be exploring some of the frameworks used for monitoring unwell adults, you may find it useful to access some of the 'further reading' at the end of this chapter to ensure that you can carry out required clinical observations in the correct manner.

In an emergency setting (e.g., the ED) the Manchester Triage System (Mackway-Jones et al., 2013) is commonly used across the UK and Europe (Table 14.3). Individuals are prioritised into one of five categories (immediate, very urgent, urgent, standard, and non-urgent). The assessing nurse uses one of several flowcharts based on the individual's symptoms and 'discriminators'. Those individuals who fall into the immediate category need instant treatment; very urgent should be treated within 10 minutes, urgent within one hour, standard within two hours and non-urgent within four hours.

Table 14.3 Manchester triage system

1	Immediate	Red	Immediately
2	Very urgent	Orange	Within 10 minutes
3	Urgent	Yellow	Within 1 hour
4	Standard	Green	Within 2 hours
5	Non-urgent	Blue	Within 4 hours

More recently, the implementation of electronic health records (EHR) has seen growing interest in the adoption of intelligent Decision Support Systems (iDSS) also known as Clinical Decision Support Systems (CDSS). These are systems designed to support clinical decision makers to make decisions relating to the management of the individuals in their care. There is evidence emerging that suggests CDSS can improve ED triage and predict the need for critical care (Fernandes et al., 2020).

Recognising deterioration in adults

Admission to hospital can be a disruptive and worrying time for individuals and their families. Once in hospital, a person ought to feel that they are safe and that they will receive optimum care throughout their stay. However, when suffering from acute illness a person may be unstable and at risk of deterioration due to their altered physiological state. Acutely ill adults will often manifest abnormal vital signs, indicating cardiovascular, respiratory, or neurological deficits. There is evidence to suggest that these changes can go unrecognised by staff, resulting in late treatment, unnecessary admission to critical and intensive care units (ICU), and even death (NICE, 2007; Department of Health, 2009; Sinha et al., 2014). In 2021, the incidence of adult cardiac arrest was at 1.5 per 1000 hospital admissions, with most cardiac arrests (85%) occurring on wards in people admitted to hospital for medical reasons (Perkins et al., 2021). Only 23.6% of those treated by the hospital resuscitation team survived to achieve hospital discharge (Perkins et al., 2021).

In recognition of growing concerns about suboptimal standards of care within the hospital environment, clinical guidelines have been published that aim to support healthcare professionals in the assessment and subsequent management of acutely ill adults (NICE, 2007). However, despite regular evidence-based guidelines on resuscitation being produced by the Resuscitation Council UK (2021) and significant amounts of time and money being spent on staff training and equipment, survival rates for cardiac arrest remain low (Intensive Care National Audit & Research Centre (ICNARC), 2020). Therefore, whilst there have been significant advances in resuscitation knowledge and practice over the decades, it is not surprising given the low survival rates, that attention has switched to focusing more on the prevention of cardiac arrest.

Regardless of the clinical setting, nurses need to be aware of the contents of the resuscitation trolley and how to use them:

- How well prepared are you to look after a deteriorating adult?
- What do you know about the contents of the resuscitation trolley?
- Would you know how to use each piece of equipment correctly?
- What checks are in place to ensure that this equipment is safe to use?

Track-and-trigger systems

Most individuals who have a serious adverse event, such as an unplanned ICU admission, cardiac arrest or even death, show signs of clinical deterioration in the preceding hours. In 2005, a report from the National Confidential Enquiry into Patient Outcome and Death (NCEPOD) focusing on people referred to ICUs, identified that ward-based recognition of acute illness and its subsequent management was suboptimal (NCEPOD, 2005). Unfortunately, a recent review of the literature suggests clinical deterioration continues to be missed by healthcare professionals, resulting in delays responding to the acutely ill adult (Al-Moteri et al., 2019).

Nice (2007) *Acutely Ill Patients in Hospital*, and Scottish Intercollegiate Guidelines Network (SIGN) *Care of Deteriorating Patients* guidelines (SIGN, 2014) address the recognition of and response to acute illness in adults in hospital. A key priority identified within the NICE (2007: 7) guideline is that *'staff caring for patients in acute hospital settings should have competencies in monitoring, measurement, interpretation and prompt response to the acutely ill patient appropriate to the level of care they are providing'.*

NICE (2007) also recommends that physiological track-and-trigger systems are used to monitor all adults in acute hospital settings, suggesting that physiological observations should be monitored at least every 12 hours. Track-and-trigger systems monitor clinical observations ('track') and, if predetermined criteria are met, a clinical response is activated ('trigger'). Track-and-trigger systems allow for individuals to be monitored for signs of clinical deterioration, which are frequently similar, regardless of the cause. NICE (2007) identifies six physiological parameters to be included in a track-and-trigger system:

1   Respiratory rate;
2   Oxygen saturations;
3   Temperature;
4   Systolic blood pressure;
5   Heart rate;
6   Level of consciousness (AVPU).

Several track-and-trigger systems exist, but NEWS2 (2017) is one of the most used in acute hospital trusts across the UK. The six essential parameters identified by NICE (2007), alongside an additional score for individuals requiring oxygen or presenting with new confusion are included in NEWS2. Deviations from normal parameters earn a score providing a total NEWS2 score, as outlined in Table 14.4. Those individuals with an elevated NEWS2 score are potentially at risk of deterioration.

In addition to the scoring system, the Royal College of Physicians (2017) provide an outline of responses to elevated NEWS2 scores and suggested frequency of monitoring, with higher scores requiring a more urgent response by a clinician or team with core competencies in the care of acutely ill adults (Table 14.5). Although the use of NEWS2 can support clinical decision making, it is important to remember that a normal NEWS2 score does not preclude calling for help when you consider that a person is unwell. NEWS2 does not replace clinical judgement.

Several technologies exist that integrate with electronic health record (EHR) systems and allow for the inputting of early warning score data (e.g., NEWS2 data) and the calculation of aggregate scores that automatically generate early warning score alerts, with the intention of improving the response to an individual at risk of deterioration.

Table 14.4 NEWS2 Score Royal College of Physicians (2017)

Physiological parameter	Score						
	3	2	1	0	1	2	3
Respiration rate (per minute)	≤8		9-11	12-20		21-24	≥25
SpO₂ Scale 1 (%)	≤91	92-93	94-95	≥96			
SpO₂ Scale 2 (%)	≤83	84-85	86-87	88-92 ≥93 on air	93-94 on oxygen	95-96 on oxygen	≥97 on oxygen
Air or oxygen?		Oxygen		Air			
Systolic blood pressure (mmHg)	≤90	91-100	101-110	111-219			≥220
Pulse (per minute)	≤40		41-50	51-90	91-110	111-130	≥131
Consciousness				Alert			CVPU
Temperature (°C)	≤35.0		35.1-36.0	36.1-38.0	38.1-39.0	≥39.1	

(Reproduced from Royal College of Physicians. National Early Warning Score (NEWS) 2: Standardising the assessment of acute illness severity in the NHS. Updated report of a working party. London: RCP, 2017. Available at: www.rcplondon.ac.uk/projects/outputs/national-early-warning-score-news-2. Please see the full-colour versions of the NEWS charts before making any clinical use of the information)

Table 14.5 Clinical response to the NEWS2 trigger thresholds

NEW score	Frequency of monitoring	Clinical response
0	Minimum 12 hourly	Continue routine NEWS monitoring
Total 1-4	Minimum 4-6 hourly	Inform registered nurse, who must assess the person Registered nurse decides whether increased frequency of monitoring and/or escalation of care is required
3 in single parameter	Minimum 1 hourly	Registered nurse to inform medical team caring for the person, who will review and decide whether escalation of care is necessary
Total 5 or more Urgent response threshold	Minimum 1 hourly	Registered nurse to immediately inform the medical team caring for the person Registered nurse to request urgent assessment by a clinician or team with core competencies in the care of acutely ill adults Provide clinical care in an environment with monitoring facilities
Total 7 or more Emergency response threshold	Continuous monitoring of vital signs	Registered nurse to immediately inform the medical team caring for the person – this should be at least at specialist registrar level Emergency assessment by a team with critical care competencies, including practitioner(s) with advanced airway management skills Consider transfer of care to a level 2 or 3 clinical care facility, i.e., higher-dependency unit or ICU Clinical care in an environment with monitoring facilities

Activity 14.4

The Royal College of Physicians, together with the Royal College of Nursing and the National Outreach Forum, have developed an online training programme in the use of NEWS2:

- Access and complete the short training course at the following website: https://news.ocbmedia.com/
- Calculate the NEWS scores on the following individuals and write down what action you think should be taken.

MARIANA AND RASHID

Mariana is 60 years old and recovering after a minor operation to remove a skin lesion. Post-operative observations are:

- Respiratory rate: 17 breaths/minute;
- Oxygen saturation: 97%;
- Blood pressure: 172/84mmHg;
- Heart rate: 74 beats/minute;
- Level of consciousness: alert ('A' on the ACVPU scale);
- Temperature 36.2°C.

The dressing is intact and there are no signs of discharge or bleeding from the wound.

Rashid is 74 years old and has been admitted with heart failure, complaining of feeling tired and short of breath. Supplementary oxygen 2 litres via nasal cannula has been commenced, with target saturations of 94-98%. Appearing drowsy, Rashid's current observations are:

- Respiratory rate: 22 breaths/minute;
- Oxygen saturation: 96% on supplemental oxygen;
- Blood pressure: 96/40mmHg;
- Heart rate: 104 beats/minute;
- Level of consciousness: responding to voice ('V' on the ACVPU scale);
- Temperature 37.4°C.

Mariana has a NEWS2 total score of 0. The outline clinical response suggested by the Royal College of Physicians (2017) would be to continue routine NEWS2 monitoring. Although it is worth noting that Mariana has a raised blood pressure, the Royal College of Physicians acknowledges that this is a risk factor for cardiovascular disease but that a low or falling blood pressure is of more significance in recognising a deteriorating adult.

On the other hand, Rashid has a NEWS2 total score of 10. The urgent or emergency response suggested by the Royal College of Physicians (2017) is outlined in Table 14.5. Although each individual component of Rashid's NEWS2 may not be considered at the extreme, when Rashid's condition is considered in its entirety it is evident that there is a considerable risk of clinical deterioration.

- What do you think are the limitations of the track-and-trigger system outlined above?
- What underpinning knowledge and understanding would you need to be able to interpret the above scores effectively?

Although track-and-trigger systems such as NEWS2 have been widely introduced across the UK, problems in identifying deteriorating adults still exist. Track-and-trigger systems rely on vital signs being monitored correctly and at the correct frequency. The nurse caring for an individual must recognise deterioration, take appropriate action and escalate appropriately, conveying the seriousness of their concerns to trigger an appropriate medical response. It has been identified that compliance with track-and-trigger systems is frequently poor and that there are often errors in early warning scoring and a failure to comply with clinical response recommendations (Odell, 2015). Additionally, Credland et al. (2018) recognise assessment and escalation of the deteriorating adult requires confidence and that individuals who are deteriorating may not be escalated due to the practitioner fearing they will instigate a false alarm and appear incompetent, often leading to delays in treatment and poorer outcomes. Coulter-Smith et al. (2013) also argue that systems such as these tend to focus on the core physiological indicators of severity and that these should be used together with sound clinical judgement based on experience rather than be seen as a replacement. Grant (2019) suggests the factors resulting in poor compliance with track-and-trigger systems are often exacerbated by the low priority given to the monitoring of vital signs and that undertaking clinical observations is a task often delegated to the lowest qualified members of staff.

The ABCDE approach to the assessment of the acutely ill adult

Although track-and-trigger systems are useful, on some occasions you might encounter an urgent or emergency situation where you are presented with a deteriorating or critically ill adult that calls for a rapid assessment to identify life-threatening problems quickly. In these circumstances, the Resuscitation Council UK (2021) advocate the use of the Airway, Breathing, Circulation, Disability, Exposure (ABCDE) approach to assessment. The order of the ABCDE facilitates the identification of the most severe life-threatening problems first. It is essential that you treat any issues that are identified as they arise, before continuing with your assessment, for example, an airway obstruction should be treated before moving onto resolving a circulatory problem. In urgent and emergency situations, it is also essential that you summon appropriate help early. Additionally, you must consider your own safety by checking the area is safe and that you 'don' personal and protective equipment as appropriate.

The steps of the ABCDE approach to assessment are briefly outlined below. You can find the full Resuscitation Council UK version at: www.resus.org.uk/library/abcde-approach

A – Airway assessment and management

Walz et al. (2007) recognise that the skill of airway management is important for any healthcare provider caring for acutely and critically ill adults. A person with a compromised airway will quickly deteriorate (Higginson et al., 2011). Problems with decreased levels of consciousness (assessed as part of Disability) can lead to airway compromise. Sandberg et al. (2013: 20) suggest that 'the awake, alert patient who is able to speak with a normal voice has no immediate threat to the airway'. The look, listen and feel approach is recommended to assess airway and breathing:

- **Look** – look at the person for signs of airway obstruction. These can include paradoxical (see-saw) breathing and cyanosis.
- **Listen** – listen for added noises that might indicate airway obstruction. This could be gurgling noises caused by liquids such as secretions, blood, or vomit; snoring, or stridor which is a high-pitched whistling sound and suggests laryngeal or tracheal obstruction.
- **Feel** – feel for breath against your cheek as you look for the chest rising and falling.
- Remove anything that might be obstructing the airway if you are confident you can do so safely. Liquid obstructions will need to be removed by suctioning, turning the person onto their side can also facilitate draining of fluids from the upper airway. Solid obstructions can be removed with your fingers or Magill's forceps **if safe to do so**, although you must be sure that you will not push the obstruction further into the airway.
- A head tilt chin lift can be used to open the airway; this manoeuvre lifts the tongue and the epiglottis away from the glottic opening.
- Airway adjuncts including nasopharyngeal, oropharyngeal airways and supraglottic airway devices are useful to help maintain a patent airway. Nasopharyngeal airways are particularly useful for people who are awake or semi-conscious; unlike oropharyngeal and supraglottic airways, they do not cause gagging.
- If the person is unconscious but breathing it might be appropriate to care for them in the lateral position whilst you closely monitor their condition.

Manage choking using the Resuscitation Council Adult Basic Life Support Guidelines (Perkins et al., 2021) available at: www.resus.org.uk/library/2021-resuscitation-guidelines/adult-basic-life-support-guidelines.

B – Breathing assessment and management

The monitoring and recording of respiratory rate is an essential nursing skill. An altered respiration rate is a significant predictor of serious health problems and life-threatening events; therefore, altered respiratory function needs to be recognised and treated early (Hill and Annesley, 2020). Ansell et al. (2014) report that nurses admit circumstances in which they miss observing respiratory rate. Taking and recording a person's respiratory rate is essential for assessing their condition and the respiratory rate should be counted for a full minute rather than trying to estimate.

- Observe the person for signs of cyanosis being mindful that people with darker skin tones might not look obviously cyanosed and you will need to check mucous membranes;
- Observe for laboured breathing and the use of accessory muscles;
- Assess the depth and pattern of breathing;
- Assess whether the rise and fall of the chest is equal on each side;
- Measure respiration rate, normal is 12-20 breaths/minute[-1;]
- Measure oxygen saturations using a pulse oximeter;
- Assess if the person can speak in full sentences;
- Listen for added breath sounds such as wheeze or rattling.

Cyanosis is a relatively late finding in an ill adult (McMullen and Patrick, 2013) and is associated with the presence or risk of serious illness requiring emergency treatment (Hill and Annesly, 2020). Moore (2007) notes that central cyanosis usually indicates circulatory or ventilatory problems whereas peripheral cyanosis usually indicates poor circulation.

- If safe to do so, consider moving the person into a position that can support their breathing, e.g., sitting upright.
- Oxygen therapy is a vital element in the care of an acutely ill adult. Oxygen is widely used in the treatment of a variety of conditions, and it is vital that nurses are safe, knowledgeable, and competent in its use. Both an inadequate or excessive oxygen dose may be potentially harmful. The British Thoracic Society (O'Driscoll et al., 2017) state that the lack of a prescription should not prevent oxygen being administered in an emergency. Give oxygen to maintain appropriate oxygen saturations. Target oxygen saturation for acutely ill adults not at risk of hypercapnic respiratory failure is 94–98%. The target oxygen saturation for individuals with known Chronic Obstructive Pulmonary Disease (COPD) or risk factors for hypercapnic respiratory failure is 88–92% (O'Driscoll et al., 2017). The oxygen therapy given must be recorded in the recipient's notes.
- If the person's breathing is inadequate or absent, administer breaths using a bag-valve mask or pocket mask if safe to do so.

Those responsible for administering oxygen need to monitor the recipient and aim to keep saturations within range by adjusting the oxygen delivery devices or flow rates. Monitoring of saturations and respiratory function after the administration of supplemental oxygen is essential.

There are several devices available for the delivery of oxygen including nasal cannula, a simple oxygen mask and a high-concentration reservoir mask (non-rebreathe mask). It is important to acknowledge that the concentration of oxygen that an individual receives depends not only on the flow rate but also on the type of mask and breathing pattern.

C – Circulation assessment and management

- Look at the colour of the person's skin and mucous membranes for signs of mottling and/or cyanosis, be aware that you might not be able to identify changes in skin colour in people with dark skin tones.
- Check the person's pulse. Although the pulse can be observed electronically, feeling the pulse manually can provide you with useful information. A weak and thready pulse potentially indicates hypovolaemia; a bounding pulse can suggest early sepsis and if the pulse is irregular the person may have a cardiac dysrythmia. Skin temperature can also be assessed while checking the pulse: is the person cool and clammy or warm to the touch?
- Monitor the person's blood pressure. An arbitrary figure of 120/80mmHg is given for a normal blood pressure, with a systolic blood pressure of less than 100mmHg or a drop of more than 40mmHg in systolic blood pressure suggesting hypotension and possible shock. A manual blood pressure using a sphygmomanometer must be taken on all individuals who have an irregular heart rhythm as inaccurate results can be obtained when using mechanical blood pressure machines in this group of people. Additionally, if an abnormal blood pressure is observed when using a blood pressure machine, this should always be rechecked manually.
- The capillary refill time (CRT) should also be assessed. CRT is measured by applying cutaneous pressure to the finger tip when held at heart level or pressing on the sternum for 5 seconds with enough pressure to cause blanching. The CRT is the time it takes for normal colour to return to the compressed skin once the pressure has been released. Normal CRT is less than 2 seconds with anything longer indicating poor perfusion, be mindful that this test might be less accurate in people with darker skin tones.
- Observe for fluid loss. Circulatory emergencies are frequently caused by hypovolaemia, observe for external haemorrhage, being mindful of the possibility of internal bleeding and other conditions such as sepsis that can cause relative hypovolamia.
- Consider 12 lead-electrocardiogram (ECG) and continuous 3-lead ECG monitoring reviewed by an appropriately trained healthcare professional. A 12-lead ECG can help identify other clinical problems such as an electrolyte imbalance (e.g., hypo-/hyperkalaemia).

The treatment of cardiovascular problems will depend on the cause but is typically directed at fluid replacement.

- Insert two large bore cannulas. IV access is important, particularly if a person is at risk of hypovolaemia or in need of fluid resuscitation. The National Institute for Health and Care Excellence (NICE, 2013) has produced guidelines for IV fluid therapy for adults in hospital. The guidelines suggest that an individual's fluid and electrolyte requirements are identified using the 5Rs: resuscitation, routine maintenance, replacement, redistribution, and reassessment. Although many of these guidelines are aimed at prescribers it is important to acknowledge that managing hydration is a fundamental nursing role (Ugboma and Cowen, 2012). Indicators that an individual may need urgent fluid resuscitation include the following:

○ Systolic blood pressure <100 mmHg;
○ Heart rate >90 beats/minute;
○ CRT >2 seconds or peripheries are cold to the touch;
○ Respiratory rate >20 breaths/minute;
○ NEWS ≥5;
○ Passive leg raising suggests fluid responsiveness (NICE, 2013).

• Take blood samples for haematological, biochemical and coagulation investigations and crossmatch blood if haemorrhage is suspected.
• If an individual is in hypovolemic shock, infuse intravenous (IV) fluid according to local or national guidelines. IV therapy is a common intervention that does not always get the attention it deserves. Although commonplace, it is easy to become complacent. NCEPOD (1999) reported that up to one in five people receiving IV fluids in hospital could experience complications or morbidity because of their inappropriate use. Urinary output and fluid balance should also be monitored carefully. A decreased urinary output can be a sign of decreased renal perfusion. NICE (2019) recognise a urinary output of less than 0.5ml/kg per hour as a clinical characteristic of acute kidney injury. Reassess the person every 5 minutes.
• Monitor the person for signs of cardiac failure (signs include dyspnoea, reduced oxygen saturations and pulmonary crackles on auscultation). If cardiac failure is suspected reduce, or stop the intravenous fluid infusion.

D – Disability assessment and management

• Assess level of consciousness. This is typically done using the ACVPU scale in an emergency situation, though the Glasgow Coma Scale (GCS) can provide additional useful information and is recommended when assessing the conscious level of individuals suspected to have sustained a traumatic brain injury. The ACVPU scale is part of NEWS2 and is performed as outlined in Table 14.6 below.

The GCS (Table 14.7) was originally developed to measure the conscious level of adults with a traumatic brain injury, but has also been adopted in other fields including neurosurgery and emergency medicine. The best possible score is 15 out of 15 and the worst 3 out of 15. When documenting the GCS it is important to record not only the total score (i.e., a GCS of 13/15) but also the components of that score (e.g., a GCS of 13/15, i.e., eyes 3, verbal 4, motor 6).

Table 14.6   ACVPU scale

A – Alert	The person is aware of their environment and opens their eyes spontaneously.
C – Confused	The person exhibits new confusion or altered mental state. The person may have a history of confusion and you will need to assess whether they are more confused than before, you might need to ask the person's friend or relative if they have noticed that the person is more confused then normal if you are unsure. You can assess whether the person is orientated to person, place and time by asking them the following questions and checking their responses. Orientated to person: Who are you? Orientated to place: Where are you? Orientated to time: What day is it/what time is it/ is it morning or afternoon?
V – Voice	The person's eyes do not open spontaneously but in response to a verbal stimulus directed towards them.
P – Pain	The person does not open their eyes spontaneously or to verbal stimuli. The person responds to pain applied by squeezing the person's trapezius muscle or applying pressure to the nail beds.
U – Unresponsive	The person does not move, open their eyes or make any sounds.

Table 14.7   The Glasgow Coma Scale

Score	Eye Opening (E)	Best verbal response (V)	Best motor response (M)
6			Obeys commands
5		Orientated to time and place	Localises to pain
4	Eyes open spontaneously	Confused	Withdrawal from pain
3	Eyes open to speech	Inappropriate words	Flexion to pain
2	Eyes open to pain	Incomprehensible sounds	Extension to pain
1	No eye opening	No verbal response	No motor response

(Source: Teasdale, G. and Jennett, B. (1974) 'Assessment of coma and impaired consciousness: a practical scale', *The Lancet*, 304(7872): 81–4)

Activity 14.5

Access and review nurse.org's page on understanding and interpreting the Glasgow Coma Scale at: https://nurse.org/articles/glasgow-coma-scale/

What conditions might cause a patient to lose consciousness?

What other tests or assessments might be useful?

Further observations that are monitored in the disability section of the ABCDE assessment include blood glucose level (BGL) and pain:

- Normal BGL is typically considered to be between 4-7mmol/L. Although hyperglycaemia should be avoided, hypoglycaemia is a more common problem in hospital patients and is associated with a reduced conscious level. For people experiencing hypo/hyperglycaemia follow local guidelines for the management. Hypoglycaemia is a serious condition and should be treated as an emergency regardless of the person's level of consciousness (Joint British Diabetes Societies for Inpatient Care, 2022).
- Pain can be a useful indicator of the cause of a person's deteriorating condition and will be discussed in detail later in this chapter.
- If the person is displaying signs of altered conscious level seek appropriate help immediately.
- Place an unconscious but breathing person in the lateral position.

E - Exposure assessment and management

- This is a head-to-toe check for anything not already discovered on the ABCD check that may suggest a cause for a person being unwell. Fully expose the person whilst maintaining their dignity;
- Perform a head-to-toe, front and back check of the person to observe for clues that might explain the person's condition (e.g., rashes, bruising, bleeding, or swelling);
- Feel the person's skin temperature;
- Measure core temperature;
- Treat any issues identified;
- Provide extra blankets if the person feels cold;
- Seek advice on treating pyrexia and screen the person for sepsis.

Evidence-Based Interventions in Acute Care

Jim

Jim, a 56 year-old, had a bowel resection to remove a tumour 3 days ago. The surgery was uneventful and the surgeons are confident that the entire tumour has been removed in time, that it has not spread and therefore that this is a curative operation. Jim has a urinary catheter, one peripheral cannula in the left forearm and a central line. You are the nurse looking after Jim this evening. You have just been given a handover. On your initial assessment you find that:

A: Jim is talking to you.

B: Jim has a slightly elevated respiratory rate (18) and is receiving 4 L/min of oxygen via nasal specs: oxygen saturations are 95%.

C: Jim's pulse rate is 92 and manual blood pressure is 135/60;

D: Jim is alert and pain free.

E: There are no obvious rashes, the wound on examination looks clean and dry, and the abdomen looks 'normal.'

Two hours later, the person in the bed next to Jim summons you over saying that Jim does not look well. You re-examine Jim and on examination you find:

A: Jim responds to questions.

B: Jim's respiratory rate is now 22, and oxygen saturations are 92% on 4 L/min via nasal specs.

C: Jim's pulse rate is now 110, and manual blood pressure is 95/40; Jim appears flushed with a temperature of 37.8°C.

D: Jim's pain score is 8/10.

E: The surgical wound looks red.

- What do you think is happening? Write down in detail the physiological responses and consider what is happening and how this has affected Jim's cardiovascular system, e.g., which component (heart, vessels, and blood) is compensating.
- What would you do next?

Sepsis

The changes to Jim's cardiovascular and respiratory function could be a result of the body's response to infection, also known as sepsis. Although the source of this infection appears to be from Jim's wound site, given the information above, Jim has several potential sites of infection that could be the cause of sepsis: the surgical procedure, the intravenous access, and the urinary catheter.

Sepsis and severe infection are the most common cause of inpatient deterioration in the UK (Daniels and Nutbeam, 2022). Sepsis is defined as *'a life-threatening organ dysfunction caused by a dysregulated host response to infection'* (Singer et al., 2016: 804). *'Septic shock is a subset of sepsis where particularly profound circulatory, cellular and metabolic abnormalities substantially increase mortality'* (Singer et al., 2016: 806).

Sepsis arises when the body's response to infection injures it's own tissues and organs, and can lead to shock, organ failure and death if not recognised and treated early (Daniels and Nutbeam, 2022). Both NICE (2017) and the UK Sepsis Trust (Daniels and Nutbeam, 2022) have developed guidance on the screening and management of individuals who are suspected to have sepsis.

They suggest any individual whose NEWS2 score triggers action should be screened for sepsis. Depending on the severity of the individual's condition, they are categorised into either 'amber flag' or 'red flag' sepsis, with 'red flag' sepsis requiring initiation of the Sepsis Six, unless contraindicated.

Activity 14.6

- Identify and familiarise yourself with the SEPSIS screening and management tool used in your clinical area.
- What underpinning knowledge and understanding do you require to use this tool?
- Do you think that there are any limitations to using this tool?

The Sepsis Six (The UK Sepsis Trust, 2018) is a set of interventions to be performed in the first hour of suspected sepsis, which can improve survival. These are as follows:

1 Ensure senior clinician attends;
2 Give oxygen if required;
3 Send blood samples including blood cultures and obtain I.V access;
4 Give intravenous antibiotics and consider source control;
5 Give IV fluids;
6 Monitor NEWS-2 and urine output.

Sepsis is a complex condition that requires prompt diagnosis and management to prevent poor outcomes associated with delays in treatment. Utilising the screening and management tools available to you and getting appropriate help quickly will facilitate the acutely unwell adult receiving timely and appropriate treatment and is likely to result in improved patient outcomes.

SBAR Communication Tool

As we have already outlined, the ABCDE assessment, track-and-trigger systems and sepsis screening aid recognition of the acutely ill adult. An appropriate response together with immediate lifesaving interventions is likely to include a call for help. Clear and effective communication is essential to provide effective care and maintain a person's safety and the 'SBAR' communication tool can aid this (NICE, 2018). SBAR is a communication tool that can be used to help provide structure to this important conversation when reporting a clinical deterioration in an acutely unwell adult. SBAR was originally used by US Navy nuclear submarine personnel; it was adapted for healthcare use by Leonard et al. (2004) and is recommended by the World Health Organization (2007b).

The SBAR acronym stands for **s**ituation, **b**ackground, **a**ssessment, and **r**ecommendation. Table 14.8 provides more detail on the five elements of the SBAR framework.

The use of SBAR may help to deliver critical information effectively and promote patient safety. Müller et al. (2018) performed a systematic review that found evidence of safety improvements through using SBAR. Beliveau (cited in Buttaro and Barba, 2012) suggests that if SBAR

Table 14.8   Example use of the SBAR Framework

SBAR element	Example
Situation: What is happening now?	Hello, my name is Derek, I am the staff nurse on ward 44 and I am calling about Prem Patel. I am concerned because the NEWS2 score has increased from 3 to 6.
Background	Prem was admitted yesterday with abdominal pain, anorexia, nausea and vomiting and was diagnosed with an acute appendicitis. Prem has no previous medical history.
Assessment: What you think is the problem?	Prem is scoring 2 for the respiration rate, 1 for SpO$_2$ scale, 1 because the systolic BP has dropped to 105mmHg and 2 for the pulse. Prem is complaining of feeling increasingly unwell, has started vomiting again and is reporting that pain has increased from moderate to severe. I have given analgesia and antiemetic as prescribed, but this does not appear to be helping. I think Prem may be developing sepsis.
Recommendation: What should be done to correct the situation?	In accordance with NEWS2 and Sepsis Trust recommendations, I would like Prem to receive an urgent review from a Specialty Trainee 3 doctor or above. How soon can you get here? I am going to take some bloods, is there anything else you would like me to do in the meantime?

Adapted from Burgess et al. (2020).

is used consistently, not only will the first responder understand how to gather, organise and report appropriate information quickly and concisely, but also the recipient of this information can anticipate how it will be conveyed. A study by DeMeester et al. (2013) found that after the introduction of SBAR across 16 hospital wards, there was an increased perception of effective communication between nurses and doctors and a reduction in unexpected deaths. It is important to remember the listening skills necessary for the receiver.

Activity 14.7

Revisit the earlier case scenario about Jim. How would you report the changes in Jim's condition to the nurse in charge or medical staff? Write down the conversation you would have using the SBAR tool as a guide.

Your response to Activity 14.7 should have included the following.

Situation

Identify yourself and where you are calling from. Identify which person you are calling about and briefly the reason for the call. Leonard et al. (2004) advocates the use of powerful 'critical language' such as 'I'm concerned, this is unsafe', or 'I'm worried' because that will have the effect of gaining the necessary attention of the receiver.

Background

You need to relay relevant information, including the reason for admission, relevant past medical/surgical history, and current management.

Assessment

Convey what you found on your ABCDE assessment of the person. You should include the NEWS-2 score and if it is helpful, bring relevant information such as the observation chart/notes to the phone when making the call to ensure that you have all the relevant information to hand. You can then state what you think is going on.

Recommendation

You should have a clear idea of what you would like to happen because of your call. Are you calling for advice? Do you want an urgent assessment? Alternatively, are you simply providing an update? Do you think that the person should be transferred to another clinical area such as ICU? You can make suggestions for actions: 'I would like you to ....'

Acute Pain Management

Pain is a common occurrence in hospitalised individuals with approximately 70% reporting pain (Wu et al., 2020).

Pain is an individual subjective sensation that not only involves a physical sensation, but is also influenced by psychological, environmental, and social factors. How an individual interprets the physiological signal depends on numerous factors and includes the type and site of tissue damage, previous experience of pain, age, gender, psychological factors, such as anxiety, and social and environmental influences (Gregory, 2017). The International Association for Pain (IASP, 2020:1) defines acute pain as *'an unpleasant sensory and emotional experience associated with, or resembling that associated with, actual or potential tissue damage'*. Acute pain is a short-term symptom often described as a warning, for example in chest pain, pancreatitis, or bone fracture. Acute pain usually resolves if treated and tends to respond to analgesia and other interventions (Macintyre and Schug, 2021). When pain occurs, a physiological stress response is stimulated leading to changes in vital signs including an increase in respiratory rate, heart rate and blood pressure. However, these changes should not be relied on when identifying pain as this stress response can be sustained for a certain length of time and will depend on the general health of the individual. The stress response also has a wider effect on bodily systems, which can cause deterioration in a person's condition if the pain is not treated effectively (Macintyre and Schug, 2021) (Table 14.9).

Table 14.9 The effects of unrelieved pain

Bodily system	Effects of pain stress response
Respiratory	Increased respiratory rate – shallow breathing Avoidance of deep breaths and coughing Increase risk of chest infection Increased risk of pulmonary embolism
Cardiovascular	Increased heart rate and raised BP Increased need for oxygen for cardiac tissue
Gastro-intestinal	Slow gastric emptying and peristalsis Nausea and vomiting Constipation Poor nutrition
Muscular skeletal	Immobility Loss of muscle tone Joint stiffness Increased risk of moisture lesions and deep vein thrombosis
Sleep and rest	Insomnia Poor recovery Reduced ability to cope, irritability
Psychological	Increased anxiety and fear Depression Anger Loss of confidence in healthcare professionals' ability
Long term	Increased risk of chronic pain is associated with poorly controlled acute pain

Effects of unrelieved pain

Pain is recognised as the fifth vital sign. As such, pain scores are incorporated into vital sign monitoring, although is not included in scoring systems used to identify a deterioration in individuals such as the NEWS2 (RCP, 2017). A high pain score and altered vital signs should prompt interventions to reduce pain, leading to a return to the individual's usual physiological measures and prevent potential complications that can occur because of the stress response (Schug et al., 2015; Swift, 2018).

Previously in this chapter, enhanced recovery after surgery (ERAS) was described. ERAS protocols and pathways recognise the importance of controlling pain and have incorporated pain management strategies into the preoperative and postoperative pathways to reduce the pain experience, preventing deterioration and facilitating rapid recovery after surgery.

Assessment of pain

Lukas et al. (2013) describe the assessment of pain as fundamental to ensuring appropriate and effective pain interventions to improve care outcomes, with the pain management process beginning with the recognition and assessment of pain followed by analgesia and/or non-pharmacological interventions which are evaluated with the recipient to ensure that they are effective and appropriate (Macintyre, 2021). Pain scales or tools provide a standard means of assessing and measuring pain. Using assessment tools and reassessing an individual's report of pain regularly can aid the evaluation and planning of treatment (Wood, 2008). Many pain assessment scales that ask individuals to rate their pain exist and these have been found to be easy to use and are described as highly valid and reliable. The successful use of these pain scales depends on a person's ability to use them as well as the accurate interpretation of the scores.

- How is pain assessed in your current clinical practice area?
- Have you observed the use of observational pain assessment tools?
- How effective are the tools in identifying and assessing pain?

The identification and assessment of pain is more complex than obtaining a pain score by simply asking someone 'have you any pain today?' According to Hjermstad et al. (2011), pain intensity is the most clinically relevant dimension of the pain experience; hence, it is the most assessed element of pain using the one-dimensional scales described in Table 14.10.

Table 14.10 Self-report pain assessment scales

The pain assessment tool or scale	Description	Strengths	Limitations
Visual analogue scale (VAS).	Consists of a 10cm line with anchor words at each end of the line from 'no pain' to 'worst pain imaginable'. A mark on the line is made by the individual experiencing pain with a pen or pencil and is measured on the line A plastic or metal slide-ruler may be used as an alternative to paper.	Provides an accurate measure of pain. Used in research studies. Can be written in different languages.	Complicated and requires cognitive skills. Time-consuming. Requires special equipment. Difficult to use for people with visual impairment and dexterity problems Inappropriate for people with cognitive impairment.
Numerical rating scale (NRS).	Pain is rated as a number (0-10) with 0 indicating no pain and 10 the worse pain imaginable.	Quick and easy to use for people who can communicate effectively. Suitable for all ages. Highly valid and reliable. The numbers are sensitive to small changes in pain. The NRS can overcome problems of visual and physical impairment associated with VAS.	Difficult to use with language barriers. Some people have difficulty rating their pain as a number. Inappropriate to use with an individual who is cognitively impaired.

(Continued)

Table 14.10   Self-report pain assessment scales (*Continued*)

The pain assessment tool or scale	Description	Strengths	Limitations
Verbal descriptor scale (VDS).	Individuals are asked to indicate which descriptor describes their pain. Examples of descriptors are: No pain. Mild pain. Moderate pain. Severe pain.	Quick and easy to use. Valid and fits with the WHO analgesic ladder. Often the preferred scale for use in older people. Royal College of Physicians, British Geriatrics Society and British Psychological Society suggest it is useful for older people with mild-to-moderate cognitive impairment.	The ratings are subject to a person's interpretation of the words. Lacks the sensitivity of NRS.
Numerical verbal descriptor scale (NVDS).	The individual with pain is asked to indicate which descriptor describes their pain, as above, and this is then given a numerical score by the nurse/carer. For example: No pain = 0. Mild pain = 1. Moderate pain = 2. Severe pain = 3.	As above for VDS. Quick and easy to use. The numerical score enables quick documentation.	The ratings are subject to a person's interpretation of the words. Lacks the sensitivity of NRS. Some nurses ask a person to rate their pain between 0 and 3 rather than asking them to describe the pain. The numbers can be confused with an NRS.

A more comprehensive assessment would also include several factors, such as how pain affects the individual's activities of daily living. To explore pain in more depth you could use one of the mnemonics described earlier, such as OLD CARTS or SOCRATES.

When an individual cannot communicate and describe their pain (e.g., those with a learning disability, cognitive impairment, or dementia), pain may be assessed through observing behaviours. Numerous observational behavioural pain assessment tools have been devised, for example the Critical Care Pain Observation Tool (CPOT; Gelinas et al., 2006); in addition to observing facial expression and agitation, the CPOT relies on physiological changes to help identify pain. The Abbey Scale (Abbey et al., 2004) and the Pain Assessment in Advanced Dementia Scale (Warden et al., 2003) have been developed for people living with dementia. The tools devised for people with dementia include verbalisation, facial expression, body movements, changes in interaction, and changes in their activities of living and mental status changes. The Abbey Tool also includes physiological changes and any physical damage that may be causing pain.

Activity 14.8

Precious

Precious, a 65 year-old who has fallen downstairs at home, is admitted into A&E complaining of severe right ankle pain. On admission observations are as follows:

A: Precious can speak to you in full sentences.

B: Respiratory rate is 28, respirations are shallow and oxygen saturations are 95% on room air.

C: Pulse is 112, strong and regular, and blood pressure is 185/90.

D: Precious is alert and orientated but very distressed and the pain score is 9/10.

E: Precious is clammy and sweaty. There is minimal bruising observed to Precious's right arm and ankle but you are aware that bruising in individuals with darker skin is often more difficult to see than bruising in individuals with lighter skin. You can see swelling to the ankle.

- What do you think is Precious' main problem?
- What might happen if this is not resolved?

The A&E doctor has requested an X-ray of Precious' ankle, As the nurse responsible for the provision of care in this instance:

- Would you be happy to send Precious straight to radiology?
- What care would be appropriate before transfer?

Precious is prescribed the following analgesia:

- Morphine IV, 10 mg PRN.
- Morphine orally, 10-20 mg 2-4 hourly.
- Paracetamol 1 gram, orally or IV, QDS.

What do you feel is the most appropriate analgesia, and by which route would you administer it?

Describe how and what you would monitor for Precious: how frequently would you do this?

What other possible side-effects would you monitor?

Is there any other analgesia that may help?

Once Precious' pain is controlled, how would you expect the ABCDE observations to alter?

Pain Management Interventions

Once pain is identified and assessed, it is managed using pharmacological and/or non- pharmacological interventions, often in combination. It is important that adult nurses understand the pain management options available. We have established that pain is an individual experience and, as such, the effectiveness of interventions can vary between individuals, with wide differences in the reaction to interventions

Pharmacological pain management

There is a choice of analgesic drugs available, depending on the nature and severity of the pain and the individual's reaction to medication. It is important that you advise people of the benefits of reducing their pain and reiterating that analgesia needs to be taken regularly to prevent pain rather than waiting for pain and then taking analgesia. This is because waiting for pain leads to 'chasing the pain' rather than managing or controlling it.

The WHO's analgesic ladder

The use of analgesia for all types of pain has been based on the WHO's (1986) analgesic ladder which was initially introduced for palliative care. It has steps that guide us in the use of analgesia. There are three main classes of analgesic medication - paracetamol (simple analgesia), non-steroidal anti-inflammatory drugs (NSAIDs) and opioids/opiates. These medications are well established and are incorporated into the WHO's analgesic ladder. The analgesic ladder relates to the intensity of pain:

Step 1 = mild pain, paracetamol and NSAID;
Step 2 = moderate pain, paracetamol, NSAID and mild opiate;
Step 3 = severe pain, paracetamol, NSAID and strong opiate;

For acute severe pain it is appropriate to start at Step 3, but if the assessment indicates mild pain, Step 1 would be appropriate followed by reassessment of the pain to evaluate the effectiveness of the analgesia administered.

Simple analgesia

Paracetamol can be administered IV, orally as tablets, capsules, syrup, or soluble preparations or rectally (although it should be avoided in active liver disease). The daily maximum dose of 4 grams should never be exceeded because it can cause liver damage and/or failure. The IV dose of paracetamol should be calculated on weight at 15mgs/kg. It is important to check that a person is not taking any other medication that may contain paracetamol, such as cough and flu remedies, or combination analgesia.

Non-steroidal anti-inflammatory drugs

Ibuprofen, diclofenac, and naproxen are examples of non-steroidal anti-inflammatory drugs (NSAIDs). They can be taken orally, IV, rectally or applied as a gel for mild-to-moderate musculoskeletal pain. They act by blocking the prostaglandins responsible for some of the inflammatory response to tissue damage (Bond and Simpson, 2006). Systematic reviews of randomised controlled trials of NSAIDs have found them to be very effective for the mild to moderate pain associated with many conditions including dysmenorrhea, joint and muscle pain, post-surgical pain, and toothache.

Opioid analgesia

Opioid analgesia is derived from the opium poppy and is regulated under the *Misuse of Drugs Act*. Strong opioids are classed as controlled drugs (CDs; see Chapter 6). A prescription is therefore always required for opioid analgesia. Opiates are agonist-type drugs that combine with opiate receptors distributed throughout the central nervous system (Bond and Simpson, 2006). They interfere with the transmission of the pain signal within the spinal cord and change an individual's perception of the pain (Williams and Salerno, 2012). Systematic reviews have found opioids to be more effective when used in combination with paracetamol and NSAIDs (Doherty et al., 2011).

When caring for a person using opioid analgesia it is important to consider potential side effects and carefully monitor their reaction to the medication. Anticipate constipation and inform the individual of this potential side effect and that laxatives may be required. Antiemetics may also be required initially, and antihistamines can help with itchiness and any rash caused by opioids. Many healthcare professionals and members of the public fear addiction and will avoid using opioid analgesia as a result. However, addiction is rare when analgesia is required and the importance of good pain control should always be emphasised (Gregory, 2014).

Morphine is considered the cornerstone of pain relief for severe pain. It is cheap and available in many forms, orally and parentally. The dose of morphine required for individuals varies in its ability to provide similar pain relief. The dose needs to be adjusted according to the person's reaction (Bond and Simpson, 2006). Patient-controlled analgesia (PCA) is a system commonly used after surgery, which aims to overcome some of this individual variation. PCA is a device (usually electronic) that enables the individual to deliver a small, predetermined dose of opioid intravenously via a demand button or handset. There is a 'lockout' safety feature, which means a person does not receive the selected opioid more than every five minutes.

Inhaled analgesia

Nitrous Oxide 50% and Oxygen 50% (Entonox) is a medical gas indicated for procedural pain. It has been traditionally used in maternity and emergency departments, and increasingly in hospital wards and departments for painful procedures such as wound care. Effects are quick, within a few deep breaths; it is easy to use and provides an individual with an element of control and distraction from the procedure. Nitrous Oxide is safe to use with other analgesics, and is considered safe for all age groups. It's main side effect is nausea (Gregory, 2008).

Methoxyflurane (penthrox) is another form of inhaled analgesia; however, it is only licensed for use in moderate to severe pain associated with trauma and should only be administered under close medical supervision (Joint Formulary Committee, 2022).

Non-pharmacological pain interventions

Pain is not just a physical event. It responds to a variety of treatments and often a combination of strategies is used to provide pain relief. This section examines some of the non-pharmacological and less invasive interventions that may be used alongside analgesia to help pain.

Psychological interventions help people to cope with pain and are also known as cognitive-behavioural therapies. These can be simple or complex interventions. The aim of these interventions is to decrease or change an individual's perception of pain. It is important to remember that an ability to distract someone from pain does not indicate that the pain is not real; believing the person during the assessment and encouraging the use of distraction are therapeutic. Some of the strategies include the use of distraction, music therapy, meditation, guided imagery, and relaxation.

Physical therapy can help reduce pain. Exercise helps to maintain joints and muscles, and it stimulates the body's natural pain relief - endorphins. The use of hot or cold can help alleviate pain. Heat in the form of a heat pad or a warm bath can help an individual to relax. Heat increases vasodilation and increases the blood supply to the affected area. Cold packs have the opposite effect and cause constriction of the blood vessels; in acute inflammation, this can reduce swelling and pain. A trans-electrical nerve stimulation (TENS) machine stimulates touch sensations which can override some of the pain stimulus; it also acts as a distraction. Complementary therapies can also be helpful for some people and include acupuncture, aromatherapy, and reflexology; these therapies can be provided only by therapists who have undergone approved training programmes.

Evaluation of pain management

Evaluation or reassessment of pain to establish the effectiveness of interventions is as important as the initial assessment. Has the pain score reduced? Is the person able to complete their normal activities of daily living (ADLs)? It is important to monitor side effects such as gastric irritation and constipation as part of the evaluation to ensure they continue with their medication. If nausea and vomiting are experienced, they are likely to refuse to continue with analgesia because they can tolerate the pain better than vomiting. Alternative medications may be required, and/or if the analgesia is not effective then a gradual increase or titration of the dose may be necessary to provide adequate pain relief with less severe side effects. The use of non-pharmacological interventions can be suggested and encouraged once the pain has become tolerable. For many individuals, an increase or improvement in activity may be as important as the reduction of pain intensity and should be included in the evaluation of pain management interventions.

Caring for a Group of Adults

Aston et al. (2010: 108) identify a series of items that the nurse needs to consider when caring for a group of adults:

- How you utilise information that has been handed over to you by previous staff;
- Deciding if you need more information;
- Assessing or reassessing people in your care;
- Prioritising care;
- Planning care;
- Deciding what to delegate and to whom you can delegate;
- How to manage time efficiently;
- How to respond to changes/incidents/issues that arise;
- Adapting your initial plans.

Indeed, there are several factors to consider in prioritising care for a group of people or just one individual. Time management and prioritising care are interlinked. Although you should always have a person-centred approach to care and avoid considering care provision as simply 'tasks to be done,' a 'to-do list' can help you focus. Making a list can also make it easier to prioritise and delegate. This prioritisation can lead to a plan of care. As you will now be aware, it is important to plan care in collaboration with recipients of care because what the person you are caring for considers most important may vary from your perspective on what is important. **It is the person and not the task that is the priority**. It is important that any plan of care is not considered a fixed or permanent schedule, because priorities can and do change.

In thinking about how to manage time effectively you should consider if there is the potential for multi-tasking. It is important that you use the best evidence available to support your decision making. Priority setting is based on assessment. As a nurse, you will need to be flexible and able to adapt to changing priorities and demands. You should remember that you are providing care as part of a team and that effective teamwork can positively impact care outcomes. A nurse must work in a collaborative manner to ensure the safe provision of care.

Enhancing a Person-Centred Experience

Within the NHS there has been a progression in the way that the quality of the care being provided is assessed. Although traditional measures looking at clinical effectiveness (e.g., standardised mortality ratios) and safety have unquestionable significance, the importance of the service-user experience is now recognised. The National Institute for Health and Care Excellence (2012a, 2012b) has produced clinical guidance and a set of quality standards on improving the experience of care for people using adult NHS services. These documents contain some key themes, including providing an individualised service, family, and carer involvement, getting the basics right and clear communication.

Access some of the friends and family test data from the website below:

www.england.nhs.uk/fft/friends-and-family-test-data/

As an adult nurse working in an acute care setting, what could you do to try to enhance the experience of those you care for?

Chapter Summary

Nurses have a significant role in ensuring safe care provision. This chapter has discussed the knowledge, skills and attributes needed by adult nurses working in an acute care setting. We have also focused on the knowledge and skills needed in the assessment, recognition and management of acutely ill adults. The signs of clinical deterioration can happen many hours before a cardiac arrest. Early detection of deterioration gives an opportunity to improve care outcomes by providing timely and appropriate intervention. NEWS2 is a valuable tool in achieving this, but it is important to remember that if you are concerned about a person's safety and are not sure what to do, you should call for help. A comprehensive assessment using the ABCDE approach and use of the SBAR communication tool can help you in these situations.

Medical technology is part of the modern healthcare environment and is not limited to critical care areas. Although the 'technical' aspects of nursing may be appealing to nurses working in acute care, these cannot and must not be promoted at the expense of providing compassionate nursing care. A nurse should use appropriate technology for the benefit of all individuals but also be aware of the potential of over reliance. For example, a nurse should not have to rely on pulse oximetry to be able to identify that a person with an increased respiratory rate, who is cyanotic, using accessory muscles and unable to talk in complete sentences with an audible wheeze, is unwell.

Pain assessment and management are also fundamental aspects of the registered nurse's role. Sometimes this can be difficult, particularly when dealing with acutely ill and vulnerable people. However, there are tools and strategies available to help us to manage pain effectively, thereby improving the overall experience of acute care.

The profile of adults cared for in an acute setting and the way that care is provided are changing. Individuals who have a greater level of acuity tend to be older and have more co-morbidity. Acute care environments need to adapt to these changes. It is important to remember that the acute care environment can be a scary place for individuals and their families.

Further Reading

Adam, S., Odell, M., Welch, J. (2010) *Rapid Assessment of the Acutely Ill Patient*. Chichester: John Wiley and Sons.

Bickley, L.S. (2020) *Bates' Guide to Physical Examination and History Taking*, 13th edn. Philadelphia, PA: Lippincott, Williams & Wilkins.

British Geriatric Society (2021) *Quality urgent care for older people (Silver Book II)*. Available at: www. bgs.org.uk/resources/resource-series/silver-book-ii (last accessed 12 August 2022).

British Geriatric Society/Centre for Peri-operative Care (2021) *Care for People living with Frailty Undergoing Elective and Emergency Surgery*. Available at: www.bgs.org.uk/cpocfrailty. (last accessed 12 August 2022).

Clarke, D. and Ketchell, A. (2016) *Nursing the Acutely Ill Adult*. London: Palgrave Macmillan.

Page, K. and Mckinney, A. (2012) (eds), *Nursing the Acutely Ill Adult Case Book*. Oxford: Oxford University Press.

Peate, I. (2020) *Alexander's Nursing Practice: Hospital and Home*, 5th edn. London: Churchill Livingstone.

Resuscitation Council UK (2021) *Immediate Life Support Manual*, 5th edn. London: Resuscitation Council UK.

References

Abbey, J.A., Piller, N., DeBellis, A., Esterman, A., Parker, D., Giles, L. and Lowcay, B. (2004) 'The Abbey Pain Scale: a 1-minute numerical indicator for people with late-stage dementia', *International Journal of Palliative Nursing*, 10(1): 6–13.

Al-Moteri, M., Plummer, V., Cooper, S. and Symmone, M. (2019) 'Clinical deterioration of ward patients in the presence of antecedents: a systematic review and narrative synthesis', *Australian Critical Care*, 32(5): 411–20.

Aning, J., Neal, D., Driver, A. and McGrath, J. (2010) 'Enhanced recovery: from principles to practice in urology', *BJU International*, 105(9): 1199–201.

Ansell, H., Meyer. A. and Thompson, S. (2014) 'Why don't nurses consistently take patient respiration rates?' *British Journal of Nursing*, 23 (8): 414-418'

Aston, L., Wakefield, J. and McGown, R. (eds) (2010) *The Student Nurse Guide to Decision Making in Practice*. Maidenhead: Open University Press.

Blomaard, L.C., de Groot, B., Lucke, J.A., de Gelder, J., Booijen, A.M., Gussekloo, J. and Mooijaart, S.P. (2021) 'Implementation of the acutely presenting older patient (APOP) screening program in routine emergency department care. A before and after study,' *Zeitschrift für Gerontologie und Geriatrie*, 54(2): 113–21.

Bond, M.R. and Simpson, K.H. (2006) *Pain: Its Nature and Treatment*. Edinburgh: Churchill Livingstone.

Burgess, A., van Diggele, C., Roberts, C. and Mellis, C. (2020) 'Teaching clinical handover with ISBAR', *BMC Med Educ*, 20, 459. Available at: https://bmcmededuc.biomedcentral.com/articles/10.1186/s12909-020-02285-0 (last accessed 2 August 2022).

Buttaro, T.M. and Barba, K.M. (eds) (2012) *Nursing Care of the Hospitalized Older Patient*. Oxford: Wiley-Blackwell.

Casey, A., Coen, E., Gleeson, M. and Walsh, R. (2016) *Setting the Direction – a development framework supporting nursing practice skills and competencies in acute medical assessment units (amaus) and medical assessment units (maus)*. Dublin: HSE. Available at: www.hse.ie/eng/about/who/cspd/ncps/acute-medicine/developmental-framework-acute-medicine-nursing.pdf (last accessed 6 May 2022).

Conroy, S. and Cooper, N. (2010) *Acute Medical Care of Elderly People*. London: British Geriatric Society.

Conroy, S. and Thomas, M. (2021) 'Urgent care for older people', *Age and Ageing,* 51(1). Available at: https://doi.org/10.1093/ageing/afab019 (last accessed 1 August 2022).

Coulter-Smith, M.A., Smith, P. and Crow, R. (2013) 'Critical review: a combined conceptual framework of severity of illness and clinical judgement for analysing diagnostic judgement in critical illness', *Journal of Clinical Nursing*, 23: 784–98.

Corrado, O., Swanson, B., Hood, C., Morris A., Ofili, S., Capistrano, J., Butler, J. and Bourke, L. (2019) *National Audit of Dementia Care in General Hospitals 2018–2019 Round Four Audit Report*. Available at: www.hqip.org.uk/wp-content/uploads/2019/07/ref-113-national-audit-of-dementia-round-4-report-final-online-v4.pdf (last accessed 1 August 2022).

Credland, N., Dyson, J., and Johnson, M.J. (2018) 'What are the patterns of compliance with Early Warning Track and Trigger Tools: A narrative review', *Applied Nursing Research*, 44: 39–47. Available at: www-sciencedirect-com.manchester.idm.oclc.org/science/article/pii/S0897189718304993 (last accessed 2 August 2022).

Daniels, R. and Nutbeam, T. (2022) *The Sepsis Manual,* 6th edn. Available at: https://sepsistrust.org/professional-resources/education-resources/ (last accessed 1 August 2022).

DeMeester, K., Verspuy, M., Monsieurs, K.G. and Van Bogaert, P. (2013) 'SBAR improves nurse–physician communication and reduces unexpected death: a pre and post intervention study', *Resuscitation*, 84: 1192–6.

Department of Health (2009) *Competencies for Recognising and Responding to Acutely Ill Patients in Hospital*. Leeds: DH.

Doherty, M., Hawkey, C., Goulder, M., Gibb, I., Hill, N., Aspley, S. and Reader, S. (2011) 'A randomised controlled trial of ibuprofen, paracetamol or a combination tablet of ibuprofen/paracetamol in community-derived people with knee pain', *Annals of Rheumatic Disease*, 70: 1534–41.

Dwyer, A.J., Thomas, W., Humphry, S. and Porter, P. (2014) 'Enhanced recovery programme for total knee replacement to reduce the length of hospital stay', *Journal of Orthopedic Surgery (Hong Kong)*, 22(2): 150–4.

Ellis, G., Gardner, M., Tsiachristas, A., Longhorne, P., Burke, O., Harwood, R.H., Conroy, S.P., Kircher, T., Somme, D., Saltvedt, I., Wald, H., O'Neill, D., Robinson, D. and Shepperd, S. (2017) 'Comprehensive geriatric assessment for older adults admitted to hospital', *Cochrane Database Syst Rev*, 9(9): Cd006211. Available at: DOI: 10.1002/14651858.CD006211.pub3. (last accessed 1 August 2022).

Enhanced Recovery Partnership Programme (2010) *Delivering Enhanced Recovery: Helping Patients to Get Better Sooner After Surgery*. Available at: www.gov.uk/government/publications/enhanced-recovery-partnership-programme (last accessed 1 August 2022).

Fernandes, M., Vieira, M., Leite, F., Palos, C., Finkelstein, S., and Sousa, J.M.C. (2020) 'Clinical decision support systems for triage in the emergency department using intelligent systems: a review', *Artificial Intelligence in Medicine*, 102: 101762.

Gelinas, C., Fillion, L., Puntillo, K., Viens, C. and Fortier, M. (2006) 'Validation of a critical care pain observational tool in adults', *American Journal of Critical Care*, 15(4): 420–7.

Grant, S. (2019) 'Limitations of track and trigger systems and the National Early Warning Score. Part 3: cultural and behavioural factors', (4): 234–41 Available at: https://pubmed.ncbi.nlm.nih.gov/30811231/ (last accessed 27 July 2022).

Gregory, J. (2008) 'Using nitrous oxide and oxygen to control pain in primary care', *Nursing Times*, 104(37): 24–6.

Gregory, J. (2014) 'Dealing with acute and chronic pain: part one – assessment', *Journal of Community Nursing*, 28(5): 83–6.

Gregory, J. (2017) 'Assessing pain for cognitive impaired patients in acute care', *Nursing Times*, 113(10): 18–21.

Higginson, R., Jones, B. and Davies, K. (2011) 'Emergency and Intensive care: assessing and managing the airway', *British Journal of Nursing*, 20(16): 973–7.

Hill, B. and Annesly, S.H. (2020) 'Monitoring respiratory rate in adults', *British Journal of Nursing*, 29(1): 14–16. Available at: doi.org/10.12968/bjon.2020.29.1.12 (last accessed 12 August 2022).

Hjermstad, M.J., Fayers, P.M., Haugen, D.T. and Caraceni, A. (2011) 'Studies comparing numerical rating scales, verbal rating scales and visual analogue scales for assessment of pain in adults: a systematic literature review', *Journal of Pain and Symptom Management*, 41: 1073–93.

Ibrahim, M.S., Alazzawi, S., Nizam, I., and Haddad, F.S. (2013) 'An evidence-based review of enhanced recovery interventions in knee replacement surgery', *Annals of the Royal College of Surgeons England*, 95(6): 386–9.

International Association for Pain (2020) *IASP Terminology. IASP Revises Its Definition of Pain for the First Time Since 1979*. Available at: www.iasp-pain.org/wp-content/uploads/2022/04/revised-definition-flysheet_R2.pdf (last accessed 1 August 2022).

Intensive Care National Audit & Research Centre (ICNARC) (2021) *Key Statistics from the National Cardiac Arrest Audit 2020/21*. Available at: www.icnarc.org/Our-Audit/Audits/Ncaa/Reports/Key-Statistics. (last accessed 12 August 2022).

Joint British Diabetes Societies for Inpatient Care (2022) *The Hospital Management of Hypoglycaemia in Adults with Diabetes Mellitus*. Available at: https://abcd.care/sites/abcd.care/files/site_uploads/JBDS_Guidelines_Archive/JBDS_01_HypoGuideline_4th_edition_FINAL_Archive.pdf (last accessed 2 August 2022).

Joint Formulary Committee. (2022) *British National Formulary 83*. London: BMJ Publishing and the Royal Pharmaceutical Society.

Jones, R., White, P. and Armstrong, D. (2010) *Managing Acute Illness*. London. Available at: www.kingsfund.org.uk/sites/default/files/field/field_document/managing-acute-illness-gp-inquiry-research-paper-mar11.pdf (last accessed May 2022).

King's Fund (2014) *Making Our Health and Care Systems Fit for an Ageing Population*. London: The King's Fund.

Leonard, M., Graham, S. and Bonacum, S. (2004) 'The human factor: the critical importance of effective teamwork and communication in providing safe care', *Quality Safety Healthcare*, 1(Suppl 1): i85-90. doi: 10.1136/qhc.13.suppl_1. i85. PMID: 15465961; PMCID: PMC1765783.

Lukas, A., Niederecker, T., Günther, I., Mayer, B. and Nikolaus, T. (2013) 'Self- and proxy report for the assessment of pain in patients with and without cognitive impairment: experiences gained in a geriatric hospital', *Zeitschrift für Gerontologie und Geriatrie*, 46(3): 214–21.

Macintyre, P. and Schug, S. (2021) *Acute Pain Management. A Practical Guide*, 5th edn. Boca Raton. CRC Press.

Mackway-Jones, K., Marsden, J. and Windle, J. (2013) *Emergency Triage*. Manchester Triage Group.

McMullen, S.M. and Patrick, W. (2013) 'Cyanosis', *American Journal of Medicine*, 126 (3): 210–12.

Moore, T. (2007) 'Respiratory assessment in adults', *Nursing Standard*, 21(49): 48–56.

Müller, M., Jürgens, J., Redaèlli, M., Klingberg, K., Hautz, W.E. and Stock, S. (2018) 'Impact of the communication and patient hand-off tool SBAR on patient safety: a systematic review', BMJ Open. Available at: https://bmjopen.bmj.com/content/8/8/e022202. (last accessed 1 August 2022).

National Confidential Enquiry into Patient Outcome and Death (NCEPOD) (2005) *An Acute Problem?* Available at: www.ncepod.org.uk/2005report/summary.pdf (last accessed 1 August 2022).

NHS Digital (2020) *Hospital Admitted Patient Care Activity 2019-20: National statistics.* Available at: https://digital.nhs.uk/data-and-information/publications/statistical/hospital-admitted-patient-care-activity/2019-20 (last accessed 6 May 2022).

NHS Digital (2021a) *Hospital Accident & Emergency Activity 2020-21: Official statistics.* Available at: https://digital.nhs.uk/data-and-information/publications/statistical/hospital-accident–emergency-activity/2020-21/introduction (last accessed 6 May 2022).

NHS Digital (2021b) *A&E Attendances and Emergency Admissions 2020-2.* Available at: www.england.nhs.uk/statistics/statistical-work-areas/ae-waiting-times-and-activity/ae-attendances-and-emergency-admissions-2020-21/ (last accessed 6 May 2022).

NHS Improving Quality (2013) *Enhanced Recovery Care Pathway: A Better Journey for Patients Seven Days a Week and a Better Deal for the NHS.* Progress review (2012/2013) and level of ambition (2014/2015). London: NHS.

National Institute for Health and Care Excellence (2007) *Acutely Ill Patients in Hospital: Recognition of and Response to Acute Illness in Adults in Hospital*, NICE Clinical Guideline 50. London: NICE.

National Institute for Health and Care Excellence (2012a) *Patient Experience in Adult NHS Services: Improving the Experience of Care for People using Adult NHS Services*, NICE Clinical Guidance 138. London: NICE.

National Institute for Health and Care Excellence (2012b) *Quality Standard for Patient Experience in Adult NHS Services*, NICE Quality Standards (QS15). London: NICE.

National Institute for Health and Care Excellence (2013) *Intravenous Fluid Therapy in Adults in Hospital*, Clinical Guideline 174 (updated May 2017). Available at: www.nice.org.uk/guidance/cg174 (last accessed 11 August 2022).

National Institute for Health and Care Excellence (2016) *Sepsis: Recognition, Diagnosis and Early Management.* Available at: www.nice.org.uk/guidance/NG51/chapter/Recommendations# identifying-people-with-suspected-sepsis (last accessed 2 August 2022).

National Institute for Health and Care Excellence (2018) *Chapter 32 Structured Patient Handovers: Emergency and acute medical care in over 16s: service delivery and organization.* Available at: www.nice.org.uk/guidance/ng94/evidence/32.structured-patient-handovers-pdf-172397464671#:~:text=The%20World%20Health%20Organisation%20goes,local%20adaptations%20may%20be%20needed. (last accessed 2 August 2022).

National Institute for Health and Care Excellence (2019) *Acute Kidney Injury [NG148]*. London: NICE. Available at: www.nice.org.uk/guidance/ng148/chapter/Recommendations (last accessed 1 August 2022).

National Institute for Health and Care Excellence (2020) *Perioperative Care in Adults [NG180]*. London: NICE. Available at: www.nice.org.uk/guidance/ng180 (last accessed 1st August 2022).

NHS Modernisation Agency (2004) *10 High Impact Changes for Service Improvement and Delivery: A Guide for NHS Leaders*. Available at: https://www.england.nhs.uk/improvement-hub/publication/10-high-impact-changes-for-service-improvement-and-delivery/ (last accessed 29th March 2023).

Nursing and Midwifery Council (2018) *Future Nurse: Standards of Proficiency for Registered Nurses*. London: NMC.

Odell, M. (2015) 'Detection and management of the deteriorating ward patient: An evaluation of nursing practice', *Journal of Clinical Nursing*, 24 (1–2): 173–82.

O'Driscoll, B., Howard, L., Earis, J. and Mak, V. (2017) 'BTS guideline for oxygen use in adults in healthcare and emergency settings', *Thorax*, 72 (Suppl 1): ii1–ii90.

Office for National Statistics (2022) *Overview of the UK Population: 2020*. Available at: www.ons.gov.uk/peoplepopulationandcommunity/populationandmigration/populationestimates/articles/overviewoftheukpopulation/2020 (Last accessed 1 August 2022).

Organisation for Economic Co-operation and Development (2021). *Hospital beds- acute care*. Available at: https://www.oecd.org/coronavirus/en/data-insights/hospital-beds-acute-care (last accessed 09 June 2023).

Parker, S.G., et al. (2017) 'What is comprehensive geriatric assessment (CGA)? An umbrella review,' *Age and Ageing*, 47(1): 149–55. Available at: https://doi.org/10.1093/ageing/afx166 (last accessed 8 January 2022).

Perkins, G.D., Nolan, J.P., Soar, J., Hawkes, C., Wyllie, J., et al. (2021) *Epidemiology of Cardiac Arrest Guidelines*. Available at: www.resus.org.uk/library/2021-resuscitation-guidelines/epidemiology-cardiac-arrest-guidelines (last accessed 27 July 2022).

Resuscitation Council UK (2021) *The ABCDE Approach*. Available at: www.resus.org.uk/library/abcde-approach (last accessed 1 August 2022).

Royal College of Physicians (2007) *Acute Medical Care: The right person, in the right setting, first time*. Available at: www.rcpmedicalcare.org.uk/designing-services/specialties/acute-internal-medicine/services-delivered/acute-medical-unit/ (last accessed 12 August 2022).

Royal College of Physicians (2016. *New RCP Advice Aims to Reduce Inpatient Injury from Trips and Falls*. Available at: www.rcplondon.ac.uk/news/new-rcp-advice-aims-reduce-inpatient-injury-trips-and-falls (last accessed 1 August 2022).

Royal College of Physicians (2017) *National Early Warning Score (NEWS) 2. Standardising the Assessment of Acute-illness Severity in the NHS*. Available at: www.rcplondon.ac.uk/projects/outputs/national-early-warning-score-news-2 (last accessed 1 August 2022).

Royal College of Physicians (2018) *Acute Internal Medicine Services: Acute medical unit*. Available at: www.rcpmedicalcare.org.uk/designing-services/specialties/acute-internal-medicine/services-delivered/acute-medical-unit/#:~:text=The%20term%20acute%20medical%20unit,medical%20illness%20while%20in%20hospital'. (last accessed 6 May 2022).

Sandberg, M., Nalstad, A., Berlac, P., Hyldmo, P.K., and Boylan, M. (2013) 'Airway assessment and management'. In T. Nutbeam and Boylan (eds), *ABC of Prehospital Emergency Medicine*. London: BMJ Books,

Scott, I., Vaughan, L. and Bell, D. (2009) 'Effectiveness of acute medical units in hospitals: a systematic review', *International Journal for Quality in Healthcare*, 21(6): 397–407.

Scottish Intercollegiate Guidelines Network (SIGN) (2014) *Care of Deteriorating Patients*. Available at: www.sign.ac.uk/assets/sign139.pdf (last accessed 1 August 2022).

Singer, M., Deutschman, C.S., Seymour, C.W., Shankar-Hari, M., Annane, D., Bauer, M., Bellomo, R., Bernard, G.R., Chiche, J.D., Coopersmith, C.M. and Hotchkiss, R.S. (2016) 'The third international consensus definitions for sepsis and septic shock (Sepsis-3)', *Jama*, 315(8): 801–10.

Sinha, S., Ozdemir, B.A., Khalid, U., Karthikesalingam, A., Poloniecki, J.D., Thompson, M.M., and Holt, P.J.E. (2014) 'Failure-to-rescue and interprovider comparisons after elective abdominal aortic aneurysm repair', *Journal of British Surgery*, 101(12): 1541–50.

Swift, A. (2018) 'Understanding the effect of pain and how the human body responds', *Nursing Times*, 114(3): 22–6.

Teasdale, G. and Jennett, B. (1974) 'Assessment of coma and impaired consciousness: a practical guide', *The Lancet*, 304(7872): 81–4.

The King's Fund (2020) *NHS Hospital Bed Numbers: Past, present, future*. Available at: www.kingsfund.org.uk/publications/nhs-hospital-bed-numbers (last accessed 6 May 2022).

The UK Sepsis Trust (2018), *ED & AMU Sepsis Screening and Action Tool*. Available at: https://sepsistrust.org/wp-content/uploads/2018/06/ED-adult-NICE-Final-1107.pdf (last accessed 16 July 23)

Ugboma, D. and Cowen, M. (2012) 'Managing hydration'. In I. Bullock, J. Clark, and J. Rycroft-Malone (eds), *Adult Nursing Practice: Using Evidence in Care*. Oxford: Oxford University Press, pp. 328–42.

UK National Guideline Centre (2020) *Evidence Review for Enhanced Recovery Programmes*. Available at: www.ncbi.nlm.nih.gov/books/NBK561974/ (last accessed 1 August 2022).

Walz, J.M., Zayaruuzny, M. and Heard, S.O. (2007) 'Airway management in critical illness', *Chest*, 131(2): 608–20.

Warden, V., Hurley, A.C. and Volicer, L. (2003) 'Development and psychometric evaluation of the Pain Assessment in Advanced Dementia (PAINAD) Scale', *Journal of the American Medical Directors*, Jan/Feb: 9–15.

West Midlands Quality Review Service and the Society for Acute Medicine (SAM) (2012) *Quality Standards for Acute Medical Units (AMUs)*. Available at: www.acutemedicine.org.uk/wp-content/uploads/clinical_quality_indicators_for_acute_medical_units_v18.pdf (last accessed 29 March 2023).

Williams, C. and Salerno, S. (2012) 'The patient in pain'. In D. Tait, D. Barton, J. James, and C. Williams (eds), *Acute and Critical Care in Adult Nursing*. London: Sage, pp. 88–101.

Wood, S. (2008) 'Assessment of pain', *Nursing Times* [Online] Available at: www.nursingtimes.net/clinical-archive/pain-management/assessment-of-pain-18-09-2008/ (last accessed 1 August 2022).

World Health Organization (1986) *Cancer Pain Relief*. Geneva: WHO.

World Health Organization (2007a) *Policy Brief. Day Surgery: Making it Happen.* Available at: https://apps.who.int/iris/bitstream/handle/10665/107831/WHO-EURO-2007-866-40602-54591-eng.pdf?sequence=4&isAllowed=y (last accessed 1 August 2022).

World Health Organization (2007b) Collaborating Centre for Patient Safety Solutions. *Communication during patient handovers.* Available at: www.who.int/patientsafety/solutions/patientsafety/PS-Solution3.pdf. (Last accessed 1 August 2022).

World Health Organization (2022). *Falls.* Available at: www.who.int/news-room/fact-sheets/detail/falls (last accessed 1 August 2022).

Wu, C., Hung, L. and Yeh, T. (2020) 'Pain prevalence in hospitalized patients at a tertiary academic medical centre: Exploring severe persistent pain'. Available at: https://pdfs.semanticscholar.org/fd96/f431425b4d29bd8ce0b8528d53395b5a99ad.pdf. (last accessed 11 August 2022).

Zhuang, C.L., Ye, X.Z., Zhang, X.D., Chen, B.C., and Yu, Z. (2013) 'Enhanced recovery after surgery programs versus traditional care for colorectal surgery: a meta-analysis of randomised controlled trials', *Diseases of the Colon and Rectum*, 56(5): 667–78.

15

CARING FOR THE CRITICALLY ILL ADULT

Samantha Freeman, Colin Steen, and Greg Bleakley

Chapter Objectives

- Critically discuss the comprehensive assessment of a critically ill adult;
- Recognise and respond to critically ill adults using appropriate evidence-based strategies;
- Appreciate the importance of using medical devices safely;
- Demonstrate a critical understanding of legal and ethical issues relating to critically-ill adults in acute care settings, including consent, confidentiality, and best interest principles.

Introduction

Chapter 14 focused on the care of the 'acutely ill' adult. This chapter will explore the care of adults who require specialist treatment within a critical care environment.

The critical care environment is a constantly changing field and as an adult nurse you will be required to understand and recognise the need to respond to those requiring critical care, ensuring that you assess a person thoroughly, identify their problems and devise and critically review a plan of care based on their needs. To support a person who is critically ill, a multidisciplinary team is needed with the emphasis on team working. The coordination of the different disciplines is often the responsibility of the nurse who can constantly observe and interact with the person receiving care. By exploring the evidence base for the management of critical illness we will provide you with the underpinning knowledge necessary to be able to assist in the safe and effective care for such people. However, we will only give a brief insight into caring for someone who is critically ill. Should you wish to extend your knowledge and understanding further, please refer to the suggested reading at the end of this chapter.

Related Nursing and Midwifery Council (NMC) Proficiencies for Registered Nurses

The overarching requirements of the Nursing and Midwifery Council (NMC), are that all nurses must use information obtained during clinical assessments to identify the priorities and requirements for evidence-based nursing interventions, prioritising the needs of people. They must ensure that the care they provide and delegate is person-centred and of a consistently high standard. Nursing assessments must consider mental, physical, and spiritual needs to ensure people receive truly holistic care of the highest standard. The multidisciplinary critical care team need to consult and work in partnership with individuals, their families, carers, and significant others to ensure that their care is provided in line with their wishes and desired outcomes a nurse must also be able to evaluate whether care is effective, and the goals of care have been met (NMC, 2018).

━━━━━━━ TO ACHIEVE ENTRY TO THE NMC REGISTER
YOU MUST BE ABLE TO ━━━━━━━

- Demonstrate the ability to accurately process all information gathered during the assessment process to identify needs for individualised nursing care and develop person-centred, evidence-based plans for nursing interventions with agreed goals;
- Demonstrate an understanding of co-morbidities and the demands of meeting individual complex nursing and social care needs when prioritising care plans;
- Interpret results from routine investigations, taking prompt action when required by implementing appropriate interventions, requesting additional investigations, or escalating to others;
- Demonstrate the knowledge and ability to respond proactively and promptly to signs of deterioration or distress in mental, physical, cognitive, and behavioural health, and use this knowledge to make sound clinical decisions;
- Demonstrate knowledge of when and how to refer people safely to other professionals or services for clinical intervention or support;
- Effectively assess a person's capacity to make decisions about their own care and to give or withhold consent and understand and apply the principles and processes for making reasonable adjustments and best interest decisions where people do not have capacity;
- Demonstrate the knowledge, communication and relationship management skills required to provide people, families and carers with accurate information that meets their needs before, during and after a range of interventions;
- Effectively and responsibly use a range of digital technologies to access, input, share and apply information and data within teams and between agencies;

- Understand and recognise the need to respond to the challenges of providing safe, effective, and person-centred nursing care for people who have co-morbidities and complex care needs;
- Demonstrate the ability to coordinate and undertake the processes and procedures involved in routine planning and management of safe discharge home or transfer of people between care settings;
- Understand how to monitor and evaluate the quality of people's experience of complex care.

(Adapted from NMC, 2018)

Admission to an adult critical care unit (ACCU) is a traumatic and potentially life-altering event that can lead to lifelong physical and mental ill health. The main rationale for admission is that the individual is experiencing serious life-threatening illness so severe that without intensive specialist treatment their life would be in danger.

The classification of severity of illness and interventions required are set out in the Faculty of Intensive Care Medicine/Intensive Care Society (2022) guidelines which are endorsed by numerous organisations as a useful means of defining the varying needs of a critically ill person.

Activity 15.1

Access the following Faculty of Intensive Care Medicine/Intensive Care Society website and look at the guidelines for the provision of intensive care services

https://www.ficm.ac.uk/standardssafetyguidelinesstandards/guidelines-for-the-provision-of-intensive-care-services

1) What are the levels of care provided within an intensive care setting?
2) What knowledge, experience and skills are required by nurses working in such settings?
3) Identify the recommended nursing staffing ratios for individuals requiring intensive care.
4) Make a list of the various other healthcare professionals involved in intensive care delivery.

In 2021, the 'Levels of Adult Critical Care' classifications were redefined in response to changes in delivery and demand with levels 2 and 3 identified as 'Critical Care' (Faculty of Intensive Care Medicine/Intensive Care Society, 2022: 9). The UK uses a National Competency Framework for Registered Nurses in Adult Critical Care which has a 3-stage competency programme. Step 1 starts when the nurse starts in critical care with no experience of the specialty and works up to step 3 which describes working independently within critical care (The Critical Care National Network Nurse Leads Forum (CC3N), 2018). In addition to the nursing requirement, a complex multidisciplinary team works together to provide care to individuals within a critical care setting, including doctors, advanced critical care practitioners, physiotherapists, dieticians, infection control and microbiology specialists, and pharmacists and those from other specialisms such as renal or burns, occupational therapy, speech and language therapy, and clinical psychology, all supported by a network of administration staff, domestic, catering and portering staff.

Outreach Services

Critical care needs to be viewed as more than a dedicated unit and as a resource that supports individuals within the wider hospital environment (Department of Health [DH]/Emergency Care, 2005). The introduction of critical care outreach services developed from the 'critical care without walls' (DH, 2000) concept of care focusing on a person's needs rather than their location. As a result of this document two key developments occurred: first, early warning scoring systems (as discussed in Chapter 14); second, critical care outreach services were introduced. The National Institute for Health and Care Excellence (NICE, 2018) guideline on the effectiveness of outreach services suggests that critical care outreach teams may provide a benefit in increased numbers of 'Do Not Attempt Resuscitation' (DNAR) orders issued, but there is no clear evidence that the service improved in-hospital mortality, avoidable adverse events such as cardiac arrest or unplanned intensive care unit (ICU) admissions. The current research exploring the effectiveness of outreach services is of low or medium quality, which may be why there can be significant variations in the composition, and names for, critical care outreach teams (Pattison and Eastham, 2011).

Activity 15.2

Research the outreach service within your placement area.

- Who is on the team?
- How would you contact them?
- What is their aim and what services do they provide?

Medical Technology

Critical care areas utilise an extensive range of medical technology for nurses to contend with. Adult nurses are responsible for ensuring that all the medical devices and equipment they are likely to use are checked regularly to ensure that everything is in working order. You will need to be aware of the potential pitfalls of using medical devices and equipment, and the impact that these can have on the safety of those we care for.

- What medical devices have you already used in clinical practice?
- Do you know how to use them safely? If not, how would you rectify this?

Airway

Activity 15.3

Before reading the next section, you may want to refresh your knowledge and understanding of the respiratory system. It is important to understand normal respiratory function before we care for those who need respiratory support.

It would also be worth identifying all the required clinical competencies (Annexes A and B) within the NMC (2018) *Standards of Proficiency* document. Within a critical care environment how could you ensure that you are able to develop your clinical skills to meet the required competencies outlined?

When an airway problem is identified, if standard interventions and basic manoeuvres are not successful then a person will require more advanced airway care using artificial airways such as an endotracheal tube (ETT) or a tracheostomy tube. Mechanical ventilation is one of the various interventions a person may encounter during their admission (Chen et al., 2014). Nursing someone with an artificial airway in place presents many challenges in maintaining their safety through ensuring the patency of the artificial airway, preventing aspiration of any secretions, and decreasing potential trauma to the trachea.

Endotracheal intubation

Intubation involves inserting a tube directly into the trachea with the aid of a laryngoscope. The tube is secured using cotton tape (or similar) tying the tube in position, and inflating a balloon, the 'cuff,' which is situated and integral to, the distal end of the Endotracheal Tube (ETT). It is important to measure the pressure in the cuff to detect over-inflation which may cause tracheal damage. The recommended range for ETT cuff pressure is 20–30 cm H_2O (Lazy 2014). Once inserted and secured the nurse's role is to monitor and maintain the position and patency of the ETT.

The length of the tube visible should be noted at either the lips or the teeth. This gives a baseline position and you will need to check frequently to see whether it has moved or become dislodged, particularly after moving or re-positioning a person. Diligent mouth care and suction of oral secretions are vital to maintain the person's comfort and hygiene and to reduce the risk of ventilator-associated pneumonia (Hellyer et al., 2016).

Endotracheal suctioning is one of the most common procedures performed in individuals with artificial airways. There are many things you need to consider before, during and after endotracheal suctioning.

Activity 15.4

For further information on suctioning look at this guidance: https://resources.acls.com/free-resources/knowl-edge-base/respiratory-arrest-airway-management/basics-of-suctioning and read the paper *Endotracheal suctioning of the intubated adult –what is the evidence?* https://pubmed.ncbi.nlm.nih.gov/18632271/

There may be post-intubation complications you need to be aware of such as:

- Hypoxia;
- Trauma to lips, teeth, and vocal folds;
- Transient cardiac arrhythmias due to vagal nerve stimulation;
- Hypertension, tachycardia or raised intracranial pressure;
- Aspiration;
- Missed placement: potential oesophageal intubation;
- Infection;
- Reduced cough reflex;
- Bronchial and tracheal ulceration or stenosis;
- Laryngeal oedema;
- Bronchospasm;
- Discomfort and anxiety;
- ETT kinked or damaged;
- Measurement of cuff pressure.

Tracheostomy

This is a tube that is inserted through the anterior wall of the trachea just below the larynx and cricoid cartilage.

The indications for a temporary tracheostomy are (Intensive Care Society, 2008):

- To protect the airway;
- To aid the removal of excessive secretions;
- To aid weaning from mechanical ventilation.

For further information you are advised to visit the following website: www.tracheostomy.org.uk

Many individuals in need of critical care will have a temporary tracheostomy sited. They may require this to remain *in situ* when discharged from the ICU to another clinical area. Often a person with a tracheostomy is nursed in another clinical environment such as a community setting (Freeman, 2011). As an adult nurse you will need to be aware of the additional equipment required, the risks and management.

Jan

Jan, a 42 year-old, was admitted to the ICU with respiratory failure. Jan had a prolonged recovery which required a temporary tracheostomy to be inserted. Jan no longer requires ventilation, is breathing unsupported via a tracheostomy with 35% humidified oxygen and is transferred to your clinical area.

- What additional equipment do you think you will need at Jan's bedside to ensure Jan's safety?
- In relation to caring for someone with a temporary tracheostomy, what are the nursing implications?
- What are the potential complications of a tracheostomy?
- What symptoms of complications would you look for?

According to the Intensive Care Society (2008), when caring for an individual with a temporary tracheostomy it is important that staff are familiar with and able to use the following additional equipment, which should be immediately available:

- An operational suction unit, which should be checked at least daily, with suction tubing attached;
- Appropriately sized suction catheters;
- Non-powdered, latex-free gloves, aprons, and eye protection;
- Spare tracheostomy tubes of the same type as inserted: one the same size and one a size smaller;
- Tracheal dilators;
- Re-breathing bag with tubing and a connection to an oxygen supply;
- Catheter mount or connection;
- Tracheostomy disconnection wedge;
- Tracheostomy tube holder and dressing;
- 10-ml syringe (if tube cuffed);
- Artery forceps;
- Resuscitation equipment;
- Manometer to measure cuff pressure.

The potential complications of a temporary tracheostomy are (Intensive Care Society, 2008):

- Airway occlusion;
- Displaced tubes;
- Blocked tubes;
- Air leaks;
- Impaired cough;
- Impaired swallow reflex which increases the risk of aspiration;

- Surgical emphysema;
- Infection wound/chest;
- Haemorrhage;
- Tracheal stenosis;
- Ulcerated tissue damage;
- Altered body image.

You should note that there are some differences in resuscitation procedures for individuals who have a temporary tracheostomy. If effective ventilation can be provided with a bag/valve, then continual chest compressions should be carried out and the person ventilated with approximately 10 breaths/minute (Resuscitation Council (UK, 2021).

If not, then check the following:

- Is the tube patent?
- Can a suction catheter be passed down?
- Can you change the inner cannula? (Some tracheostomies have an inner cannula);
- If the tracheostomy is occluded or displaced, remove and cover stoma and ventilate via the person's mouth.

Breathing

Normal respiration is quiet, effortless and rhythmical. It happens automatically without any conscious effort and any changes indicate abnormal breathing. For gas exchange to occur there needs to be a neurological stimulus from the respiratory centre in the brain. This stimulus triggers contraction of the diaphragm downwards and contraction of the intercostal muscles drawing the rib cage upwards and outwards. The overall effect is an increase in intrathoracic space resulting in a decrease in intrathoracic pressure. The pressure in the thoracic cavity is now less than atmospheric pressure and this results in air being drawn into the lungs. For air to reach the alveoli) air sacks of the lungs where gas exchange takes place) a patent airway is needed along with a patent respiratory tree. This means that, as both lungs expand, there is no obstruction to gas flowing into the lungs.

When caring for someone in need of respiratory support, consider what you can do to improve chest expansion to aid air entry into all areas of the lungs.

What could be the reasons for an obstruction in airflow?

What might cause an obstruction to the airflow to the alveoli?

Activity 15.5

Mary is 48 years old and has been admitted with shortness of breath and low oxygen saturations. Mary was being treated by a GP (General Practitioner) for a chest infection and has no other medical history. Mary is diagnosed with type 1 respiratory failure.

- Why is Mary's oxygen saturation low?
- What could act as a barrier to the gas exchange in the lungs?
- What can you do about this to improve Mary's breathing?

Respiratory assessment

A person experiencing critical illness may have a multitude of symptoms, some specific to the respiratory system. It is important to ascertain a good history to diagnosis respiratory problems or disease correctly. In addition to the physical examination, a detailed respiratory assessment can help focus the correct plan of care. Whilst a person receiving mechanical ventilation support it is important to conduct frequent breathing assessment. A principal element of the respiratory assessment is to inspect the chest for symmetry of movement. The nurse closely observes the chest wall for symmetrical movement during each respiration. Abnormal chest wall expansion during respiration, for example only one side of the chest wall inflating could indicate underlying pathology, including previous surgical removal of lung or pneumothorax (collapsed lung) (Arshad et al., 2016).

Enhanced respiratory assessment includes chest auscultation but this skill is often challenging in a busy and noisy critical care environment. Normally, chest auscultation occurs with the person in a sitting position but this may not be possible during critical illness. With use of a stethoscope, chest auscultation allows the nurse to detect normal airflow sounds which change if airways are blocked, narrowed, or filled with fluid (Singh, 2016).

Arterial blood gas interpretation

An Arterial Blood Gas (ABG) provides a lot of information, we are just focusing on respiratory function which includes four elements:

1. The pH;
2. Partial pressure of oxygen (PaO_2);
3. Partial pressure of carbon dioxide ($PaCO_2$);
4. Bicarbonate (HCO_3^-).

The pH is the measure of acidity or alkalinity of a substance; the normal range for blood is 7.35–7.45. During normal cellular metabolism CO_2 carried in the blood to the lungs combines with H_2O to give carbonic acid H_2CO_3. Therefore, the blood pH changes according to the level of carbonic acid present and this allows the person to compensate for any changes. Compensation can either be quick by increasing or decreasing respiratory function or slow as the kidney either retains or excretes bicarbonate (HCO_3^-) to maintain pH in a normal range. It is worth remembering that when a person is unwell the body will respond by trying to maintain normal homoeostasis through compensation. Detecting these compensatory mechanisms provides vital information that illness is present and its severity.

The reading of the partial pressure of oxygen (PaO_2) dissolved in arterial blood should be >10 kPa (kilopascals) and the partial pressure of carbon dioxide ($PaCO_2$) dissolved in arterial blood should be between 4.5 kPa and 6.1 kPa. The bicarbonate (HCO_3^-) reading should be between 22 mmol/L and 26 mmol/L.

There are some basic steps to interpreting a simple ABG result. However, prior to interpreting ABGs it is important to understand the context i.e., what oxygen therapy if any, the person is receiving. There is a difference between the levels of oxygen we breathe in and the partial pressure (PaO_2) of oxygen dissolved in arterial blood. The difference is normally around 10 kPa. In a person with damage to their lungs (by either infection or illness) this difference will be bigger. The larger the gap between what concentration of oxygen the person inhales and their PaO_2 the more the degree of damage. This difference is referred to as the alveolar–arterial (A–a) gradient. For example, we would expect a person with healthy lungs receiving 60% oxygen to have a PaO_2

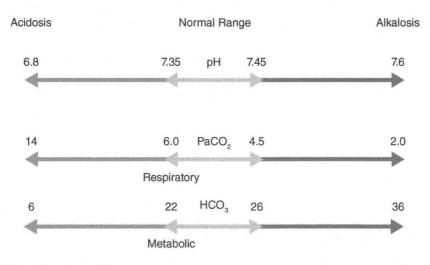

Figure 15.1   Plot the results

of approximately 50 kPa (60 – 50 = 10). Once we have all the information we need, we can then start to interpret the ABG using five questions:

1. Is the person hypoxic?
2. How does this relate to the inspired O_2?
3. Do they have acidosis or alkalosis (the pH level)?
4. Is the cause respiratory or metabolic (determined by $PaCO_2$ and HCO_3^-)?
5. Is there any attempt at compensation (determined by $PaCO_2$ and HCO_3^-)?

These last two questions can sometimes be more challenging. If the result is marked on the same side as the pH then it is the cause of the deterioration; if the result is on the opposite side, it is the compensatory mechanism trying to correct the pH. Read the scenario below and mark the results on Figure 15.1.

Activity 15.6

68 year-old Jose presents in the emergency department complaining of increased breathlessness and low oxygen saturations. The paramedics have applied an oxygen mask to give 40% oxygen.

Significant findings on your examination are that Jose is drowsy with:

- A respiratory Respiratory rate of 28;
- O_2 saturation of 85%;
- Widespread coarse crackles on auscultation.

Arterial blood gas analysis reveals:

- PaO_2: 7.0;
- pH: 7.25;
- $PaCO_2$: 8.9;
- HCO_3^-: 35.

Invasive ventilation

Invasive or mechanical ventilation assists with the movement of gases into and out of a person's lungs while minimising the effort of breathing (Scholz et al., 2011). Most mechanical ventilators used in the UK today are positive-pressure ventilators, where lung volumes and gas exchange are achieved by applying oxygen/air in a positive pressure through the trachea via an artificial airway (Higginson et al., 2011), effectively blowing gas into the lungs inflating them.

There are numerous types of positive-pressure ventilation strategies and ventilator modes. It is important that the nurse understands the different modes of ventilation and why a person is receiving a particular mode. Different modes affect the pattern of breathing to optimise gas exchange while reducing the risk of lung injury. Some modes also permit people to breathe spontaneously through the ventilator.

Nurses also need to be aware of the complications of mechanical ventilation and the interventions that can minimise the risk. Common complications associated with mechanical ventilation include ventilator-induced lung injury, ventilator-associated pneumonia (VAP), blocked artificial airways and unplanned extubations.

VAP is a life-threatening nosocomial infection and a major complication of mechanical ventilation. To ensure consistency in care delivery, there is a VAP evidence-based care bundle that nurses should deliver to reduce the risk of a person developing VAP.

Recommended bundle of interventions for the prevention of VAP (Hellyer et al., 2016; Neuville et al., 2017; Zhao et al, 2020): include

- Elevation of head of bed (30–45°);
- Daily sedation interruption and assessment of readiness to extubate;
- Use of subglottic secretion drainage;
- Avoidance of scheduled ventilator circuit changes;
- Oral hygiene with chlorhexidine;
- Stress ulcer prophylaxis;
- Thromboembolism prophylaxis.

Positioning

Individuals experiencing critical illness are often immobile due to therapeutic interventions and sedation. Body positioning is one of the most important nursing considerations to prevent complications of immobility (Alcan et al., 2016). Unless cervical spine injury or lesion is suspected, critically ill individuals are nursed with 30–45° head of bed elevation to prevent aspiration of gastric contents (Hellyer et al., 2016). Moreover, aspiration of gastric contents is linked to the pathogenesis of VAP. Prolonged periods of immobility are known to cause thromboembolic occlusion, muscle weakness, pressure ulcer development and pulmonary insufficiency (Makic, 2015). Critically ill individuals are at increased risk of developing chest infection because endotracheal intubation and mechanical ventilation bypass normal anatomical defences (Benson et al., 2013). Consequently, Acute Respiratory Failure (ARF) is a common phenomenon within the critical care setting since prolonged mechanical ventilation increases the risk of VAP (Scaravilli et al., 2015).

To prevent further cellular hypoxia, prone positioning during mechanical ventilation has been demonstrated to enhance arterial oxygenation in the most severe cases of acute respiratory distress syndrome (ARDS). Prone positioning i.e., (lying a person on their front) is often instigated when, despite elevated levels of ventilation, the person continues to have poor gas exchange in the lungs (Drahnak and Custer, 2015). In addition, prone positioning can be used to aid surgical procedures and improve lymphatic drainage and secretion removal. However, prone positioning risks dislodging an ETT and specialised airway securement devices should be considered (Drahnak and Custer, 2015). Furthermore, nursing individuals in prone positions is problematic as access to the person's front is reduced and there is an increased risk of pressure sores, including facial sores and facial oedema. Often the absorption of nasogastric feed is also disrupted resulting in malnutrition. There was a rapid increase in the use of prone positioning during the Covid-19 pandemic and yet research remains inconclusive regarding the benefit or harm from universal application of proning in mechanically ventilated adults with hypoxaemia (Bloomfield et al., 2015).

Non-invasive ventilation

Non-invasive ventilation refers to the administration of ventilatory support without using an invasive artificial airway.

- CPAP - continuous positive airway pressure;
- BiPAP - bilevel positive airway pressure.

These are types of non-invasive modes of ventilation requiring an individual to wear a very tightly fitting mask. They can find this difficult to cope with because the oxygen is humidified and therefore warm. They may also find the mask uncomfortable and claustrophobic. Both treatments are for individuals who are breathing spontaneously.

CPAP delivers oxygen via a continuous one pressure setting with the aim to:

- Increase oxygen levels;
- Recruit redundant alveoli.

Throughout the whole respiratory cycle, CPAP maintains a positive pressure within the respiratory circuit as a pressure higher than atmospheric pressure. It increases intrathoracic pressure which reduces venous return to the heart. This can lower blood pressure, increasing the workload of the heart. The improved blood oxygen levels should compensate for this increase in workload. However, it may be a treatment of choice to manage a person with left ventricular failure because CPAP can reduce the workload of the left ventricle by reducing the resistance against which the left ventricle has to pump - known as the afterload.

BiPAP uses CPAP but also provides extra support to reduce the work of breathing. As the person breathes in, the machine supports this effort by blowing gas under positive pressure to improve the volume of air inspired, oxygen levels and reduce the $PaCO_2$ and respiratory workload.

It is important to understand normal circulatory functions before we care for those with abnormal circulatory functions. See Cooke et al. (2020) in the further reading section of this chapter if needed.

Circulation

For the heart to function normally it must have three main systems functioning in unison. It requires an electrical system, a mechanical pump, and a valve system.

The electrical system

The electrical system is recorded using an electrocardiograph (ECG). This shows the route the electricity flows through the cells that make up the muscle of the heart. Where there is any damage to these cells, the route the electricity must take is either delayed or deviates and these changes can be seen in the ECG. The electricity is generated by the movement of positively and negatively charged electrolytes passing into and out of the cell. This shift in charged electrolytes creates an electrical impulse that results in contraction of the muscle. If there is an imbalance in the electrolytes in the body then the electrical system may become unstable and disrupted, causing either minor symptoms or a risk to life.

Jolanka

Jolanka, a 72 year-old, is complaining of chest palpitations stating that it feels as though the heart is racing with extra strong, pounding beats. Jolanka also complains of tiredness and occasional dizziness.

- What could be causing these symptoms?
- What investigations could be done to determine whether there is an electrical problem with the heart?
- What simple observations could you make to detect an abnormal heart rhythm?
- How could an imbalance in electrolytes be diagnosed?

There are various electrical disorders of the heart, some of which are simple and some imminently life threatening. Atrial fibrillation is a major electrical disorder of the heart that is linked to a variety of co-morbidities and the incidence increases with age. This occurs when there is erratic electrical flow through the upper chambers, the atria of the heart. The consequence of this is that these chambers do not contract or pump properly and this creates turbulent blood flow through the heart. The result of turbulent blood flow is blood clots, which leave the heart and affect other parts of the body, especially the brain, causing stroke. Untreated, atrial fibrillation is a major contributing factor to the cause of stroke in the UK (NICE, 2021).

- Have you cared for someone with an arrhythmia? Reflect on what could have been the cause of this arrhythmia, and how it was diagnosed and monitored. What observations did you perform to help with the diagnosis and monitoring?

ECG monitoring

There are six basic steps to assist you in interpreting a basic ECG:

1. Is there a pulse?
2. Is there any electrical activity?
3. What is the ventricular (QRS) rate?

When recording speed and calculating the rate, check that the ECG is recorded at the standard UK paper speed of 25 mm/s for 1 minute of recording = 300 large squares. Each large square (5 mm) = 0.2 s, each small square (1 mm) = 0.04 s.

Regular rhythm: count number of large squares between two consecutive R waves then divide 300 by the number, e.g., if there are 5 large square intervals between R waves, heart rate = 300/5 = 60 beats/min or b [m.

Irregular rhythm: count the number of QRS in 30 large squares (QRS in 6 s) × 10 = rate/min (bpm).

4. Is the QRS rhythm regular or irregular?
5. Is the QRS width normal or broad?
6. Is atrial activity present?

If so:

- Is it regular?
- Is there more than one P wave?
- Is there any other atrial activity?
- How is atrial activity related to ventricular activity?
- Does it appear in front of every QRS complex?
- Is there any delay between the P wave and the QRS complex?

Activity 15.7

Look at the following website for further information: https://bjcardio.co.uk/2014/03/my-top-10-tips-for-ecg-interpretation.

The heart as a mechanical pump

The heart is a muscle and therefore requires a blood supply to the muscle itself so that it can contract and relax. The efficiency in the contraction of the heart is dependent on the muscle of the heart being undamaged, the amount of blood that is flowing into the heart and the resistance against which the heart must pump the blood out. It is reliant on the valves that separate the four chambers of the heart working efficiently.

The amount of blood that flows into the heart is an indication of an individual's level of hydration. If the person is dehydrated there is insufficient blood entering the heart, the efficiency of the contraction of the heart is reduced and consequently the volume and pressure of blood leaving the heart are reduced, resulting in poor oxygen and nutrient delivery to the cells of the body.

To determine whether a person is dehydrated or not there are several measurements that nurses can make:

1. Measure the fluid intake and urine output, i.e., the fluid balance;
2. Measure the pulse rate (heart rate)- as the blood volume declines the heart rate increases to compensate and maintain a normal oxygen and nutrient supply to the cells;
3. Feel the person's skin to determine whether they are cold and peripherally shut down. This is an autonomic compensation system the body uses to maintain oxygen and nutrient supply to the cells of the vital organs;
4. Measure the person's blood pressure. Please note that a low blood pressure is a late indication of the person being short of blood or fluid;
5. They may state that they are thirsty;
6. Their eyes may appear sunken;
7. Their skin loses its elasticity;
8. Their mucous membranes, (i.e., their tongue and mouth) will appear dry and coated;
9. In some more severe cases they may become confused.

All the above are simple observations that nurses can make to determine whether a person is dehydrated.

Ahmed

Ahmed, 74 years old, has been admitted to hospital feeling unwell. Ahmed is confused and has been feeling unwell for a few days. Ahmed lives alone and has been struggling to manage recently.

- How would you assess Ahmed's hydration status?
- Which of your observations would tell you that Ahmed may be dehydrated?
- How would you help to rehydrate Ahmed?
- What records would you need to make to continue the management of Ahmed's hydration?

Where a person is unable to take sufficient fluids orally or through an alternative enteral feeding system, an intravenous drip can be used to administer fluids and electrolytes where necessary. In these circumstances a clear and accurate record of the person's fluid balance is vitally important. A detailed record of all fluids and diet taken orally and through an intravenous drip should be documented along with all their outputs such as urine, vomit, the nature and consistency of faeces, and whether they are sweating excessively. The difference between intake and output should be calculated every 24 hours and the result used to inform the next 24-hour fluid management. Regular testing of the person's blood electrolyte levels will determine whether specific electrolytes need to be added to the intravenous fluid.

In critical care, the assessment of circulation is invasive and detailed. It uses both central venous lines and arterial lines to assess the hydration status of the person, the function of the heart and the vascular tone, i.e., vasoconstriction, vasodilation.

What are the factors that influence the flow of blood around the body and the diseases or conditions that may affect this?

In critical care, some individuals may suffer acute renal failure because of poor fluid management before admission. These individuals will receive a gentle form of dialysis called haemofiltration. This form of dialysis is less likely to cause major shifts in blood volume adversely affecting blood pressure.

In addition to IV fluid, blood and blood product transfusions are frequently administered to critically ill adults. Transfusions can help increase oxygen delivery to the tissues and improve the oxygen demand/supply balance but may also have some harmful effects (Vincent et al., 2018). The various blood products that you may see administered are:

- Packed red blood cells;
- Platelets;
- Fresh frozen plasma;
- Albumin;
- Cryoprecipitate.

Activity 15.8

Globally, there are clear differences in transfusion practice (Vincent et al., 2018).

- What is your organisation's policy on blood and blood product transfusion?
- What are the risk factors and what safety measures are taken to manage these risks during transfusion?

Consider the needs of those who do not wish to receive blood or blood products. How have you seen this managed? Look at the NICE guidelines on alternatives to blood products:

www.nice.org.uk/guidance/ng24/chapter/Key-priorities-for-implementation#alternatives-to-blood-transfusion-for-patients-having-surgery.

Nutrition

During an episode of critical illness most people are unable to eat due to the presence of an artificial airway and the need to be sedated. The nutritional needs of critically ill adults are often poorly understood and can vary at different stages of illness. During critical illness profound metabolic changes occur and malnutrition is associated with impaired immune function and muscle weakness, resulting in increased ventilator-dependent days and length of stay in intensive care (McDonald et al., 2012). Nutrition support refers to enteral or parenteral provision of calories, protein, electrolytes, vitamins, minerals, trace elements and fluids. Enteral feeding, either through an oral or a nasal tube, or directly into the gastrointestinal tract via a gastrostomy or jejunostomy is the preferred method in critical care (McDonald et al., 2012).

Activity 15.9

What are the differences between *enteral* nutrition and *parenteral* nutrition?
What are the advantages and disadvantages of each method?
What are the nursing implications?

Discuss your findings with a dietician.

Sedation

The care and treatments provided in critical care can often be painful and invasive. To ensure that the level of intervention is tolerated, sedation is administered and is deemed an essential component of care (Whitehouse et al., 2014). In some cases, a paralysing agent is also required to aid a person's ventilation. As they recover, the level of sedation is reduced enabling them to breathe, allowing a decrease in the dependency on mechanical ventilation (Intensive Care Society, 2008). The level and type of sedation will vary from person to person with the most common sedative agents being opioids, benzodiazepines, intravenous, occasionally inhaled, general anaesthetic agents, neuroleptic drugs, phencyclidine derivatives, phenothiazines, α agonists and barbiturates (Whitehouse et al., 2014). The main aim of the sedation strategy is to use the minimal dose to ensure treatment compliance. The Intensive Care Society (2014) stated that the following were indications for the use of sedation:

- To alleviate pain;
- To facilitate the use of an otherwise distressing treatment and minimise discomfort, e.g., tolerance of ETTs and ventilation;
- To augment the effectiveness of a treatment, e.g., inverse ratio ventilation;
- As a treatment, e.g., seizure control or management of intracranial pressure;
- To reduce anxiety;
- To control agitation;
- For amnesia during neuromuscular block.

Assessment of sedation

There are many sedation scoring tools available but the most used are the Ramsay Sedation Scale (RSS) and the Richmond Agitation Sedation Score (RASS). Using a sedation scoring tool, doses of sedation can be titrated to achieve a pre-prescribed sedation score. Table 15.1 illustrates the RASS scoring system.

There are many complications with continuous sedation and the clinical team will often give a critically ill person a break from sedation.

Table 15.1 The Richmond Agitation Sedation Score (RASS)

Score	
+4	Combative, violent, danger to staff
+3	Pulls or removes tube(s) or catheters; aggressive
+2	Frequent non-purposeful movement, fights ventilator
+1	Anxious, apprehensive, but not aggressive
0	Alert and calm
−1	Awakens to voice (eye opening/contact) >10 s
−2	Light sedation, briefly awakens to voice (eye opening/contact) <10 s
−3	Moderate sedation, movement or eye opening. No eye contact
−4	Deep sedation, no response to voice, but movement or eye opening to physical stimulation
÷5	Unrousable, no response to voice or physical stimulation

(Adapted from Barr et al., 2013)

Activity 15.10

Review the Standards and Guidelines on sedation breaks issued by the Intensive Care Society at: www. ics.ac.uk

Legal and Ethical Considerations in Critical Care

Nurses in critical care environments may be faced with several situations or decisions that have ethical or legal considerations and they must approach such situations with due care and deliberation.

Consent

Although we covered the concepts of consent and mental capacity in Chapter 3, it is worthwhile revisiting these here as applied within the context of critical care provision. Consent should be obtained by any healthcare professional before any examination, treatment or care is provided. It is based on the fundamental principle of autonomy, whereby a person has the right to choose what happens to his or her own body. The Department of Health (DH, 2009: 9) guidance on consent considers that,

> *"For consent to be valid, it must be given voluntarily by an appropriately informed person who has capacity to consent to the intervention in question (this will be the person themselves or someone with parental responsibility for person under the age of 18, someone authorised to do so under a Lasting Power of Attorney (LPA) or someone who has the authority to make treatment decisions as a court appointed deputy)".*

Considering this statement, three key questions need to be considered:

1. Does the person have capacity?
2. Has consent been given voluntarily?
3. Has the person received sufficient information?

Does the person have capacity?

The assessment of a person's capacity to give or withhold consent is considered in relation to a specific decision. Although they may not have the capacity to make some decisions they may still retain capacity for other decisions. For example, a person may not have the capacity to decide about a surgical procedure but could retain the capacity to consent (or not) to having their clinical observations (e.g., blood pressure) checked. The Mental Capacity Act 2013 (see www.gov.uk/government/publications/mental-capacity-act-code-of-practice) provides guidance on the issue of capacity and has five key principles;

1 Every person has the right to make his or her own decisions and must be assumed to have capacity to make them unless it is proved otherwise;

2 A person must be given all practicable help before anyone treats them as not being able to make their own decisions;

3 Just because someone makes what might be seen as an unwise decision they should not be treated as lacking capacity to make that decision;

4 Anything done or any decisions made on behalf of someone who lacks capacity must be done in their best interest;

5 Anything done for or on behalf of someone who lacks capacity should be the least restrictive of their basic rights and freedoms.

If somone lacks capacity a decision may be made in their best interest. The Code of Practice (The Stationery Office, 2007) of the Mental Capacity Act 2013 also provides guidance on how best to establish a person's best interests. This will include trying to establish their previous wishes and feelings, and may involve consulting carers, family, or friends.

Is the consent given voluntarily?

Consent should be obtained voluntarily without coercion. Healthcare providers could be considered as being in a position of power whereas the person who is critically unwell may be in a vulnerable or stressed state. Likewise, family members can place undue pressure on the person's decision-making process and this needs to be considered. Ideally, someone should not feel pressurised into deciding quickly, without having had adequate time to consider their options. They also have the right to withdraw consent at any time.

Has the person received sufficient information?

Information should be provided to someone in a way that they can readily understand. The use of highly technical or medical jargon should be avoided. Information should be balanced, outlining potential benefits and the risks along with potential alternatives (if any). The use of interpreting services should be considered when appropriate.

In an emergency situation consent should still be sought from competent individuals but if this is not possible (e.g., a person who is unconscious) care can be provided that is in the person's *best interests*, i.e., that which is lifesaving or aimed at preventing serious deterioration.

Rueben

70 year-old Rueben is suffering from type II respiratory failure and is continuing to deteriorate. He has had a previous admission to the ICU and is refusing artificial ventilation. Some colleagues believe Rueben is delirious, which is affecting the decision-making process.

Jot down your thoughts about this case in relation to the following:

- Complexity in care delivery;
- Complexity in care management;
- Complexity in ethical decision making.

Do you know the difference between type I and type II respiratory failure?

Rueben has type II respiratory failure, which refers to poor carbon dioxide excretion from the lungs. Type I respiratory failure relates to low oxygen levels passing through the lungs into the bloodstream. Type I is referred to as hypoxaemia and type II as hypercapnia, but some people can have both. Rueben will require increased observation and as noted earlier, due to the potential for the need for advanced respiratory support, may need to be moved to a higher level of care. Rueben's wish not to be artificially ventilated may be due to impaired decision making because of deteriorating respiratory function or past ICU experience. This will need to be assessed carefully to establish if he does have the capacity to make an informed decision. The team will need to support and advocate for someone in situations such as this, and the involvement of family members is also key to ensuring that treatment and care are in the best interests of the individual concerned.

Pain, agitation and delirium in critical care settings

Delirium is a frequent problem in the acute setting, with Ryan et al. (2013) estimating that it may affect one in five of those receiving care. It is defined by Maldonado (2008) as an acute change in cognition, inattention, and a disturbance of consciousness. Delirium can develop over a brief period of hours or days and fluctuate over time (Griffiths and Jones, 2007). The NICE (2010) guidelines for delirium identify those at risk as:

- Aged 65 years or older;
- Having cognitive impairment (past or present) and/or dementia;
- Having a current hip fracture;
- Having a severe illness.

Ely et al. (2001) noted that individuals receiving care within an intensive care setting have a high probability of developing delirium due to multi-system illness, their co-morbidities, the use of psychoactive medications and age. Delirium is the most common neurological diagnosis among adults within ICU (Guenther et al., 2012) and yet is often missed by staff due to individuals with delirium displaying different clinical symptoms. A person with delirium can be restless, agitated, aggressive, and can try to remove a line and catheters. This is often referred to as *hyperactive* delirium (NICE, 2010). Those with hyperactive delirium are easily identified; however, a group who are often missed are those experiencing *hypoactive* delirium. These individuals become quiet, withdrawn, and sleepy (NICE, 2010). It is vital that this specific group of individuals are adequately assessed, diagnosed, and treated. The Confusion Assessment Method for the Intensive Care Unit (CAM-ICU) tool is one of the most common tools for identifying delirium in the ICU, which can be used by nurses and has been found to be a valid and reliable measure (Krahne et al., 2006; Nishimura et al., 2016).

Promotion of a Natural Sleep

Poor sleep is a frequent occurrence in the ICU and people cared for within such settings are known to have disrupted sleep and circadian rhythms (Ding et al., 2017). Reasons for sleep disruption may include the underlying illness, uncomfortable therapy, psychological stress, or the environment (Hu et al., 2015).

One of the challenges is to restore an individual's normal sleep–wake cycle and this can involve pharmacological and non-pharmacological interventions. Non-pharmacological interventions may include noise reduction strategies such as the use of earplugs, grouping of care activity to minimise disruption, music therapy, eye masks, complementary therapy, and using social and family support. Pharmacological approaches may include the use of melatonin and regular review of medication which may have a negative impact on someone's ability to sleep.

- How can you reduce the light and noise levels within a clinical environment?
- How do you plan your nursing interventions to reduce the number of interactions?

Decisions about CPR

Although most people would prefer to die in their own home, currently most who die in the UK die in hospital (Clark, 2022). Acknowledging this, there are issues about decision making at the end of life including those encompassing cardiopulmonary resuscitation (CPR). The British Medical Association (BMA), the Resuscitation Council (UK) and the Royal College of Nursing's (2016) decisions relating to CPR provide some guidance. Some of the main points identified in the document are as follows:

1 'Where no explicit decision about CPR has been considered and recorded in advance, there should be an initial presumption in favour of CPR';
2 'Every decision about CPR must be made on the basis of a careful assessment of each individual's situation';

3 'Clear and full documentation of decisions about CPR, the reasons for them, and the discussions that informed those decisions are an essential part of high-quality care';

4 'Each decision about CPR should be subject to review based on the person's individual circumstances';

5 'Any decision about CPR should be communicated clearly to all those involved in the person's care';

6 'A DNACPR (Do Not Attempt CPR) decision does not override clinical judgement in the unlikely event of a reversible cause of a person's respiratory or cardiac arrest that does not match the circumstances envisaged when that decision was made and recorded. Examples of such reversible causes include but are not restricted to choking, a displaced tracheal tube or a blocked tracheostomy tube';

7 'Deciding not to attempt CPR that has no realistic prospect of success does not require consent of the individual or of those close to them. However, there is a presumption in favour of informing an individual patient of such a decision.'

Activity 15.11

Access the following website and read the guidance related to CPR:

www.resus.org.uk/library/publications/publication-decisions-relating-cardiopulmonary

Access and read the following document: Joyce, T. (2007) *Best Interests Guidance on Determining the Best Interests of Adults who Lack the Capacity to Make a Decision (or Decisions) for Themselves (England and Wales)*. Leicester: The British Psychological Society.

• How could you use the guidance above to inform the decision-making process when considering Rueben's 'best interests'?

Organ and Tissue Donation

There were 586,334 deaths registered in England and Wales in 2021 (Office for National Statistics [ONS] 2023). A small group of individuals being cared for in critical care environments have the potential to become organ donors after death. During 2021–22, 1397 people donated their organs to help others with lifesaving and life-enhancing transplant operations (NHS Blood and Transplant, 2022). However, the number of people waiting for an organ transplant far outstripped the number of donated organs. On 31 March 2022, 6269 people were on the active transplant waiting list, which included a high proportion of people from ethnic backgrounds for whom those from the same ethnic group were more likely to be a good match. Although increases over the last few years are encouraging, BAME communities are still under-represented among those donating (NHS Blood and Transplant, 2019).

Many must wait months, even years, for their transplant and sadly, some die while waiting. On average, three people on the transplant waiting list die every day because no suitable donor organ had been identified (NHS Blood and Transplant, 2022).

The three categories of organ donation include donation following brainstem death (DBD), donation following circulatory death (DCD) and living donation. Deceased organ donation is only possible from the DBD and DCD route - usually within the critical care areas. Clinically, the individual is often on mechanical ventilation and vasoactive drugs. DBD arises when brainstem death testing confirms the absence of brainstem reflexes (Academy of Medical Royal Colleges, 2008; Bleakley, 2017). DCD occurs following the withdrawal of life-sustaining treatment. Living donation occurs when a healthy person donates an organ to an identified recipient as either a directed donation (the donor may have genetic or pre-existing emotional relationship) or a directed altruistic donation, whereby the donor and recipient have no qualifying genetic or pre-existing emotional relationship (Human Tissue Authority, 2017).

Activity 15.12

The Organ Donation and Transplantation (ODT) clinical website provides online learning resources that are useful and informative. Access the website below and search for the distinct types of organs and tissue that can be donated: www.odt.nhs.uk.

A clinical plan to perform brainstem death testing or planned withdrawal of life-sustaining treatment on a critically ill person should trigger an urgent referral to the on-call specialist nurse–organ donation (SNOD). The SNOD is specifically trained to facilitate all aspects of the donation process including initiating donation conversations with distressed relatives/carers. The refusal rate for organ donation in the UK is 42% (significantly higher than other European countries). Refusal of family consent for organ and tissue donation is the single greatest barrier to lifesaving and life-enhancing transplants (Hulme et al., 2016). Consent rates for donation are significantly higher if the approach is made by the SNOD, working collaboratively with the clinical team.

There are slightly different laws in the UK that relate to consent to organ donation. In May 2020 in England, the law has changed so that all adults in England are considered to have agreed to be an organ donor when they unless they have recorded a decision not to donate, the 'opt out' system. Some people will not be able to be considered and they are in an excluded group. In Wales, the process is similar, there is 'deemed consent,' unless the person has objected and in Scotland it is 'deemed authorisation' for donation if the person has not stipulated a preference. The change for Scotland came into effect in 2021 and in Wales the relevant legislation was introduced in 2015. In Northern Ireland, the change in legislation can into effect in 2023 and is the same as England, the 'opt out' process.

NHS Blood and Transplant have produced guidance on how best to approach a relative/carer with an organ donation request. As identified by Kübler-Ross (1969), normal grief response observes the relative/carer enter a primary state of denial after the delivery of bad news. Nurses need to be mindful of the inner turmoil experienced by relatives/carers before making an approach. Best practice encourages nurses to make a referral to the on-call SNOD and gain expert advice (Bleakley, 2010; NICE, 2011). Critical care areas often have extensive resources regarding organ and tissue donation, including the pager/telephone number for the on-call specialist. Figure 15.2 provides a suitable structure to plan for difficult donation discussions.

Organ donation occurs with a specific and small number of deaths in critical care areas, but almost every other death in a hospital or community setting has the potential for tissue donation. It is helpful to establish known wishes before initiating donation discussion. This requires nurses to routinely check the organ donor register (ODR) after the death of an individual. The ODR is a confidential NHS database that can be accessed 24 hours a day, 7 days a week, allowing clinical staff to assess whether a person has already made their donation wishes known. Even if the person has a known absolute contraindication to donation, it is helpful to inform the relative/carer that donation was not possible due to a specific clinical reason. This approach ensures that donation is embraced as a normal part of end-of-life care within the clinical setting and, more importantly, does not leave the relative/carer wondering whether donation was possible (DH, 2008). Many clinical settings are specialised, with intricate disease processes contributing

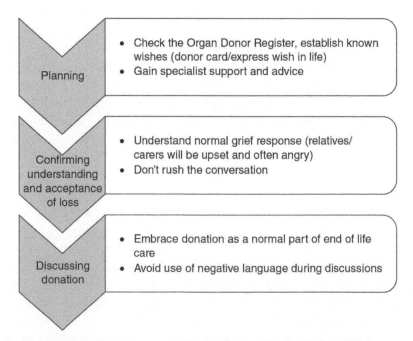

Figure 15.2 Consent: the family approach. (Adapted from NHS Blood and Transplant, 2017). Available at: www.odt.nhs.uk/deceased-donation/best-practice-guidance/consent-and-authorisation

to the death of a person. It is important that nurses do not make any judgement on whether the person is a suitable candidate for organ and tissue donation. They must remember to gain specialist advice from the SNOD or specialist nurse in the National Referral Centre (NRC) for tissue donation and allow these professionals to use their clinical judgement on suitability.

Activity 15.13

Access the following link and identify the process for contacting the NHS Blood and Transplant Duty Office to check the Organ Donor Register (ODR): www.organdonation.nhs.uk/register-your-decision/check-registration

Identify the contact details for the SNOD who can be contacted for professional advice, training, and further support.

George

You are working on the acute medical unit (AMU) and admit George who has increasing shortness of breath (dyspnoea) with underlying ischaemic heart disease (IHD). George's clinical condition rapidly deteriorates and results in a cardiorespiratory arrest. Despite advanced life support (ALS) from the resuscitation team, the decision is taken to stop CPR and death is confirmed. Following your involvement with the cardiac arrest, you discuss care after the death process with clinical colleagues. You think that tissue donation might be an option. No one has considered donation as an end-of-life option and notice that George's partner is tearful and distressed at the bedside. You raise the issue of donation with other team members who agree to support you with a donation request.

- How would you check the Organ Donor Register to establish if George has made the wishes to donate clear?
- What are your immediate plans to initiate the donation discussion with George's partner?
- What words are you going to use during the donation request?

Supporting the Families of Critically Ill Adults

When a person is acutely unwell the psychological distress within family members is an inherent factor that a nurse needs to be mindful of and they should do their utmost to provide appropriate support. Informing an individual that their loved one is acutely unwell and moving to a department such as an ICU can illicit the same response outlined elsewhere in the book when breaking bad news. The ability to calm feelings of panic and distress felt by critically ill adults, family and friends is an important aspect of care that cannot be over-looked and will place significant demands on your communication skills and ability to dem-onstrate empathy, compassion and understanding. For example, the society we currently live in is diverse and as a nurse you will encounter various types of 'family.' In fact, due to this the term 'significant other' is often used. A lot of high care areas such as ICUs have extremely strict visiting rules related to family only, and yet as adults we have more than 'family' mem-bers who may want to visit and offer support These restrictions can put increased strain on an already stressed individual trying to visit. In addition, families may be left waiting while interventions are carried out, such as a line insertion or X-rays. Nurses must remain vigilant in updating families and visitors about the reasons why they have been asked to wait.

The families of those admitted to an ICU are often in a highly anxious state and are con-fronted with a highly technical environment with their loved one at the centre, so it is vital they are adequately supported. Families can provide a crucial contribution to the person's care. After receiving care in an ICU setting, many individuals have problems recalling ele-ments of their illness and care and families can provide this insight into the experience. More importantly, families can be provided with reassurance and support. A study conducted by Kean (2014), which explored how ICU nurses perceived families, found that families made notable contributions to an individual's care; however, the nurses felt they needed to remain in control of that involvement.

If the critically ill adult or their 'significant other' is happy to receive a visitor, do you think nurses should be able to act as 'gatekeepers' in this way?

What factors would influence your decision to limit visiting?

How do you feel about families witnessing resuscitation? Find out what the policy is in your place-ment area in relation to families witnessing resuscitation.

You may want to read the guidance from the Resuscitation Council (UK) 2021 at www.resus.org.uk.

What sort of reception do families and visitors get in your current clinical area?

Access and read the Intensive Care Society's (1998) *Guidelines for Bereavement Care in Intensive Care Units*.

After critical care

Individuals and their families can often feel anxious and apprehensive about the move from critical care to a ward environment. They will need lots of reassurance and may have many questions about the care provided. Recipients of critical care may be experiencing significant changes in their body image or mobility, appetite, and sleep as well as the physiological impact of surviving a critical illness. Many have difficulty remembering their time during their critical illness, and some departments use diaries compiled by family and staff to support and address these gaps in memories. To ensure continuity of care, the person's rehabilitation care pathway should be coordinated and communicated to the new nursing team.

The NICE (2017) document on rehabilitation after critical illness in adults states that:

Quality statement 1: Rehabilitation goals: adults in critical care at risk of morbidity have their rehabilitation goals agreed within 4 days of admission to critical care or before discharge from critical care, whichever is sooner;

Quality statement 2: Transfer from critical care to a general ward: adults at risk of morbidity have a formal handover of care, including their agreed individualised structured rehabilitation programme, when they transfer from critical care to a general ward;

Quality statement 3: Information on discharge from hospital: adults who were in critical care and at risk of morbidity are given information based on their rehabilitation goals before they are discharged from hospital;

Quality statement 4: Follow-up after critical care discharge: adults who stayed in critical care for more than 4 days and were at risk of morbidity have a review 2–3 months after discharge from critical care.

(Reproduced with permission under the NICE UK Open Content Licence)

Although the guidelines are clear and useful, they address the care and rehabilitation of an adult only within an acute care setting. Stepping down from critical care is challenging for the individual, their family members, and staff. The needs of a person post-critical illness are complex, and they are often vulnerable. It is well documented that some adults experience intense anxiety when being discharged from the critical care unit (Kauppi et al., 2018). Readmission to critical care is associated with increased mortality. Discharging someone too quickly, without appropriate resources and poor communication, contributes towards poor healthcare outcomes. Stepping down from critical care must be planned, controlled and appropriate (Kauppi et al., 2018).

Nasar

54 year-old Nasar has had a 3-month stay in ICU admission due to sepsis, requiring the insertion of a temporary tracheostomy, sedation, and ventilation for several weeks. Weaning from the ventilator was prolonged. Nasar was transferred to a different clinical area for a further two weeks. During this time, the tracheostomy was removed; however, Nasar remained weak with a significant loss of muscle

mass and experienced nightmares and flashbacks from the ICU admission. Nasar also has residual renal impairment following the illness but is now fit for discharge.

Consider the implications of Nasar being discharged home. What do the community team need to be aware of?

How effective do you think our current strategies of communicating a person's clinical history across services are?

Chapter Summary

Nurses have a leading role in ensuring safe, person-centered care is provided. This chapter has discussed some of the knowledge, skills and attributes needed by adult nurses working in a critical care setting. Medical technology is part of the modern healthcare environment and is not limited to critical care areas. A nurse should use appropriate technology for the benefit of those under their care but also be aware of the potential of over-reliance. It is important to remember that the critical care environment can be a scary place for individuals and their families, so the importance of compassion in nursing cannot be over-emphasised. An admission to a critical care environment can be the result of a vast range of reasons that we are unable to cover in this chapter, but we hope this will provide a springboard for your interest in critical care nursing.

Useful Websites

For information on distinct types of arrhythmias, their causes, and treatments, see the following websites:

www.nhs.uk/conditions/arrhythmia/Pages/arrhythmia.aspx

www.bhf.org.uk/informationsupport/publications/heart-conditions/heart-rhythms

www.bhf.org.uk/publications/heart-conditions/m111a-inherited-heart-conditions—sudden-arrythmic-death-syndrome

www.heartrhythmalliance.org/aa/uk

British Association of Critical Care Nurses (BACCN): www.baccn.org/Intensive Care Society: https://ics.ac.uk/

Faculty of Intensive Care Medicine: www.ficm.ac.uk/

NHS Blood and Transplant Organ Donation and Transplantation: www.odt.nhs.uk/

Further Reading

Bickley, L.S. (2021) *Bates' Guide to Physical Examination and History Taking*, 13th edn. Philadelphia, PA: Lippincott, Williams & Wilkins.

Bleakley, G. (2017) 'Understanding brainstem death testing,' *British Journal of Neuroscience Nursing*, 13(4): 172–7.

Boore, J., Cook, N. and Shepard, A. (2016) *Essentials of Anatomy and Physiology for Nursing Practice*. London: Sage.

Brooker, C. and Nichol, M. (2019) *Alexander's Nursing Practice*, 5th edn. London: Churchill Livingstone.

Cooke, N., Shepherd, A and Boore, J. (2020) 'Cardiovascular and Lymphatic Systems: Internal Transport', Chapter 12. In *Essentials of Anatomy and Physiology for Nursing Practice*, 2nd edn. London: Sage.

Freeman, S., Steen, C. and Bleakley, G. (2021) *Essentials of Nursing Critically Ill Adults*. London: Sage.

National Institute for Health and Care Excellence (2021) *Patient Experience in Adult NHS Services: Improving the Experience of Care for People Using Adult NHS Services*. NICE Clinical Guidance 138. London: NICE.

O'Driscoll, B.R., Howard, L.S., Earis, J. on behalf of the BTS Emergency Oxygen Guideline Development Group, et al. (2017) 'British Thoracic Society Guideline for oxygen use in adults in healthcare and emergency settings', *BMJ Open Respiratory Research*, 4: e000170. doi: 10.1136/bmjresp-2016-000170

Resuscitation Council (UK) (2021) *2021 Resuscitation Guidelines*. Available at: www.resus.org.uk/library/2021-resuscitation-guidelines

Tait, D., James, J., Williams, C. and Barton, D. (2022) *Acute and Critical Care in Adult Nursing*, 3rd edn. London: Sage.

References

Academy of Medical Royal Colleges (2008) *A Code of Practice for the Diagnosis of Death*. Portsmouth: PPG Design and Print Ltd.

Alcan, A., Giersbergen, M.Y., Dinscarslan, G., Hepcivici, Z., Kaya, E. and Uyar, M. (2016) 'Effect of patient position on endotracheal cuff pressure in mechanically ventilated critically ill patients', *Australian Critical Care*, 30(5): 267–72.

Arshad, H., Young, M., Adurty, R. and Singh, A.C. (2016) 'Acute pneumothorax', *Critical Care Nursing*, 39(2): 176–89.

Barr, J., Fraser, G.L., Puntillo, K., Ely, E.W., Gélinas, C., Dasta, J.F., Davidson, J.E., Devlin, J.W., Kress, J.P., Joffe, A.M. et al. (2013) 'Clinical practice guidelines for the management of pain, agitation, and delirium in adult patients in the intensive care unit', *Critical Care Medicine*, 41(1): 263–306.

Benson, S., Johnson, A. and Petera, C. (2013) 'VAP Free for 1000 days, it can be done', *Critical Care Nursing*, 36(4): 421–4.

Bleakley, G. (2010) 'Implementing minimum notification criteria for organ donation in an acute hospital's critical care units', *Nursing in Critical Care*, 15(4): 185–91.

Bleakley, G. (2017) 'Understanding brainstem death testing', *British Journal of Neuroscience Nursing*, 13(4): 172–7.

Bloomfield R, Noble DW, Sudlow A. (2015), Prone position for acute respiratory failure in adults. *Cochrane Database of Systematic Reviews* 11. Art. No.: CD008095. DOI: 10.1002/14651858. CD008095.pub

British Medical Association, the Resuscitation Council (UK) and the Royal College of Nursing (2016) *Decisions Relating to Cardiopulmonary Resuscitation*, 3rd edn. (Guidance from the British Medical Association, the Resuscitation Council (UK) and the Royal College of Nursing [previously known as the 'Joint Statement']). Available at: www.bma.org.uk/advice-and-support/ethics/end-of-life/decisions-relating-to-cpr-cardiopulmonary-resuscitation. (last accessed 26 August 2022).

Chen, H.-B., Liu, J., Chen, L.-Q. and Wang, G.-C. (2014) 'Effectiveness of daily interruption of sedation in sedated patients with mechanical ventilation in ICU: a systematic review', *International Journal of Nursing Sciences*, 1(4): 346–51.

Critical Care 3 Network (2018) *National Competency Framework (steps 1–4)*. Available at: www.cc3n.org.uk/step-competency-framework.html (last accessed 25 June 2023).

Clark, D. (2022) *Death in the UK - Statistics & Facts*. Available at: www.statista.com/topics/6656/death-in-the-uk/. (last accessed 26 August 2022).

Department of Health (2000) *Comprehensive Critical Care. A Review of Adult Critical Care Services*. London: DH.

Department of Health (2008) *Organs for Transplant: A Report from the Organ Donation Taskforce*. London: DH.

Department of Health (2009) *Consent for Examination, Treatment or Care*. London: DH. Available at: www.health-ni.gov.uk/articles/consent-examination-treatment-or-care (last accessed 30th August 2022).

Department of Health/Emergency Care (2005) *Quality Critical Care – Beyond 'Comprehensive Critical Care'*. London: DH/Emergency Care. Available at: http://webarchive.nationalarchives.gov.uk/20130124071030/http://www.dh.gov.uk/prod_consum_dh/groups/dh_digitalassets/@dh/@en/documents/digitalasset/dh_4121050.pdf (last accessed 26 August 2022).

Ding, Q., Redeker, N.S., Pisani, M.A., Yaggi, H.K. and Knauert, M.P. (2017) 'Factors influencing patients' sleep in the intensive care unit: perceptions of patients and clinical staff', *America Journal of Critical Care*, 26(4): 278–86.

Drahnak, D.M. and Custer, N. (2015) 'Prone positioning of patients with acute respiratory distress syndrome', *Critical Care Nurse*, 35(6): 29–37.

Ely, E.W., Inouye, S.K., Bernard, G.R., Francis, J., May, L., Truman, B., Speroff, T., Gautam, S., Margolin, R., Hart, R.P. and Dittus, R. (2001) 'Delirium in mechanically ventilated patients: validity and reliability of the Confusion Assessment Method for the Intensive Care Unit (CAM-ICU)', *Journal of the American Medical Association*, 286: 2703–10.

The Faculty of Intensive Care Medicine/Intensive Care Society (2022), *Guidelines for the Provision of Intensive Care Services*. Available at: https://www.ficm.ac.uk/standardssafetyguidelinesstandards/guidelines-for-the-provision-of-intensive-care-services. (last accessed 10 July 2023)

Freeman, S. (2011) 'Care of adult patients with a temporary tracheostomy', *Nursing Standard*, 26(2): 49–56.

Griffiths, R.D. and Jones, C. (2007) 'Deliriums, cognitive dysfunction and posttraumatic stress disorder', *Current Opinion in Anaesthesiology*, 20(2): 124–9.

Guenther, U., Weykam, J., Andorfer, U., Theuerkauf, N., Poop, J., Ely, W. and Putensen, C. (2012) 'Implications of objective vs subjective delirium assessment in surgical intensive care patients', *American Journal of Critical Care*, 21(1): 12–20.

Hellyer, T.P., Ewan, V. and Wilson, P. (2016) 'The Intensive Care Society recommended bundle of interventions for the prevention of ventilator-associated pneumonia', *Journal of the Intensive Care Society*, 17(3): 238–43.

Higginson, R., Jones, B. and Davies, K. (2011) 'Emergency and intensive care: assessing and managing the airway', *British Journal of Nursing*, 20(16): 973–7.

Hu, R.-F., Jiang, H.R.F., Chen, J., Zeng, Z., Chen, X.Y., Li, Y., Huining, X. and Evans, D.J. (2015) 'Nonpharmacological interventions for sleep promotion in the intensive care unit', *Cochrane Database of Systematic Reviews*, doi: 10.1002/14651858.CD008808.pub2.

Hulme, W., Allen, J., Manara, A.R., Murphy, P., Gardiner, D. and Poppitt, E. (2016) 'Factors influencing the family consent rate for organ donation in the UK', *Anaesthesia*, 17(9): 1053–63.

Human Tissue Authority (2017) *Types of Living Donation*. Available at: www.hta.gov.uk/guidance-public/living-organ-donation/types-living-organ-donation (last accessed 26 August 2022).

Intensive Care Society (1998) *Guidelines for Bereavement Care in Intensive Care Units*. London: The Intensive Care Society.

Intensive Care Society (2008) *Standards for the Care of Adult Patients with a Temporary Tracheostomy*. London: The Intensive Care Society.

Intensive Care Society (2014) *Review of Best Practice for Analgesia and Sedation in Critical Care*. London: Intensive Care Society.

Kauppi, W., Proos, M. and Olausson, S. (2018) 'Ward nurses' experiences of the discharge process between intensive care unit and general ward', *Nursing in Critical Care*, 23(3): 127–33.

Kean, S. (2014) 'How do intensive care nurses perceive families in intensive care? Insights from the United Kingdom and Australia,' *Journal of Clinical Nursing*, 23(5–6): 663–72.

Krahne, D., Heymann, A. and Spies, C. (2006) 'How to monitor delirium in the ICU and why it is important', *Clinical Effectiveness in Nursing*, 269–79.

Kübler-Ross, E. (1969) *On Death and Dying*. London: Tavistock Publications.

Lazy C. Swinnnen W. Labeau S. et al (2014) Cuff Pressure of Endotracheal Tubes After Changes in Body Position in Critically Ill Patients Treated with Mechanical Ventilation. *American Journal of Critical Care*. 23(1): e1-e8.

McDonald, K., Page, K., Brown, L. and Bryden, D. (2012) 'Parenteral nutrition in critical care', *Continuing Education in Anaesthesia Critical Care & Pain*, 13(1): 1–5.

Makic, M.B.F. (2015) 'Rethinking mobility and intensive care patients', *Journal of Perianesthesia Nursing*, 30(2): 151–2.

Maldonado, J.R. (2008) 'Delirium in the acute care setting: characteristics, diagnosis and treatment', *Critical Care Clinics*, 24: 657–722.

National Institute for Health and Care Excellence (2010) *Delirium: Diagnosis, Prevention and Management* (last updated 14 March 2019). London: NICE.

National Institute for Health and Care Excellence (2011) *Organ Donation for Transplantation: Improving Donor Identification and Consent Rates for Deceased Organ Donation*, Clinical Guidance 135 (last updated 21 Dec 2016). London: NICE. Available at: www.nice.org.uk/Guidance/CG135 (last accessed 26 August 2022).

National Institute for Health and Care Excellence (2017) *Rehabilitation after Critical Illness*, Clinical Guidance QS158. London: NICE. Available at: www.nice.org.uk/guidance/QS158. (last accessed 26 August 2022).

National Institute for Health and Care Excellence (2021) *Atrial fibrillation: diagnosis and management (NG196)*. Available at: www.nice.org.uk/guidance/ng196. (last accessed 26 August 2022).

National Institute for Health and Care Excellence (2018) *Critical Care Outreach Teams Emergency and Acute Medical Care in Over 16s: Service Delivery and Organisation* London: NICE. Available at: www.nice.org.uk/guidance/ng94/evidence/27.critical-care-outreach-teams-pdf-172397464640 (last accessed 26th August 2022).

National Institute for Health and Care Excellence (2021) *Atrial Fibrillation: Diagnosis and management*, Clinical Guidance CG180. Available at: www.nice.org.uk/guidance/ng196. (last accessed 26 August 2022).

Neuville, M., Mourvillier, B., Bouadma, L. and Timsit, J.-F. (2017) 'Bundle of care decreased ventilator-associated events: implications for ventilator-associated pneumonia prevention', *Journal of Thoracic Disease*, 9(3): 430–3.

NHS Blood and Transplant (2017) *Consent: The Family Approach*. Available at: www.odt.nhs.uk/deceased-donation/best-practice-guidance/consent-and-authorisation-the-family-approach/. (last accessed 26 August 2022).

NHS Blood and Transplant (2019) *Organ Donation and Transplantation data for Black, Asian, and Minority Ethnic (BAME) communities Report for 2018/2019* (1 April 2014-31 March 2019). Available at: www.odt.nhs.uk/statistics-and-reports/ (last accessed 26 August 2022).

NHS Blood and Transplant (2022) *Transplant Activity Report*. Available at: https://nhsbtdbe.blob.core.windows.net/umbraco-assets-corp/27107/activity-report-2021-2022.pdf (last accessed 2 August 2022).

NICE (2018), Critical care outreach teams Emergency and acute medical care in over 16s: service delivery and organisation, Chapter 27. Available at: www.nice.org.uk/guidance/ng94/evidence/27.critical-care-outreach-teams-pdf-172397464640 (last accessed 25 June 2023)

Nishimura, K., Yokoyama, K., Yamauchi, N., Koizumi, M., Harasawa, N., Yasuda, T., Mimura, C., Igita, H., Suzuki, E., Uchiide, Y., Seino, Y., Nomura, M., Yamazaki, K., and Ishigooka, J (2016), Sensitivity and specificity of the Confusion Assessment Method for the Intensive Care Unit (CAM-ICU) and the Intensive Care Delirium Screening Checklist (ICDSC) for detecting post-cardiac surgery delirium: A single-centre study in Japan *Heart & Lung: The Journal of Cardiopulmonary and Acute Care*, Volume 45, Issue 1, 15 – 20

Nursing and Midwifery Council (2018) *Future Nurse: Standards of Proficiency for Registered Nurses*. London: NMC.

Office for National Statistics (2023) "Deaths registered in England and Wales: 2021 (refreshed populations) Registered deaths by age, sex, selected underlying causes of death, leading causes of death. Death rates and registrations by residence area, single year of age." Available at: (last accessed June 2023).

Pattison, N. and Eastham, E. (2011) 'Critical care outreach referrals: a mixed-method investigative study of outcomes and experiences', *Nursing in Critical Care*, 17(2): 71–82.

Resuscitation Council (UK) (2021) *Immediate Life Support Manual*, 8th edn. London: Resuscitation Council (UK).

Ryan, D.J., O'Regan, N.A., Caoimh, R.Ó., Clare, J., O'Connor, M., Leonard, M., McFarland, J., Tighe, S., O'Sullivan, K., Trzepaczk, P.T. et al. (2013) 'Delirium in an adult acute hospital population: predictors, prevalence and detection', *BMJ Open*, 3: e001772. doi:10.1136/bmjopen-2012-001772.

Scaravilli, V., Grasselli, G., Castagna, L., Zanella, A., Isgro, S., Lucchini, A., Patroniti, N., Bellani, G. and Pesenti, A. (2015) 'Prone positioning improves oxygenation in spontaneously breathing nonintubated patients with hypoxemic acute respiratory failure: a retrospective study', *Journal of Critical Care*, 30(6): 1390–4.

Scholz, A.W., Weiler, N., David, M. and Markstaller, K. (2011) 'Respiratory mechanics measured by forced oscillations during mechanical ventilation through a tracheal tube', *Physiological Measures*, 32(5): 571–83.

Singh, S. (2016) 'Respiratory symptoms and signs', *Medicine*, 44(4): 205–12.

Stationery Office, The (2013) *Mental Capacity Act Code of Practice*. London: TSO. Available at: www.gov.uk/government/publications/mental-capacity-act-code-of-practice (last accessed 30 August 2022).

Vincent, J.-L., Jaschinski, U., Wittebole, X., Lefrant, J.-Y., Jakob, S.M., Almekhlafi, G.A. et al., on behalf of the ICON Investigators (2018) 'Worldwide audit of blood transfusion practice in critically ill patients', *Critical Care*, 22: 102.

Whitehouse, T., Snelson, C., Grounds, M., Willson, J., Tulloch, L., Linhartova, L., Shah, A., Pierson, R. and England, K. (2014) *Review of Best Practice for Analgesia and Sedation in Critical Care*. Available at: www.ics.ac.uk/Society/Guidance/PDFs/Analgesia_and_Sedation. (last accessed 26 August 2022).

Zhao, T., Wu, X., Zhang, Q., Li, C., Worthington, H.V. and Hua, F. (2020) 'Oral hygiene care for critically ill patients to prevent ventilator-associated pneumonia', *Cochrane Database of Systematic Reviews* 2020, 12. Art. No.: CD008367. DOI: 10.1002/14651858.CD008367.pub4

16

PALLIATIVE CARE

Laura Green and Joanne Timpson

Chapter Objectives

- Describe the way in which palliative care for adults has been developed in the UK;
- Explain the principles of palliative care and identify key policies and standards which underpin an evidence-based approach;
- Highlight the importance of effective communication and therapeutic relationships in exploring individual choice and preferences in end-of-life care;
- Explore the legal and ethical issues associated with end-of-life care and advanced planning decisions;
- Define what constitutes a good death for individuals, their family members and health practitioners;
- Examine the role of the nurse in meeting the needs of informal caregivers;
- Define effective end-of-life care for individuals and their family members, illustrating how to initiate, implement and carry out culturally competent care effectively and sensitively.

Introduction

Although palliative care is often described as a specific clinical field provided by specialists and sometimes within dedicated institutions, this chapter addresses the broader scope of generalist palliative care. We propose that a palliative approach to care transcends clinical specialisms. Developing skills in palliative care is relevant to nurses in all clinical areas. No matter where you work, you will encounter people affected by life-limiting illness or grief. Nurses frequently encounter people at transitional points in their lives which may be characterised by uncertainty and loss of independence. Living with, and dying from life-limiting illness presents complex, existential challenges to individuals, their carers and professionals. This chapter intends to provide an overview of the context of palliative care in the United Kingdom, illustrated by case studies and reflection points throughout. Whilst it can only present an introduction to the vast field of caring for the dying and bereaved, we hope that we manage to communicate something of the richness and diversity of palliative care nursing.

Related Nursing and Midwifery Council (NMC) Proficiencies for Registered Nurses

Nursing people at the end of life is a uniquely sensitive area or practice that requires demonstration of the full range of NMC competencies. All nurses must act in the best interests of people, putting them first and ensuring that care is safe and compassionate. Working in partnership with individuals and their families is vital in palliative care, as is effective multidisciplinary team collaboration. Proficiency 3.2 states that nurses will: *'recognise and respond compassionately to the needs of those who are in the last few days and hours of life'* (NMC, 2018). Of course, end-of-life care is not restricted to this very last part of life, the period often referred to as 'active dying.' This chapter seeks to broaden the concept of end-of-life care and addresses a range of ways in which nurses can develop their skills and competencies.

━━━━━ TO ACHIEVE ENTRY TO THE NMC REGISTER

YOU MUST BE ABLE TO ━━━━━

- Take appropriate action to always ensure privacy and dignity;
- Understand and apply DNACPR (Do Not Attempt Cardiopulmonary Resuscitation) decisions and verification of expected death;
- Engage in difficult conversations, including breaking bad news and support people who are feeling physically vulnerable or in distress, conveying compassion and sensitivity;
- Identify and assess the needs of individuals and their families for care at the end of life, including requirements for palliative care and decision making related to their treatment and care preferences;
- Understand and apply advance planning decisions, living wills and health and Lasting Power of Attorney;
- Assess and review preferences and care priorities of the dying person, and their family and carers;
- Demonstrate the knowledge and skills required to prioritise what is important to individuals and their families when providing evidence-based, person-centred nursing care at the end of life, including the care of people who are dying, their families, the deceased and the bereaved;
- Provide care for the deceased person and the bereaved, respecting cultural requirements and local protocols.

(Adapted from NMC, 2018)

Palliative care in the UK originated with the work of Dame Cicely Saunders, who established the world's first hospice in 1967 (Clark, 2016). St Christopher's Hospice was built to provide care for the dying, at a time when cancer was a much-feared diagnosis and pain was not managed well. Saunders trained as a nurse, then a social worker. Her work with people dying from cancer led her to develop the concept of 'total pain,' the notion that suffering comprises physical, psychological, social, and spiritual elements, and that therapeutic engagement with an individual requires a professional to address the person in their entirety. This holistic view of care provision is the foundation of palliative care and continues to provide the framework for nursing assessment of those facing the end of life.

Since that time, palliative care has become available across the globe, albeit to varying degrees. In 1987, palliative medicine was recognised as a medical sub-speciality through the work of Balfour-Mount (Clark, 2016). In 1993, the first textbook on the subject was published – the *Oxford Textbook of Palliative Medicine* is now in its fifth edition (Cherny et al., 2015).

In 2015, *The Economist* published the Quality of Death Index, a ranking of palliative care across the world. For those countries ranking highly, there were several shared characteristics including having a strong national palliative care policy framework and high levels of public spending on healthcare services. Additionally, the quality of dying was influenced by the availability of opioids, public awareness of palliative care and financial support for people with life-limiting illnesses (The Economist Intelligence Unit, 2015). However, here in the UK there is no room for complacency. There are many areas in which the quality of care is thought to be less than ideal. For example, several recent investigations have highlighted concerns about the quality of hospital based end-of-life care, particularly for older adults (Parliamentary and Health Service Ombudsman, 2011; Francis, 2013; Parliamentary and Health Service Ombudsman, 2015). Care homes have also come under scrutiny with issues around inappropriate hospital admissions, lack of clarity about advance care planning and 'do not resuscitate' orders, and communication and continuity of care. Whilst strong opioids and other medications may be readily available, this is not the case across the country. Variations in services and issues with accessibility still mean that an unacceptable number of people experience delays in symptom management and palliative care which can often precipitate an unplanned admission to hospital. The role of the nurse is crucial to the development and provision of good palliative care.

Concepts and Controversies

The term 'palliative' is derived from the medieval Latin 'palliare,' meaning 'to cloak.' The term is often misunderstood, even by healthcare professionals. It is important to be clear about what is meant when a 'palliative' approach to care is indicated. Whilst as a nurse you are unlikely to be the first person to mention palliative care directly to an individual or their family, you may well find yourself in the role of interpreter when someone has been given bad news, or of speaking to a worried family member who has found out information online about their loved one's condition. This can be a source of anxiety for inexperienced nurses; worries about 'saying the wrong thing' or 'not knowing what to say' are often described by students faced with these kinds of situations.

Later in the chapter, we will briefly touch upon some approaches to communication that can help reassure students that not only are they well equipped to support people and their families at this distressing time, but that they are often the healthcare professionals who have the most time to spend with them to talk, without the responsibilities of the registered nurse. This means that spending time with people receiving palliative care whilst you are still a student can provide a valuable opportunity to develop and refine your skills of sensitive communication and active listening.

Many individuals are concerned that adopting a 'palliative' approach means that nothing more can be done. It is important to dispel that myth. One helpful way to view the transition from active to palliative care is to consider a change in gear, where the priority shifts from cure to comfort. Palliative care is provided when there are significantly diminished opportunities for cure. It is no longer restricted to those with malignant conditions but can be an appropriate form of care right from the point of diagnosis in some instances. Further, palliative care is often given concurrently with curative treatment where there are significant issues such as symptom problems or where the chances of cure are remote. It is unsurprising then that this causes so much confusion in practice. The following case study about David illustrates a typical scenario.

David

David has advanced chronic obstructive pulmonary disease (COPD) and has recently been admitted to hospital with an acute infective exacerbation for the fourth time this year. Each time, antibiotics, oxygen, and steroids have been administered and David has managed to return home. David's case is mentioned at the GP practice's Gold Standards Framework meeting as someone who might benefit from some additional support as they are deteriorating. The District Nurse (DN) is unable to attend the meeting but a referral has been made to the District Nursing Service from one of the GPs (General Practitioner) to visit David to undertake an introductory palliative assessment. You accompany the DN on this visit. David welcomes you both in but looks distinctly anxious. You introduce yourselves and explain that you are there to do a 'palliative support visit.' David becomes visibly distressed and expresses concern about being 'put on the rubbish heap.' David informs you that a close relative was 'made palliative' just before they 'put up a pump that killed them.'

Activity 16.1

- How might you turn this conversation into something more therapeutic?

- How might a palliative approach to David's care improve his quality of life?
- What palliative care needs do you think David has now? And in the future?
- What key information do you think David needs to aid understanding of the use of a continuous subcutaneous infusion (CSCI, or syringe pump) in the previous care episode that David refers to?

In your reflections you may have suggested exploring David's understanding of the word palliative. Discussing David's recent hospital admission can help with this. Many individuals do not want to have prolonged burdensome treatment, but they also do not want to feel as though they are not receiving care at all, or that they have somehow been deprioritised. It is important to emphasise that palliative care does not preclude treatment, and if there is a reversible clinical condition there is no reason that David will not be offered treatment for this. Even with a palliative approach hospital admission may be appropriate.

In some areas, palliative care is referred to as the best supportive care. However, this term is also problematic as it does not specify the approach in the same way as the word palliative. Indeed, one might argue that all care should be 'best supportive' care.

A further source of confusion is the term end-of-life care. In the UK this came into common usage with the publication of the *End of Life Care Strategy* (DoH, 2008), in which it referred to care in the last year of life. Nevertheless, this term is frequently used in practice, particularly in the acute clinical setting, to describe people who are actively dying.

Core Principles of Palliative Care

Palliative care is an approach that aims at improving the *'quality of life of individuals and that of their families, who are facing challenges associated with life-threatening illness, whether physical, psychological, social, or spiritual'* (World Health Organisation, 2020). Central to this definition is the notion of suffering. Effective palliative care means identifying suffering early, appropriate assessment of pain or other problems, and multidisciplinary management.

Although symptom management forms a crucial component of palliative care, suffering is not solely a physical concern. In palliative care, multidisciplinary teamwork is paramount. This enables a holistic approach to care from the point of identification of palliative needs until death and into the bereavement period. The Department of Health's current guidance, *One Chance to Get it Right* (Leadership Alliance for the Care of Dying People, 2014) stipulates that when a person is thought to be in the last hours or days of life, there are five principles of care.

1   The possibility (that a person is sick enough to die) is recognised and communicated clearly, decisions made, and actions taken in accordance with the person's needs and wishes, and these are regularly reviewed, and decisions revised accordingly.
2   Sensitive communication takes place between staff and the dying person, and those identified as important to them.

3   The dying person and those identified as important to them are involved in decisions about treatment and care to the extent that the dying person wants.

4   The needs of families and others identified as important to the dying person are actively explored, respected, and met as far as possible.

5   An individual plan of care, which includes food and drink, symptom control and psychological, social, and spiritual support, is agreed, coordinated, and delivered with compassion.

Contemporary challenges

Since the inception of the National Health Service in 1948, there have been significant changes in the demography of the British population. This has presented a set of challenges to the ideals of palliative care, illuminating several tensions and controversies which are addressed below.

1. Increased life expectancy.

People are living longer, but not necessarily in good health. Mortality and morbidity associated with infectious diseases have reduced but we are seeing a worrying increase in antimicrobial resistance that may herald problems to come. Certain unhealthy lifestyle choices have reduced (i.e., smoking) whilst others have increased (i.e., diets high in fat and sugar). This has altered the aetiology of chronic disease, making cardiovascular disease the second most common cause of mortality in the UK (National Institute for Clinical Excellence, 2020).

2. Increasingly complex healthcare system and advancing medical technologies

We can diagnose and treat an ever greater number of illnesses, and the number of specialisms within medicine has expanded exponentially so that now there are 61 distinct specialisms recognised in the UK and over 150 in the USA. This fragmentation can make the ideals of multidisciplinary palliative care particularly challenging. It is vital that the goals of care are commensurate with a person's wishes and that there is concordance between the various professionals and disciplines that may be involved in their care. As people can be treated for far longer for illnesses that were once associated with a short prognosis, the journey through treatment and the transition between curative and palliative, has become increasingly unpredictable. The availability of advanced medical technologies brings with it a series of important ethical dilemmas, including that of whether to proceed with treatments that may have burdensome side effects or require gruelling interventions, particularly where the outcome of such treatments is uncertain.

3. Changing demographics

Palliative and end-of-life care take place in an increasingly culturally and ethnically diverse society. This can present challenges in practice and requires adaptable approaches to care - whereby palliative care is provided according to a person's needs. When Dame Cicely Saunders established the world's first hospice at St Christopher's, London, it was a vision born from a Christian paradigm. People with terminal diseases received exceptional nursing and spiritual care but there was little medical input as it was believed that the role of the physician was primarily to cure. Individuals admitted to the hospice were likely to remain there until they died and there was no palliative care provision within the home. Most had a diagnosis of cancer.

Although cancer remains the most common cause of death in hospices there has been a gradual increase in admissions for people with non-malignant conditions. Unfortunately, this increase is far from commensurate with the corresponding increase in non-malignant conditions across the population. Hospices tend to serve those from more affluent backgrounds and far fewer people from deprived backgrounds access hospice inpatient services. This gap appears to have grown over time. This is a worrying trend as it implies there is an inequality in access (Sleeman et al., 2016). Palliative care is now generally viewed as being applicable in all life-limiting illnesses.

The needs of the LGBTQ+ community have been identified as an area for development in palliative care. Among the issues identified, lack of awareness by healthcare professionals has been found to contribute to poor psychosocial care, inadequate advance care planning, and a disproportionately increased rate of emotional and psychological suffering in the LGBTQ+ community (Shiu et al., 2016; Stinchcombe et al., 2017). An important part of our role is to ensure that those we care for stay safe but this does not just refer to physical safety. Emotional safety is paramount, particularly when people are highly vulnerable, such as when living with advanced life-limiting disease.

Evidence has shown that there are inequalities in access to palliative care from people from black and minority ethnic (BAME) groups. The cultural background of a person will inform the shape of palliative care. As nurses, you must always consider an individual's cultural background and beliefs. Being alert to the nuances of cultural preferences can be a rewarding aspect of care and can enhance the effectiveness and acceptability of palliative care. Understanding this can also help you to support families and loved ones with the adjustment required over the process of dying. There are several barriers to accessing palliative care, such as a lack of understanding as to what it entails and difficulties in decision making. There may be important beliefs around taking medications at the end of life, or cardiopulmonary resuscitation, or care of the dead person.

Tender Conversations

Traditional clinical education has focused on how healthcare professionals can engage in 'difficult' or 'challenging' conversations. In recent years, there has been a move away from this, with Mannix (2019) suggesting that 'tender conversations' might be a better way to think about these interactions. Mannix argues that this suggests that distress may be nearby but we act in such a way as to seek to minimise pain. Approaching death with trepidation may be the traditional approach, but there is a compelling case to enhance our therapeutic power through seeking openness, honesty and understanding with the people we care for. Speaking with people who are dying, and with their families, is known to be a source of anxiety for inexperienced nurses (Hussain, 2020) and that this can be further compounded by a lack of appropriate education and support. Ensuring that you are aware of the common themes facing individuals and their families can be useful in preparing you to undertake these tender conversations. Consider the following case study about Kateryna.

Kateryna

You are visiting a small flat in the middle of a noisy part of town, where Kateryna lives with sister Daryna, and teenage daughter Olga. Kateryna has been living with Parkinson's disease for several years, becoming increasingly dependent on Daryna for support with many activities of daily living. On the few occasions that Kateryna gets out of bed, a wheelchair is needed as safe mobility is increasingly unpredictable. Kateryna has a urinary catheter. Daughter Olga is spending more time staying with friends, often not returning home for several days. Kateryna complains of feeling tired all the time and states that when Olga is home they often argue about various things. Further, Kateryna's difficulties with speech result in a tendency to avoid contact with Olga. Kateryna also experiences severe tremors and problems with 'freezing.' Olga tells you that friends are not invited to visit due to the embarrassment caused by Kateryna's appearance. 'I just want to have a normal family, and this is not normal at all. I hate it, I hate this.' Daryna appears tired and withdrawn, although when you mention this, Daryna's responds with 'I'm fine, I have no choice. My sister would do this for me. I just wonder how long we can last like this.'

The ambivalence and relationship issues apparent in this case study are not unusual. Particularly with illnesses with a prolonged trajectory of decline, informal caregivers may experience great strain, and with this comes difficult feelings of guilt. Some people report that they often feel like a burden on their loved ones. Ruptures in relationships such as those between Kateryna and Olga are common.

As a nurse, it is important that as well as considering your own skills and role, you are also aware of the function of the wider multidisciplinary team. The above example is complex, and Kateryna and family members are likely to benefit from specialist input here. However, you still have a vital role in identifying concerns and referring appropriately. Further, your therapeutic role does not end once someone is being seen by another professional. Every time you see Kateryna, you will be building rapport and building your relationship. For people to discuss their difficulties, it is vital that they trust you. Speaking empathically and honestly, and ensuring you prioritise listening over speaking can help you in this endeavour. Often, nurses are the closest healthcare professionals to a person and their family, and this can mean that you are in the privileged responsible position of hearing what is most important to them.

Table 16.1 SPIKES framework

Step 1 [S] SETTING UP the interview - *where are you speaking with this person? Is it by the bedside separated from neighbours by only a curtain? Is it in a noisy corridor? How can you create a calm and conducive environment?*

Step 2 [P] Assessing the person's PERCEPTION - *what does the person already know about the situation? Before you tell, ask.*

Step 3 [I] Obtaining the person's invitation - *whilst many individuals wish to be fully informed and involved in discussions about their care, some do not. Avoiding details of illness is a valid response to distressing news. You might wish to ask whether the person wishes to talk about the situation, or perhaps whether they might prefer you to speak to a friend or relative.*

Step 4 [K] Giving KNOWLEDGE and information to the person - *using what is commonly termed a 'warning shot' can help to lessen the shock of hearing distressing information. Phrases such as 'I am so sorry to tell you…' or 'I think this might be difficult for you to hear…' are examples. However, it is important for you to develop your own style of communication; authenticity is much more important than a script.*

Step 5 [E] Addressing EMOTIONS with empathy - *conveying empathy involves four steps. First, observe closely for signs of emotion. Does the person look shocked, or tearful, or blank? Second, try to identify the emotion, perhaps using open questions. Third, check with the person whether their response is related to the conversation you are having, perhaps again using open questions to find out more. Finally, allow time for the person to express their feelings and acknowledge them. Do not feel under pressure to fill the space with words.*

Step 6 [S] STRATEGY and SUMMARY - *it can be very helpful for people to have a way forwards. This may relate to a treatment plan or it might be a conversation about plans for the future. Sharing responsibility for decisions helps to convey to the person that, in the words of Cicely Saunders, 'you matter because you are you, and you matter to the end of your life' (Saunders, 2006).*

Several models exist that can help nurses to engage in these conversations. An example is the 'SPIKES' model (Baile et al., 2000) shown in Table 16.1, which offers a concise number of steps to take to provide a framework for the conversation.

Advance Care Planning

Advance care planning (ACP) is a structured conversation with an individual and those that are important to them, about their wishes and preferences for future care. It enables exploration of concerns about approaching the end of life and can be reassuring as it allows people to think ahead and to make plans that are realistic. A tangible benefit of ACP is that it can reduce the chance that someone will receive burdensome or futile treatments or interventions at the end of life, increasing the likelihood of a dignified death in their preferred place of care.

EVA

Eva has a recent diagnosis of dementia and is living at home with partner, Kez, who has longstanding mental health problems, including depression and anxiety. Eva has expressed concerns about the future, particularly about when the illness advances and Kez needs to provide care as Eva feels this is an unrealistic expectation.

Activity 16.2

Look at the following document:
www.goldstandardsframework.org.uk/advance-care-planning

- Now reflect on how the process of advance care planning might be helpful to Eva and Kez, and how you as a nurse could facilitate this discussion.
- What development needs can you identify in your own clinical practice to give you confidence in approaching a sensitive topic such as deteriorating health, and the kinds of issues that might be facing Eva and Kez?

ACP has been defined as:

"a process that supports adults at any age or stage of health in understanding and sharing their personal values, life goals, and preferences regarding future medical care. The goal of advance care planning is to help ensure that people receive medical care that is consistent with their values, goals, and preferences during serious and chronic illness". (Sudore et al., 2017: 826)

When undertaking ACP, it is important that you are familiar with the core principles of the Mental Capacity Act, 2005 (www.legislation.gov.uk/ukpga/2005/9/contents). It is common for someone with an advanced life-limiting illness to lose capacity at some point. An ACP can be a valuable indicator of their personal preferences and concerns and can inform, if not dictate, the balance and direction of care.

As a nurse, you are likely to be involved at some point in ACP with an individual. Although clinical treatment decisions may not be part of the nursing role, nurses are in a prime position to support people to think about the wider context of ACP on account of their therapeutic relationship. The nurses' role in ACP is varied and vital. The NMC *Code* (2018b: 2.3) stipulates that nurses must *'encourage and empower people to share decisions about their treatment and care'* and their value as advocates for individuals and families is particularly important when it comes to putting down plans in advance of losing capacity. Sometimes, an ACP will include refusal of a particular kind of care or a certain treatment such as hospital admission for intravenous antibiotics. Nurses are ideally placed to facilitate and support these kinds of decisions as well as ensuring that a person possesses sufficient evidence-based information to help them to make empowered choices. Some aspects of ACP involve careful working with other members of the multidisciplinary team.

Fatima

Fatima is taken to A&E one night with worsening breathlessness and 2 litres of oxygen via a nasal cannula is administered prior to being transferred to the Medical Assessment Unit. Following further review, the medical registrar informs Fatima that the maximal drug therapy for heart failure has already been prescribed and suggests referral to the palliative care team. When you see Fatima at home, you are told by relatives that Fatima does not want to be admitted to hospital for treatment again 'if there is nothing else that they can do'.

Activity 16.3

1   How might advance care planning help Fatima in the coming months?
2   Why do you think that people with non-malignant diseases like heart failure tend to receive less palliative care support at the end of life?
3   What services might be available to support Fatima and family at home?
4   What questions might you ask Fatima to help to formulate a plan?

Fatima's case study highlights several key issues. ACP is often much less likely to be carried out by people with non-malignant conditions. This is thought to relate to difficulties prognosticating for this group of people when compared with those with cancer. The following images show the typical 'disease trajectories' for people with different conditions. As is apparent, it can be challenging to plan for someone who has an illness that is typically characterised by multiple exacerbations and potential hospital admissions.

The ACP process should be a clear balance of personal issues and clinical issues. A straightforward way to remember this is to think about 'what matters to me' (psychosocial view) as well as 'what is the matter with me' (medical view), shown in Table 16.2.

Table 16.2 The Advanced Care Planning (ACP) Process

'What Matters to Me'	'What's the Matter with Me'
A person's ideas, concerns and expectations (ICE)	Pathology, differential diagnosis
An individual may wish to document their priorities, feelings and thoughts	Emergency plans (eg ReSPECT – see next section)
It is important that the person's perspective and understanding of their illness experience is captured, which may incorporate spiritual and social concerns.	Treatment options including any Advanced Decisions to Refuse Treatment (ADRT)
The importance of communication skills in palliative care cannot be overstated. Conversations may be fraught with difficult emotions.	Symptoms (either current or anticipated)

ACP in practice: Recommended Summary Plan for Emergency Care and Treatment

Currently, in the UK the ReSPECT document is an agreed format for the purpose of basic advance care planning. Even where this actual document is not in use, the information it contains is considered good practice (Perkins and Fritz, 2019) and should be clearly identified in a person's medical record.

Activity 16.4

Take a closer look at the contents of the ReSPECT form and review further information via the link below:

www.resus.org.uk/sites/default/files/2020-09/ReSPECT%20v3-1-formSPECIMENFINAL_0.pdf

- What are your thoughts on the information being sought in the ReSPECT form?
- How useful do you think this information would be to all the healthcare professionals providing care?

The aim of completing a ReSPECT document is to provide healthcare professionals with details of what is important to a person if they are unable to communicate this at a critical time – for example, when they are acutely unwell. The goal of planning in this way is to ensure that they receive appropriate treatment, at the appropriate time and in the appropriate place of care. It can provide reassurance for individuals, families, and professionals, that even if that person is unable to speak for themselves their wishes and preferences can still be honoured. The process begins with a conversation between a healthcare professional and a person and their loved ones, to produce a plan about what to do in case of an emergency. The following is an overview of the information contained in the document.

- *Shared understanding of health and current condition* – may include diagnosis, previous/ present condition, prognosis, communication difficulties and how to overcome them, any other relevant care planning documents such as ADRTs (Advanced Decisions to Refuse Treatment) and whether a legal healthcare proxy has been appointed.
- *Personal priorities for end-of-life care.* In this section, the individual marks their position on the scale shown in Table 16.3:

Table 16.3 Template for ReSEPCT document

Living as long as possible matters most to me	Quality of life and comfort matters most to me

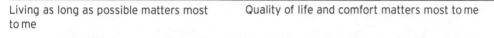

What I most value	What I most fear / wish to avoid

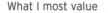

- *Clinical recommendations for emergency care and treatment.* This section enables documentation of priorities following a conversation about the preference documented above. The clinician completing the document signs one of three sections relating to the goal of care: (1) prioritise extending life, (2) balancing extending life with comfort and valued outcomes, (3) prioritise comfort.
- *Specific realistic interventions* that may or may not be wanted, e.g., hospital admission, intensive care.
- *CPR recommended or not recommended.* Note that the presence of a ReSPECT document does not automatically mean that the person is not for cardiopulmonary resuscitation.
- *Mental capacity and representation.*
- *Which people were involved in making the ReSPECT plan?*

It is not somewhere to document resuscitation status but enables a focus on what treatments would be acceptable as well as important contextual information such as whether a legal healthcare proxy has been appointed.

Leah

Leah has advanced recurrence of metastatic breast cancer and lives with Beti who had a stroke two years ago. Leah is Beti's full-time carer and attends outpatient day therapy at the local hospice once a week. Leah has considered completing a ReSPECT form but felt it did not apply in their current situation. However, one of Leah's friends who attended the day therapy unit has recently died and Leah has been affected emotionally by this experience. In conversation with a nurse, Leah reveals the wish to not die at home, worrying about the impact of this on Beti. Further, Leah shares worries about what would happen to Beti when either of their conditions worsen. The nurse asks Leah for permission to capture some of these concerns and preferences so that any healthcare professionals providing care now or in the future would be aware of them, and Leah agrees.

Leah personally decides that quality of life and comfort matter more to than living as long as possible but that emergency treatment such as intravenous antibiotics would be acceptable if the benefits outweigh the burden. Leah was also able to document personal concerns about Beti on the form. The nurse scanned the form and kept a copy within Leah's medical records, and Leah was given a copy to take home to facilitate a discussion with Beti about it.

Some weeks later, Leah wakes up in the night confused and disorientated and falls when trying to go to the bathroom. Beti calls an ambulance and the paramedics assess that Leah is pyrexial and dehydrated. Leah expresses a wish to go to hospital for treatment. Once in the ward Leah is diagnosed with a urinary tract infection and treated with fluids and antibiotics. Leah hands the ReSPECT document to a ward nurse who can recognise that there are concerns about Beti being at home alone and contacts the social worker to alert them of this.

Unfortunately whilst in hospital, Leah continues to deteriorate and stops eating and drinking. On the reSPECT form Leah has stated that comfort should be prioritised over prolonging life. The multidisciplinary team agrees with Leah to withdraw treatment. The social worker arranges transport to bring Beti to the bedside as it is felt that Leah is too unwell to cope with a discharge home. Leah is moved to a side room and can spend the last few precious hours of life with Beti.

Activity 16.5

Can you identify the distinct roles of the multidisciplinary team in the above case study?
What might the consequences have been if the ReSPECT document had not been completed?

Gold Standards Framework

The Gold Standards Framework (GSF) is a model first developed for use in the community setting by Keri Thomas, a General Practitioner (GP) in the North of England who was concerned about the lack of coordinated care for those in the last year of life who were living at home (Shaw et al., 2010). GPs and community nursing teams are in a key position to identify and support those approaching the end of life. The framework is intended to be adapted and used according to need and provides teams with a foundation upon which to continually improve and develop their practice. There are three key components of the GSF: (1) identification of those who may need palliative care, (2) assessment of needs and preferences, and (3) planning of care. The GSF outlines seven key tasks, also known as the seven Cs:

- *Communication:* all members of the multidisciplinary team are aware of the status of the person and a supportive care register is maintained and used to plan and monitor care;
- *Coordination:* a nominated coordinator of care acts as a hub for the person. This may be a District Nurse, Care Home matron, or palliative care Nurse Specialist;

- *Control of symptoms:* Symptoms are holistically assessed and appropriately managed;
- *Continuity:* Information is conveyed to out-of-hours services so that no matter what time of day or night, a congruent plan of care can be followed that has been developed with the person concerned;
- *Continued learning:* Staff are supported to continually stay up to date in matters related to end-of-life care. This is a key part of the role of specialist palliative care teams;
- *Carer support:* Carers frequently need emotional and practical support. They also may need follow up into the bereavement period;
- *Care in the dying phase:* Individuals in the last days of life are given appropriate care and their dignity is maintained. Non-essential interventions are discontinued and comfort is prioritised. Medications are reviewed frequently and protocols are followed for notification and actions to take after death. Care of the deceased person maintains dignity and personhood.

Activity 16.6

There is an argument that the phrase *'do not attempt resuscitation'* is a negative one, with critics saying that it sounds like you are abandoning someone and giving a death sentence. One alternative that has been suggested is *'allow natural death'*.

- Write down your thoughts about the phrases above.
- What might be problematic with the suggested alternative term?

What is a Good Death?

Death is not a failure of medicine. It is an inevitable event and countless philosophers, scholars and religious thinkers have reminded us of the value of contemplating our mortality. Illich (1982) suggested that as death and dying have become increasingly medicalised, society has become further removed from the experience of witnessing death. Now, most people in technologically developed countries die in hospitals.

Although we have abundant data on the place and cause of death of our population, we have little information as to the quality of dying. Anecdotal evidence and case studies suggest that hospices and palliative care input can improve the quality of end-of-life care. However to date, there is no robust metric by which we can definitively state what works in this complex, multidisciplinary domain of care. Research has begun to examine what a 'good death' might look like and this is an important consideration for nurses as they advocate for people at the end of life. Of course, everybody's perspective will differ slightly and applying the findings of research must be done judiciously. A literature review by (Meier et al., 2016) identified several themes across 36 studies that included individuals receiving care, their families and health-care professionals. Life completion was considered important by over half of the respondents, and this included issues such as saying goodbye, feeling that life was well lived and accept-ance of death. Treatment preferences included a wish not to prolong life, whilst simultane-ously feeling assured that all available treatments had been used. Respondents also valued control over treatment choices. The theme of dignity included feeling respected as an indi-vidual and maintaining independence. In relation to the dying process, comfort – such as the absence of pain – is of paramount importance to those receiving care, families and healthcare professionals alike. Finally, the theme of 'family' included family support and preparedness, and not feeling a burden to loved ones.

Being aware of what the research shows can help nurses to anticipate potential challenges and raise subjects for discussion where individuals and/or families may not. Creative approaches to supporting a person at the end of life can involve such activities as the creation of memory boxes or other legacy items and supporting people to put their affairs in order.

Diagnosing Dying

Identifying that someone may be sick enough to die is the first step in being able to provide effective end-of-life care. Yet evidence suggests that many individuals are diagnosed as dying with extraordinarily little time before death to put plans into place. This can lead to several undesirable outcomes, such as dying in hospital when one prefers to die at home or having burdensome treatment or interventions that will not change the ultimate outcome. Whilst it is not the role of a nurse to make a clinical diagnosis, nurses are in a prominent position by vir-tue of their proximity to the individual and their families. The use of effective communication skills when liaising with clinicians is vital. Ensure that you are aware of the signs of deteriora-tion and that you are familiar with the clinical history, in order that you might contribute to multidisciplinary discussions.

It is vital that healthcare professionals can recognise the point at which a person begins to die. If this is not done it can be difficult to provide effective, compassionate, and person-centred care in the last hours and days of life. Diagnosing dying enables us to focus on comfort and dig-nity and to avoid futile interventions. Further, it can assist us to put into practice the person's expressed prior wishes, whether captured in an advance care plan or otherwise known. Finally, recognising dying allows us to acknowledge it. This is a fundamental part of supporting people and families to prepare for what is to come. It is usually the role of the medical team to identify dying. However, at times this relies on accurate information being relayed by the nurses who are caring for that person. Evidence continues to suggest that identifying dying, particularly in the hospital setting, happens extremely late – often giving little time for people and families to prepare (Kennedy et al., 2014).

Consider the following case study about Violet and think about what you might do in this situation.

Violet

Megan is working on the medical ward when Violet is admitted, having had a stroke. On admission Violet is unconscious and unresponsive to pain. Megan notices that Violet's lower limbs have swollen and that breathing sounds are a little 'rattly.' Violet is diagnosed as having a chest infection and is started on intravenous antibiotics. Unfortunately, Violet's urinary output decreases significantly over the next 24 hours despite intravenous fluids and the lower limb swelling appears to be getting worse. The doctor decides that due to poor kidney function it would not be in Violet's best interests to be prescribed diuretics. Violet's son Mark, tells you that Violet was always so full of energy and would have hated wearing an incontinence pad with no idea of what is going on.

You might have noticed that this case study does not state with any certainty whether Violet is dying, or whether her condition is reversible. This is highly typical of clinical reality, particularly where an individual has multiple comorbid conditions. One of the challenges to diagnosing dying is that there are several reversible reasons for clinical deterioration and it is of course vital that these are excluded before confirming that death is imminent.

Diagnosing dying is more straightforward in some diseases than in others. Figure 16.1 illustrates some typical 'disease trajectories' and demonstrates why there is variation in the accuracy of prognostication in different clinical conditions.

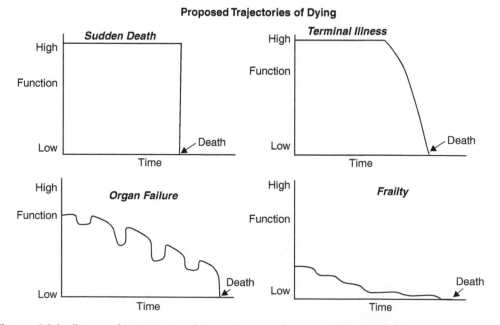

Figure 16.1   Proposed trajectories of dying (Lunney, Lynn and Hogan, 2002)

"These days, swift catastrophic illness is the exception; for most people, death comes only after long medical struggle with an incurable condition—advanced cancer, progressive organ failure (usually the heart, kidney, or liver), or the multiple debilities of very old age. In all such cases, death is certain, but the timing isn't. So, everyone struggles with this uncertainty—with how, and when, to accept that the battle is lost. As for last words, they hardly seem to exist anymore. Technology sustains our organs until we are well past the point of awareness and coherence. Besides, how do you attend to the thoughts and concerns of the dying when medicine has made it almost impossible to be sure who the dying even are? Is someone with terminal cancer, dementia, incurable congestive heart failure dying, exactly?" (Gawunde, 2010)

To aid the process of recognising dying, nurses can ensure that they fully document the changes that are observed in an individual including any expressions of discomfort. Continuity of care can be invaluable in terms of keeping track of subtle changes in condition. It may be useful to make use of existing prognostic aids (Shaw et al., 2010). Further, in conversations with other members of the team as well as with families, it is important to avoid euphemisms such as 'very poorly'. If someone is sick enough to die, then say so. Finally, and perhaps most significantly, it is vital that the entire healthcare team acknowledge the uncertainty inherent in prognosticating and in diagnosing dying. Recognising uncertainty enables plans to be put in place even when this is against a backdrop of potential recovery. Tools such as the Amber Care Bundle allow for this dual planning process (Bristowe et al., 2015).

Uncertainty

The uncertainty that surrounds end-of-life care can often present obstacles to care. However, there are important steps that the nurse can take to ensure that care is compassionate and person-centred, as well as being adaptable for when a person's condition changes. Ensure that documentation is clear and detailed and includes any significant changes that you have observed. Ensure that you are aware of the support offered by other members of the multidisciplinary team – for example, physiotherapists can provide excellent support for those struggling with respiratory symptoms or mobility issues. Occupational therapists can help to maximise a person's independence, even in the presence of advancing disease.

Hetty

Hetty has been living with dementia for 8 years and currently lives in a nursing home. This morning Hetty woke up even more disorientated than usual and fell while trying to get out of bed, though she did not sustain any injuries. However, Hetty is much less conscious of surroundings, seems uncomfortable and has now gone back to sleep. You notice that Hetty breathing is noisy and 'bubbly' sounding.

Activity 16.7

If you were on placement in the nursing home when this occurred, what would your concerns be? How might you make use of ethical principles to think about what to do next? Who would you need to speak with?

The nurse's role in scenarios like this one is to be a compassionate advocate. There is a balance to be struck between the potential for Hetty to have sustained an unidentified injury, confounded by an inability to clearly express herself. It is well known that expression of pain may be altered in people with advanced dementia (Lawrence et al., 2011). Furthermore, the symptoms Hetty is manifesting may be a sign of a respiratory tract infection, which can cause altered levels of consciousness, particularly if oxygen levels are reduced. However, there is an alternative view to this situation. Hetty is in a worsening physical state with a diminished level of consciousness. There are audible respiratory secretions, which might suggest a chest infection. It is vital that discussions about care include family members or next of kin, as well as any prior statement of preferences of care that Hetty may have written (such as an ACP). Additionally, the doctor will be able to evaluate whether Hetty's current condition could be treated at home, as there are significant risks associated with older people with dementia being admitted to hospital.

Symptom Assessment and Management

Central to the WHO (World Health Organization) definition of palliative care is the *'identification and impeccable assessment and treatment of pain and other problems'* (World Health Organization, 2020).

It is certainly beyond the scope of this chapter to provide detailed instructions on the wide array of physical symptoms experienced by people with advanced life-limiting illness. Indeed, the most recent version of the *Oxford Textbook of Palliative Medicine* (Cherny et al., 2015) listed over 50 unique symptoms. However, it is possible to consider a set of core principles for assessment of symptoms that can be developed and applied in several different settings.

Activity 16.8

What is a symptom? How does it differ from a sign?

When you identify a symptom that is causing a problem, consider the following prompts:

1. What is causing this?
2. What else could be causing this?
3. Who can I ask?
4. What has the person tried already?

A holistic nursing assessment will provide vital information for the multidisciplinary team in deciding the best approach to managing care. A useful mnemonic when assessing symptoms you may remember from previous chapters is PQRST:

> **P** – palliative/provocative factors. What makes the symptom better or worse? For example, is nausea worse before or after eating? Is pain helped by application of heat or cold?
> **Q** – quality. What does the symptom feel like? For example, if it is pain, is it 'stabbing,' 'aching,' 'gnawing' or 'tingling'? Using the individual's' own words can convey a lot about the underlying aetiology (cause) of the symptom.
> **R** – radiation. Does the symptom travel anywhere? For example, if it is back pain, is it also felt down the leg?
> **S** – severity. Can the individual rate it? Perhaps using a simple numerical scale such as 0-10, where 0 is no pain at all and 10 is the worst pain ever? Or more simply, an individual could rate a pain as absent (0), mild (1), moderate (2) or severe (3).
> **T** – timing. When does the symptom arise and pass? Does the person wake with anxiety but feel settled during the day?

If the individual is unable to understand or communicate, perhaps because of a language barrier, the use of visual rating scales could help, such as the Wong 'smiley faces' scale (Baker and Wong, 1987) which provides a scale of facial expressions ranging from smiling through to extreme distress. Although this was originally developed for use in children, it has since been validated for pain assessment in multiple settings with a wide variety of people. For those unable to engage in self-assessment at all there are useful assessment scales developed for this purpose such as the Abbey Pain Scale for people with cognitive impairment (Abbey et al., 2004).

Activity 16.9

Pain assessment scale – activity

John is 45 years old. He has Down's Syndrome and also suffers from chronic arthritis. He lives in a supported living environment with carers visiting daily. He has been in a cheerful mood in the past, but recently he seems more withdrawn and agitated. John does not communicate verbally and communicates mostly through sign language, facial expressions, and body language. He appears to have limited ability to express his pain through sign language and often communicates through actions such as refusing assistance with tasks he normally accepts help with.

There are a variety of assessment tools that might be used with John. Each has advantages and disadvantages.

Reflect on the appropriateness and feasibility of using the Wong-Baker FACES Pain Rating Scale in assessing John's pain levels. Consider his cognitive and communication abilities, his understanding of symbolic representation, and the likelihood of him being able to relate the facial expressions to his own pain.

How might you modify or supplement the use of this scale to better suit John's needs? Could any potential challenges arise in its application? Reflect on how using such a tool might enhance your ability to assess pain in non-verbal patients and improve patient outcomes.

Activity 16.9

Jerome

Jerome is a 78 year-old who was referred to the heart failure nurse following an acute hospital admission. Jerome had gradually become more fluid overloaded and breathless which was tolerated until waking suddenly in the night panicking and ringing for an emergency ambulance. Jerome has had several similar past admissions at 3-monthly intervals.

On referral to the heart failure nurse Jerome was sleeping downstairs as he could not manage the stairs.

- What might the heart failure nurse do?

One month later, Jerome developed worsening oedema in both legs extending up to the thighs. Oral Bumetanide was increased without any improvement so Jerome was readmitted to hospital. On admission, his Glomerular Filtration Rate (GFR) was 30ml/min (previously stable at 40ml/min for the past 2 years) and fluid retention responded well to IV Furosemide but then the GFR fell further to 25ml/min.

- What do you think Jerome's prognosis is and why?

In view of the poor renal function, Jerome's frequent hospital admissions and the fact that optimal therapy was already being administered, it was considered likely that Jerome was in end stage heart failure (with a prognosis of months). Digoxin was commenced with some benefit and a palliative care approach was suggested. Following this hospital admission, the heart failure nurse talked to Jerome and his wife (they have no children) about future care options.

- What issues would you discuss?

Jerome really did not want to go into hospital again. Prior to the visit from the heart failure nurse, Jerome was unaware that the condition was not 'curable' and was searching for answers. Now he no longer felt the need to do this and wanted to have time with his wife.

- What could you do to increase his chances of being able to avoid a hospital admission?

Over the following weeks Jerome gradually became more tired and breathless and found it difficult to get out of bed. The district nurses began visiting daily. Jerome complained of a loss of appetite and feeling continuously nauseated.

- What do you think is happening?
- What would you do about his medications and symptoms?

Supporting Informal Caregivers

Informal caregivers are essential to end-of-life care and yet their support is often overlooked (Ewing et al., 2018). Whether you are visiting a person at home or caring for them in an acute hospital setting, do not forget to consider the needs of caregivers when planning and implementing care. Carer burnout is a frequent reason for unplanned admissions to hospital at the end of life. There may also be significant financial burdens, particularly where carers are unable to work because of their caregiving role. Involving other members of the multidisciplinary team such as social workers can help to ensure that care is holistic.

Freya

Freya a 54 year-old with advanced motor neurone disease is living at home with partner Dec. Freya's mobility has deteriorated significantly over the last few weeks and spends most of the time in bed. The district nurses have arranged for a hospital bed to be delivered and set up in the living room. Freya has also been catheterised as skin integrity was a concern and had expressed pain when being hoisted onto the commode. Dec also supports another close relative who has dementia and lives about an hour away, resulting in the need to take long-term leave from work and is currently receiving Carer Support Allowance. During a routine visit you notice that Freya is uncomfortable having slipped down the bed trapping a foot in the cot side. There is a small, reddened area on Freya's ankle. You draw it to Dec's attention who immediately starts to cry saying 'I can't do this anymore".'

- What emotions do you think Dec is experiencing? How might you offer support as a nurse?

The role of the nurse

As we have emphasised throughout this book, the development of therapeutic relationships with people and their loved ones is a vital component of the role of the nurse with a specific focus on the provision of holistic and person-centred care. This requires that the nurse not only understands aspects of the disease and its progression but is also aware of their own emotions and able to develop emotional intelligence. Looking after people at the end of life can be both upsetting and rewarding and it is essential that nurses draw on the support of their team to ensure resilience. In some clinical settings there are opportunities for clinical supervision to discuss experiences of death. One of the main responsibilities is to assess and manage the ongoing physical and emotional needs of the person and their family members. This may include assessing symptoms and managing both pharmacological and non-pharmacological interventions. At times, the role is one of advocacy, facilitating clear communication between individuals, families and health and social care providers. At a more advanced level, nurses may play a role in coordinating care. For example, a clinical nurse specialist may support people with life-limiting illness in the community and act as key worker to help them to navigate transitions in care and multiple care providers such as general practitioners, district nurses, pharmacists, hospital teams and out-of-hours services. Finally, the nurse can be instrumental in educating and informing individuals and families about issues relating to end-of-life care such as advance care planning and may play a role in supporting them to make several important decisions over the course of their illness.

Chapter Summary

This chapter has provided an overview of some of the contemporary challenges in palliative care, outlining the role of the nurse and offering an overview of approaches to care. Whilst palliative care is certainly a challenging aspect of nursing, developing your skills in end-of-life care will benefit those you care for and their families, regardless of the clinical setting in which you are working. People with life-limiting illnesses will need care in many contexts and settings and the impact of bereavement is far reaching throughout our society. Developing the therapeutic relationship required in these situations will profoundly enhance your nursing practice. Palliative care is underpinned by fundamental principles of holistic assessment, compassionate care, and effective working across institutional, professional, and clinical boundaries.

Further Reading

Cherny, N., Fallon, M., Kaasa, S., Portenoy, R. and Currow, D. (2015) *Oxford Textbook of Palliative Care.* Oxford: Oxford University Press.

Parliamentary and Health Service Ombudsman (2011) *Care and Compassion? Report of the Health Service Ombudsman on ten investigations into NHS care of older people.* Available at: www.ombudsman.org.uk/sites/default/files/2016-10/Care%20and%20Compassion.pdf (last accessed 17 February 2023).

Parliamentary and Health Service Ombudsman (2015) *Dying Without Dignity. Investigations by the Parliamentary and Health Service Ombudsman into complaints about end of life care.* Available at: www.ombudsman.org.uk/sites/default/files/Dying_without_dignity.pdf (last accessed 17 February 2023).

Pryde, N. (2022) (ed.), *Enhanced Palliative Care. A Handbook for Paramedics, Nurses, and Doctors.* Somerset: Class Professional Publishing.

Walshe, C., Preston, N. and Johnston, N. (2018) (eds), *Palliative Care Nursing. Principles and Evidence for Practice,* 3rd edn. London: Open University Press.

References

Abbey, J., Piller, N., Bellis, A.D., Esterman, A., Parker, D., Giles, L. and Lowcay, B. (2004) 'The Abbey pain scale: a 1-minute numerical indicator for people with end-stage dementia', *International Journal of Palliative Nursing,* 10: 6–13.

Baile, W., Buckman, R., Lenzi, R., Glober, G., Beale, E. and Kudelka, A. (2000) 'SPIKES—A six-step protocol for delivering bad news: application to the patient', *The Oncologist,* 5: 302–11.

Baker, C. and Wong, D. (1987) 'Q.U.E.S.T.: A process of pain assessment in children', *Orthopaedic Nursing,* 6: 11–21.

Bristowe, K., Carey, I., Hopper, A., Shouls, S., Prentice, W., Caulkin, R., Higginson, I.J. and Koffman, J. (2015) 'Patient and carer experiences of clinical uncertainty and deterioration, in the face of limited reversibility: a comparative observational study of the AMBER care bundle', *Palliative Medicine,* 29: 797–807.

Cherny, N., Fallon, M., Kaasa, S., Portenoy, R. and Currow, D. (2015) *Oxford Textbook of Palliative Care.* Oxford: Oxford University Press.

Clark, D. (2016) *To Comfort Always: A history of palliative medicine since the nineteenth century.* Oxford: Oxford University Press.

Department of Health (2008) 'End of Life Care Strategy: promoting high quality care for adults at the end of their life'. In CARE, D. O. H. A. S. (ed.). London.

Ewing, G., Austin, L., Jones, D. and Grande, G. (2018) 'Who cares for the carers at hospital discharge at the end of life? A qualitative study of current practice in discharge planning and the potential value of using The Carer Support Needs Assessment Tool (CSNAT)' Approach', *Palliat Med,* 32: 939–49.

Francis, R. (2013) *Report of the Mid Staffordshire NHS Foundation Trust Public Inquiry.* Available at: https://assets.publishing.service.gov.uk/government/uploads/system/uploads/attachment_data/file/279124/0947.pdf (last accessed 17 February 2023).

Gawunde, A. (2010) Letting Go: What should medicine do when it can't save your life? *The New Yorker.* New York.

Hussain, F. (2020) 'Managing conversations with patients about death and dying', *British Journal of Nursing,* Mar 12;29(5): 284–9.

Illich, I. (1982), *Medical Nemesis: The Expropriation of Health.* New York: Pantheon.

Kennedy, C., Brooks-Young, P., Brunton Gray, C., Larkin, P., Connolly, M., Wilde-Larsson, N.B., Larsson, M., Smith, T. and Chater, S. (2014) 'Diagnosing dying: an integrative literature review', *BMJ Support Palliat Care,* 4: 263–70.

Lawrence, V., Samsi, K., Murray, J., Harari, D. and Banerjee, S. (2011) 'Dying well with dementia: qualitative examination of end-of-life care', *Br J Psychiatry,* 199: 417–22.

Leadership Alliance for The Care of Dying People (2014) *One Chance to Get it Right.* London: UK Gov.

Lunney, J., Lynn, J. and Hogan, C. (2002) 'Profiles of older medicare decedents', *Journal of the American Geriatrics Society,* 50(6): 1108–12.

Mannix, K. (2019) *With the End in Mind: How to Live and Die Well.* London: HarperCollins Publishers Limited.

Meier, E.A., Gallegos, J.V., Thomas, L.P., Depp, C.A., Irwin, S.A. and Jeste, D.V. (2016) 'Defining a good death (successful dying): literature review and a call for research and public dialogue', *Am J Geriatr Psychiatry,* 24: 261–71.

National Institute for Clinical Excellence (2020) *Clinical Knowledge Summary: What is the impact of CVD?* London: NICE.

Nursing and Midwifery Council (2018) *Future Nurse: Standards of proficiency for registered nurses.* Available at: www.nmc.org.uk/globalassets/sitedocuments/standards-of-proficiency/nurses/future-nurse-proficiencies.pdf (last accessed 19 January 2023).

Parliamentary and Health Service Ombudsman (2011) *Care and Compassion? Report of the Health Service Ombudsman on ten investigations into NHS care of older people.* Available at: www.ombudsman.org.uk/sites/default/files/2016-10/Care%20and%20Compassion.pdf (last accessed 17 February 2023).

Parliamentary and Health Service Ombudsman (2015) *Dying Without Dignity. Investigations by the Parliamentary and Health Service Ombudsman into complaints about end of life care.* Available at: www.ombudsman.org.uk/sites/default/files/Dying_without_dignity.pdf (last accessed 17 February 2023).

Perkins, G.D. and Fritz, Z. (2019) 'Time to change from do-not-resuscitate orders to emergency care treatment plans', *JAMA Netw Open,* 2, e195170.

Saunders, C. (2006), *Selected Writings 1958-2004.* Oxford: Oxford University Press.

Shaw, K., Clifford, C., Thomas, K. and Meehan, H. (2010) 'Improving end-of-life care: a critical review of the Gold Standards Framework in primary care', *Database of Abstracts of Reviews of Effects (DARE): Quality-assessed Reviews.*

Shiu, C., Muraco, A. and Fredriksen-Goldsen, K. (2016) 'Invisible care: friend and partner care among older lesbian, gay, bisexual, and transgender (LGBT) adults', *J Soc Social Work Res,* 7: 527–46.

Sleeman, K.E., Davies, J.M., Verne, J., Gao, W. and Higginson, I.J (2016) 'The changing demographics of inpatient hospice death: population-based cross-sectional study in England, 1993-2012', *Palliat Med,* 30, 45–53.

Stinchcombe, A., Smallbone, J., Wilson, K. and Kortes-Miller, K. (2017) 'Healthcare and end-of-life needs of lesbian, gay, bisexual, and transgender (LGBT) older adults: a scoping review', *Geriatrics (Basel),* 2.

Sudore, R.L., Lum, H.D., You, J.J., Hanson, L.C., Meier, D.E., Pantilat, S.Z., Matlock, D.D., Rietjens, J.A.C., Korfage, I.J., Ritchie, C.S., Kutner, J.S., Teno, J.M., Thomas, J., McMahan, R.D. and Heyland, D.K. (2017) 'Defining advance care planning for adults: a consensus definition from a multidisciplinary Delphi panel', *J Pain Symptom Manage,* May;53(5): 821–832.e1.

The Economist Intelligence Unit (2015) *The 2015 Quality of Death Index: Ranking palliative care across the world.* London: Economist Intelligence Unit.

World Health Organization (2020) *Factsheets: Palliative Care* [Online]. Available at: www.who.int/news-room/fact-sheets/detail/palliative-care (last accessed 2 July 2022).

17

MANAGING THE TRANSITION TO REGISTERED NURSING PRACTICE

Karen Heggs and Samantha Freeman

Chapter objectives

- Consider how best to approach your final practice learning experience;
- Describe the process of application for employment and explain how best to promote yourself to prospective employers;
- Begin to develop and enhance a personal statement;
- Consider strategies for self-care and personal development;
- Explain how preceptorship can support you in your transition from student nurse to registrant;
- Outline the process of revalidation.

The transition from nursing student to registered nurse can be a daunting and exciting time. This transition period can sometimes feel challenging and stressful, and you may feel apprehensive about your pending change in role. This chapter will explore the challenge of managing role transition and help you to prepare for the start of your professional career. We will explore the theory and evidence base around role transition as well as practical aspects of:

- Your final practice learning experience;
- Applying for employment;
- Self-care;
- Becoming a registered nurse;
- Preceptorship;
- Nursing and Midwifery Council (NMC) revalidation.

The primary shift is that you will have developed skills of leadership, management and decision making and yet conducted them only in the role as a supervised student. Your concerns may stem from feelings of needing to know everything. Within this chapter, you should find useful guidance to support you during this time and the reassurance that none of us know everything!

TO ACHIEVE ENTRY TO THE NMC REGISTER

YOU MUST BE ABLE TO

- Act as an ambassador, upholding the reputation of your profession and promoting public confidence in nursing, and healthcare services;
- Understand the demands of professional practice, acknowledge the need to accept and manage uncertainty, and demonstrate an understanding of strategies that develop resilience in self and others;
- Understand and maintain the level of health, fitness and wellbeing required to meet people's needs for mental and physical care;
- Demonstrate how to recognise signs of vulnerability in yourself or your colleagues and the action required to minimise risks to health;
- Take responsibility for continuous self-reflection, seeking and responding to support and feedback to develop their professional knowledge and skills;
- Support and supervise learners in the delivery of nursing care, promoting reflection, and providing constructive feedback, and evaluating and documenting their performance;
- Contribute to supervision and team reflection activities to promote improvements in practice and services;
  a Demonstrate effective supervision, teaching and performance appraisal with clear instructions and explanations when supervising, teaching or appraising others;
  b Provide unambiguous, constructive feedback about strengths and weaknesses and potential for improvement;
  c Provide encouragement to colleagues that helps them to reflect on their practice;
  d Demonstrate active listening when dealing with team members' concerns and anxieties;
- Understand the role of registered nurses and other health and care professionals at various levels of experience and seniority when managing and prioritising actions and care in the event of a major incident.

(Adapted from NMC, 2018a)

Approaching the End of Your Nursing Programme

It may seem at the start of your nursing degree programme that the point of registration is a long way off. But time will pass quickly and before you know it, you are approaching the end of your programme and at the point of registration.

This can be an exciting time providing the opportunity to begin to develop your own practice and move forward in your career, with a wealth of opportunities available to you. However, it can also be a time of apprehension, uncertainty and worry as the responsibility of becoming a registrant becomes a reality. Often, students can worry that they are not ready to become registrants; they do not feel prepared and are concerned that they may not have the skills that they need to begin their role as a newly registered nurse.

Expectations of Yourself and Others

Do the expectations below reflect the reality of what is expected of you as a newly registered nurse?

- Confidence in own abilities;
- Competent in skills specific to your new role;
- Knowledge base specific to your new role;
- Highly skilled;
- An ability to 'hit the ground running.'

Whilst there will be an expectation that you are able to perform safely and competently, it is important to remember to be kind to yourself as you approach the end of your degree programme, acknowledging the skills and knowledge that you have acquired throughout your programme and the value that this has to your future employers. Overall, you will be expected to demonstrate confidence and competence in your own abilities and to be able to demonstrate that you can meet *all* the required proficiencies for entry to the NMC register as an adult nurse. However, there would normally be no expectation that you have specific knowledge related to a new role or that you will already be highly skilled in that area. A willingness to ask someone more experienced for help or advice with something that is unfamiliar or new is considered as a strength not a weakness! Employers of newly qualified adult nursing registrants seek individuals who:

- Can think critically;
- Are adaptable;
- Are open to development and change;
- Can work collegiately with others;
- Are professional in their approach.

You will be supported in your development as a newly qualified nurse through the completion of a preceptorship programme. We will discuss this in more detail later in this chapter.

The Beginning of Your Journey of Lifelong Learning

A key factor to consider as you approach the end of your degree programme is that life-long learning is an important key aspect of your new role as a professional. In line with *The Code* (NMC, 2018b), it is essential that you continue to engage in learning and development throughout your career. Therefore, it is helpful to view your educational journey to registration as the foundation for your lifelong learning and consider your learning, growth and development throughout your undergraduate studies as the roots and trunk of your nursing career (Figure 17.1). They are vital to provide you with deep-rooted knowledge and skills, and the stability to begin to grow and develop as a registered nurse.

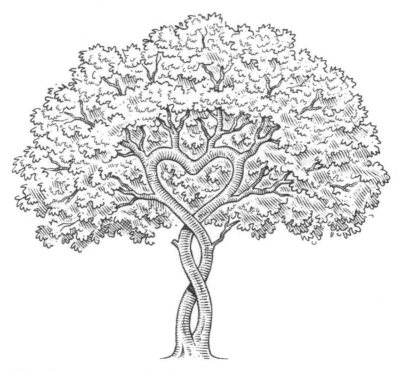

Figure 17.1   What do you consider to be the roots and trunk of your nursing career?
Source: iStock

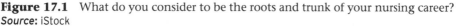

Activity 17.1

1   Look at the NMC proficiencies for 'Entry to the NMC register' (NMC, 2018a) pages at the front of this book and begin to map these to any evidence you have from your own learning journey (e.g., experiences in practice, theoretical knowledge and skills gained, etc.).

2 Can you identify any gaps in your knowledge, understanding or skills required at this point?

3 Now consider how you can address these gaps and develop a personal development plan (e.g., how might the gaps you have identified be addressed in your remaining practice learning experiences as you approach the end of your programme?)

It is good to ask questions of yourself and to not be frightened to admit it if you do not know something. Developing skills in clinical judgement and decision making are guided by our experiences and by seeking information on which to base these decisions.

Earlier in this book (Chapter 8), we identified the role of the theory developed by the seminal work of Benner (1984) in the development of the experiential learner and the skills of clinical judgement and decision making. It would be appropriate to consider the work of Benner here again but in the context of your identity as a student and as a newly qualified nurse.

In her intuitive–humanistic theory, Benner (1984) identifies stages of development from novice through to expert via the development of knowledge base and experience. It is useful to consider this model in the context of your current identity as a student and your upcoming new identity as a qualified registered nurse. There is no expectation that you will complete your degree programme and be an expert in your identified field of nursing since this takes time and experience. But you may have knowledge and experience that you bring with you from before the commencement of your programme, through study and exposure to the role of the nurse. You will also have skills, knowledge and experience that you gain from the programme itself and the range of exposure to both practice learning and theoretical experiences offered to you. Finally, you may have supplementary knowledge, skills and experience that you gain through your life – for example your hobbies, personal life and interests or voluntary work. All of these add to the rich and unique map that is your own identity as a registered nurse.

Activity 17.2

Consider Benner's model (Figure 17.2) and your perception of yourself.

Think about your skills, knowledge, and experiences that you bring to your role as a student nurse and about your future identity as a registered nurse.

Where do you see yourself within the context of Benner's model?

Take time to identify the value that you bring to the nursing role. Does this match your previous expectations of where you feel you should be?

As you may have found when completing the previous activities, it is incredibly helpful to look back and consider your learning and experiences so far to help you in identifying any gaps. Looking back through any reflections that you have developed would be an interesting and insightful exercise and offers the opportunity to consider how far you have come and how and what direction you want to progress to in the future. This may also help you to consider your learning needs for your final practice learning experience. One tool that can facilitate you in this process is the use of a SWOT analysis (Figure 17.3); thought by some to have been originally developed in the 1960s by Albert Humphrey, the SWOT analysis has been developed further over time and is utilised in a wide range of different contexts such as decision making, evaluation and change management.

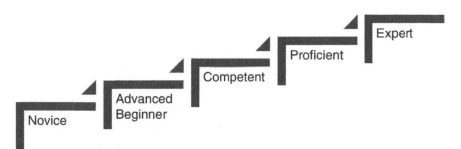

Figure 17.2   Novice to expert stages 1–5 (Adapted from Benner, 1984)

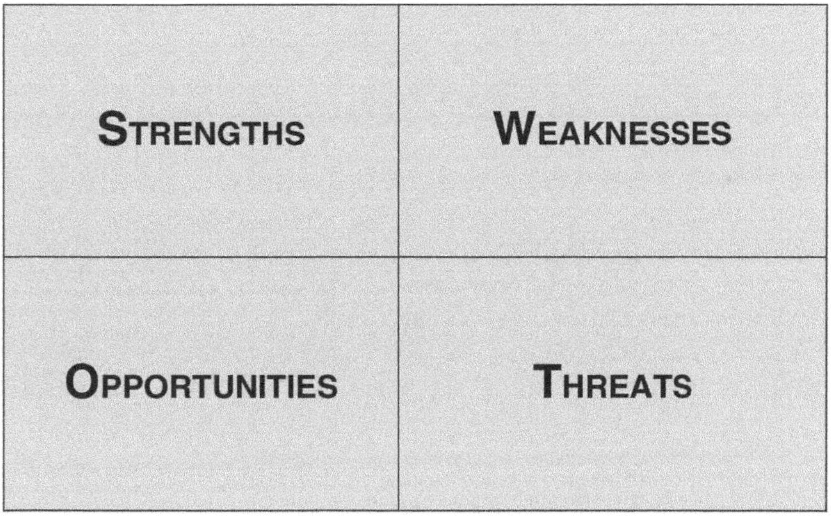

STRENGTHS	**WEAKNESSES**
OPPORTUNITIES	**THREATS**

Figure 17.3   SWOT analysis tool

Taking the time to consider your own strengths and opportunities, alongside areas for development and threats to this, may support you to consider how best to utilise the remaining learning opportunities available to you.

It may also be helpful to link your SWOT analysis to a Personal Development Plan (PDP) to support you in identifying any specific personal learning needs for your final practice learning experiences. A good PDP will require you to develop SMART objectives so that your action plan objectives are:

Specific

Measurable

Achievable

Relevant

Time-based

You may remember that we introduced the idea of SMART objectives in previous chapters and it is worth recognising that these can be applied in a wide range of contexts. For example, you may find that your employer encourages you to use SMART objectives in an annual professional development review (PDR) or appraisal, or you may have considered using SMART objectives when implementing a change in practice or a service improvement. Using this same approach here helps you to identify your own personal objectives and can help ensure that you maintain motivation and focus on your development.

The completion of SWOT and PDP may also support you in identifying your career plans and moving forward into your preceptorship and beyond, which we will consider later in this chapter.

Activity 17.3

Using the SWOT analysis framework highlighted in Figure 17.3, complete your own SWOT analysis of the nursing knowledge and skills you have developed so far, and then reflect on how you may address your own areas for development and the potential threats to this.

Now use your completed SWOT analysis to support you in creating a short-term PDP for the next 12 months. What do you feel you *need* to achieve? What do you *want* to achieve? How will you do this?

Opportunities for Multi-Professional Learning and Development

One key factor to consider as you approach the end of your nursing programme is your future role as a core member of the multi-professional team. As a registered nurse you will be pivotal in leading and supporting the multi-professional team and their collaborative work in managing the provision of care. It is vital that you have a good understanding of the roles of other health and social care professionals to ensure the delivery of effective and safe person-centered care.

The *Five Year Forward View* (NHS England, 2014) highlighted the need to break down barriers that have prevailed in the context of health and social care across a range of care settings to ensure that the care provided is coordinated, effective, safe, and ultimately individualised and person-centred. These core values of multidisciplinary working remain current today and form the foundations of the NHS long-term plan (NHS England, 2019). As a qualified nurse, you will play a pivotal role in this vital service development. Therefore, utilising opportunities in your practice learning experiences to work with other members of the team is incredibly valuable.

In Chapter 4 we encouraged you to identify and explore the roles and responsibilities of other multi-professional team members with whom you had the opportunity to work within a variety of practice learning environments. We now encourage you to consider these again, this time as a registered nurse since you will be required to facilitate inter-professional collaboration, the assessment, management and evaluation of care provision, collaborating with colleagues to successfully and significantly, impact on the safe delivery of care and positive outcomes for individuals within your care (Martin et al., 2010).

Your own exposure to the expertise and valuable input of wider team members will vary dependent on your individual practice learning experience, your new role and where you choose to work. Nevertheless, by now you will no doubt have recognised that it is essential that you take the time to work and learn alongside each member of the team in order that you respect the value of the input that they offer. Learning from each other in practice is a valuable part of development as a healthcare professional. Later in this chapter, we will again consider the importance of self-care and reflective practice, but it is important here also to highlight the value of engaging the wider team in group reflection – this is particularly valuable after involvement in a stressful or demanding situation such as a major trauma. There is a growing body of evidence to support this as a valuable learning opportunity for all. One example is that of 'Schwartz rounds' which are supported by the Point of Care Foundation in the UK and are being utilised across many organisations nationally. Schwartz rounds are an excellent example of the value of supported group reflection where teams come together to discuss a situation and share their experiences, learning about the input and role of each team member and the value of their involvement. A greater appreciation of roles and experiences can lead to more effective team working, improved staff health and wellbeing. This in turn, can have a significant impact on the quality-of-care provision and patient experience (Point of Care Foundation, 2015: 13). Goodrich (2012: 120) also identified that by sharing experiences team members have a greater understanding, appreciation, and respect for each other.

Activity 17.4

Make a list of all professionals you work with and consider your understanding of their contribution to the wider multi-professional team.

Now, imagine yourself as a leader of this team. How would you apply what you know about their role and responsibilities to assist you in leading the team to provide safe and effective care?

Can you identify any gaps in your knowledge here? If so, consider how you plan to find out more about the role of each member of the wider multi-professional team.

Getting the Most from Your Practice Learning Experiences

As you should be aware by now, your practice learning experiences provide an opportunity for you to apply the theoretical elements of your degree programme to your own nursing practice. It is important to take on board any feedback you receive from those you work with in practice in order to have the opportunity to enhance and build on your prior learning and identify your future learning needs as you approach registration. It is also important to be aware that you will have the opportunity to learn from many other members of the wider multi-professional team Therefore, we recommend that you take ownership of your learning and lead in the facilitation of this, consider your learning needs and link this to your ongoing personal development plan to strengthen your learning and overall development.

Embracing your learning opportunities

As you have continually progressed through your nursing programme you will have completed a range of learning experiences and acquired a learning journey that is unique to you. It may be the case that your final practice learning experience is not your preferred area of employment on registration. However, it is important to consider that this is your final experience as a student nurse and to take every learning opportunity offered to you. The skills, knowledge and experience you gain from this experience are transferable into any area of nursing practice, alongside those achieved and gained throughout your nursing education.

When you begin your new post as a registered nurse, your employer and team will support you in developing the skills, knowledge and experience that will be specific to your new role; you may not have encountered these during your nurse education depending on your practice learning journey, but you will have a solid grounding of core skills, knowledge and experience (Figure 17.4) that will be a foundation on which to build, adapt and develop as you progress through your career.

Application for Employment

You may have already started to think about your career plans. This may have been influenced by your experiences in practice to date or you may have had a clear idea of your career direction from the very start of the programme. Whatever your thoughts on your career plans, you may consider applying for employment as you approach the end of your undergraduate programme. It is worth remembering here when considering your career path: your first job might not be your forever job! Be mindful that there is an incredible amount of flexibility and multiple career routes within nursing as a profession, and you may make the decision to change your specialty as you progress through your career. Many skills in nursing are transferable and can be utilised and developed in a wide range of areas including various clinical specialisms, healthcare management, education, and research.

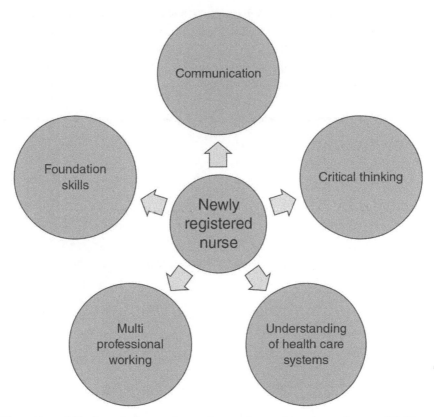

Figure 17.4   Core skills, knowledge, and experience of a newly registered nurse (NMC, 2018a)

You may wish to take some time at the end of the programme to have a break after years of study, to travel or to consider further your career plans (see 'Further reading' at the end of this chapter about working internationally). If this is the case, you will need to check to ensure that you register to practice with the NMC within the required timescales. The NMC provides clear and up-to-date guidance about the process of registration on its website:

www.nmc.org.uk/registration/joining-the-register/

Developing your curriculum vitae and a personal supporting statement

Your curriculum vitae (CV) is a fluid tool that will develop with you throughout your career. You may already have a developed CV from your employment prior to commencing your degree programme, or you may have never developed a CV. Whatever your situation, it is useful to begin to structure and develop your CV before beginning to look for employment. It can take time to pull together all the relevant information, so you are advised to allow yourself some protected time to complete or update your CV in preparation for your new role. Once you have the basic outline structure, your CV will then grow and develop with you as you progress through your nursing career journey, wherever that may take you.

The basic outline structure for a CV has not changed over many years. The key is to keep it clean and simple and to keep it to a minimum length. Writing in a succinct manner is a valuable skill and this will reflect well to prospective employers. Ideally, your initial CV should be no longer than two sides of A4 paper. Ensure that you check for spelling and grammatical errors – prospective employers will notice this.

Box 17.1 CV Template

This list below should help you to develop your CV structure:

1   Title and name
2   Address
3   Date of birth and age
4   A brief statement about yourself, including key drivers and positive statements (this is an opportunity to really sell yourself!)
5   Education:
   a   Institution attended (school/college/further education/higher education)
   b   Qualifications gained
   c   Grades/outcome
6   Details of relevant courses attended
7   Details of employment (starting with the most recent)
   a   Organisation
   b   Job title
   c   Dates of employment
   d   Brief outline of key roles and responsibilities
8   A brief overview of activities that you enjoy out of work
9   Contact details of two referees

The initial information will remain the same as you progress through your career, with additions to qualifications and details of employment that can be added and amended as you progress and move along. Investment in your CV now is an investment in your future.

Activity 17.5

Think about the information that you will need to begin to populate or update your nursing CV. Do you have access to certificates and contact details for any previous employment? Begin to develop your CV by asking tutors, trusted critical friends, peers and practice supervisors/assessors to review this for you.

    Do you need to make any changes, updates, or amendments?

Your personal statement is a key aspect of the job application process; it is another opportunity to sell yourself to your prospective employer, to stand out from the crowd and to highlight the reasons why they should consider you for employment. Again, it is important that you take time to develop your personal statement and that this links clearly to both the person specification and the role description that are linked to the job itself. You will normally find both attached to the advertisement for the job and it is vital that you read these thoroughly since the key to successfully applying for posts is knowing what the employer wants and knowing what you can offer.

Depending upon the role advertised, the employing organisation and the organisational environment, there may be some variation in the person specification and the job description, but there are common factors that employers identify as key in their search for an employee. Bright et al. (2014: 70) have identified what they feel are the eight key qualities that are identified in person specifications:

1 Effective communication skills: both verbal and written;
2 The ability to contribute as an effective team member.
3 The ability to work under pressure;
4 The ability to use your own initiative;
5 Attention to detail;
6 Enthusiasm and passion;
7 Energy and drive;
8 Evidence of potential leadership skills.

When you have reviewed the job description and person specification, take time to consider how you can demonstrate your suitability for the job, what skills and attributes you can bring to the role through reflection on your experiences in practice, theory, and extracurricular activities which you have engaged in.

The use of a simple spider diagram is a helpful tool (Figure 17.5) to begin the development of your personal statement.

You may also find that reviewing and revisiting any reflections on your experiences will be a huge help to you in the development of your personal statement.

Activity 17.6

1 Look through the specification for a job in an area of practice you are interested in. You can source these on organisational web pages and/or recruitment sites.
2 Now take some time to read your written reflections on practice and the feedback you have received from those you have worked alongside. What do these tell you about your experience and professional development?

Are there any key reflections that you feel will contribute towards your personal statement?
Have you had feedback that could be incorporated to strengthen your personal statement?

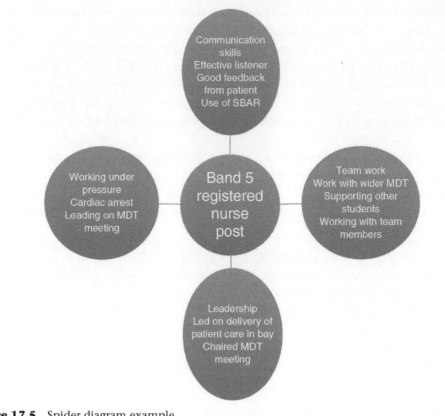

Figure 17.5 Spider diagram example

Organisations now utilise online websites to facilitate the process of application, seeking references and offering jobs. For example, if applying for a post within the NHS in England, Scotland and Wales, websites such as the ones highlighted in the box below offer a good opportunity to search for posts that may be of interest to you and may also offer the option to receive notifications when posts are advertised on the site, which is a useful tool to support you in your search for posts.

Box 17.2

www.jobs.nhs.uk (England and Wales)
https://jobs.hscni.net/ (Northern Ireland)
https://apply.jobs.scot.nhs.uk/ (Scotland)
www.nhsjobs.com/ (Independent of the NHS and Department of Health)

You will need to ensure that you have your outline CV to hand and that you have an outline personal statement available. If you see a post that interests you, it is best to apply sooner rather than later since you may miss the opportunity to apply if the advert is closed before the deadline due to a high number of applicants.

You will find that many online systems also offer the opportunity to save relevant information that you may need again for future applications. Although it may take time to collate information on the system in the first instance, you will save time when submitting any applications in the future because much of the information can be taken from that which you have previously submitted.

Not all employers use online systems for applications for employment and some may use paper-based application processes. In these situations, it is important that you use black ink to complete your form (unless otherwise indicated) and that you do not complete the form when you may be rushed or have little time. Nothing looks worse to prospective employers than a poorly completed application form. If you do have to complete a handwritten form, ensure that you have the time and space to undertake the task in hand and all the relevant information to hand. Use clear writing and ensure that you read the form thoroughly.

Attending open days

There have been some changes over recent years in the methods of application for employment for nurses, with many organisations now offering open days and opportunities to interview 'on the spot' for posts within the organisation.

If you have worked within an organisation, ward or specific team during your degree programme and enjoyed your experience, you may be interested to attend an open day at the organisation to find out more about employment and development opportunities. This is a chance to meet informally with senior nursing staff and to make an initial good impression that could prove to be beneficial for any future employment opportunities. Open days also offer the chance to ascertain what benefits and opportunities the organisation can offer you.

It is important to remember when attending an open day that you have a good understanding of the organisation and their values before the day. Access the organisation's website and take time to read about the organisation so you are well prepared as this may prompt questions for further information on your part.

Wear smart clothing and bring along relevant information (e.g., a copy of your current CV) so that prospective employers can view this (if you are happy for them to do so) should the opportunity for an interview arise on the day.

Interview skills

You have submitted a successful application and have been invited to attend an interview. What do you do now? At this stage it would be useful to ask practice colleagues, other students, your practice supervisors, and assessors, what questions they think might be asked at an interview. You may want to start collating a bank of questions and consider how you will respond to them. As you attend interviews make a note of the questions that form part of the interview; revisiting how you might approach the question if asked again. Many universities will have a career support service so seek this out and find out what general interview support is available. One key element of learning from an interview is to seek feedback from the interview panel; successful or not in the interview, there is so much that you can learn from the process and take forward to any future interviews that you may have. It is a valuable part of your personal growth and development.

Box 17.3 Interview Tips

- Read around and demonstrate that you understand the organisation's mission or goal;
- Be aware of your body language. You want to convey that you are enthusiastic, positive, and energetic. Try to keep fidgety hands still and smile appropriately;
- Make eye contact with all members of the interview panel. Try not to just focus on the person who has asked the question you are answering;
- Be clear and concise in your responses;
- If your mis-hear something, do not understand the question, or lose your train of thought do not panic, just say so. Ask for the question to be repeated;
- Link any question topics back to your own experience. An effective way to succinctly sell yourself is to provide examples of how you have achieved positive outcomes or overcome challenges using the **CAR** (providing a summary of the **C**ontext of the situation, the **A**ctions you took and the **R**esult you achieved) or **STAR** (**S**pecific situation, **T**ask, **Action,** and **R**esult) frameworks.

You will be offered the opportunity to ask questions as part of the interview process so try to prepare a question to ask the interview panel. Having questions to ask helps demonstrate that you are keen, you are interested in the job and that you have readily prepared for your interview. For example, you may ask about working patterns, developments in the organisation and support offered to your personal development.

Accepting a post

Following the process of application and interview, you may find that you are in a position where you have more than one offer of employment. At this point, you will have a choice to make about whether you want to accept the job being offered or not. It is important to be considerate of your potential employers in this situation and to inform them as soon as possible of your decision, so they can offer the position to an alternative suitable candidate or re-advertise the position in a timely manner, if necessary, in order that the vacancy can be filled as soon as possible.

Be mindful of your professional responsibility in this situation and the need to consider the needs of the wider service. Although it can sometimes be difficult to make a final decision for your first post as a registered nurse, as we have identified, this may not be your 'forever' role and there are a wide range of opportunities available to you in your career. The decision to accept a role and then to decline this at the last minute could lead to a missed opportunity for the organisation to fill a post and may impact on the service that they provide.

Starting your role as a registered nurse

Once you have successfully completed your programme of study, your university will inform the Nursing and Midwifery Council (NMC). There may be a slight delay in you completing your studies and receiving your personal identification number (PIN), but once you receive your PIN number, you will need to alert your employer and you can then practice as a registered nurse.

Preceptorship

There is a growing body of evidence to support the need to ensure that healthcare practitioners have a clear plan of support in the transition period, to facilitate their growth and development as a practitioner and to help them identify their ongoing learning needs as a developing practitioner.

'Preceptorship' is the term used to outline the structured period in which you are supported in your new employment as a newly registered nurse. The NMC (2006) suggests that this period will allow for the development of confidence and competence in practice and allows the newly qualified nurse to be supported to practice in line with *The Code* (NMC, 2018b). There have been many developments in the drive for preceptorship over recent years. The NMC *'Principles of Preceptorship'* document acknowledges the importance of a robust preceptorship to facilitate transition from student to registered professional; emphasising the importance of the ongoing learning and development throughout the career of the nurse (NMC, 2020). In response, new preceptorship frameworks have been launched in Scotland (NHS Education for Scotland, 2021), England (NHS England, 2022) and Northern Ireland (Northern Ireland Practice and Education Council for Nursing and Midwifery, 2022).

Activity 17.7

1   Find out more about available 'Preceptorship' by accessing the following websites:
    https://learn.nes.nhs.scot/42348/preceptorship (Scotland)
    https://learn.nes.nhs.scot/735/flying-start-nhs (Scotland)
    https://nipec.hscni.net/service/ni-preceptorship-framework- (Northern Ireland)

www.nwssp.wales.nhs.uk/sitesplus/documents/1178/Final%20Report%20for%20Preceptorship.pdf (Wales)

www.england.nhs.uk/publication/national-preceptorship-framework-for-nursing/ (England)

2 Consider how preceptorship might assist you in your transition into registered practice. What elements of preceptorship would be particularly important to you?

Utilising preceptorship to support your development

Through the completion of your degree programme, you will be required to meet the *Standards of Proficiency for Registered Nurses* (NMC, 2018a). Throughout this book, so far you have been introduced to a range of these standards in the openings to each chapter.

Embracing learning through the process of preceptorship will allow you the opportunity to build on your developing knowledge and skill base, through the support of your preceptor and your employing organisation as your transition from student to registered nurse

The aim of preceptorship is to support your development as a newly registered practitioner in several ways:

- Increase your confidence in applying evidence-based practice;
- Develop your self-awareness;
- Assist you in implementing the code of professional values;
- Increase your knowledge and clinical skills;
- Help you to integrate prior learning into practice;
- Help you to better understand policies and procedures;
- Enhance your reflective abilities and your responses to receiving feedback;
- Help you to develop an outcome-based approach to continuing professional development;
- Enhance your interpersonal and advocacy skills;
- Help you to managing risk effectively;
- Better understand issues of equality and diversity;
- Enhance your leadership and management skills including negotiation and conflict resolution;
- Enhance team working and decision-making skills.

Of course, throughout your time on your nursing programme you will have experienced and already been exposed to many of these aspects. However, preceptorship allows to you to continue to build and reflect on your prior learning, growth, and development, acknowledging that you will continue to develop all these aspects of your professional practice as you move through your nursing career.

The utilisation of a period of preceptorship will also feed forward into your first revalidation with the NMC and will encourage you to maintain supporting evidence of your achievements.

Nursing and Midwifery Council: Revalidation

Revalidation (NMC, 2021) is the way in which nurses demonstrate to the NMC that they have continued to practice safely and effectively via a process of gathering feedback and facilitating reflection on one's own practice. Registrants are required to apply critical reflective skills to continually develop as a practitioner, with clear links to *The Code* (NMC, 2018b) and its application to professional practice. This is evidenced via a professional portfolio and is required to be formally reviewed every three years.

The NMC have developed a useful microsite that contains all the information you will need to undertake revalidation and provides templates that will support you in the building and development of your professional portfolio from the point of registration. During your preceptorship, your new employer should also be able to give you guidance on how the process of revalidation is managed within the organisation.

Activity 17.8

Take some time to visit the NMC's Revalidation webpage and read the guidance provided on revalidation. Look through and familiarise yourself with the documentation/templates provided and consider how you would start to create and further develop and enhance your professional portfolio to support you in your revalidation.

http://revalidation.nmc.org.uk/welcome-to-revalidation
http://revalidation.nmc.org.uk/download-resources/forms-and-templates

---

Self-care and the Demands of Professional Practice

By now, you will no doubt have recognised that adult nursing is a demanding role, both physically and emotionally. This is acknowledged by the NMC (2018a:8) when they require that as a registered nurse you must be able to:

> "Understand the demands of professional practice and demonstrate how to recognise signs of vulnerability in themselves or their colleagues and the action required to minimise risks to health".

In addition, *The Code* (NMC, 2018b: 19) also identifies that, as a nurse, you '*maintain the level of health you need to carry out your professional role'*.

The Royal College of Nursing (RCN, 2018) campaign *Rest, Rehydrate and Refuel* provides some useful tips on what you can do to help yourself stay well at work. In addition, although we have explored the need for emotional resilience in previous chapters, it is worth revisiting the important aspects again as you begin your role as a registered nurse.

Resilience is often considered to be an important attribute in healthcare professionals (McGowan and Murray, 2016). However, there is little agreement on what being resilient entails, and how we develop into resilient practitioners. What it is not is absorbing all that you witnessed or experienced and just 'getting on with it.' It is important that you share your experiences with your colleagues, have open dialogue and seek support from your peers and senior colleagues. Remember that you should not have to feel that you must manage everything on your own. Looking after yourself allows you to remain healthy and well, so that you can practice safely and effectively. If you do feel that you are finding things difficult and recognise vulnerability in yourself, there is value in sharing this with your peers and knowing that you will be supported. In turn, too, it is important that you also look out for your colleagues and encourage them to seek support and help if you feel that they are finding things difficult.

- Can you remember some of the things you might be able to do to increase your resilience?

As a newly registered nurse you may be working in an unfamiliar environment, faced with change and reorganisation, and you will have to be able to deal with this, in addition to the role and responsibility of providing care to individuals and their families. A multifaceted approach will help you cope with this potentially challenging time. Jackson et al. (2007) identified key strategies in the development of resilience:

- Positive relationships;
- A sense of humour;
- Self-awareness;
- A sense of balance;
- Developing as a reflective practitioner.

The benefits of working in a team and developing effective working relationships with your peers are a valuable approach to ensuring support and a sense of belonging throughout your nursing career.

Reflection and self-care

Earlier in this chapter, the use of Schwartz rounds (Point of Care Foundation, 2015) was identified as a positive model to facilitate effective team working and to enhance respect and communication through reflective discussion. In addition to this there are other ways in which you can engage in supportive reflection.

You may recall at the very start of this book, we introduced you to the concept of reflection as a process to facilitate understanding, knowledge and development, and the varying models that may support this process. In addition to this, it is also appropriate to consider here how the process of reflection can be utilised in the facilitation of self-care and, in some cases, the engagement of others, so this is a shared process where learning and support are encouraged within the wider team.

Through the process of revalidation, the NMC (2021) encourages nurses to engage in written reflection to demonstrate learning and development through experiences in practice. There are several ways in which you can engage in written reflection, and you will have undertaken this as part of your nursing degree programme. Some will enjoy the process of written reflection, taking the time to focus on their learning through experiences. Others may find written reflection a challenge and acknowledge that the skill of written reflection takes time to develop and hone. It is important to acknowledge that, through the process of reflective writing, it is not simply a case of recording an event, but that the writing itself is the process of reflection (Bolton and Delderfield, 2018). There are a range of ways that reflective writing can be developed. The use of a journal or diary is often the most common method, and some may find that the structure of a model (e.g., Driscoll, 2007; Jasper, 2013) can help in the development of reflection. Bolton and Delderfield (2018) discuss in detail the practice of reflective writing identifying the process of developing your reflective writing and the value of time and space to develop this practice. This would be a valuable activity to begin to develop as a student and as a registered nurse.

Activity 17.9 Six-Minute Writing Task

1   Write whatever is in your head – do not edit this;
2   Write for 6 minutes – do not stop writing during this time, let the words flow;
3   Do not stop, re-read or be critical during these 6 minutes;
4   Do not worry about spelling, grammar, punctuation;
5   Allow yourself the permission to write anything;
6   Importantly, whatever you write is right: it belongs to you, and you do not have to share it with anyone.

(Bolton and Delderfield, 2018: 160)

Clinical supervision

Clinical supervision is the process of reflection through discussion with an identified colleague or an independent professional. In 2013, the Care Quality Commission (CQC) acknowledged the value of clinical supervision in the delivery of safe and effective patient care, identifying the purpose of clinical supervision to be:

"a safe and confidential environment for staff to reflect on and discuss their work… The focus is on supporting staff in their personal and professional development and in reflecting on their practice".

(CQC, 2013: 4)

Clinical supervision can be on a one-to-one basis or as part of a group and is a valuable aspect of support for nurses. Bifarin and Stonehouse (2017) acknowledge the incredible value that effective clinical supervision can offer to each nurse who engages with the activity, but it can have a significantly positive impact on working relationships and care provision through stress reduction, and a feeling of value and satisfaction in the role of the nurse.

The value of supervision has been further highlighted through the development of the Professional Nurse Advocate (PNA) programme, with the launch of the new role of the PNA to assure restorative supervision for nurses, recognising the importance of supervision not just for the health and wellbeing of nurses, but also for the delivery of good quality care. The role is supported through the development and delivery of an evidence-based model called 'A-EQUIP.' Launched in 2021, the model focuses on the importance of restorative supervision to enhance personal development, the quality of care and hearing the voice of the service user and the nurse (NHS England, 2021). As a newly registered nurse, you will have the opportunity to engage with restorative supervision and embrace the valuable learning opportunities that come from this supported reflective discussion process.

Your Future Career

Consider how you felt about becoming a nurse at the beginning of your degree programme.
Do you feel that your professional identity has changed?

By engaging with the content of this book you will have been introduced to the many potential roles and pathways of your future nursing career. You will also have had exposure to the vast array of options open to you from your own experiences in practice learning environments, and through the theoretical context of your nursing degree programme.

Figure 17.6 depicts the overlapping spheres of the four key aspects of the registered nurse's role. As you can see, none are in isolation and there is overlap between the varying aspects of the role.

Activity 17.10

Consider your reading from the book so far and your experiences from your degree programme, and apply this to the four key aspects of the nurse's role identified as:

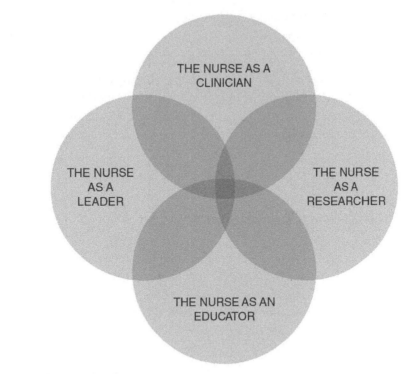

Figure 17.6 The nurse's role

1   Clinician;
2   Educator;
3   Researcher;
4   Leader.

Identify examples of nurses whom you have met and how they fit within the various aspects of the role identified above.

Think about which aspects are of interest to you.

Continuing your professional development

Nursing requires lifelong commitment to personal learning and development to ensure that the best nursing care is provided, and it is a vital activity as it is how we continue to learn and develop throughout our careers to ensure our skills and knowledge are up to date.

As a registered nurse, you will develop skills and experience new professional responsibilities, developing relationships and becoming part of a team. There will be opportunity to access a range of continuing professional development opportunities:

- Organisational education and training;
- Education relating to your specific role;
- Further Postgraduate study.

This can further enhance and extend your clinical and leadership skills to maintain and develop the delivery of high-quality care across a range of settings. You should be guided by your continuing professional development needs through your annual performance development review (PDR) or appraisal, the process of revalidation and the identification of areas of specific interest for you as a nurse.

Supporting and Supervising Others in Practice

As a qualified nurse and a registrant, you will be involved and engaged in the process of supporting learners in practice. *The Code* (NMC, 2018b) stipulates the professional responsibility of nurses to engage in the education and support of learners and colleagues. As a nurse, you should support learners and colleagues to help them develop their professional competence and confidence. You will know from your own experience as a student that engagement with learners provides an excellent opportunity to share knowledge and engagement in the process of supporting learners as a registered nurse will serve to support your own continuing professional development.

As you have moved through your own degree programme, you may have supported other learners within the practice learning environment. These may be new to the area, and may have not had similar experiences to you or may be at an earlier point in their own degree programme. You may also meet learners from other professions whom you can support in your role.

Peer support is incredibly valuable in your learning and can allow the opportunity to share knowledge and experiences from your learning in both practice and theory. It could be argued that the utilisation of peer support lends itself well to the concept of coaching; that being so, it promotes problem solving and learning through experience. In some situations, clinical supervision can be peer led, and can allow registered nurses and teams to work through and learn from challenging situations in practice.

Coaching is defined as *'unlocking a person's potential to maximise their own performance'* (Whitmore, 2009: 10). Rather than teaching, showing, and telling; the coach supports the learner to identify their learning needs and to achieve those through empowerment and with the use of a nurturing approach. This approach to supporting learners not only serves to enhance and develop the autonomous practitioner, but also lends itself to the development of self-esteem and self-belief.

- Have you ever been coached?
- If so, in what context were you coached? Was this during your nurse education, in a sport activity, at school?
- What skills do you think you need to have to be an effective coach?

There are a range of ways in which you can engage in the support and development of others in the practice learning environment, which have been clearly identified by the NMC (2018c; 2023). As a registered nurse, you will engage in the support and supervision of students as a practice supervisor and may undertake the role of practice assessor as you progress in your career and after suitable preparation for the role (Box 17.4). It is important to remember that students are valuable team members, working and learning alongside the team. There is also a significant opportunity to learn from students who bring with them developing knowledge and understanding. Through reciprocity in the relationship between student and supervisor and assessor, there is immense value in acknowledging that we can all learn from each other.

Box 17.4 Roles of practice supervisor and assessor

Practice supervisor

- A role model
- Supporting learning
- Working within own scope of practice
- Current knowledge and experience
- Contributing to assessment via feedback to assessor and recording experience of observing learners in practice

Practice assessor

- Assessing achievement and providing feedback
- Working in partnership with the academic assessor and practice supervisors
- Gathering and coordinating feedback from the wider team
- Understanding a students' learning needs and outcomes
- Current knowledge and experience
- Undertaking preparation or evidence of prior experience that would facilitate the role.

NMC (2018c)

Activity 17.11

Visit NMC (2019) and read *Part 2: Standards for Student Supervision and Assessment*

How could you develop an effective practice environment for learners?
Consider how you could be involved in the supervision of learners in practice as a newly qualified nurse.
What requirements would you need in the future to become an assessor?

Major Incident Response: Your Responsibilities as a Registrant

A major incident is defined by the Joint Emergency Service Interoperability Programme (JESIP) as 'beyond the scope of business-as-usual operations, and is likely to involve serious harm, damage, disruption or risk to human life or welfare, essential services, the environment or national security' (JESIP, 2016). It is widely accepted that major incidents such as terrorist attacks, natural disasters, traumatic events, or industrial accidents with multiple casualties cannot be managed within routine service arrangements. Most organisations have contingency plans in place so that they can respond appropriately in the event of a major incident. As a registered nurse you have a professional responsibility to be aware of such plans and the expectations placed upon you in the overall response to a major incident (NMC, 2018a).

In the event of a serious emergency or major incident, it is quite possible that as a registered nurse you could be called upon to provide first aid or basic life support. Examples of first aid include performing cardiopulmonary resuscitation (CPR), helping choking victims, taking a person's vital signs, cleaning and applying bandages to minor cuts and wounds or applying a tourniquet to a severely injured limb if needed. It is quite clear that effective initial help in these situations can assist victim recovery. However, it is important to remember that, even in such situations, you must act only within the limits of your knowledge and competence (NMC, 2018b) and always follow the local major incident policies. If an incident happens away from your normal place of work, you are advised to follow current NMC guidance (NMC, 2017). In addition, witnessing or being involved in a major incident can be a highly traumatic experience. Talking about your experiences within a supportive environment is one of the strongest predictors of recovery after psychological trauma (Brewin et al., 2000) and the NMC (2017) advocate seeking support and help from your employer or GP (General Practitioner) if needed.

Activity 17.12

Access and read the following documents and guidelines:

1 Resuscitation Council UK (2021) *Adult Basic Life Support Guidelines*. Available at: www.resus.org.uk/library/2021-resuscitation-guidelines/adult-basic-life-support-guidelines.
2 NHS/Public Health England (2020) *Clinical Guidelines for Major Incidents and Mass Casualty Events*. Available at: www.england.nhs.uk/wp-content/uploads/2018/12/B0128-clinical-guidelines-for-use-in-a-major-incident-v2-2020.pdf
3 30 NHS (2022) *First Aid*. Available at: www.nhs.uk/conditions/first-aid/
   Now locate and access the major incident policy or plan for your employer organisation.
   How well prepared are you? How might you be called upon to contribute to a major incident response?
   Find out what support services might be available for staff affected.

Chapter Summary

The transition from student to registered nurse is supported through the process of preceptorship. It is acknowledged that this period of transition can be a period of challenge and uncertainty, but, with the support of peers and the wider team, the period of transition can be facilitated in a nurturing and safe environment. It is important that newly qualified nurses continue to engage in personal development, through the process of preceptorship and moving into revalidation. It is also important to engage in reflective activities and you will encounter a range of ways to facilitate this. As a registered nurse, you will also be expected to support and eventually assess learners in the practice environment; you are best placed to consider your own experiences as a student and the influence of this on your own enactment of this aspect of your role. As someone approaching the end of your degree programme, you are encouraged to consider the many options available to you, but importantly acknowledging your own self-care and supporting those around you in what is a challenging but incredibly rewarding career. As you begin your journey as a registered nurse, you will have a wide range of career options available to you and your career journey will be unique to you, taking on board the four aspects of the role of the nurse within this.

Useful Websites

www.rcn.org.uk/Professional-Development/Your-career/Nurse/Career-Crossroads
/Career-Progression
www.nursingandmidwiferycareersni.hscni.net/career-pathways/career-specific-pathways/
www.careers.nhs.scot/careers/explore-our-careers/nursing/adult-nurse/
www.prospects.ac.uk/careers-advice/what-can-i-do-with-my-degree/nursing

Further Reading

Bolton, G. and Delderfield, R. (2018) *Reflective Practice: Writing and Professional Development*, 5th edn. London: Sage.

Chen, F., Liu, Y., Wang, X. and Dong, H. (2021) 'Transition shock, preceptor support and nursing competency among newly graduated registered nurses: a cross-sectional study', *Nurse Education Today*, 102(2021): 104891.

Higgins, G., Spencer, R.L. and Kane, R. (2010) 'A systematic review of the experiences and perceptions of the newly qualified nurse in the United Kingdom', *Nurse Education Today*, 30(6), Aug: 499–508.

Horsburgh, D. (2013) 'Care and compassion: the experiences of newly qualified staff nurses', *Journal of Clinical Nursing*, 22 (7-8), April: 1124–32.

Royal College of Nursing (2016) *Students: Thinking about Your Career*. London: RCN.

Royal College of Nursing (2017) *Working Internationally. A Guide to Humanitarian and Development Work for Nurses and Midwives*. London: RCN.

Whitehead, Owen, P., Holmes, D., Beddingham, E., Simmons, M., Henshaw, L., Barton, M. and Walker, C. (2013) 'Supporting newly qualified nurses in the UK: a systematic literature review', *Nurse Education Today*, 33(4), April: 370–7.

References

Benner, P. (1984) *From Novice to Expert: Excellence and Power in Cli*nical Nursing Practice. Melno Park, CA: Addison-Wesley.

Bifarin, O. and Stonehouse, D. (2017) 'Clinical supervision: an important part of every nurse's practice', *British Journal of Nursing*, 26(6): 331–5.

Bolton, G.E.J. and Delderfield, R. (2018) *Reflective Practice: Writing and Professional Development*, 5th edn. London: Sage.

Brewin, C.R., Andrew, B. and Valentine, J.D. (2000) 'Meta-analysis of risk factors for posttraumatic stress disorder in trauma-exposed adults', *Journal of Consulting Clinical Psychologists*, 68(5): 748–66.

Bright, J., Earl, J. and Winter, D. (2014) *Brilliant Graduate CV: How to Get Your First CV to the Top of the Pile*. Harlow: Pearson Education.

Care Quality Commission (2013) *Supporting Information and Guidance: Supporting Effective Clinical Supervision*. Available at: https://work-learn-live-blmk.co.uk/wp-content/uploads/2018/04/CQC-Supporting-information-and-guidance.pdf (last accessed 20 October 2022).

Department of Health (2010) *Preceptorship Framework for Newly Registered Nurses, Midwives and Allied Health Professionals*. Available at: www.networks.nhs.uk/nhs-networks/ahp-networks/documents/dh_114116.pdf (last accessed 25 August 2022).

Driscoll, J.J. (2007) Practising Clinical Supervision: A Reflective Approach for Healthcare Professionals (2nd edition). London: Bailliere Tindall.

Goodrich, J. (2012) 'Supporting hospital staff to provide compassionate care: do Schwartz rounds work in English hospitals?', *Journal of the Royal Society of Medicine*, 105: 117–22.

Jackson, D., Firtko, A. and Edenborough, M. (2007) 'Personal resilience as a strategy for surviving and thriving in the face of workplace adversity: a literature review', *Journal of Advanced Nursing*, 60(1): 1–9.

Jasper, M. (2013) *Beginning reflective practice* (2nd edition). Andover: Cengage Learning

Joint Emergency Service Interoperability Programme (JESIP) (2016) *Definitions of Terms Used: Glossary*. Available at: www.jesip.org.uk/ (last accessed 20 October 2022).

Martin, J.S., Ummenhofer, W., Manser, T. and Spirig, R. (2010) 'Interprofessional collaboration among nurses and physicians: making a difference in patient outcome', *Swiss Medical Weekly*, 140: w13062. https://doi.org/10.4414/smw.2010.13062.

McGowan, J.E. and Murray, K. (2016) 'Exploring resilience in nursing and midwifery students: a literature review', *Journal of Advanced Nursing*, 72(10): 2253–68.

NHS Education for Scotland (2021) *Scotland's Preceptorship Framework*. Available at: www.nes.scot.nhs.uk/nes-current/scotland-s-preceptorship-framework/. (last accessed 20 October 2022).

NHS England (2014a) *Five Year Forward View* [online]. Available at: www.england.nhs.uk/wp-content/uploads/2014/10/5yfv-web.pdf (last accessed 25 August 2022).

NHS England (2019) *The NHS Long Term Plan*. [online]. Available at: www.longtermplan.nhs.uk/ (last accessed 30 May 2022).

NHS England (2021) Professional Nurse Advocate A-EQUIP Model - A model for clinical supervision for nurses version 1. (last accessed 25 August 2022).

NHS England (2022) *National Preceptorship Framework for Nursing*. Available at: www.england.nhs.uk/publication/national-preceptorship-framework-for-nursing/. (last accessed 20 October 2022).

Northern Ireland Practice and Education Council for Nursing and Midwifery (2022) *Preceptorship: What's it all about?* Available at: https://nipec.hscni.net/service/ni-preceptorship-framework-2022/ (last accessed 20 October 2022).

Nursing and Midwifery Council (2006) *Preceptorship Guidelines*. NMC Circular 21/2006, published 4 October 2006. Available at: www.nmc.org.uk/globalassets/sitedocuments/circulars/2006circulars/nmc-circular-21_2006.pdf (last accessed 25 August 2022).

Nursing and Midwifery Council (2017) *Information for Nurses and Midwives on Responding to Unexpected Incidents or Emergencies*. Available at: www.nmc.org.uk/news/news-and-updates/information-for-nurses-and-midwives-on-responding-to-unexpected-incidents-or-emergencies (last accessed 20 October 2022).

Nursing and Midwifery Council (2018a) *Future Nurse: Standards of Proficiency for Registered Nurses*. London: NMC. Available at: www.nmc.org.uk/globalassets/sitedocuments/education-standards/future-nurse-proficiencies.pdf (last accessed 20 October 2022).

Nursing and Midwifery Council (2018b) *The Code: Professional Standards for Practice and Behaviour for Nurses and Midwives*. London: NMC. Available at: www.nmc.org.uk/globalassets/sitedocuments/nmc-publications/nmc-code.pdf (last accessed 20 October 2022).

Nursing and Midwifery Council (2018c) *Realising Professionalism: Standards for Education and Training. Part 2: Standards for Student Supervision and Assessment*. Available at: www.nmc.org.uk/globalassets/sitedocuments/education-standards/student-supervision-assessment.pdf (last accessed 20 October 2022).

Nursing and Midwifery Council (2020) *Principles for Preceptorship*. Available at:.nmc.org.uk/globalassets/sitedocuments/nmc-publications/nmc-principles-for-preceptorship-a5.pdf (last accessed 25 August 2022).

Nursing and Midwifery Council (2021) *Revalidation*. Available at: www.nmc.org.uk/revalidation/(last accessed 20 October 2022).

Nursing and Midwifery Council (2023) *Realising Professionalism: Standards for Education and Training. (Part 1)*. Available at: www.nmc.org.uk/education-framework/ (last accessed 30 March 2023).

Point of Care Foundation (2015) *Staff Care: How to Engage Staff in the NHS and Why it Matters*. Available at: https://s16682.pcdn.co/wp-content/uploads/2014/01/POCF_FINAL-inc-references.pdf. (last accessed 20 October 2022).

Royal College of Nursing (2018) *Rest, Rehydrate, Refuel*. London: RCN.

Whitmore, J. (2009) *Coaching for Performance: GROWing People, Performance and Purpose*, 4th edn. London: Nicholas Breale.

Index